UNDERSTANDING ALZHEIMER'S DISEASE

Edited by **Inga Zerr**

Understanding Alzheimer's Disease
http://dx.doi.org/10.5772/46004
Edited by Inga Zerr

Contributors

Christian Gonzalez-Billault, Daniel A. Borquez, Ismael Palacios-Garcia, Isidre Ferrer, Jose Luna-Muñoz, Charles R. Harrington, Claude M. Wischik, Paola Flores-Rodríguez, Jesús Avila, Sergio Zamudio R., Fidel De La Cruz, Raul Mena-López, Benjamín Florán-Garduño, Takahide Matsushima, Yuhki Saito, Toshiharu Suzuki, Halil Murat Sen, Sibel Cevizci, Fahri Günes, Elif Karaahmet, Weili Xu, Camilla Ferrari, Hui-Xin Wang, Francesca Mangialasche, Gordon Glazner, Brandon Ally, Emily Mason, Manus Donahue, Genaro Ortiz, Fermín Pacheco-Moisés, L Javier Flores-Alvarado, Miguel A Macías-Islas, Irma E Velázquez-Brizuela, Ana C Ramírez-Anguiano, Erandis D Tórres-Sánchez, Eddic W Morales-Sánchez, José A Cruz-Ramos, Genaro E Ortiz-Velázquez, Fernando CortésEnríquez, Mei Sian Chong, Tih-Shih Lee, Klemens Wild, Ulrike Mueller, Rita Moretti, Kohzo Nakayama, Lucia Pastorino, Asami Kondo, Kun Ping Lu, Armand Perret-Liaudet, Aline Dorey, Yannick Tholance, Benoit Dumont, Isabelle Quadrio, Harish C. Pant

Published by InTech

Janeza Trdine 9, 51000 Rijeka, Croatia

Publishing Process Manager Iva Lipovic
Technical Editor InTech DTP team
Cover InTech Design team

Additional hard copies can be obtained from orders@intechopen.com

Understanding Alzheimer's Disease, Edited by Inga Zerr
p. cm.
ISBN 978-953-51-1009-5

For EU product safety concerns:
IN TECH d.o.o., Prolaz Marije Krucifikse Kozulić 3, 51000 Rijeka, Croatia,
info@intechopen.com or visit our website at intechopen.com.

Meet the editor

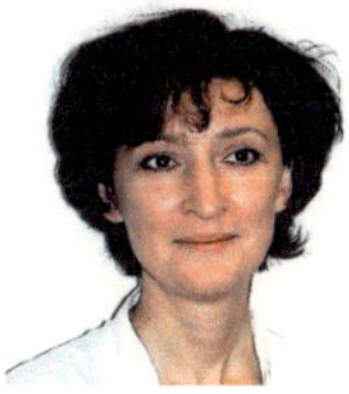

Inga Zerr is Professor at the Department of Neurology and Chair of the Clinical Dementia Center at the University Medical School, Göttingen. She received her habilitation (venia legendi for neurology) in 2001 for her work on cerebrospinal fluid in human prion diseases. With over 180 publications, Inga Zerr's current research interests include clinicopathological characterisation of molecular disease subtypes in neurodegenerative dementia (such as prion diseases, Alzheimer's disease) and the understanding of the molecular basis which leads to the phenotypic diversity in these pathological conditions.

Contents

Preface

This book spans a variety of approaches to address the complex problem of Alzheimer's disease - what is the cause, is there a single pathogenetic pathways or are there many of them, how can we address the whole clinical spectrum of the disease, how can the disease be diagnosed early and reliable and which perspectives we have for prevention and treatment. The collection covers actual topics of interest for basic researcher, clinicians, epidemiologists and provides insight to various aspects of the disease.

Inga Zerr, MD
Department of Neurology
Cliical Dementia Center
Georg August University Göttingen
Germany

Section 1

Pathogenesis

Chapter 1

Structure and Function of the APP Intracellular Domain in Health and Disease

Ulrike Müller and Klemens Wild

Additional information is available at the end of the chapter

http://dx.doi.org/10.5772/54543

1. Introduction

Talking about Alzheimer's disease (AD) on a biochemical level needs to highlight the molecular „*corpus delicti*": the amyloid or senile plaques [1]. These plaques are extracellular fibrillar deposits in the cortex and hippocampus mainly composed of a single proteinaceous compound, the Aβ peptide comprising predominantly 40 or 42 amino acid residues (Aβ40, Aβ42) [2]. The Aβ peptides originate by sequential ectodomain shedding and regulated intramembrane proteolysis (RIP) of the amyloid precursor protein (APP), a type I integral membrane protein highly expressed in neurons including synaptic compartments. The responsible proteases, the famous β- and γ-secretase respectively, have been reviewed in detail and will not be part of this paper [3, 4]. Since the cloning of APP 25 years ago, more than 9,000 publications (about one per day!) are listed for this protein in the PubMed database indicating its pivotal position in the amyloid cascade hypothesis [5], which constitutes the widely accepted pathogenic cascade ultimately leading to AD. While some years ago the plaques themselves were thought to be the primary cause of disease, it is nowadays well recognized that soluble Aβ oligomers are responsible for many of the neurotoxic properties causing memory dysfunction and finally dementia.

Despite intense research efforts AD can so far only be insufficiently treated in a purely symptomatic way and disease-modifying drugs are most wanted but are still not available [6]. In order to get a glimpse of understanding AD pathology at a biochemical level, we therefore have to understand the molecular structure of the key-player APP and its connected protein network. The structure, however, needs to be correlated with the physiological functions and the deregulating mechanisms causing toxicity, cell death, and disease [7, 8]. Bearing this in mind, the simultaneously generated sister peptides of Aβ deserve a major focus, namely the amino-terminal fragment (N-APP286) derived from sAPPβ as a ligand for the death receptor

6 (DR6) [9], and the APP intracellular domain as created by the ε-cut of γ-secretase during the RIP process [3], which is the topic of this paper. We will start by getting the architecture of APP into place.

2. Architecture of the APP protein

APP can be divided into three domains (Figure 1). As a single pass type I membrane protein, the N-terminal ectodomain of APP (residues 18 to 624 neglecting the signal peptide, numbers refer to the neuronal splice form APP695, UniPROT entry: P05067-4) locates to the extracellular space. The single hydrophobic transmembrane domain (TMD, residues 625 to 648) is followed by the rather short APP intracellular domain (AICD, residues 649 to 695). More important than this topological classification is the distinction according to the fragments produced by secretase cleavage events [10]. The products produced by ectodomain shedding are sAPPα (residues 18 to 612; cleaved by α-secretases, members of the ADAM family of zinc metalloproteases) and sAPPβ (residues 18 to 596; cleaved by β-secretase, an aspartic protease also known as BACE1 in the nervous system and BACE in peripheral tissue). The C-terminal fragments (CTFs) generated by ectodomain shedding are the still membrane embedded αCTF (CTF83) and βCTF (CTF99), respectively. The CTFs are subsequently cut in the RIP process by the intramembrane aspartate protease presenilin (1 or 2) as part of the γ-secretase complex, with αCTF being split into the p3 peptide and the AICD (residues 646 to 695) and βCTF into the Aβ peptide (Aβ40: residues 597 to 636; Aβ42: residues 597 to 638) and again the AICD.

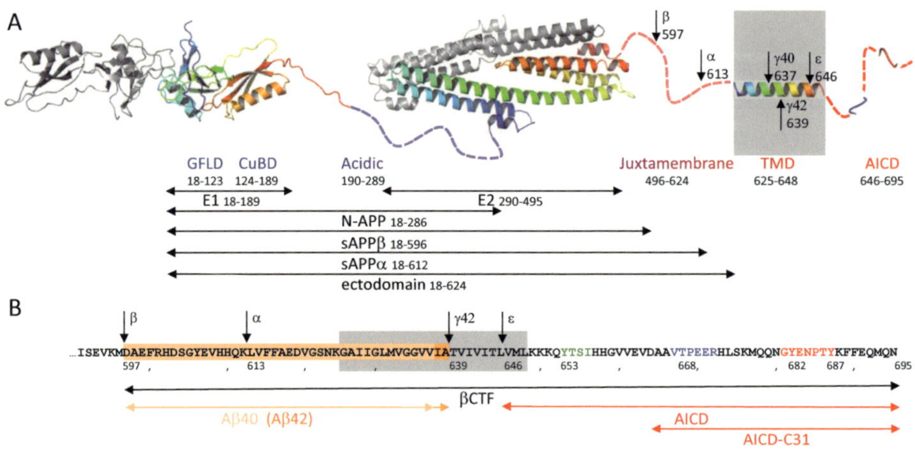

Figure 1. Architecture of APP and of its proteolytic fragments. A. Domain architecture of the neuronal splice variant APP695. Domains with known atomic structures (E1 and E2) and the TMD are shown as ribbon diagrams in a colour code from blue (N-terminus) to red (C-terminus). Dashed lines give structurally unknown regions. Proposed homodimeric interactions within E1 and E2 are shown in gray. Positions of secretase cleavage events and the respective breakdown products are labeled. B. Sequence and proteolytic fragments within βCTF. Aβ peptides, the TMD (gray), and sequence fingerprints within the AICD are colour coded.

In terms of three-dimensional structure, only substructures within the large APP ectodomain have been solved as independently folded subdomains. The N-terminal E1 domain is a two-lobe structure consisting of the growth factor like domain (GFLD, residues 18-123) and a copper-binding domain (CuBD, residues 124 to 189), both comprising mixed $\alpha\beta$ topologies rigidified by disulfide bridges [11-13]. The E1 domain is followed by a highly acidic, and probably unfolded, stretch of about 100 residues that passes on to the E2 domain (residues 290 to 495), consisting of two coiled-coils connected through a continuous central helix and resembling a spectrin family fold [14]. E1 and E2 domains have been implicated in APP dimerization [14-16], which is reported to be modified by the extracellular matrix [17], and to have significant impact on localization and cleavage events. In addition, dimerization might also involve the TMD region [16]. Besides dimerization, APP architecture (and likely function) is also influenced by a series of post-translational modifications, mainly by N- and O-glycosylation and phosphorylation [18], which will be discussed in detail below. The reminder of the ectodomain between E2 and the TMD, the so-called juxtamembrane region (residues 496 to 624), is again intrinsically disordered based on secondary structure prediction and contains the cleavage sites for the α- and β-secretases. The single TMD is clearly α helical, although with partial propensity in forming β structures. This propensity extends also to the juxtamembrane region with the fatal consequence, that after secretase cleavage the amyloid peptide folds into a β hairpin structure and aggregates to form the toxic oligomers and finally the amyloid fibrils. Finally, the AICD itself is again intrinsically disordered as shown by NMR and CD experiments [19, 20]. Importantly however, this small C-terminal stub has recently been shown to adopt different conformations reflecting its versatile functions. The structure-function relationship of the AICD shall be described in the following.

3. Biology of the AICD: Tales of a tail

When talking about the AICD, a clear distinction has to be made: the function (and probably also the structure) is different for AICD as part of APP at the membrane and for AICD as peptide generated by ε-cleavage of γ-secretase and first described by Passer *et al.* [21]. Within the AICD three sequence motifs have been identified to be of functional relevance. The first one is the ^{653}YTSI sequence, which has been implicated in the basolateral sorting of APP in polarized MDCK cells [22] and which is reminiscent to the YXXΦ (X: any residue; Φ: aromatic or large hydrophobic residue) consensus motif as tyrosine-based and clathrin-mediated endocytic sorting signal [23]. Indeed, when Tyr653 is mutated to alanine, APP is equally distributed on apical and basolateral membranes in MDCK cells [24]. Somewhat surprisingly, in neurons polarized sorting occurs independently of this signal [25]. Subcellular trafficking and neuronal APP sorting is still poorly understood [26] and remains a topic of intense investigation. This first motif contains three phosphorylatable residues (YTS), and it has been reported that at least Thr654 and Ser655 are phosphorylated in the adult rat brain under physiological conditions [27].

Much more attention has been drawn to the second fingerprint ^{667}VTPEER, as this site seems to be also critically involved in pathophysiological processes. While the function of the residues has remained elusive prior to the availability of structural data, Thr668 has since been established as the major phosphorylation site of APP and its physiological function has been investigated in the adult rat brain, post mitotic differentiating neurons and dividing cells [18]. Whereas pT668 in neurons is dominant in the fully-glycosylated mature APP, in differentiating cells the purely N-glycosylated immature protein as present in the endoplasmic reticulum and the early Golgi is of relevance. Accordingly, different kinases are responsible for Thr668 phosphorylation. In neurons, it is glycogen synthase kinase-3β (GSK3β) and cyclin-dependent kinase 5 (Cdk5), while Cdk1 and cdc2 kinase phosphorylate this residue in dividing cells. Moreover, when cells are exposed to stress, phosphorylation is taken over by c-Jun N-terminal kinase (JNK) [28].

Phosphorylation on Thr668 of APP depends on the presence of Pro669 and strongly affects Aβ production [29]. This is reminiscent of the Tau protein, where the phosphorylation of certain serine and threonine residues depends on adjacent proline residues and leads to tangle formation [29]. A first molecular explanation for the proline-dependency was revealed by studies showing that the prolyl isomerase Pin1, catalyzing the *cis-trans* isomerization of the Thr-Pro peptide bond, increases amyloidogenic APP processing and selectively elevates Aβ42 levels. Intriguingly, Pin1 is down regulated and/or inhibited by oxidation in neurons of Alzheimer's disease patients and *Pin1* knockout causes neurodegeneration (and tauopathy). Pin1 binds to Thr668-phosphorylated APP and accelerates Pro669 isomerization (by a factor of 10^3). Thus, the AICD swaps between two conformations, as visualized by NMR [29]. This conformational switch may in turn have crucial consequences with regard to the AICD protein interacting network, as shown for the neuronal adaptor protein Fe65 (Figure 2 and see below) [20, 30]. To evaluate in as much the phosphorylation state of Thr688 controls APP processing *in vivo*, knockin mice were generated in which Thr668 was changed to alanine ($APP_{TA/TA}$) [31, 32]. The $APP_{TA/TA}$ mutation, and thus absence of phosphorylation, did not significantly alter APP localization, processing, and Aβ generation, thus questioning the i*n vivo* role of Thr668 phosphorylation. However, these studies cannot rule out the possibility that a pathological increase in Thr668 phosphorylation, as found in AD patients [33], will also modulate its function. In line with this notion, Thr668 phosphorylation has also been reported to influence APP cleavage by caspases between residues Asp664 and Ala665, producing the cytotoxic AICD-C31 fragment, a process that has been strongly implicated in AD pathogenesis [34].

The third and most intensely studied fingerprint within the AICD is the ^{681}GYENPTY sequence containing an NPXY motif, a well-established internalization signal for membrane proteins [35]. NPXY is a classical tyrosine-based sorting signal for transmembrane proteins to endosomes and lysosomes [23]. However, the signal has been shown to only mediate rapid internalization of a subset of type I membrane proteins, including APP as well as members of the low-density lipoprotein (LDL) receptor family and integrin β. These proteins are internalized via clathrin-coated pits. Nevertheless evidence for a direct interaction of NPXY motifs with the coat or the AP-2 adaptor is weak.

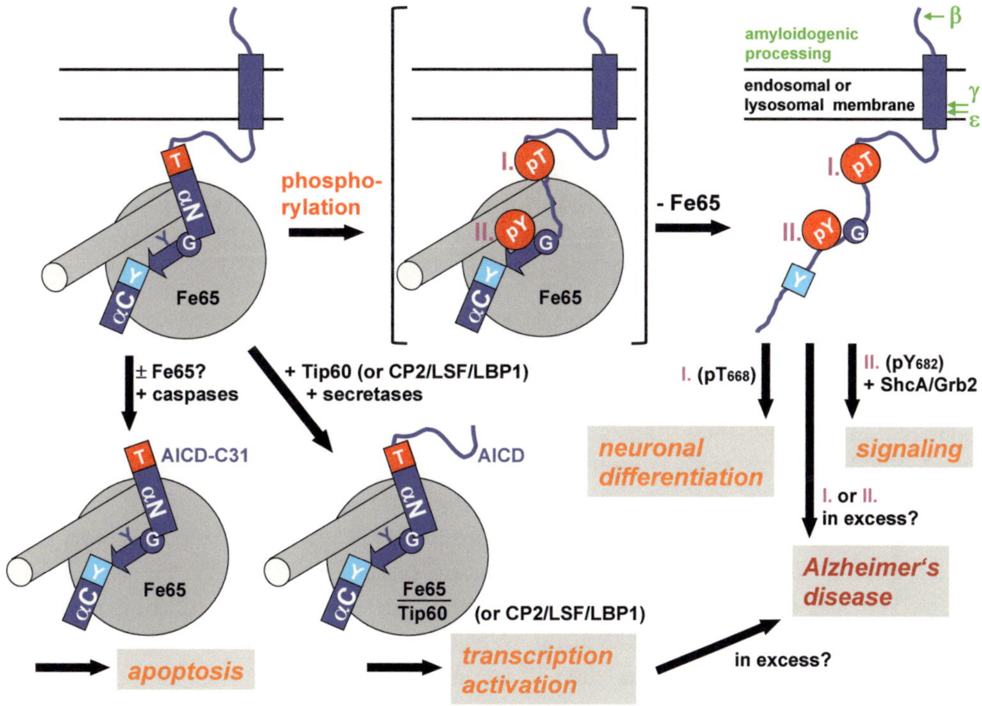

Figure 2. AICD in health and disease. Different fates of the AICD are exemplified for the main AICD interaction with Fe65-PTB2 (red T-box: TPEE, cyan Y-box: NPTY, G: glycine hinge, gray cylinder: C-terminal helix of Fe65-PTB2). In the non-phosphorylated state, AICD forms a stable complex with Fe65-PTB2 that assembles in ternary complexes with i.e. Tip60 or CP2/LSF/LBP1 via Fe65-PTB1. Upon cleavage by the secretases, the liberated complexes are involved in transcription activation. Alternatively, caspase cleavage within the AICD results in cytotoxic AICD-C31, which might compete with AICD for Fe65-PTB2 binding and induce apoptosis. Phosphorylation of either Thr668 (I.) or Tyr682 (II.) results in a destabilization of the Fe65-PTB2/AICD interaction (shown in brackets) and results in complex dissociation. Phosphorylation stimulates (I.) neuronal differentiation or (II.) initiates signaling cascades. Deregulation of the Fe65-PTB2/AICD interactions is strongly implicated in Alzheimer's disease progression.

Instead, the NPXY motif is well known to interact with adaptor proteins containing a domain known as phosphotyrosine-binding (PTB) or phosphotyrosine-interacting domain (PID) [36]. PTB domains reveal a fine tuned plasticity in ligand recognition, and besides recognizing phosphorylated NPXpY motifs, most PTB adaptor proteins can also bind to their ligand in a pY-independent manner. Accordingly, *in vitro* phosphorylation of Tyr687, which does not seem to occur in the brain [18], does i.e. not alter the binding affinity of AICD to its major PTB-containing adaptor protein Fe65.

In APP, the NPXY signal is extended by three residues at the N-terminal side (GYE), with especially Tyr682 being most critical for function [31, 37, 38]. The motif is present in many lysosomal glycoproteins that are endocytosed and targeted to the lysosomes [39]. In cell-culture studies, Tyr682 can be readily phosphorylated by the nerve growth factor receptor TrkA and the tyrosine kinases Abl and Src [40]. In brains of AD patients, it is known that at least βCTF is phosphorylated, whereas this is not the case for αCTF [41]. In addition, phosphorylation regulates both AICD peptide formation and AICD-dependent cellular responses (Figure 2). These data point to a sorting function regulated by Tyr682 phosphorylation, with non-phosphorylated APP kept at the plasma membrane and therefore processed by α-secretase, and a phosphorylation-dependent re-localization resulting in β-cleavage. Sorting implies docking to respective intracellular trafficking machineries and their adaptors, including PTB domain containing proteins. Consistently, an $APP_{YG/YG}$ mutation introduced into the endogenous APP locus by knock-in led to a marked shift toward the non-amyloidogenic pathway in brain with increased levels of full length APP, sAPPα, αCTF, unaltered βCTF and reduced sAPPβ and Aβ40 levels [31].

Sorting due to differentially phosphorylated residues is one side of the medal, signaling is the other [40]. Two signaling proteins are well known to require Tyr682 phosphorylation for binding to APP-CTFs, namely ShcA and Grb2. ShcA is a member of a family of cytoplasmic adaptor proteins (ShcA, ShcB, ShcC) that interacts with its PTB and Src homology2 (SH2) domains with receptor tyrosine kinases (RTKs) and activated growth factor receptors, which is the case also for SH2/SH3 domains containing Grb2 [42]. The initiated cascades are involved both in cell proliferation and gene transcription events, like i.e. the MAP kinase pathway. Again, binding occurs only to pTyr682 of βCTFs but not of αCTFs [41] (Figure 2). Whereas the reasons for the different binding preferences remain elusive, the underlying structural transitions within the AICD itself modulating sorting and signaling have been studied in some detail.

4. Structural transitions within the AICD

First structural insights on the AICD peptide came from NMR experiments, revealing most of the AICD to be unstructured. The transient structure (also termed intrinsic disorder: ID) of cytoplasmic domains of membrane proteins is well suited for the molecular recognition in intracellular signaling events for a number of reasons [43]: (i) modulation of the structural propensity provides ID proteins with the capability to combine high specificity with low affinity; (ii) binding diversity in which one region specifically recognizes differently shaped partners by structural accommodation at the binding interface, a phenomenon known as one-to-many signaling; (iii) binding commonality in which distinct sequences recognize a common binding site (with eventually different folds); (iv) the formation of large interaction surfaces as the ID region wraps up or surrounds its binding partner, making it possible to overcome steric restrictions; (v) faster rates of association by reducing dependence on orientation factors and by enlarging target sizes; (vi) faster rates of dissociation by unzipping mechanisms; (vii) the precise control and simple regulation of the binding thermodynamics; and (viii) the reduced life-time of ID proteins in the cell, possibly representing a mechanism of rapid turnover of important regulatory molecules. A prominent example of intrinsically disordered proteins is α-synuclein, a protein critically involved in Parkinson's disease, which binds to a multitude of partners differentially by alternative folding [44], a feature that equally applies to the intracellular domain of APP.

http://dx.doi.org/10.5772/54543

Although NMR experiments revealed the AICD to be intrinsically disordered, the TPEE and NPTY motifs where found to form type I β-turns and TPEE forms part of a helix-capping box [19] (Figure 3). Type I turns are the most frequent reverse turns in protein structures, which in total involve about 1/3rd of all residues. Turns usually occur on the exposed protein surfaces and represent molecular recognition sites. In a capping box, the side chain of the first helical residue forms a hydrogen bond with the backbone of the fourth helical residue and, reciprocally, the side chain of the fourth residue forms a hydrogen bond with the backbone of the first residue [45]. These boxes are known to stabilize the N-termini of α-helices, and preordering of the elements is thought to guide recognition of the intracellular protein network and to reduce the entropic costs for complex formation, a feature that applies as well for APP. In addition, the conformation of the TPEE motif and the propensity of forming the N-terminally capped α helix critically depend on the phosphorylation status of Thr668 [20, 46]. This structure-function relationship can be explored by the study of the AICD with its cytoplasmic interaction partners.

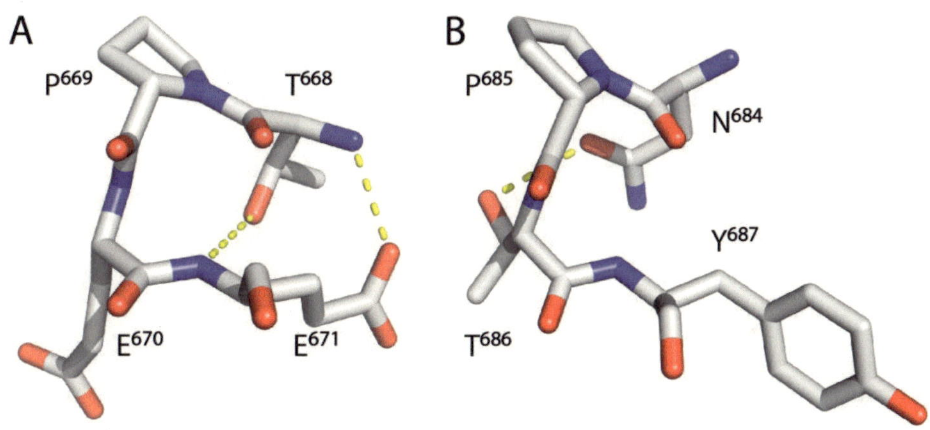

Figure 3. The TPEE and NPTY motifs. A. The TPEE motif forms a type I β-turn and a helix capping box with two characteristic hydrogen bonds (dashed yellow lines). B. The NPTY motif forms a similar type I β-turn.

5. Interaction partners of the AICD

More than 20 proteins have been reported to interact with the AICD [47] (Table 1). However, little is known whether these complexes occur also *in vivo* and what relevance they may have for cell physiology or AD pathogenesis. Basically, they can be classified in modifying, sorting, or signaling interactions. The modifying enzymes have been already mentioned and account for phosphorylation and prolyl *cis/trans* isomerization events. Basolateral sorting is guided by the protein PAT1, which is the only protein that has been shown to directly interact with the ^{653}YTSI motif and is associated with microtubules [48].

Knowledge about the interaction partners for the [667]VTPEER motif is similar scarce. Major binder for the motif, and as well for the complete AICD, are the multi-domain adaptor/scaffolding proteins of the Fe65 family (Fe65, Fe65L1, and Fe65L2) [49]. The only additional binding partner to the [667]VTPEER motif is the dimeric adaptor protein 14-3-3γ, which seems to stabilize the AICD/Fe65 interaction [50]. Fe65 is enriched in brain, whereas Fe65L1 and Fe65L2 are more widely expressed. All three members contain a WW domain and two PTB domains (PTB1 and PTB2). Through the PTB2 domain, they interact with the AICD and can alter APP processing. After proteolytic processing of APP and release of the AICD to the cytoplasm, Fe65 can translocate to the nucleus to participate in gene transcription events (Figure 2), which is modulated by 14-3-3γ. This role is further mediated by interactions of Fe65-PTB1 with the transcription factors CP2/LSF/LBP1 [51] and Tip60 [52] and the WW domain with the nucleosome assembly factor SET [53]. Possible target genes identified by reporter assays include GSK3β, Neprilysin, KAI1, and the low-density lipoprotein receptor-related protein 1 (LRP1), but the physiological relevance for endogenous transcriptional regulation has been discussed controversially [54]. Fe65-PTB1 also interacts with two cell surface lipoproteins receptors, namely LRP1 [55] and ApoEr2 [56], forming trimeric complexes with APP. The Fe55 WW domain further binds to mammalian Ena (mEna) [57], through which it functions in regulation of the actin cytoskeleton, cell motility, and neuronal growth cone formation [49]. The interaction has been implicated in a role for AICD signaling, in synaptic plasticity and memory [58]. Moreover, Fe65 family proteins have attracted attention, as Fe65 or Fe65L1 double knockout mice revealed defects in cortical development with neuronal mispositioning and ectopia, resembling human lissencephaly type 2 [59]. Interestingly, very similar cortical defects were also found in APP-/-APLP1-/-APLP2-/- triple knockout mice lacking all APP family members, suggesting a lack of APP/Fe65 dependent signaling as the underlying cause of defects in both mouse mutants [60].

Fe65 binding to the AICD is unique, as its extended binding interface ranges from the [667]VTPEER up to the [681]GYENPTY motif and thus includes almost the entire AICD-C31 fragment (Figures 2 and 4A). Most other AICD interacting proteins recognize the [671]GYENPTY motif and neighbouring residues, with the interaction site spanning only about 10 residues. As [681]GYENPTY is essential for APP trafficking, the respective complexes can also alter APP processing. Like Fe65, the binders for this motif are PTB-containing proteins including members of the X11/Mint, JIP, Dab, and Shc families, as well as the Numb protein.

Mints consist of a divergent N-terminal region and conserved C-terminal sequences composed of one PTB domain and two tandem PDZ domains. Although their regulatory role for APP metabolism and transport is unresolved, it seems that they slow cellular APP processing and reduce Aβ40 and Aβ42 secretion [61] by suppressing translocation of APP into BACE- and γ-secretase-rich detergent-resistant membrane (DRM) domains, the so-called rafts [62, 66]. In addition, there is evidence for a functional role of the AICD interaction with X11/Mints for synapse formation [62, 67] and synaptic neurotransmitter release [68]. c-Jun N-terminal kinase (JNK) interacting protein-1 (JIP1), a scaffolding protein for the JNK kinase cascade, has been suggested to mediate anterograde transport of APP by the molecular motor kinesin-1. However, this initial view has been challenged recently, as in contrast to this model, APP

http://dx.doi.org/10.5772/54543

constructs lacking the AICD are still transported to the nerve terminal by the fast axonal transport mechanism [63].

Protein	Interacting domain	Interacting region within AICD	Function	Processing*	Selected citations
PAT1	n.a.	YTSI	Basolateral sorting	α↑, β↓**	[48]
Fe65,	PTB2	AICD-C31:	Endocytosis, signaling and	β↓	[49]
Fe65L1, -L2	n.a.	VTPEER + GYENPTY	transcription activation, ...	n.a.	[50]
14-3-3-γ	PTB	VTPEER	AICD/Fe65 stabilization	β↓	[61] [62]
X11/Mint		GYENPTY	Exocytosis, synapse formation, ...		
JIP1	PTB	GYENPTY	Transport	β↓	[63]
Dab1	PTB	GYENPTY	Transport, signaling	α↑, β↓	[64]
ShcA/Grb2	PTB/SH2	G(pY)ENPTY	Signaling	-	[42]
Numb	PTB	GYENPTY	Notch crosstalk	***	[65]

Table 1. Selected interaction partners of the AICD. *Data depend on cell line studied and are sometimes conflicting. **Due to basolateral sorting and independent of PAT1 binding. Pat1 binding as such increases Aβ levels [48]. ***Numb isoform dependent. ↓ denotes changes of non-amyloidogenic (α) or amyloidogenic (β) APP processing.

The Dab family member Dab1 regulates neuronal migration in mammals as an essential component of the Reelin signaling pathway. Dab1 binds not only to APP family proteins [64] but is well known to also bind to ApoE receptors (ApoEr2, VLDLR, and LRP) [69]. Dab1 increases cell surface expression of APP and ApoEr2, increases α-cleavage of APP and ApoEr2, and decreases APP βCTF formation and Aβ production in transfected cells and in primary neurons. The Dab family represents a prototype of PTB domains that bind their ligands in a pY-independent manner [36]. In addition Dab proteins bind specifically to the phosphoinositide (PI) PI-4,5-P_2, which is predominantly located at the cellular membrane [70]. Binding of PTB domains to PIs is a common principle to locate and orientate the adaptors at the target membrane and to facilitate downstream events that accompany NPXY peptide binding. Since PTB domains structurally belong to the pleckstrin homology (PH) superfold family and PH domains are the prototypical PI binding domains, this function seems to be evolutionarily conserved within PTB domains [36]. The crystal structures of ternary complexes of Dabs bound to ApoEr2 [71] or APP [72] peptides and lipid revealed the lipid head group (IP_3) to be recognized by a large basic patch opposite the peptide-binding groove (Figure 4A). This patch, also termed as "phospholipid binding-crown", is conserved in many PTB domains [36].

Finally, binding of the AICD to the Numb PTB domain has been found to inhibit Notch signaling [65], thereby establishing a crosstalk between the APP family and Notch in the development of the peripheral nervous system (PNS) [73]. Like APP, the Notch receptor undergoes a series of proteolytic cleavages that release the Notch intracellular domain (NICD) that functions in transcriptional activation and subsequent signal transduction events, including proliferation, differentiation, or apoptotic cues [74]. Similar to the NICD, the AICD has been also found to regulate PI-mediated calcium signaling through a γ-secretase dependent pathway [75, 76]. Cells lacking APP were shown to exhibit deficits in calcium storage that could be reversed by transfection with APP constructs containing an intact AICD. Constructs lacking the AICD were not able to rescue the phenotype, strongly indicating that this domain is critically involved in endoplasmic reticulum (ER) calcium filling [76]. The multitude of interactions with the AICD raises the question of the spatial and temporal regulation of all these complexes, which needs a detailed structural analysis and a thorough biochemical characterization.

6. Structure-function relationship of AICD complexes

The structure-function relationship of AICD complexes is governed by the one-to-many principle with the intrinsically disordered AICD folding onto its manifold adaptor proteins, in particular the PTB domain containing proteins. The recurrent interaction pattern includes the recognition of the ^{681}GYENPTY sequence, which shall be described in the following. High resolution structures for this interaction are known for Dab1 and 2 [72], X11α [77], and the Fe65-PTB2 domains [30] (Figure 4A). All PTB domains comprise a pleckstrin homology (PH) fold consisting of a central β sandwich structure and a C-terminal α helix. Overall, complex formation can be described as an induced-fit docking of the AICD to a rigid PTB domain scaffold. Common to all the complexes is the binding of the ^{681}GYEN sequence to the β5 strand of the respective PTB domain by a mechanism called β completion, where a (antiparallel) β sheet is created between two polypeptide chains (*in trans*) (Figure 4D). This interaction occurs between the protein backbones and therefore strong sequence conservation is not present on the PTB domain side. The conservation of AICD Gly681 is explained as longer side chains would cause steric clashes with the PTB domains, as shown for the Fe65-PTB2/AICD interaction, where a G681A mutation abolishes the binding and Gal4-Tip60-dependent transactivation [78]. The importance of the flexible glycine becomes evident when comparing the solved PTB/AICD complexes (Figure 4B), revealing that Gly681 forms a hinge that allows for different AICD conformations in the N-terminal direction. The hinge function correlates with a peptide-flip of the glycine [30].

The side chain of Tyr682 is accommodated in the center of the interface and faces the C-terminal helix of PTB domains (Figures 3A and 3D). In all complexes it lays in a hydrophobic pocket, however, the conformations between the Fe65-PTB2 and Dab1 in respect to X11α and Dab2 complexes are different. The hydrophobic nature of the pocket explains the general conservation of a tyrosine or phenylalanine in this position in the context of NPXY sequences. All crystallized complexes are specific for non-phosphorylated Tyr682, which can be readily explained, as there is no space available to accommodate the extra phosphate moiety. This is in contrast to ShcA, where the binding site is more open [79], which apparently allows for binding of a phosphorylated Tyr682 (although no structure of this complex is available). The readout of the conserved glutamate is again different in the PTB complexes, although its function as selectivity filter seems to be minor. Whereas it forms i.e. a salt bridge with an arginine of X11α, in the Fe65-PTB2 complex it is fixed *in cis* to Lys688 following the NPTY motif.

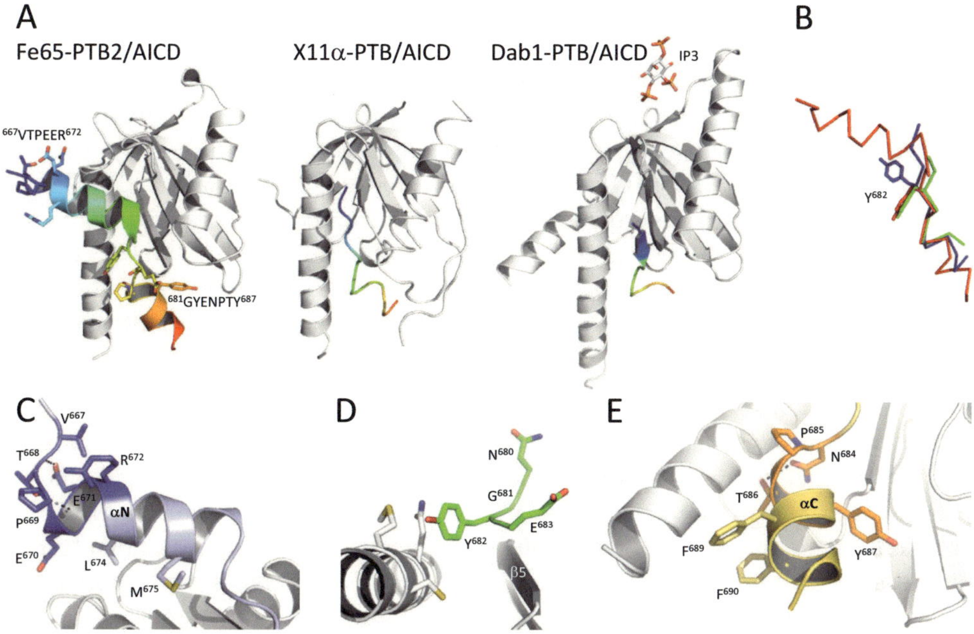

Figure 4. Structure of the AICD in PTB domain complexes. A. Crystal structures of AICD peptides in complex with PTB domains: Fe65-PTB2/AICD (PDB code 3DXC), X11α-PTB/AICD (1X11), and Dab1-PTB/AICD (1OQN). AICD peptides are colour coded from blue (N-terminus) to red (C-terminus) and PTB domains are given in gray. In Fe65-PTB2/AICD, the visible AICD structure corresponds to AICD-C31 and includes both the ^{667}VTPEER and the ^{681}GYENPTY sequences. Dab1 is also bound to the polar head group of the lipid PI-4,5-P_2 (IP3: inositol-1,4,5-triphosphate). B. Superposition of the three AICD fragments as shown in Figure 3A (complex with Fe65-PTB2: red; X11α: blue; Dab1: green). The alternative side chain conformations of Tyr682 are highlighted. C. Close-up view on the AICD helix αN in complex with Fe65-PTB2. The ^{667}VTPEER motif is highlighted in blue and hydrogen bonds within the capping box are given as dashed lines. D. Interaction of the ^{680}NGYE motif with Fe65-PTB2. The AICD stretch forms a β sheet *in trans* with strand β5 from the PTB domain. The side chain of Tyr682 is accommodated in a hydrophobic pocket created by the C-terminal helix of the PTB domain. E. Interaction of the ^{684}NPTY motif and helix αC of the AICD with Fe65-PTB2. Tyr687 is rather solvent exposed and helix αC is fixed to the PTB domain by hydrophobic interactions of two subsequent phenylalanines.

As already described, the ^{684}NPTY sequence is forming a type I β-turn structure, which is retained within the complexes and forms the N-terminal cap of an induced α-helix at the very C-terminus of AICD (helix αC) (Figure 4E). Asn684 has a conserved structural role, with the carboxamide of the side chain hydrogen bonding to the main chain of Thr686. As the carboxamide is also tightly bonded to the PTB domains, the preformed NPTY conformation is a major determinant and probably also a starting point for AICD folding and complex formation. The conserved proline initiates and stabilizes the subsequent helix as found in many α helices. The most prominent residue, however, is Tyr687, as the tyrosine at this position is the discriminator for the classification in pY-dependent and pY-independent PTB domains [36]. In all structurally solved AICD/PTB domain complexes the peptide is non-phosphorylated, which reflects the *in vivo* situation within neurons. The pY-independence is readily explained, as the binding pocket is rather solvent exposed, and besides some van-der-Waals interactions of the benzene ring the tyrosine is not coordinated further. The binding mode is quite different in pY-dependent Shc or IRS1 peptide complexes, where the phosphate moiety is read out by a set of conserved arginine residues and the binding pocket is much more pronounced [36].

The NPTY sequence is followed by the ^{688}KFFEQMQN^{695} sequence, which forms the C-terminus of the AICD (Figures 4A and 4E). The conformation of this region is slightly different and not always present in the structures, as the complexes have mostly been formed with truncated synthetic peptides. In the Fe65-PTB2 (which contains the entire C-terminus) and X11α complexes, the region is part of the C-terminal helix αC. The helix is fixed to the PTB domains by hydrophobic interactions of the two phenylalanines (Phe689 and Phe690) with the C-terminal helices of the respective PTB domains. These helices are three turns longer than those of Shc [79] and IRS1 [80] PTBs, and therefore the total interaction surfaces are significantly larger.

In most PTB domain complexes bound to an NPXY motif the described surfaces comprise the entire interaction, however, there is a single exception to the rule: the Fe65-PTB2/AICD complex, where the interface is about three times as large and includes an additional α helix (helix αN, ^{669}PEERHLSKMQQ^{679}) N-terminal to the ^{681}GYENPTY sequence (Figure 4C) [30]. This helix is N-terminally capped by the ^{667}VTPEER motif comprising the phosphorylatable Thr668 as already described. Like helix αC, helix αN is of amphipathic character and binds on a hydrophobic patch on the Fe65-PTB2 surface located in between strand β5 and the N-terminus of the C-terminal helix, which is almost perpendicularly crossed by helix αN. Whereas Leu674 and Met677 cover the hydrophobic patch, Glu670, His673, and Gln678 are involved in polar interactions with the PTB domain. With the exception of Glu670, the ^{667}VTPEER capping box is not touching the PTB domain, which is somewhat astonishing, as it was afore known that phosphorylation of Thr668 is detrimental to complex formation [20]. As described for free AICD, the side chain of Thr668 is hydrogen-bonded to the main chain of Glu671, and Pro668 is *in trans* configuration. Furthermore, the side chain of Glu671 is tied back to the main chain nitrogen of Thr668, and thus completing the rigid helix cap.

The most important question arising from structural data is how phosphorylation is able to regulate Fe65-PTB2/AICD complex formation in a process that is critically involved in Aβ generation and AD pathogenesis? Phosphorylation induces a *cis* configuration of Pro669 [46], which is incompatible with the formation of helix αN. As found by mutational studies [30], the destruction of the helix cap increases the entropy of the system and reduces the binding affinity, and once the helix is dissolved, the remaining interfaces are not sufficient for maintaining the complex. This molecular switch model is only valid for the Fe65-PTB2/AICD interaction, as all other PTB domains do not contact Thr668 and phosphorylation does therefore not alter their binding affinity [20]. Intriguingly, the Fe65-PTB2/AICD interface spans almost the entire AICD-C31 fragment, which has been implicated in apoptotic events. This raises the next question: what determines stability, lifetime, and eventually toxicity of the AICD?

7. AICD turnover

The turnover of APP is very fast (with a half life of cell surface APP of about 30-40 minutes only [81] and only about 10% of APP are estimated to reach the cellular membrane, whereas the majority of APP locates to the Golgi apparatus and trans-Golgi network [10]. APP not shed at the surface is internalized within minutes [82], delivered to endosomes, and if not degraded in lysosomes recycled to the cell surface [83]. AICD is even more difficult to study, as due to its small size it is rapidly degraded once it is released from the membrane by the insulin degrading enzyme (IDE) [84], that also degrades the Aβ peptide, by the proteasome [85], or by the endosomal/lysosomal system [86]. However, AICD found in the nucleus appears to be more stable, suggesting that AICD involved in signal transduction escapes rapid degradation [87]. Nuclear AICD is stabilized via interaction with Fe65 [88, 89], which accordingly has a dominant function in AICD mediated physiological and pathophysiological processes.

From a structural viewpoint it is evident that the enlarged and unique protein-protein interface coupled with high affinity binding prevents the AICD from degradation. Interestingly, AICD-C31 (starting at Ala665), which is believed to induce apoptosis and is enriched in AD brains [34], fits exactly in length with the AICD part interacting with Fe65-PTB2. Hence, two scenarios comprising a modulating role for Fe65 in AICD-C31 mediated neurotoxicity might be envisaged: (i), under physiological conditions Fe65 protects the AICD from caspase cleavage occurring at Asp664 and might therefore inhibit apoptosis as shown previously [90] and (ii), increased levels of AICD-C31 compete with AICD binding as part of full-length APP and therefore interfere with physiological Fe65 functions including nuclear signaling and trafficking of APP. In any case, modifying the protein-interacting network around the AICD seems to be a valid target for decreasing neurotoxicity and the treatment of AD.

8. Conclusion

Despite enormous efforts to develop an efficient treatment for AD, only symptomatic treatments with modest impact on the progress of the disease are available [6]. Drugs currently approved for the treatment of AD are either acetylcholine esterase inhibitors to increase the level of the neurotransmitter, which is depleted in AD brains, or antagonize the NMDA receptor to prevent abnormal neuronal stimulation [91]. None of them directly targets the amyloid cascade and would thereby allow for a disease-modifying treatment. Many current therapeutic approaches for AD focus on the reduction of the Aβ load either by inhibiting the involved secretases BACE and γ-secretase, or by augmenting the elimination of amyloid peptides, e.g. by active or passive immunotherapy [6]. Finally, a smaller number of trials have targeted ApoE4 levels or either tau phosphorylation or tau aggregation. None of the approaches was successful so far, which means that either there were not enough clinical trials or the ideas were too simplistic to be potent for a complex disease. Like for other complex diseases (i.e. hypertension or AIDS), a combination of drugs that have different modes of action could be the key to success.

In this sense, the AICD might be re-evaluated as a potential drug target. In contrast to Aβ, the AICD is a physiological highly relevant protein domain modulating a diverse set of important APP functions including trafficking and signal transduction. As both processes are also directly affecting Aβ production, upstream targeting of AICD might be beneficial as the Aβ pathology is prevented *a priori*. Moreover, the pathophysiology of the AICD and its breakdown product AICD-C31 has come into the focus of AD research and would be tackled directly. As the AICD by its nature is created intracellular, efficient compounds need to be able to pass the plasma membrane and to accumulate within neurons, as is i.e. the case for the NMDA receptor antagonist memantine [92]. However, the AICD is intrinsically disordered, and therefore the protein interaction network around the AICD might be the crucial target rather than the AICD itself. Major binding partners are the PTB domains, with their known ability to modulate Aβ production (like Fe65, ShcA, and X11α) and to specifically recognize and fold the AICD. Although protein-protein interactions are notoriously difficult to be targeted, the urgent need for a disease-modifying and efficient treatment for this devastating disease seems worth the trial.

Acknowledgements

UM and KW are supported by the Research Unit FOR1332 from the Deutsche Forschungsgemeinschaft (DFG). UM was further supported by NGFNplus and KW by DFG grant KW2649/1-4.

Author details

Ulrike Müller[1] and Klemens Wild[2*]

*Address all correspondence to: klemens.wild@bzh.uni-heidelberg.de

1 Institut für Pharmazie und Molekulare Biotechnologie, Universität Heidelberg, Germany

2 Biochemiezentrum der Universität Heidelberg (BZH), Universität Heidelberg, Germany

References

[1] Ballard, C, et al. *Alzheimer's disease.* Lancet, (2011)., 1019-1031.

[2] Masters, C. L, & Selkoe, D. J. *Biochemistry of Amyloid beta-Protein and Amyloid Deposits in Alzheimer Disease.* Cold Spring Harb Perspect Med, (2012)., a006262.

[3] Lichtenthaler, S. F, Haass, C, & Steiner, H. *Regulated intramembrane proteolysis--lessons from amyloid precursor protein processing.* J Neurochem, (2011)., 779-796.

[4] Dislich, B, & Lichtenthaler, S. F. *The Membrane-Bound Aspartyl Protease BACE1: Molecular and Functional Properties in Alzheimer's Disease and Beyond.* Front Physiol, (2012)., 8.

[5] Tam, J. H, & Pasternak, S. H. *Amyloid and Alzheimer's disease: inside and out.* Can J Neurol Sci, (2012)., 286-298.

[6] Huang, Y, & Mucke, L. *Alzheimer mechanisms and therapeutic strategies.* Cell, (2012)., 1204-1222.

[7] Muller, U. C, & Zheng, H. *Physiological Functions of APP Family Proteins.* Cold Spring Harb Perspect Med, (2012)., a006288.

[8] Pardossi-piquard, R, & Checler, F. *The physiology of the beta-amyloid precursor protein intracellular domain AICD.* J Neurochem, (2012). Suppl 1:, 109-124.

[9] Nikolaev, A, et al. *APP binds DR6 to trigger axon pruning and neuron death via distinct caspases.* Nature, (2009)., 981-989.

[10] Haass, C, et al. *Trafficking and Proteolytic Processing of APP.* Cold Spring Harb Perspect Med, (2012)., a006270.

[11] Dahms, S. O, et al. *Structure and biochemical analysis of the heparin-induced E1 dimer of the amyloid precursor protein.* Proc Natl Acad Sci U S A, (2010)., 5381-5386.

[12] Barnham, K. J, et al. *Structure of the Alzheimer's disease amyloid precursor protein copper binding domain. A regulator of neuronal copper homeostasis.* J Biol Chem, (2003)., 17401-17407.

[13] Rossjohn, J, et al. *Crystal structure of the N-terminal, growth factor-like domain of Alzheimer amyloid precursor protein.* Nat Struct Biol, (1999)., 327-331.

[14] Wang, Y, & Ha, Y. *The X-ray structure of an antiparallel dimer of the human amyloid precursor protein E2 domain.* Mol Cell, (2004)., 343-353.

[15] Soba, P, et al. *Homo- and heterodimerization of APP family members promotes intercellular adhesion.* EMBO J, (2005)., 3624-3634.

[16] Kaden, D, et al. *The amyloid precursor protein and its homologues: structural and functional aspects of native and pathogenic oligomerization.* Eur J Cell Biol, (2012)., 234-239.

[17] Gralle, M, et al. *Solution conformation and heparin-induced dimerization of the full-length extracellular domain of the human amyloid precursor protein.* J Mol Biol, (2006)., 493-508.

[18] Suzuki, T, & Nakaya, T. *Regulation of amyloid beta-protein precursor by phosphorylation and protein interactions.* J Biol Chem, (2008)., 29633-29637.

[19] Ramelot, T. A, Gentile, L. N, & Nicholson, L. K. *Transient structure of the amyloid precursor protein cytoplasmic tail indicates preordering of structure for binding to cytosolic factors.* Biochemistry, (2000)., 2714-2725.

[20] Ando, K, et al. *Phosphorylation-dependent regulation of the interaction of amyloid precursor protein with Fe65 affects the production of beta-amyloid.* J Biol Chem, (2001)., 40353-40361.

[21] Passer, B, et al. *Generation of an apoptotic intracellular peptide by gamma-secretase cleavage of Alzheimer's amyloid beta protein precursor.* J Alzheimers Dis, (2000)., 289-301.

[22] Lai, A, et al. *Signal-dependent trafficking of beta-amyloid precursor protein-transferrin receptor chimeras in madin-darby canine kidney cells.* J Biol Chem, (1998)., 3732-3739.

[23] Bonifacino, J. S, & Traub, L. M. *Signals for sorting of transmembrane proteins to endosomes and lysosomes.* Annu Rev Biochem, (2003)., 395-447.

[24] Haass, C, et al. *Polarized sorting of beta-amyloid precursor protein and its proteolytic products in MDCK cells is regulated by two independent signals.* J Cell Biol, (1995)., 537-547.

[25] Back, S, et al. *beta-amyloid precursor protein can be transported independent of any sorting signal to the axonal and dendritic compartment.* J Neurosci Res, (2007)., 2580-2590.

[26] Brunholz, S, et al. *Axonal transport of APP and the spatial regulation of APP cleavage and function in neuronal cells.* Exp Brain Res, (2012)., 353-364.

[27] Oishi, M, et al. *The cytoplasmic domain of Alzheimer's amyloid precursor protein is phosphorylated at Thr654, Ser655, and Thr668 in adult rat brain and cultured cells.* Mol Med, (1997)., 111-123.

[28] Standen, C. L, et al. *Phosphorylation of thr(668) in the cytoplasmic domain of the Alzheimer's disease amyloid precursor protein by stress-activated protein kinase 1b (Jun N-terminal kinase-3).* J Neurochem, (2001)., 316-320.

[29] Pastorino, L, et al. *The prolyl isomerase Pin1 regulates amyloid precursor protein processing and amyloid-beta production.* Nature, (2006)., 528-534.

[30] Radzimanowski, J, et al. *Structure of the intracellular domain of the amyloid precursor protein in complex with Fe65-PTB2.* EMBO Rep, (2008)., 1134-1140.

[31] Barbagallo, A. P, et al. *Tyr(682) in the intracellular domain of APP regulates amyloidogenic APP processing in vivo.* PLoS One, (2010)., e15503.

[32] Sano, Y, et al. *Physiological mouse brain Abeta levels are not related to the phosphorylation state of threonine-668 of Alzheimer's APP.* PLoS One, (2006)., e51.

[33] Lee, M. S, et al. *APP processing is regulated by cytoplasmic phosphorylation.* J Cell Biol, (2003)., 83-95.

[34] Lu, D. C, et al. *Caspase cleavage of the amyloid precursor protein modulates amyloid beta-protein toxicity.* J Neurochem, (2003)., 733-741.

[35] Chen, W. J, Goldstein, J. L, & Brown, M. S. *NPXY, a sequence often found in cytoplasmic tails, is required for coated pit-mediated internalization of the low density lipoprotein receptor.* J Biol Chem, (1990)., 3116-3123.

[36] Uhlik, M. T, et al. *Structural and evolutionary division of phosphotyrosine binding (PTB) domains.* J Mol Biol, (2005)., 1-20.

[37] Perez, R. G, et al. *Mutagenesis identifies new signals for beta-amyloid precursor protein endocytosis, turnover, and the generation of secreted fragments, including Abeta42.* J Biol Chem, (1999)., 18851-18856.

[38] Barbagallo, A. P, et al. *The intracellular threonine of amyloid precursor protein that is essential for docking of Pin1 is dispensable for developmental function.* PLoS One, (2011). , e18006.

[39] Kornfeld, S, & Mellman, I. *The biogenesis of lysosomes.* Annu Rev Cell Biol, (1989). , 483-525.

[40] Schettini, G, et al. *Phosphorylation of APP-CTF-AICD domains and interaction with adaptor proteins: signal transduction and/or transcriptional role--relevance for Alzheimer pathology.* J Neurochem, (2010). , 1299-1308.

[41] Russo, C, et al. *Signal transduction through tyrosine-phosphorylated C-terminal fragments of amyloid precursor protein via an enhanced interaction with Shc/Grb2 adaptor proteins in reactive astrocytes of Alzheimer's disease brain.* J Biol Chem, (2002). , 35282-35288.

[42] Cattaneo, E, & Pelicci, P. G. *Emerging roles for SH2/PTB-containing Shc adaptor proteins in the developing mammalian brain.* Trends Neurosci, (1998). , 476-481.

[43] Uversky, V. N, Oldfield, C. J, & Dunker, A. K. *Showing your ID: intrinsic disorder as an ID for recognition, regulation and cell signaling.* J Mol Recognit, (2005). , 343-384.

[44] Uversky, V. N. *A Protein-chameleon conformational plasticity of alpha-synuclein, a disordered protein involved in neurodegenerative disorders.* J Biomol Struct Dyn, (2003). , 211-234.

[45] Seale, J. W, Srinivasan, R, & Rose, G. D. *Sequence determinants of the capping box, a stabilizing motif at the N-termini of alpha-helices.* Protein Sci, (1994). , 1741-1745.

[46] Ramelot, T. A, & Nicholson, L. K. *Phosphorylation-induced structural changes in the amyloid precursor protein cytoplasmic tail detected by NMR.* J Mol Biol, (2001). , 871-884.

[47] Muller, T, et al. *The amyloid precursor protein intracellular domain (AICD) as modulator of gene expression, apoptosis, and cytoskeletal dynamics-relevance for Alzheimer's disease.* Prog Neurobiol, (2008). , 393-406.

[48] Kuan, Y. H, et al. *PAT1a modulates intracellular transport and processing of amyloid precursor protein (APP), APLP1, and APLP2.* J Biol Chem, (2006). , 40114-40123.

[49] Mcloughlin, D. M, & Miller, C. C. *The FE65 proteins and Alzheimer's disease.* J Neurosci Res, (2008). , 744-754.

[50] Sumioka, A, et al. *Role of 14-3-3gamma in FE65-dependent gene transactivation mediated by the amyloid beta-protein precursor cytoplasmic fragment.* J Biol Chem, (2005). , 42364-42374.

[51] Minopoli, G, et al. *The beta-amyloid precursor protein functions as a cytosolic anchoring site that prevents Fe65 nuclear translocation.* J Biol Chem, (2001). , 6545-6550.

[52] Cao, X, & Sudhof, T. C. *A Transcriptionally correction of transcriptively] active complex of APP with Fe65 and histone acetyltransferase Tip60.* Science, (2001). , 115-120.

[53] Telese, F, et al. *Transcription regulation by the adaptor protein Fe65 and the nucleosome assembly factor SET.* EMBO Rep, (2005). , 77-82.

[54] Konietzko, U. *AICD nuclear signaling and its possible contribution to Alzheimer's disease.* Curr Alzheimer Res, (2012). , 200-216.

[55] Wagner, T, & Pietrzik, C. U. *The role of lipoprotein receptors on the physiological function of APP.* Exp Brain Res, (2012). , 377-387.

[56] Bu, G. *Apolipoprotein Ea nd its receptors in Alzheimer's disease: pathways, pathogenesis and therapy.* Nat Rev Neurosci, (2009). , 333-344.

[57] Sabo, S. L, et al. *The Alzheimer amyloid precursor protein (APP) and FE65, an APP-binding protein, regulate cell movement.* J Cell Biol, (2001). , 1403-1414.

[58] Ma, H, et al. *Involvement of beta-site APP cleaving enzyme 1 (BACE1) in amyloid precursor protein-mediated enhancement of memory and activity-dependent synaptic plasticity.* Proc Natl Acad Sci U S A, (2007). , 8167-8172.

[59] Guenette, S, et al. *Essential roles for the FE65 amyloid precursor protein-interacting proteins in brain development.* EMBO J, (2006). , 420-431.

[60] Herms, J, et al. *Cortical dysplasia resembling human type 2 lissencephaly in mice lacking all three APP family members.* EMBO J, (2004). , 4106-4115.

[61] Mueller, H. T, et al. *Modulation of amyloid precursor protein metabolism by X11alpha / Mint-1. A deletion analysis of protein-protein interaction domains.* J Biol Chem, (2000). , 39302-39306.

[62] Wang, Z, et al. *Presynaptic and postsynaptic interaction of the amyloid precursor protein promotes peripheral and central synaptogenesis.* J Neurosci, (2009). , 10788-10801.

[63] Szodorai, A, et al. *APP anterograde transport requires Rab3A GTPase activity for assembly of the transport vesicle.* J Neurosci, (2009). , 14534-14544.

[64] Howell, B. W, et al. *The disabled 1 phosphotyrosine-binding domain binds to the internalization signals of transmembrane glycoproteins and to phospholipids.* Mol Cell Biol, (1999). , 5179-5188.

[65] Roncarati, R, et al. *The gamma-secretase-generated intracellular domain of beta-amyloid precursor protein binds Numb and inhibits Notch signaling.* Proc Natl Acad Sci U S A, (2002). , 7102-7107.

[66] Saito, Y, et al. *X11 proteins regulate the translocation of amyloid beta-protein precursor (APP) into detergent-resistant membrane and suppress the amyloidogenic cleavage of APP by beta-site-cleaving enzyme in brain.* J Biol Chem, (2008). , 35763-35771.

[67] Ashley, J, et al. *Fasciclin II signals new synapse formation through amyloid precursor protein and the scaffolding protein dX11/Mint.* J Neurosci, (2005). , 5943-5955.

[68] Weyer, S. W, et al. *APP and APLP2 are essential at PNS and CNS synapses for transmission, spatial learning and LTP.* EMBO J, (2011). , 2266-2280.

[69] Hoe, H. S, & Rebeck, G. W. *Functional interactions of APP with the apoE receptor family.* J Neurochem, (2008). , 2263-2271.

[70] Mclaughlin, S, et al. *PIP(2) and proteins: interactions, organization, and information flow.* Annu Rev Biophys Biomol Struct, (2002)., 151-175.

[71] Stolt, P. C, et al. *Origins of peptide selectivity and phosphoinositide binding revealed by structures of disabled-1 PTB domain complexes.* Structure, (2003)., 569-579.

[72] Yun, M, et al. *Crystal structures of the Dab homology domains of mouse disabled 1 and 2.* J Biol Chem, (2003)., 36572-36581.

[73] Merdes, G, et al. *Interference of human and Drosophila APP and APP-like proteins with PNS development in Drosophila.* EMBO J, (2004)., 4082-4095.

[74] Artavanis-tsakonas, S, Rand, M. D, & Lake, R. J. *Notch signaling: cell fate control and signal integration in development.* Science, (1999)., 770-776.

[75] Hamid, R, et al. *Amyloid precursor protein intracellular domain modulates cellular calcium homeostasis and ATP content.* J Neurochem, (2007)., 1264-1275.

[76] Leissring, M. A, et al. *A physiologic signaling role for the gamma-secretase-derived intracellular fragment of APP.* Proc Natl Acad Sci U S A, (2002)., 4697-4702.

[77] Zhang, Z, et al. *Sequence-specific recognition of the internalization motif of the Alzheimer's amyloid precursor protein by the X11 PTB domain.* EMBO J, (1997)., 6141-6150.

[78] Cao, X, & Sudhof, T. C. *Dissection of amyloid-beta precursor protein-dependent transcriptional transactivation.* J Biol Chem, (2004)., 24601-24611.

[79] Zhou, M. M, et al. *Structure and ligand recognition of the phosphotyrosine binding domain of Shc.* Nature, (1995)., 584-592.

[80] Zhou, M. M, et al. *Structural basis for IL-4 receptor phosphopeptide recognition by the IRS-1 PTB domain.* Nat Struct Biol, (1996)., 388-393.

[81] Ring, S, et al. *The secreted beta-amyloid precursor protein ectodomain APPs alpha is sufficient to rescue the anatomical, behavioral, and electrophysiological abnormalities of APP-deficient mice.* J Neurosci, (2007)., 7817-7826.

[82] Lai, A, Sisodia, S. S, & Trowbridge, I. S. *Characterization of sorting signals in the beta-amyloid precursor protein cytoplasmic domain.* J Biol Chem, (1995)., 3565-3573.

[83] Haass, C, et al. *Targeting of cell-surface beta-amyloid precursor protein to lysosomes: alternative processing into amyloid-bearing fragments.* Nature, (1992)., 500-503.

[84] Edbauer, D, et al. *Insulin-degrading enzyme rapidly removes the beta-amyloid precursor protein intracellular domain (AICD).* J Biol Chem, (2002)., 13389-13393.

[85] Nunan, J, et al. *Proteasome-mediated degradation of the C-terminus of the Alzheimer's disease beta-amyloid protein precursor: effect of C-terminal truncation on production of beta-amyloid protein.* J Neurosci Res, (2003)., 378-385.

[86] Vingtdeux, V, et al. *Intracellular pH regulates amyloid precursor protein intracellular domain accumulation.* Neurobiol Dis, (2007)., 686-696.

[87] Cupers, P, et al. *The amyloid precursor protein (APP)-cytoplasmic fragment generated by gamma-secretase is rapidly degraded but distributes partially in a nuclear fraction of neurones in culture.* J Neurochem, (2001). , 1168-1178.

[88] Kimberly, W. T, et al. *The intracellular domain of the beta-amyloid precursor protein is stabilized by Fe65 and translocates to the nucleus in a notch-like manner.* J Biol Chem, (2001). , 40288-40292.

[89] Kinoshita, A, et al. *Direct visualization of the gamma secretase-generated carboxyl-terminal domain of the amyloid precursor protein: association with Fe65 and translocation to the nucleus.* J Neurochem, (2002). , 839-847.

[90] Cao, H, et al. *Characterization of an apoptosis inhibitory domain at the C-termini of FE65-like protein.* Biochem Biophys Res Commun, (2000). , 843-850.

[91] Cummings, J. L. *Alzheimer's disease.* N Engl J Med, (2004). , 56-67.

[92] Robinson, D. M, & Keating, G. M. *Memantine: a review of its use in Alzheimer's disease.* Drugs, (2006). , 1515-1534.

Chapter 2

Mechanism of Alzheimer Amyloid β-Protein Precursor Localization to Membrane Lipid Rafts

Yuhki Saito, Takahide Matsushima and
Toshiharu Suzuki

Additional information is available at the end of the chapter

http://dx.doi.org/10.5772/54096

1. Introduction

Alzheimer's disease (AD) is a group of common neurodegenerative diseases associated with progressive dementia with aging. The principal pathological hallmarks of AD are senile plaques and neurofibrillary tangles in the brain, which are found at significantly higher frequencies in AD patients than age-matched healthy (non-AD) subjects [1]. Senile plaques consist mainly of 39–43 amino-acid amyloid-β (Aβ) peptide, which is generated by sequential proteolytic processing of amyloid β-protein precursor (APP) (Figure 1) [2]. Common Aβ species generated in the human and murine brain are Aβ40 and Aβ42. Mutations in *APP* and *Presenilin*, which have been identified as familial AD-causative genes, result in increased Aβ production and/or an increased ratio of neurotoxic Aβ42.

Aβ is generated by sequential processing of APP with β- and γ-secretase, the catalytic unit of which is presenilin. Findings reported during the late 1980s and early 1990s led to the proposal of the "Aβ cascade hypothesis" of AD onset, which states that Aβ generation is a primary cause of AD [3]. Several lines of evidence indicate that the amyloidogenic processing of APP, including Aβ generation, occurs in membrane microdomains termed lipid rafts [4]. However, the molecular mechanisms underlying APP translocation to lipid rafts remain unclear. In this chapter, regulatory mechanisms for lipid raft translocation of APP and APP C-terminal fragments (APP CTFs) generated primarily by the cleavage of APP are described.

Membrane lipid rafts are known as sites of amyloidogenic processing of APP and enriched with active β-secretase, while non-amyloidogenic cleavage of APP by α-secretase is performed outside lipid rafts. Neural adaptor protein X11-like (X11L) regulates the translocation of mature APP (mAPP), which is the *N*- and *O*-glycosylated form and real substrate of secretases in the late protein secretory pathway, to lipid rafts. APP bound to X11L preferentially localizes to sites outside of lipid rafts and escapes from active β-secretase [5]. Dissociation of the APP-X11L complex leads to APP entry into lipid rafts, suggesting that dysfunction of X11L in its interaction with APP may recruit more APP to lipid rafts and increase the generation of Aβ [5].

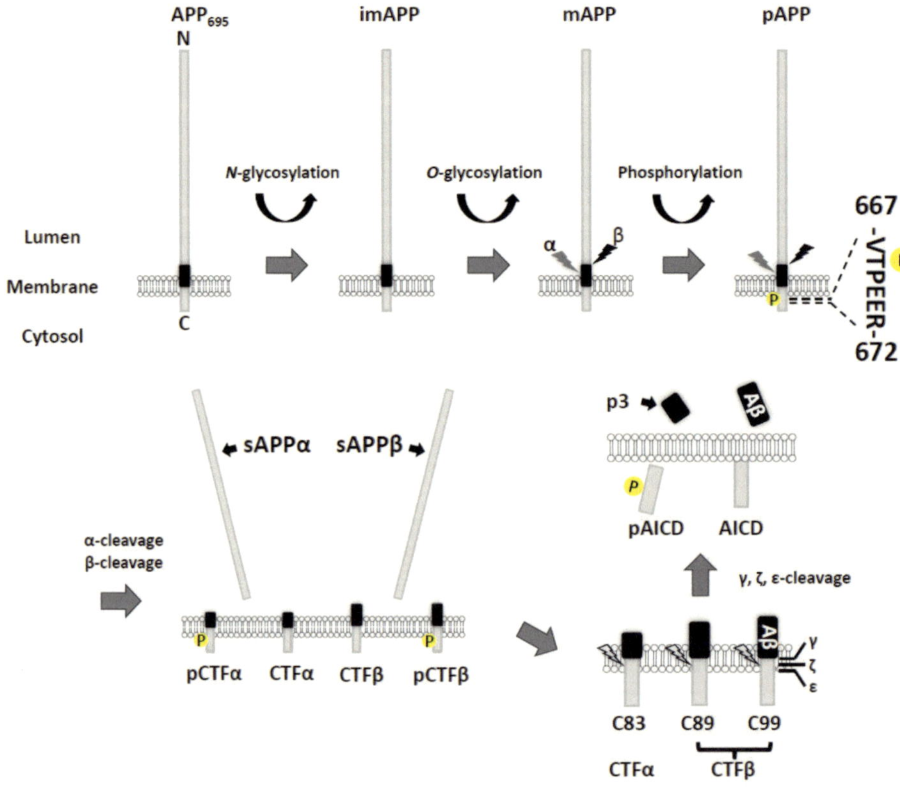

Figure 1. The schema of APP metabolism and post-translational modification of APP. APP is subjected to *N*-glycosylation at ER to form imAPP followed by *O*-glycosylation at the *medial-/trans*-Golgi apparatus to form mAPP. Residue Thr668 of mAPP is specifically phosphorylated in brain. mAPP is cleaved in sequential proteolytic events mediated by β-secretase or α-site APP cleaving enzyme, and the γ-secretase complex. β-secretase primarily cleaves APP in the luminal domain to generate sAPPβ and CTFβ (C99 and C89). C99 contains an intact Aβ sequence. γ-secretase complex mediates the cleavage of CTFβ at ε, ζ, and γ-sites to generate Aβ and AICD peptides. α-site APP cleaving enzyme generates sAPPα and CTFα (C83). CTFα cleavage by γ-secretase complex then generates p3 peptide and AICD.

In contrast to APP, APP CTF translocation to lipid rafts seems to involve another regulatory system that also includes active γ-secretase to cleave APP CTFs. The translocation of CTFs to lipid rafts is regulated by APP phosphorylation. The cytoplasmic region of APP is well known to demonstrate neuron-specific phosphorylation at Thr668 (numbering for the APP695 isoform). However, the maximum phosphorylation level of APP is 10–20% in the brain, and its physiological function is not clear [6].

http://dx.doi.org/10.5772/54096

A recent study found that the phosphorylation level of APP CTFs was much higher than that of full-length APP, and phosphorylated CTFs (pCTFs), but not nonphosphorylated CTFs (nCTFs), were preferentially located outside of detergent-resistant, lipid raft-like membrane microdomains, indicating that Thr668 phosphorylation appears to function on the APP CTF rather than full-length APP [7]. Recent analysis revealed that pCTFs are relatively movable within the membrane as integral membrane proteins, while nCTFs are susceptible to being anchored to a lipid raft by direct binding of the C-terminal tail to membrane lipids. Once in lipid rafts, nCTFs can be preferentially captured and cleaved by γ-secretase. Interestingly, phosphorylation levels of amyloidogenic CTFβ were significantly decreased in aged brain [7]. Two molecular mechanisms of APP and APP CTF translocation to ripid rafts are described in the following section.

2. Metabolism and post-translational modification of APP

APP, which is a type I membrane protein, is subjected to *N*-glycosylation at the endoplasmic reticulum (ER) to form immature APP (imAPP) followed by *O*-glycosylation at the *medial-/trans*-Golgi apparatus to form mature APP (mAPP) (Figure 1). mAPP is then transported through the *trans*-Golgi network to the plasma membrane, where it enters the late secretory pathway and is metabolized by either amyloidogenic or amyloidolytic (non-amyloiodgenic) processing [6, 8]. In the amyloidogenic pathway, APP is cleaved in sequential proteolytic events mediated by β-secretase (β-site APP cleaving enzyme 1 or BACE1) and the γ-secretase complex comprised of four core subunits, presenilins (PS1 or PS2), anterior pharynx defective 1 (APH-1), presenilin enhancer 2 (PEN2), and nicastrin. β-secretase primarily cleaves APP in the luminal domain to generate soluble APPβ (sAPPβ) and membrane-associated APP carboxyl terminal fragments (CTFβ/C99 and CTFβ'/C89). C99 contains an intact Aβ sequence (Figure 1). γ-secretase complex mediates the cleavage of CTFβ at ε, ζ, and γ-sites to generate Aβ and APP intracellular domain (AICD) peptides. Non-amyloidogenic cleavage of APP is mediated by α-site APP cleaving enzyme (α-secretase, including ADAM9, ADAM10, and ADAM17) to generate sAPPα and CTFα (C83), which contains only the carboxyl half of Aβ peptide. CTFα cleavage by γ-secretase complex then generates p3 peptide and AICD.

Residue Thr668 of the APP cytoplasmic region is located within the 667-VTPEER-672 motif and is phosphorylated (number corresponding to the APP695 isoform) in the late secretory pathway in neurons. Protein kinases such as GSK3β (glycogen synthase kinase-3β), CDK5 (cyclin-dependent kinase-5), CDK1/CDC2, and JNK (c-Jun N-terminal kinase) are thought to mediate this phosphorylation of APP [6]. APP CTFs are also phosphorylated at Thr668 and detected as phosphopeptide pC99, pC89, and pC83 by western blot analysis using a phosphorylation-state-specific anti-APP Thr668 antibody or pAPP antibody (Figure 2A). Typical APP CTF species in the brain appear as five bands: pC99, nC99, pC89, a mixture of nC89 plus pC83, and nC83. Treatment of CTFs with phosphatase is effective for the identification of the respective species. Levels of the phosphorylated CTFβ species pC99 and pC89 were significantly higher than those of their nonphosphorylated forms, nC99 and nC89, while phosphorylated CTFα, pC83, demonstrated a trend toward decreased levels in comparison to nonphosphorylated CTFα, nC83 (Figure 2B). The relative ratio of total phosphorylated CTFs was equivalent to that of nonphosphorylated CTFs (Figure 2C), although phosphorylated CTFβ and CTFβ' were predominant compared to their nonphosphorylated forms. These observations indicate that pCTFs and nCTFs are present at equal levels in the brain as potential substrates for γ-secretase.

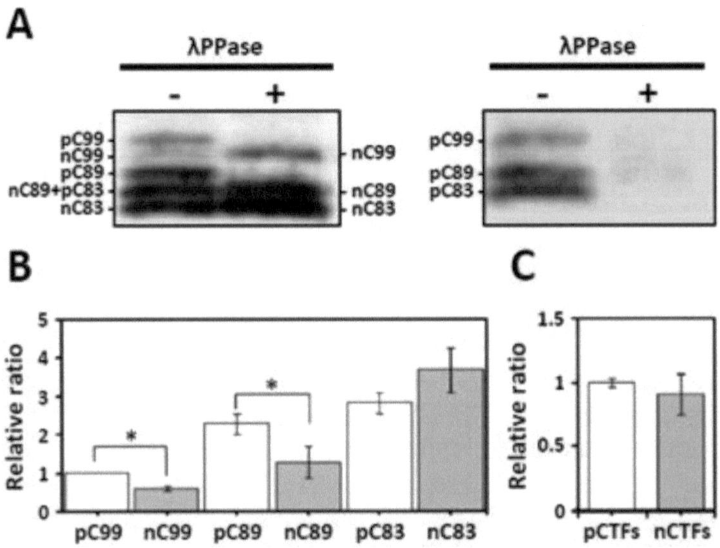

Figure 2. Level of CTF species in brain membrane fractions. (A) CTF species in brain membrane preparations. (B) and (C) Levels of CTF species in brain membrane preparations. Levels of the phosphorylated CTFβ species (pC99 and pC89) were significantly higher than those of their nonphosphorylated forms, nC99 and nC89.

The 667-VTPEER-672 motif, including the phosphorable amino acid Thr668, forms a type I β-turn and N-terminal helix-capping box structure to stabilize its C-terminal helix structure [9]. Therefore, phosphorylation of Thr668 induces significant conformational changes in the cytoplasmic region of APP (Figure 3) that affect its interaction with FE65, a neuronal adaptor protein [10]. The usual procedure to explore the function of a protein phosphorylation site is to mimic the phosphorylation state by amino acid substitutions of Asp or Glu for the appropriate Thr and Ser residues. However, this strategy may not be suitable in the case of APP phosphorylation, as the substitution of Asp for Thr668 did not alter the carboxyl terminal helix state as remarkably as phosphorylation of Thr668 (Figure 3A). By contrast, substitution of Thr668 with Ala668 in APP has been found to mimic effectively the nonphosphorylated state in the helix structure of the APP cytoplasmic domain. Figure 3B presents a schematic illustration of the Thr668-dependent conformational changes. Thr668Ala mutation mimics the nonphosphorylated state of APP, but Thr668Asp mutation did not completely mimic the phosphorylation structure of APP. Therefore, to reveal the role of APP phosphorylation at Thr668, careful analysis for the phosphorylation state of both APP and the APP metabolic fragments in the brain are described here.

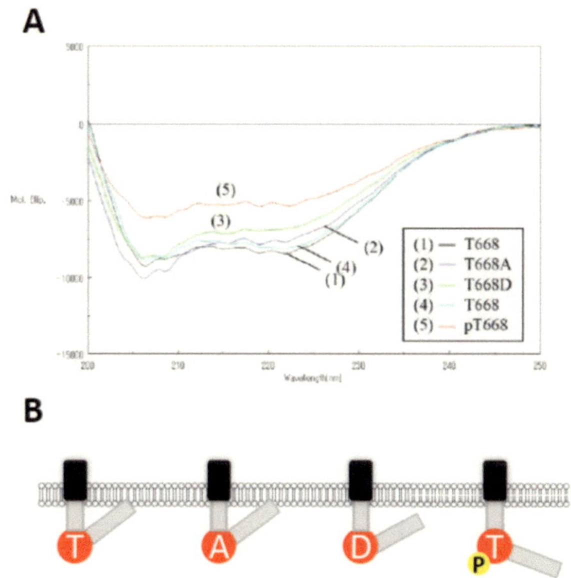

Figure 3. Circular dichroism (CD) spectra of APP cytoplasmic peptides (A) and schematic of changes to the APP cytoplasmic domain dependent on Thr668 residue modification (B). The substitution of Asp for Thr668 did not alter the carboxyl terminal helix state as remarkably as phosphorylation of Thr668. By contrast, substitution of Thr668 with Ala668 in APP has been found to mimic effectively the nonphosphorylated state in the helix structure of the APP cytoplasmic domain.

3. Lipid rafts and Alzheimer's disease

Dynamic and highly ordered membrane microdomains, termed lipid rafts, are rich in cholesterol and sphingolipids such as seramide, gangliosides, glycerophospholipids, and sterols. The average diameter of lipid rafts has been estimated at 50 nm. However, several classes of lipid rafts that vary in size and duration can exist in a cell [11]. Lipid rafts are formed in the Golgi and transported to the plasma membrane [12], where they serve as platforms for cell signaling, pathogen entry, cell adhesion, and protein sorting. Lipid rafts are biochemically defined as the detergent-resistant membrane (DRM) fraction [12]. Aβ generation and aggregation occur in lipid rafts, suggesting that lipid rafts play an important role in APP processing and subsequent AD pathogenesis. A growing body of evidence indicates that active β- and γ-secretases are located in membrane microdomains [13-15]. *S*-Palmitoylation of BACE1 at residues Cys474/478/482/485 is essential for the localization of BACE1 to lipid rafts [13,14]. *S*-Palmitoylation of nicastrin at Cys689 and of APH1 at Cys182 and Cys245 contributed to their stability and the lipid raft association of these nascent subunits, but did not affect the lipid raft localization of PS1 and PEN2 or the assembly of γ-secretase complex [15]. Taken together, lipid raft localization of secretases involved in amyloidogenic APP cleavage is regulated by their post-translational modification. However, the factors that determine lipid raft localization of APP remain unclear.

4. X11 protein regulation of APP localization to lipid rafts

X11 family proteins (X11s), consisting of X11/X11α/Mint1, X11L/X11β/Mint2, and X11L2/X11γ/Mint3, are encoded by separate genes on human chromosomes 9, 15, and 19 and mouse chromosomes 19, 7, and 10, respectively. X11s contain an evolutionarily conserved central phosphotyrosine binding/interaction (PTB/PI) domain and two C-terminal PDZ domains [16]. The PTB/PI and PDZ domains are well-characterized protein-protein interaction domains, and X11 proteins interact with various types of proteins, including APP, alcadein, apoER2, munc18, KIF17, kalirin, hyperpolarization-activated cyclic nucleotide-gated (HCN) channel, and Arfs, through their PTB/PI and PDZ domains. Interaction of X11L with APP can stabilize APP metabolism and intracellular trafficking, which induce the suppression of Aβ generation [16-18]. Metabolic analysis of APP in X11 and/or X11L knockout mice confirmed that X11s modulated APP metabolism and suppressed Aβ generation as an endophenotype *in vivo* [5, 19, 20]. X11 or X11L transgenic mice crossed to commonly used AD model mice (APPswe transgenic mice) demonstrated reduced amyloid deposition along with decreased levels of Aβ40 and Aβ42 in the brain compared to APPswe transgenic mice [21, 22].

The molecular mechanisms underlying the suppression of APP amyloidogenic metabolism by X11 and X11L have been addressed in a recent analysis. In the brains of mice lacking X11 and/or X11L, levels of CTFβ and Aβ were increased relative to wild-type animals (Figure 4) [5].

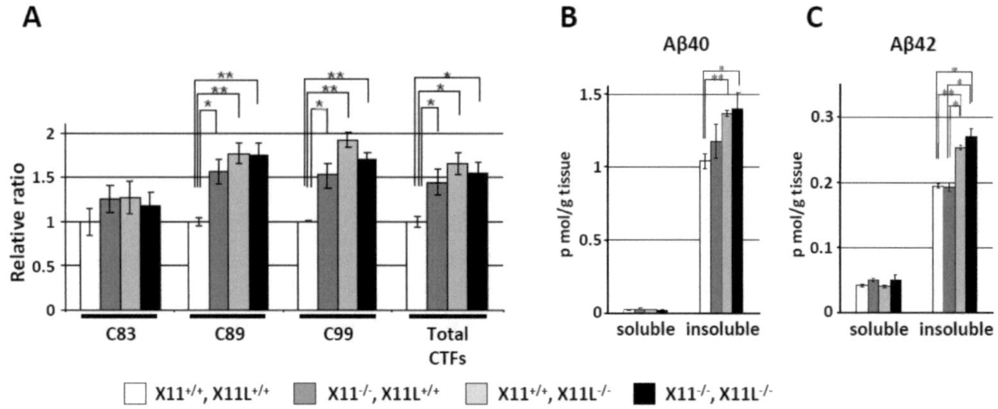

Figure 4. Quantification of APP CTFs in the hippocampus of wild-type, X11-deficient, X11L-deficient, and X11/X11L doubly deficient mice. Levels of CTFβ and Aβ were increased in X11s deficient mice, indicating that amyloidogenic metabolism of APP was enhanced in X11s deficient mice.

The absence of X11s resulted in more APP and APP CTF translocation to DRMs and enhanced colocalization of APP or APP CTFs with BACE1 in DRMs but not in non-DRMs (Figure 5A and B) [5]. Interestingly, X11s were recovered in membrane fractions, and they largely localized to non-DRMs but not DRMs (Figure 5C), indicating that APP can associate exclusively with X11s outside of DRMs to prevent APP translocation to lipid rafts, where amyloidogenic metabolism of APP occurs (Figure 6).

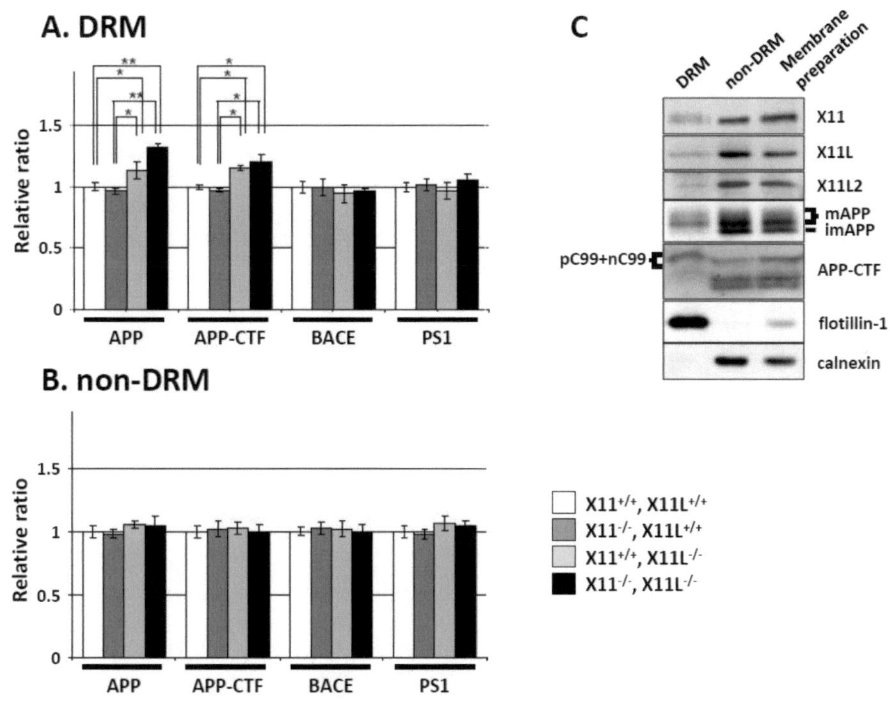

Figure 5. Quantification of APP, APP CTFs, BACE, and PS1 in (A) DRM and (B) non-DRM fractions from wild-type, X11-deficient, X11L-deficient, and X11/X11L doubly deficient mouse cortex. Higher levels of mAPP and CTFβ were recovered in DRM of the X11L-deficient and the X11/X11L doubly deficient mouse brain. (C) Localization of membrane-attached X11 proteins to DRM and non-DRM fractions. X11s were recovered in membrane fractions, and they largely localized to non-DRMs but not DRMs.

The Dysfunction of X11s in aged neurons may thus contribute to sporadic AD etiology. The dysfunction of X11s could lead to a weakening of the association between X11s and APP, resulting in greater translocation of APP to DRMs. Alteration in the lipid composition of membranes may enlarge lipid raft areas or increase the number of lipid rafts, which could also enhance APP translocation to DRMs. These qualitative alterations in X11s and/or lipid metabolism could result in increased β-cleavage of APP even if β-secretase itself is not enzymopathic.

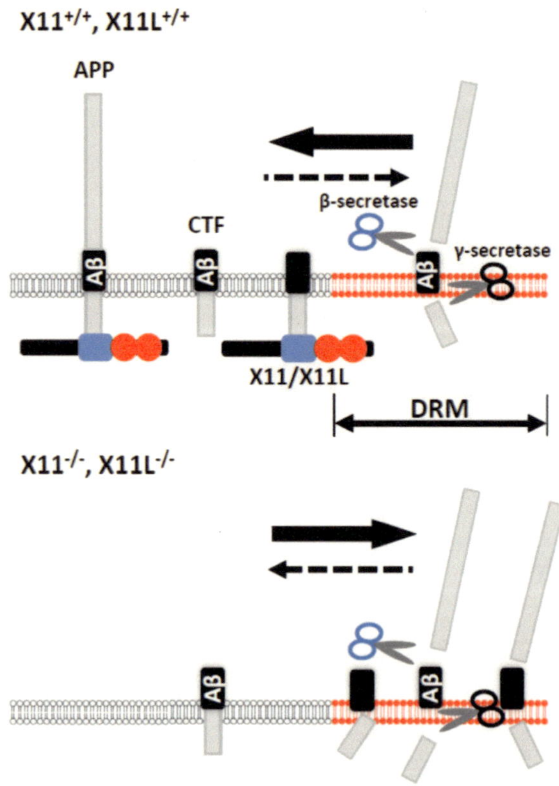

Figure 6. Possible role of X11 proteins in regulating the DRM association and β-site cleavage of APP. X11s associate with APP outside of DRMs and prevent translocation of APP into DRM. When X11L dissociates from APP, the APP translocates into DRMs, and that fraction of APP molecules is cleaved by BACE which is active in DRM (upper panel). In the absence of X11s, APP molecules are not anchored outside of DRMs, and more APP translocates into DRMs, resulting in increased β-site cleavage of APP (lower panel). The arrows indicate translocation direction of APP.

5. Regulation of APP CTF translocation to lipid rafts by Thr668 phosphorylation

Because similar amounts of nCTFs and pCTFs were found in mouse brain (Figure 2C), generation of similar levels of the APP intracellular cytoplasmic domain fragments, nonphosphorylated AICD (nAICD) and phosphorylated AICD (pAICD), is expected if γ-secretase cleaves nCTFs and pCTFs equivalently. However, membrane prepared from mouse brain generated higher levels of nAICD than pAICD in an *in vitro* γ-secretase assay (Figure 7A). Incubation of membrane preparations demonstrated a time-dependent, nearly linear increase in the generation of nAICD and pAICD during the 0–2 h time period, and the reaction essentially reached a plateau in the 2–4 h period (Figure 7B and C). Dephosphorylation and degradation of pAICD did not occur in this assay. Importantly, the ratio of pAICD to AICD generation was constant throughout the incubation time (1–4 h) with the relative ratio (amount of pAICD/amount of nAICD) measuring 0.35 ± 0.10 at the 2 h point (Figure 7D). Taken together, these *in vitro* analyses indicate that both phosphorylated and nonphosphorylated CTFs are kinetically equivalent as a substrate for γ-secretase, but the results also show that the generation of pAICD was significantly lower when compared to that of nAICD. These observations suggest that pCTFs are located at a distance from active γ-secretase in the membrane, while nCTFs are positioned nearer to the active enzyme.

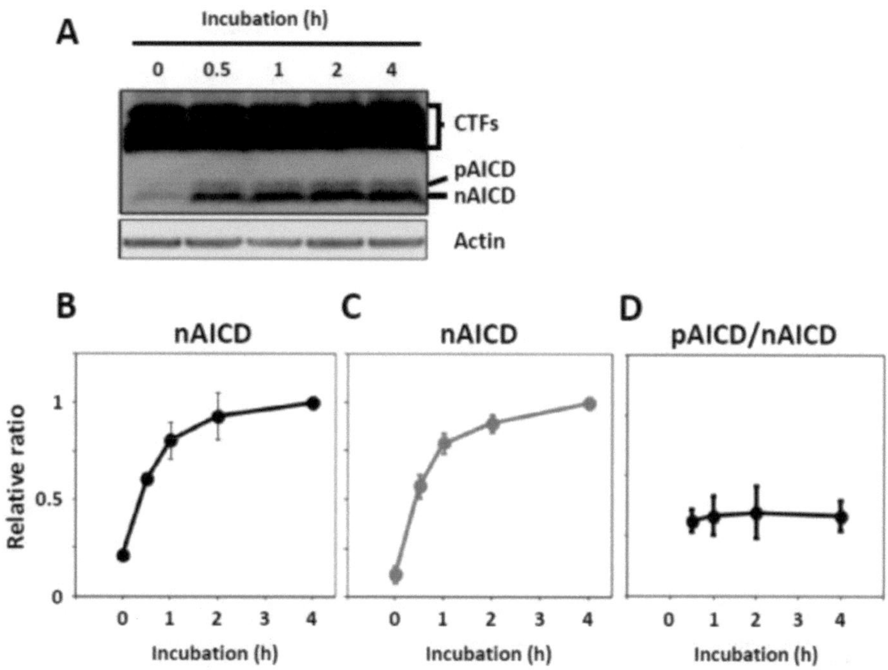

Figure 7. *In vitro* kinetic analysis of phosphorylated and nonphosphorylated CTF cleavage by γ-secretase. (A) *in vitro* γ-secretase assay with membrane preparations from wild-type mouse brain. (B) and (C) kinetic analysis of AICD generated by incubation of membrane preparations. (D) the production ratio of pAICD to nAICD (pAICD/nAICD) at the indicated times are shown. Both phosphorylated and nonphosphorylated CTFs are kinetically equivalent as a substrate for γ-secretase, but the results also show that the generation of pAICD was significantly lower when compared to that of nAICD.

Thr668 phosphorylation could regulate APP CTF translocation to the lipid raft microdomain. To examine this hypothesis, γ-secretase-enriched lipid raft-like membrane microdomains were prepared as DRMs using CHAPSO. Application of CHAPSO is preferable for the isolation of DRMs, including active γ-secretase complexes, compared to procedures using other detergents such as Triton X-100 [23, 24]. Components of the active γ-secretase complex, both PS1 N- and C-terminal fragments and PEN2, were predominantly recovered in the DRM fraction along with a small amount of APP CTFs (~20% measured) [7]. Phosphorylation levels of APP CTFs in the DRM and non-DRM fractions were examined, and the respective nCTFs and pCTFs were compared as a relative ratio in which pC99 in the DRM was set to 1.0 (Figure 8).

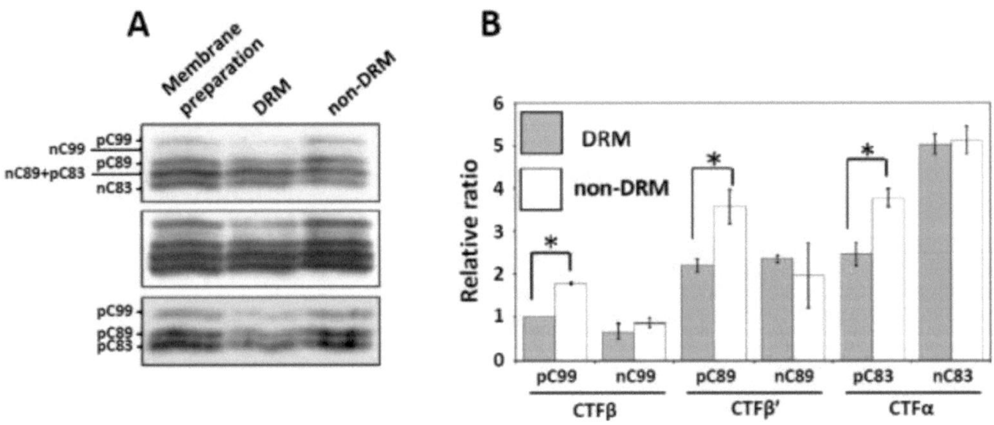

Figure 8. Quantification of pCTFs and nCTFs in DRM and non-DRM fractions. (A) Identification of APP CTFs in DRM and non-DRM fractions. (B) CTFs levels in DRM and non-DRM fractions. Significantly higher levels of the phosphorylated species pC99, pC89, and pC83 were found in the non-DRM fractions.

Significantly higher levels of the phosphorylated species pC99, pC89, and pC83 were found in the non-DRM fractions compared to the DRM fractions. Additionally, the phosphorylation level of total APP CTFs in DRM was significantly lower than that in non-DRM. These results indicate that phosphorylated CTFs are preferentially localized outside of the DRM/lipid raft-like membrane microdomain and thus prevented from cleavage by γ-secretase.

How does phosphorylation of Thr668 regulate the localization of APP CTFs between DRM and non-DRM? A recent structural analysis revealed that the cytoplasmic domain tail of APP can interact with membrane lipids [25]. Since phosphorylation of APP at Thr668 induces a significant change in its cytoplasmic domain conformation (Figure 2) [9, 10, 26], phosphorylation of the APP cytoplasmic domain at Thr668 can influence the association of the APP cytoplasmic tail with membrane lipids.

Liposomes prepared with endogenous lipids from the membrane fractions of mouse brain have been used as a model for neural membranes [27]. Synthetic cytoplasmic APP 648–695 peptide with (pC47) or without (nC47) a phosphate group at residue Thr668 was incubated with the liposomes, and the liposome-bound peptides were recovered and analyzed by immunoblotting. Notably, nonphosphorylated APP cytoplasmic peptide (nC47) bound strongly to the liposomes, while phosphorylated peptide (pC47) demonstrated no detectable association (Figure 9A) [7]. This trend was also confirmed by examining the AICD, which lacks the transmembrane domain due to ε-cleavage by γ-secretase [28, 29]. Most nAICD was recovered in the brain membrane fraction (~75%) rather than in the soluble cytoplasmic fraction (~25%), while comparatively more pAICD was found in the cytoplasmic fraction (~45%) (Figure 9B).

http://dx.doi.org/10.5772/54096

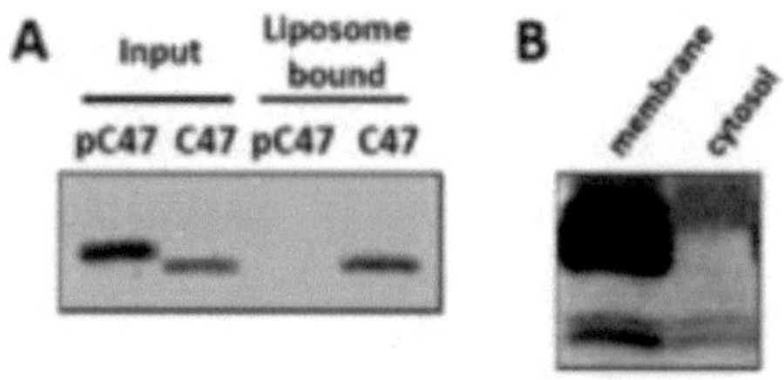

Figure 9. Liposome-binding ability of APP cytoplasmic domain and ist localization in mouse brain. (A) The binding ability of the phosphorylated APP cytoplasmic domain peptide with liposomes composed of lipids from mouse brain membranes. (B) distribution of AICD endogenously generated in mouse brain. Nonphosphorylated nC47 and AICD bound strongly to the liposome and membrane fraction.

Therefore, the nonphosphorylated forms of APP CTFs and AICD tend to bind membrane lipids, mediated by their C-termini, and phosphorylation of APP CTFs and AICD at Thr668 functions to prevent direct membrane association, apparently by changing the conformation of their cytoplasmic regions. In addition to these observations, pCTFβ levels were significantly decreased with age in cynomolgus monkey brains [7], indicating that the preservation of APP CTF phosphorylation levels correlates with the suppression of γ-cleavage.

To conclude this section, first, almost equal amounts of pCTFs and nCTFs are present in mouse brain, while lower amounts of pAICD are generated compared to nAICD. Second, both pAICD and nAICD are kinetically equivalent substrates for γ-secretase. These observations suggest that pCTFs are sequestered away from the membrane region where γ-secretase is active (DRM/lipid raft-like membrane microdomain) [15], and that pCTFs are located outside of the DRM/lipid raft-like membrane microdomain due to a change in the conformation of their cytoplasmic tail, to which the membrane lipids bind. Thus, the pCTFs can quickly disperse from the DRM/lipid raft-like membrane microdomain with their increased mobility in the membrane (Figure 10).

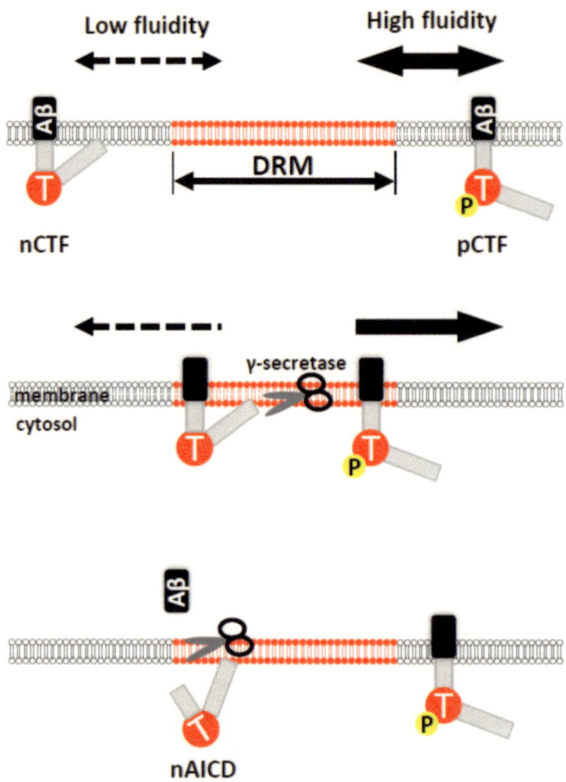

Figure 10. Possible role of APP CTF phosphorylation at Thr668 in regulating its fluidity within the membrane and its cleavage by γ-secretase.

6. Conclusions

X11L abundantly present in non-DRM traps APP outside of the DRM and prevents contact between APP and the β-secretases located within the DRM. Phosphorylation of APP at Thr668 induces conformational changes to the APP cytoplasmic domain and reduces the affinity of the APP C terminal to lipids. This change alters APP CTF fluidity and decreases the probability of APP CTF presence in lipid rafts, in which contact between APP CTFs and γ-secretase occurs. In conclusion, translocation of APP and APP CTFs to lipid rafts is regulated by neuronal adaptor protein X11L and Thr668 phosphorylation of APP CTFs.

http://dx.doi.org/10.5772/54096

Abbrevations

ADAM: a disintegrin and metalloprotease domain, APH-1: anterior pharynx defective 1, AICD: APP intracellular domain, APP: amyloid precursor protein, APP CTFs: APP C-terminal fragments, BACE1: β-site APP cleaving enzyme 1/β-secretase, CDK5: cyclin-dependent kinase-5, CD spectra: Circular dichroism spectra, DRM: detergent-resistant membrane, GSK3:βglycogen synthase kinase-3β, JNK: c-Jun N-terminal kinase, imAPP: immature APP, mAPP: mature APP, pAICD; nAICD; nonphosphorylated AICD, nCTFs; nonphosphorylated CTFs, phosphorylated AICD, pCTFs; phosphorylated CTFs, PS: presenilins, PEN2; presenilin enhancer 2, PTB/PI domain; phosphotyrosine binding/interaction domain; sAPP; soluble APP, X11L; X11-like.

Author details

Yuhki Saito, Takahide Matsushima and Toshiharu Suzuki

Laboratory of Neuroscience, Graduate School of Pharmaceutical Sciences, Hokkaido University, Sapporo, Japan

References

[1] Braak H, Braak E. Neuropathological stageing of Alzheimer-related changes. Acta. Neuropathol. 1991;82(4): 239-259.

[2] Selkoe DJ. Alzheimer's disease: genes, proteins, and therapy. Physiol Rev 2001;81(2): 741-766.

[3] Hardy JA and Higgins GA. Alzheimer's disease: the amyloid cascade hypothesis. Science 1992; 256: 184-185.

[4] Vetrivel KS and Thinakaran G. Membrane rafys in Alzheimer's disease beta-amyloid production. Biochem. Biophys. Acta. 2010; 1801: 860-867.

[5] Saito Y, Sano Y, Vassar R, Gandy S, Nakaya T, Yamamoto T. and Suzuki T. X11 proteins regulate the translocation of amyloid beta-protein precursor (APP) into detergent-resistant membrane and suppress the amyloidogenic cleavage of APP by beta-site-cleaving enzyme in brain. J. Biol. Chem. 2008;283(51): 35763–71.

[6] Suzuki T and Nakaya T. Regulation of amyloid beta-protein precursor by phosphorylation and protein interactions. J Biol Chem 2008;31(44): 29633-37.

[7] Matsushima T, Saito Y, Elliott JI, Iijima-Ando K, Nishimura M, Kimura N, Hata S, Yamamoto T, Nakaya T, Suzuki T. Membrane-microdomain Localization of Amyloid

β-Precursor Protein (APP) C-terminal Fragments is Regulated by Phosphorylation of the Cytoplasmic Thr668 Residue. J Biol Chem 2012; 287(23): 19715-24.

[8] Thinakaran G and Koo EM. Amyloid precursor protein trafficking, processing and function. J. Biol. Chem. 2008; 283 (44): 29615-29619.

[9] Ramelot TA, Gentile LN, Nicholson LK. Transient structure of the amyloid precursor protein cytoplasmic tail indicates preordering of structure for binding to cytosolic factors. Biochemistry 2000;39(10): 2714-25.

[10] Ando K, Oishi M, Takeda S, Iijima K, Isohara T, Nairn AC, Kirino Y, Greengard P, Suzuki T. Role of phosphorylation of Alzheimer's amyloid precursor protein during neuronal differentiation. J Neurosci 1999;19(11): 4421-7.

[11] Hancock JF. Lipid rafts: contentious only from simplistic standpoints. Nat Rev Mol Cell Biol 2006;7(6): 456-62.

[12] Brown DA, London E. Functions of lipid rafts in biological membranes. Annu Rev Cell Dev Biol 1998;14: 111-36.

[13] Benjannet S, Elagoz A, Wickham L, Mamarbachi M, Munzer JS, Basak A, Lazure C, Cromlish JA, Sisodia S, Checler F, Chretien M, Seidah NG. Posttranslational processing of beta-secretase (beta-amyloid-converting enzyme) and its ectodomain shedding. The pro- and transmembrane/cytosolic domains affect its cellular activity and amyloid-beta production, J Biol Chem 2001;276(14): 10879–87.

[14] Vetrivel KS, Meckler X, Chen Y, Nguyen PD, Seidah NG, Vassar R, Wong PC, Fukata M, Kounnas MZ, Thinakaran G. Alzheimer disease Abeta production in the absence of S-palmitoylation-dependent targeting of BACE1 to lipid rafts, J Biol Chem 2009;284 (6): 3793–803.

[15] Cheng H, Vetrivel KS, Drisdel RC, Meckler X, Gong P, Leem JY, Li T, Carter M, Chen Y, Nguyen P, Iwatsubo T, Tomita T, Wong PC, Green WN, Kounnas MZ, Thinakaran G. S-palmitoylation of gamma-secretase subunits nicastrin and APH-1, J Biol Chem 2009;284(3): 1373–84.

[16] Tomita S, Ozaki T, Taru H, Oguchi S, Takeda S, Yagi Y, Sakiyama S, Kirino Y, Suzuki T. Interaction of a neuron-specific protein containing PDZ domains with Alzheimer's amyloid precursor protein. J Biol Chem 1999; 274(4): 2243-54.

[17] Araki Y, Tomita S, Yamaguchi H, Miyagi N, Sumioka A, Kirino Y, Suzuki T. Novel cadherin-related membrane proteins, Alcadeins, enhance the X11-like protein-mediated stabilization of amyloid beta-protein precursor metabolism. J Biol Chem 2003; 278(49): 49448-49458.

[18] Taru H, Suzuki T. Regulation of the physiological function and metabolism of AβPP by AβPP binding proteins. J Alzheimers Dis 2009;18(2): 253-265.

[19] Sano Y, Syuzo Takabatake A, Nakaya T, Saito Y, Tomita S, Itohara S, Suzuki T. Enhanced amyloidogenic metabolism of the amyloid beta-protein precursor in the X11L-deficient mouse brain. J Biol Chem 2006;281(49): 37853-37860.

[20] Kondo M, Shiono M, Itoh G, Takei N, Matsushima T, Maeda M, Taru H, Hata S, Yamamoto T, Saito Y, Suzuki T. Increased amyloidogenic processing of transgenic human APP in X11-like deficient mouse brain. Mol Neurodegener 2010; 15;5:35.

[21] Lee JH, Lau KF, Perkinton MS, Standen CL, Shemilt SJ, Mercken L, Cooper JD, McLoughlin DM, Miller CC. The neuronal adaptor protein X11alpha reduces Abeta levels in the brains of Alzheimer's APPswe Tg2576 transgenic mice. J Biol Chem 2003; 278(47): 47025-29.

[22] Lee JH, Lau KF, Perkinton MS, Standen CL, Rogelj B, Falinska A, McLoughlin DM, Miller CC. The neuronal adaptor protein X11beta reduces amyloid beta-protein levels and amyloid plaque formation in the brains of transgenic mice. J Biol Chem 2004;279(47): 49099-104.

[23] Wahrle S, Das P, Nyborg AC, McLendon C, Shoji M, Kawarabayashi T, Younkin LH, Younkin SG,. Golde TE. Cholesterol-dependent gamma-secretase activity in buoyant cholesterol-rich membrane microdomains. Neurobiol Dis 2002;9(1): 11-23.

[24] Vetrivel KS, Cheng H, Lin W, Sakurai T, Li T, Nukina N, Wong PC, Xu H, Thinakaran G. Association of gamma-secretase with lipid rafts in post-Golgi and endosome membranes. J Biol Chem 2004;279(43): 44945-54.

[25] Beel AJ, Mobley CK, Kim HJ, Tian F, Hadziselimovic A, Jap B, Prestegard JH, Sanders CR. Structural studies of the transmembrane C-terminal domain of the amyloid precursor protein (APP): does APP function as a cholesterol sensor? Biochemistry 2008; 47(36): 9428-46.

[26] Ramelot TA, Nicholson LK. Phosphorylation-induced structural changes in the amyloid precursor protein cytoplasmic tail detected by NMR. J Mol Biol 2001; 307(3): 871-884.

[27] Sumioka A, Yan D, Tomita S. TARP phosphorylation regulates synaptic AMPA receptors through lipid bilayers. Neuron 2010; 66(5): 755-67.

[28] Gu Y, Misonou H, Sato T, Dohmae N, Takio K, Ihara Y. Distinct intramembrane cleavage of the beta-amyloid precursor protein family resembling gamma-secretase-like cleavage of Notch. J Biol Chem 2001;276(38): 35235-38.

[29] Qi-Takahara Y, Morishima-Kawashima M, Tanimura Y, Dolios G, Hirotani N, Horikoshi Y, Kametani F, Maeda M, Saido TC, Wang R, Ihara Y. Longer forms of amyloid beta protein: implications for the mechanism of intramembrane cleavage by gamma-secretase. J Neurosci 2005; 25(2): 436-45.

Chapter 3

The Amyloidogenic Pathway Meets the Reelin Signaling Cascade: A Cytoskeleton Bridge Between Neurodevelopment and Neurodegeneration

Daniel A. Bórquez, Ismael Palacios and
Christian González-Billault

Additional information is available at the end of the chapter

http://dx.doi.org/10.5772/54038

1. Introduction

Reelin is an extracellular matrix glycoprotein of ~400 kD, expressed in mammals during neurodevelopment by the Cajal-Retzius (CR) neurons, which are located in the marginal zone of the cortex and hippocampus [1], and by the cerebellar granule cells [2]. In adult stages, CR neurons degenerate in both structures [3], limiting Reelin production and secretion to GABAergic interneurons [4]. Meanwhile, the expression in the cerebellum remains being exclusive of granule cells [5]. During development, Reelin synthesis also occurs in structures like the hypothalamus, the olfactory bulb, the basal ganglia and the amygdale. In these last two brain regions, Reelin expression continues into adulthood but at low concentrations [1].

Reelin gene encompasses 450 kb of genomic DNA located on human chromosome 7q22 and in murine chromosome 5. Both genes contain 65 exons that encode a protein sharing a 94,2 (%) of identity [6-7]. The transcription initiation region and the exon 1 of the reelin gene is enriched in CG nucleotides, forming a large CpG island [8], which is associated with a methylation-dependent negative regulation of reelin transcription [9]. In fact, DNA methyltransferases and histone deacetylases inhibitors increase Reelin protein expression, most likely due to decreased reelin promoter methylation [10-11].

In addition to the epigenetic regulation, reelin gene show multiple *cis* elements, which contain binding sites for transcription factors involved in neurodevelopment such as Sp1, Tbr-1 and Pax6, and elements involved in cytoplasm-to-nucleus signal transduction as CREB and NF-κB [7,12]. Tbr-1 deficient mice show a clear disruption of cortical organization, accompanied by decreased Reelin levels [13]. On the other hand, retinoic acid, a known inducer of neuronal growth and differentiation, increase Pax6 and Sp1 levels leading to the activation of the reelin promoter and a subsequent increased Reelin protein synthesis [14].

The full length Reelin protein contains 3461 amino acids, organized from N- to C-terminal by the following domains and motifs: 1.- A signal peptide, 2.- F-spondin-like motif, 3.- 8 repeat domains, composed of a region A and region B spaced by EGF motif, and 4.- A region enriched in basic amino acids [2].

Reelin may undergo proteolytic cleavage at the beginning of the 3rd and 7th A-EGF-B repeat generating many fragments including the N-terminal, the intermediate segment and the C-terminal fragment. Cleavage may be precluded by zinc chelators, known inhibitors of metalloproteinases [15]. Recently a putative protease had been identified as p50 and p70 isoforms of a disintegrin and metalloproteinase with thrombospodin motif 4 (ADAMTS-4). The p50 isoform cleaves at N-terminal only, and p70 cleaves the N- and C-terminal sites [16]. The importance of the proteolytic processing remains unclear, however; several reports showed that the internalization of Reelin at target cells is independent of its cleavage. In turn, only the central region seems to be sufficient for Reelin functions. Reelin cleavage would be required to enable Reelin secretion, allowing the release of a central, active fragment from the extracellular matrix-attached full length protein [17-18]. In contrast to this notion, there are many studies showing that the N-terminal region is important for Reelin secretion (due to the presence of a signal peptide on this region) [19], and to promote the formation of homopolymers, which are essential for proper signal transduction [20]. There is still little evidence about the function of the C-terminal region. The *reeler* Orleans mutation characterized by a deletion of 220 nucleotides at the C-terminal, prevents the secretion of Reelin, suggesting a possible role for this region in normal Reelin functions [21].

2. Reelin in neurodevelopment

As outlined in the previous section, Reelin is a glycoprotein, which is expressed in CR neurons starting at embryonic day 11 (E11), mainly in the cortex, hippocampus and cerebellum. It expression remains high until day E18, when CR neurons begin to degenerate [1,3]. The importance of Reelin to neurodevelopment had been elucidated through numerous studies using a mice model exhibiting a spontaneous mutation (partial deletion) in the reelin gene, called the *reeler* mice [22]. These mice had pronounced defects in the correct neuronal positioning in the laminar structures of the brain. At day E11, postmitotic neurons located in the ventricular zone, migrate toward the pial surface to form the preplate. On E13, a new cohort of migrating neurons originated at the proliferative region separate the pre-plate. Pre-plate splitting originates two regions, the marginal zone and the sub-plate, which are positioned adjacent to the pial surface and near the ventricular zone, respectively. The marginal zone is rich in CR neurons, which are the primary source of Reelin during neurodevelopment. Several waves of postmitotic migrating neurons are positioned between the marginal zone and the sub plate, leading to the formation of the cortical plate. During the E14-E18 time lapse,

http://dx.doi.org/10.5772/54038

four successive waves of postmitotic neurons migrate from the ventricular zone, through the sub-plate and neurons already positioned, to reach the marginal zone where the Reelin secreted by the CR neurons acts as a "stop signal" inducing the termination of the neuronal migration. This process is termed as "radial migration", and occurs through an inside-out mechanism, where early migrating neurons are placed at the inner aspects of the cortex [23]. Mechanistically, cortical neurons migrate using two different mechanisms, a glial-dependent process termed locomotion; and a glial-independent one termed nuclear translocation. During migration across the cortical plate, the neurons adopt morphology characterized by the presence of a cytoplasmic extension oriented toward the most outer aspect of the cortex, the leading process. A secondary cytoplasmic extension emerge orthogonally from the leading process and is termed the trailing process. While the leading process will be further developed as the dendritic arbor, the trailing process will become the axon [24].

The *reeler* mutant shows a clear disruption of the cortical layers, characterized by the absence of pre-plate splitting, generating a structure called the superplate [25]. Additionally, migrating neurons fail to establish an inside-out pattern of cortical layers [26]. Thus, in the *reeler* mutant, neurons that migrate earlier during development are placed in the outer aspect of the cortex, leading to an outside-in pattern of cortical layers [23,27-29].

Abnormal neuronal migration is not exclusively for the *reeler* mice cortex. Purkinje neurons in the cerebellum are also aberrantly organized. After birth, the Purkinje cell layer is absent, and a reduction of granule cells number is appreciated, these alterations result in a dramatic reduction of foliation pattern and diminished cerebellar size [30]. At the hippocampal region, the *reeler* mutant is characterized by the presence of non-compacted dentate gyrus and disorganized pyramidal layer [31].

Summarizing, Reeler brain shows smaller size and larger ventricles, the distribution of the dorsal, medial and ventral hippocampus is altered, the cortex display an inverted array of neurons in their layers and the cerebellum shows no foliation and alterations in the organization of its layers [32].

At the molecular level, the Reelin signaling pathway control several processes required for proper neuronal migration. For example, Reelin stabilize the leading process by inducing cofilin phosphorylation at Ser3, which regulates actin dynamics [33]. Furthermore, Reelin can also induce MAP1B phosphorylation through GSK-3β activation. MAP1B function is involved in formation of brain laminated areas, therefore, Reelin can modulate neuronal guidance through post-translational modifications of MAP1B [34]. These two examples show how Reelin can act coordinately to locally regulate the assembly of actin microfilaments and microtubules (Figure 1A).

In addition to its role in neurodevelopment, Reelin controls the formation of neural circuits, promoting the growth and branching of dendrites in hippocampal neurons [35]. Moreover, Reelin can enhance the formation of dendritic spines, supporting a role at the post-synaptic compartment [36].

Most of these cellular functions are dependent on a signaling pathway, triggered by the binding of Reelin to its two main receptors, the very-low density lipoprotein receptor

(VLDLR) and the ApolipoproteinE receptor 2 (ApoER2) [37]. The binding of Reelin to its receptor induce the phosphorylation of the adapter protein mDab1 on tyrosine residues [38]. mDab1 phosphorylation lead eventually to the modulation of cytoskeleton effectors molecules such as MAP1B and cofilin [23].

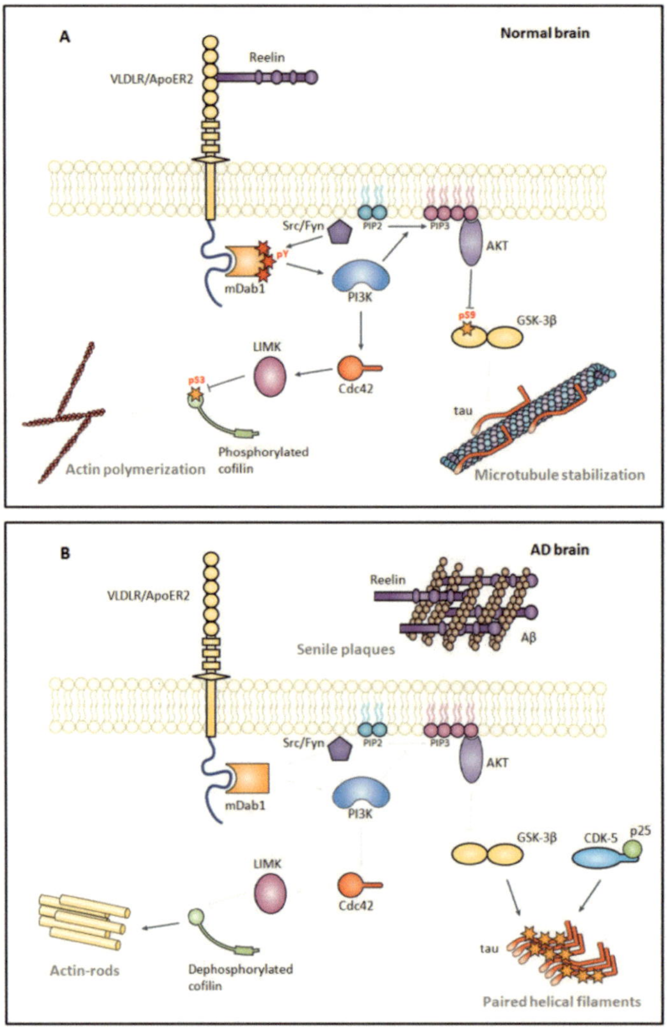

Figure 1. Reelin signaling pathway in normal brain and its impairment in AD brains. The panel A show the intracellular events triggered by the binding of Reelin to its canonical membrane receptors, ApoER2 and VLDLR. mDab1 protein is specifically phosphorylated at tyrosine residues, which concomitantly with the activation of PI3K, regulate actin and microtubule dynamic behavior. LIMK-mediated phosphorylation of cofilin and the Akt inhibitory phosphorylation of GSK-3β are essential to this regulation. On the other hand, in AD brains, diminished Reelin expression and its aggregation in amyloid-like deposits, induce impairment in its signaling pathway (represented by gray lines). Decreased Reelin signaling triggers the dephosphorylation of cofilin, promoting the formation of actin-rods. On the other hand, the activation of GSK-3β and CDK-5, lead to hyperphosphorylation of tau protein inducing its aggregation into PHFs (panel B).

http://dx.doi.org/10.5772/54038

3. Reelin in the adult brain

Although Reelin function is mainly related to neurodevelopment, several recently studies assign roles in the adult brain, such as the development of dendrites and dendritic spines [36], modulation of synaptogenesis [39], modulation of synaptic plasticity [40-43] and neurotransmitter release [44]. The mechanism by which Reelin can modulate the synaptic transmission is not fully elucidated. Currently it is strongly suggested that Reelin acting through its canonical signaling pathway facilitates the phosphorylation of NR2A and NR2B subunits of the NMDA receptor, favoring the calcium influx into the postsynaptic neuron.

This intracellular calcium increase causes the insertion of the GluR1 subunit of AMPA receptors, allowing the phosphorylation and nuclear translocation of CREB [45]. CREB phosphorylation is required to elicit the formation of dendritic spines. In addition, Reelin reduces the number of silent synapses, facilitating the exchange of subunit NR2B by NR2A of NMDA receptor [46]. Therefore, Reelin modulates synaptic plasticity events involved in learning and memory processes in adults. Consistently with a role for Reelin in the control of neurotransmission, *reeler* mice show diminished expression of presynaptic (SNARE, SNAP-25) [44] and postsynaptic (PSD-95, PTEN) markers [43]. These defects cause failures in the release of neurotransmitters, impairing synaptic transmission.

4. Animals models for neuropsychiatric diseases

Owing to the importance that Reelin have in the correct structuration and lamination of the brain during development and in neuronal connectivity and synaptogenesis in the adult brain, its dysfunction has been directly related to the generation or susceptibility to acquire neuropsychiatric conditions such as depression and schizophrenia, or neurodegenerative diseases such as Alzheimer's disease (AD) [45].

The most tangible evidence supporting these putative relationships was obtained through studies of human brains derived from neuropsychiatric and neurodegenerative conditions. Decreased levels of Reelin are shown in postmortem samples from prefrontal cortex of patients with schizophrenia and bipolar disorders [47]. This decrease may be explained in schizophrenic patients by an abnormal hypermethylation of the *reelin* promoter, an epigenetic modification involved in gene silencing [48]. Furthermore, immunohistochemistry experiments in depressive and schizophrenic patients show decreased Reelin expression at the hippocampus [49]. On the other hand, diminished Reelin levels in the hippocampus of patients with AD had been reported, suggesting a direct correlation between the severity of the disease and the extent of decreased Reelin expression [50]. All of these antecedents provide evidence enough to feature a molecular link between decreased Reelin levels and neurodegenerative/psychiatric diseases.

In order to understand the etiology of neurodegenerative/psychiatric diseases, different animal models had been developed. A widely paradigm is the "two hit" model, which suggests that genetic and environmental factors may affect the development of central nervous system, acting as "the first hit". These early disorders are linked to long-term vulnerability, which after a "second hit" could cause the symptoms for a disease [51-52]. For diseases such as depression, autism and schizophrenia, the heterozygous *reeler* mice had been used as the genetic "first hit", while stress events after the birth or in adulthood are used as the environmental "second hit". The results indicate that heterozygous *reeler* mice, after a stressful event, such as maternal deprivation or corticosterone injection, exhibit significantly increased depressive or schizophrenic behaviors as compared with wild type littermates [53-54]. Indeed, *reeler* heterozygous animals in the absence of a stressful event, display a phenotype indistinguishable from control animals [55].

The "two hit" model has also been used to study the molecular mechanisms leading to the AD [56]. It is proposed that both oxidative stress and failures in mitotic signaling can independently triggers the onset of the disease; however both are necessary for their progression [57]. In addition, a correspondence had been established between the Reelin expression in the entorhinal cortex of aged rats with their cognitive abilities. A study revealed that aged "cognitively disabled" rats show a significant decreased of Reelin in neurons on layer II of the entorhinal cortex. Such a reduction in Reelin expression was not observed in juvenile or elderly "cognitively able" rats [58].

Since Reelin is expressed from development to adult stages, is conceivable that alterations in Reelin expression, induced by genetic or environmental factors generate a vulnerable stage, and a secondary factor, present in normal aging, may trigger the onset and progression of a pathological condition.

The Reelin-activated signaling pathways, which may be involved in the generation and development of AD are still unclear and will be discussed in next sections. In the last part of this section, we present some of the evidences that correlate altered levels of Reelin and AD. Pyramidal neurons placed in layer II of the entorhinal cortex and the hippocampus derived from AD patients brains exhibit decreased Reelin expression [50]. On the other hand, an increase in the full length and 180 kD proteolytic fragment of Reelin had been observed in the frontal cortex of AD derived samples [59]. The increase of this proteolytic fragment is attributed to problems with the proteolysis of Reelin, associated with decreased Rab11-endocytosis of full length Reelin [60]. In the other hand, an increase of Reelin is also observed in the frontal cortex of AD patients, which may involve a compensatory mechanism in response to the lower expression in disease-related most vulnerable areas like the entorhinal cortex and hippocampus [50].

The CR neurons participation in AD is a controversial issue. While electronic microscopy analysis suggested that CR neurons of the temporal cortex were dramatically reduced in AD patients [61], another study showed no difference between AD patients and normal, healthy subjects [62]. On the other hand, there are some polymorphisms in the Reelin gene which had been associated with AD. Seripa and colleagues reported significant differences in two analyzed polymorphisms in the Reelin gene, in a group of 223 Caucasians AD patients. These differences were exacerbated in female patients [63].

Finally, Reelin had been associated with the pathological hallmarks for AD, the senile plaques and the neurofibrillary tangles (NFT). Reelin can modulate tau phosphorylation, the core protein of NFT [38]. It is also associated with senile plaques, large extracellular aggregates mainly formed for β-amyloid peptide (Aβ). Immunohistochemical studies revealed that Reelin colocalizes with the amyloid precursor protein (APP) in the neuritic component of typical AD plaques, at the hippocampus and cortex of mice expressing a mutant version of APP [64]. Additionally, a reduction of Reelin-producing cells had been observed in older mice and primates. This reduction is accompanied by the presence of Reelin aggregates and memory deficits. Mice harboring APP with AD-associated mutations also showed Reelin aggregates, which co-localized with non-fibrillar amyloid plaques [65]. In addition, Reelin forms oligomeric or protofibrillary deposits during aging, potentially creating a precursor condition for Aβ plaque formation [66].

A direct relationship between decreased Reelin expression and increased levels of Aβ peptide and plaque accumulation was provided by studies using transgenic mice carrying the APP Swedish and *reeler* mutation. The absence of Reelin expression resulted in an age-dependent exacerbation of plaque pathology and increased NFTs in double mutants as compared with the single APPsw mutant [67]. Finally, recent studies demonstrated a feedforward mechanism by which Reelin would favor the formation of senile plaques; and the subsequent Aβ peptide production would increase the Reelin levels by altering its proteolytic processing in the cortex of mice and humans with AD [68].

5. Cytoskeletal abnormalities in Alzheimer's disease

5.1. Tau protein and neurofibrillary tangles

Neurofibrillary tangles are amongst the standard characteristics of AD brains. These structures were firstly described by Alois Alzheimer more than a century ago and are composed of a densely packed array of fibers of 20 nm in diameter, called paired helical filaments (PHF), which at the core are mainly composed by the microtubule-associated protein, tau [69-70]. Tau protein stabilizes and enhances microtubule polymerization. It is a heterogeneous protein giving rise to 6 isoforms derived from alternative splicing [71]. It contains 3 or 4 imperfect repeats of 31 or 32 amino acids each in tandem which confers the microtubule-binding properties of the protein. These repeats are enriched in basic aminoacids that interact electrostatically with the mostly acidic C-terminal of β-tubulin subunit [72]. Tau protein is highly phosphorylated in fetal brain [73], but minimally phosphorylated in normal adult brain [74]. The abnormal phosphorylation state of several residues in tau protein plays an important role modulating the affinity to microtubules and promoting its aggregation [75] forming the core of PHFs [69,76-77]. Tau protein can be phosphorylated by many protein kinases such as calcium-calmodulin dependent kinase [78]; PKA [79-81] and PKC [82-83]. Interestingly, many of these residues are hyperphosphorylated in AD brains mainly due to an imbalance in the activity of kinases belongs to the family of proline-directed Ser/Thr protein kinases (PDPKs), such as mitogen-activated protein kinases (MAPK) [84], the glycogen synthase kinase (GSK)-3β [85], JNK [84], p38 [86] and Cyclin-dependent kinase (Cdk)-5 [87]. The abnormal phosphorylation state of tau protein is not only contributed by protein kinases, but also by deregulated protein phosphatases functions [88]. (Figure 1B)

5.2. Cofilin and actin-rods

NFTs are not the only intraneuronal cytoskeletal protein aggregates found in the brains of patients affected by AD. Hirano´s bodies and actin-rods are two closely related aggregates primarily composed of actin and the actin binding protein, cofilin. Cofilin concertedly with the actin depolymerizing factor (ADF) constitutes the major modulators of actin dynamic assembly.

Hirano's bodies were originally described in 1965 and are defined as paracrystalline structures, eosinophilic intracellular arrangements resembling rod-shaped filaments of 7 nm. The actin-rods differ from Hirano´s bodies by it smaller size, so it is hypothesized that these structures could be precursors of Hirano's bodies.

The formation of actin-rods in neurons seems to be the result of several neurodegenerative insults, such as ATP depletion, excitotoxic levels of glutamate, oxidative stress [89], and $A\beta_{1-42}$ oligomers [90]. A common event to all these stimuli triggers the formation of rods is the dephosphorylation (activation) of cofilin [89]. Cofilin/ADF is inactivated by phosphorylation of a highly conserved serine (Ser3), which precludes its binding to actin filaments and, therefore, its role as promoters of filament severing and actin subunits turnover at the minus end of filaments.

The Ser3 of ADF/cofilin is the only known substrate for the two isoforms of LIM domain kinases (LIM, an acronym for three *Caenorhabditis elegans* genes, *lin-11*, *isl-1* and *mec-3*). LIMKs is activated by phosphorylation at the Thr508, mediated by PAK or ROCK, two kinases that act as effectors for small GTPases Rac1 and RhoA respectively [91]. The regulation of signaling cascades, which target the functions of small GTPases, connect the dynamic control of the actin cytoskeleton with extracellular signals. In AD, different components of the signaling cascade involved in cofilin phosphorylation are altered, including decreased phosphorylation of PAK at Ser141, which is necessary for activation. Although a decrease in phosphorylation and activity of PAK is observed in large areas of cortex and hippocampus of AD brains, neurons located near to amyloid plaques exhibit strong staining for pSer141 PAK, suggesting that while the dephosphorylation is predominant in the brain of patients with AD, the amyloid fibrils present in amyloid plaques increases the activity of PAK [92].

Consistently, hippocampal neurons treated with fibrillar $A\beta_{1-42}$ show increased activity of PAK and its downstream substrate LIMK1 [93-94], most likely through a Rac1 and Cdc42 dependent mechanism [95]. Moreover, the treatment with oligomers of $A\beta_{1-40}$ has the opposite effect, decreasing the phosphorylation of PAK, indicating that oligomeric forms may be responsible for the overall reduction in PAK phosphorylation [92].

http://dx.doi.org/10.5772/54038

Similarly, cofilin dephosphorylation and the subsequent formation of actin-rods seem to be also a spatial-restricted phenomenon. In example, actin-rods occur in a subpopulation of neurons in organotypic slices treated with Aβ [96]. (Figure 1B)

The mechanisms involved in the Aβ-mediated cofilin dephosphorylation are dependent on changes in the activity of its upstream kinase, LIMK [90], and the activity of two known cofilin phosphatases, chronophin [97] and slingshot [94].

Interestingly, ATP depletion induces chronophin activation in a mechanism involving the dissociation of chronophin-HSP90 complex. This mechanism would be responsible for the formation of actin-rods under energy deprivation conditions [97].

6. Is the AD-associated Reelin reduction a major factor involved in the neuronal cytoskeleton pathology?

6.1. Reelin reduction in AD brains

There is an increasing body of evidence indicating that a deficiency in Reelin signaling may play a major role in the progression of AD. First, decreased Reelin expression is early observed in brains of AD transgenic mice model, even before Aβ deposition. Accordingly, Reelin expression is also decreased in brains of patients at the presymptomatic stages of AD. The progression of the disease causes in both cases, potentiate the Reelin deficiency from the hippocampus to the entorhinal cortex in mice and from the frontal cortex to the hippocampus and entorhinal cortex in humans [50,98]. The decrease in Reelin expression is linked to a reduction in CR cells at the cortical layer I in AD brains [61].

Reelin itself can form amyloid deposits in advanced stages of AD, which can or cannot be associated with Aβ senile plaques [64-66]. However, Aβ pathology seems to be a prerequisite for the formation of Reelin aggregates, as these only occur after formation of senile plaques [98].

On the other hand, the proteolytic fragments of Reelin showing aberrant glycosylation pattern are increased in the cerebrospinal fluid of patients with AD [59,99]. Altogether these antecedents support the hypothesis that the Reelin intracellular signaling is impaired at early stages of AD.

6.2. Cytoskeletal pathologies and Reelin signaling

Reelin signaling is triggered by the binding of Reelin to two members of the lipoprotein receptor family, the very low density lipoprotein receptor (VLDLR) and the ApoE receptor 2 (ApoER2)[100]. The signal is then transduced by a cytoplasmic adapter protein, the mammalian homologue for the *Drosophila* protein *disabled* (mDab)-1, which interacts with the NPXY motifs of the intracellular domain of several members of the LDL receptor family, including VLDLR and ApoER2.

As VLDLR/ApoER2 or mDab1 deficient mice exhibit a phenotype indistinguishable from *reeler* mice, it is suggested that both receptors and the adapter protein can be linearly placed on the same signal transduction pathway [37,101].

The binding of Reelin to its receptors induces mDab1 tyrosine phosphorylation, mediated by non-receptor tyrosine kinases from the Src family [102]. The mutation of these tyrosines residues by phenylalanines in a *knockin* mouse recapitulates several features of the *reeler* mouse, supporting that these phosphorylation events are required for proper Reelin signaling [103].

Several genetic models suggest that canonical Reelin signaling plays an essential role in controlling the phosphorylation state of tau and, therefore, modulating a critical event in the progression of AD (Table 1).

Mice deficient in various components of the Reelin signaling pathway, including Reelin itself, VLDLR, ApoER2 and Dab1 show increased tau phosphorylation in several AD-associated epitopes, such as those recognized by the antibodies AT8 (pSer202/205) and PHF1 (pSer396/404) [38,104-106].

The increase in tau phosphorylation is caused by increased activity of two main kinases, Cdk5 and GSK-3β [105], suggesting that Reelin is playing a negative control over the activities of these kinases.

GSK-3β is normally inhibited by phosphorylation at its N-terminal region by the protein kinase Akt, mainly at the Ser9. Reelin signaling in turn, activates Akt through its recruitment to membrane domains rich in phosphatidylinositol 3-phosphate (PIP3), whose formation is involved the activity of the phosphatidilinositol 3-kinase (PI3K). Reelin activates PI3K by potentiating the interaction between tyrosine phosphorylated-mDab1 and the p85α subunit of PI3K [107-108].

Moreover, it has been proposed that the increased activity of Cdk5 in Dab1 or Reelin deficient mice may be due to a remarkable increase of the proteolyzed form of a Cdk5 activator, called p25 [105]. This fragment induces a non-physiological activation of Cdk5, which is present mainly in pathological conditions, including brains of patients with AD [109]. Since the proteolysis of the Cdk5 activator is due to the activity of calpain, it may be hypothesized that the Reelin signaling pathway could regulate calpain-dependent proteolysis of p35.

It has been proposed that Cdk5 could not be directly regulated by the Reelin signaling cascade, because cortical neurons treated with Reelin do not exhibit any significant change in the Cdk5 activity [107] or a diminished phosphorylation state of Cdk5-dependent substrates [110]. However, it may not be ruled out that a subset of substrates still not analyzed can be phosphorylated by Cdk5 due to impairment in Reelin signaling.

Protein	Functions in Reelin signaling	Association with Alzheimer´s disease	References
Reelin	Extracellular matrix glycoprotein	Diminished levels in restricted areas of AD brain. Reelin-deficient mice show increased tau phosphorylation	[50, 98]
ApoER2	Reelin receptor	VLDLR and ApoER2 dKO mice present elevated levels of phosphorylated tau	[38]
VLDLR	Reelin receptor	VLDLR and ApoER2 dKO mice present elevated levels of phosphorylated tau	[38]
mDab1	Intracellular adapter for Reelin receptors	mDab1-deficient mice show increased tau phosphorylation and early death.	[106]
PI3K	Lipid kinase essential for membrane recruiting of Akt	Impairment in PI3K-Akt pathway was observed in aged APP-PS1 transgenic mice.	[112]
Akt	Phosphorylates and inhibits GSK-3β	Impairment in PI3K-Akt pathway was observed in aged APP-PS1 transgenic mice.	[112]
GSK-3β	Major tau kinase	Phosphorylates tau at AD-associated epitopes	[85]
tau	Microtubule-associated protein. Promotes microtubule assembly and stabilization	Hyperphosphorylated tau constitutes the core of NFTs	[77]
Cdc42	Small GTPase associated with actin dynamics	A lesser Aβ-induced actin-rod formation is observed in cdc42 null neurons	[96]
LIMK1	Major effector of Rho-family GTPases. Phosphorylates and inactivates cofilin	The expression of constitutively active LIMK1 reduces Aβ-induced actin-rods in hippocampal slices	[90]
Cofilin	Actin binding protein with F-actin depolymerizing activity	Ser3 dephosphorylation triggers its aggregation into actin-rods	[89]

Table 1. Association of Reelin signaling pathway with Alzheimer´s disease

The Reelin signaling pathway can target not only microtubule cytoskeleton, but also the actin microfilament formation. Acting through its canonical signaling pathway that involve receptors VLDLR and ApoER2, the adapter protein Dab1 and activation of PI3K, Reelin is able to activate the small GTPases Rac1 and Cdc42, increasing actin polymerization. These changes in small Rho GTPases are responsible of increased mobility of growth cones and promote the appearance of filopodia in the axon of cortical neurons in culture [111]. The stabilization of actin filaments is mediated directly by an increase in activation of LIMK and phosphorylation of cofilin Ser3 [33]. LIMK and cofilin phosphorylation are two key events that regulate actin microfilament turnover in a Rac-dependent manner. Currently, there are no studies showing a causal relationship between impaired Reelin signaling and molecular changes affecting cofilin phosphorylation that could regulate the formation of actin-rods. However, it is tempting to speculate that further studies may solve a linkage between the decreased Reelin signaling observed in AD brains and abnormal actin dynamics.

Acknowledgements

Supported by Fondecyt 1095089 to CG-B.

Author details

Daniel A. Bórquez, Ismael Palacios and Christian González-Billault

*Address all correspondence to: chrgonza@uchile.cl

Cell and Neuronal Dynamics Laboratory, Faculty of Sciences, Universidad de Chile, Santiago, Chile

References

[1] Alcantara S, Ruiz M, D'Arcangelo G, Ezan F, de Lecea L, Curran T, Sotelo C, Soriano E. Regional and cellular patterns of reelin mRNA expression in the forebrain of the developing and adult mouse. Journal of Neuroscience 1998;18(19) 7779-7799.

[2] Tissir F, Goffinet AM. Reelin and brain development. Nature Reviews Neuroscience 2003;4(6) 496-505.

[3] Ringstedt T, Linnarsson S, Wagner J, Lendahl U, Kokaia Z, Arenas E, Ernfors P, Ibanez CF. BDNF regulates reelin expression and Cajal-Retzius cell development in the cerebral cortex. Neuron 1998;21(2) 305-315.

[4] Pesold C, Impagnatiello F, Pisu MG, Uzunov DP, Costa E, Guidotti A, Caruncho HJ. Reelin is preferentially expressed in neurons synthesizing gamma-aminobutyric acid in cortex and hippocampus of adult rats. Proceedings of the National Academy of Sciences of the United States of America 1998;95(6) 3221-3226.

[5] Lacor PN, Grayson DR, Auta J, Sugaya I, Costa E, Guidotti A. Reelin secretion from glutamatergic neurons in culture is independent from neurotransmitter regulation.

Proceedings of the National Academy of Sciences of the United States of America 2000;97(7) 3556-3561.

[6] DeSilva U, D'Arcangelo G, Braden VV, Chen J, Miao GG, Curran T, Green ED. The human reelin gene: isolation, sequencing, and mapping on chromosome 7. Genome Research 1997;7(2) 157-164.

[7] Royaux I, Lambert de Rouvroit C, D'Arcangelo G, Demirov D, Goffinet AM. Genomic organization of the mouse reelin gene. Genomics 1997;46(2) 240-250.

[8] Chen Y, Sharma RP, Costa RH, Costa E, Grayson DR. On the epigenetic regulation of the human reelin promoter. Nucleic Acids Research 2002;30(13) 2930-2939.

[9] Matrisciano F, Tueting P, Dalal I, Kadriu B, Grayson DR, Davis JM, Nicoletti F, Guidotti A. Epigenetic modifications of GABAergic interneurons are associated with the schizophrenia-like phenotype induced by prenatal stress in mice. Neuropharmacology 2012.

[10] Mitchell CP, Chen Y, Kundakovic M, Costa E, Grayson DR. Histone deacetylase inhibitors decrease reelin promoter methylation in vitro. Journal of Neurochemistry 2005;93(2) 483-492.

[11] Kundakovic M, Chen Y, Costa E, Grayson DR. DNA methyltransferase inhibitors coordinately induce expression of the human reelin and glutamic acid decarboxylase 67 genes. Molecular Pharmacology 2007;71(3) 644-653.

[12] Grayson DR, Chen Y, Costa E, Dong E, Guidotti A, Kundakovic M, Sharma RP. The human reelin gene: transcription factors (+), repressors (-) and the methylation switch (+/-) in schizophrenia. Pharmacology & Therapeutics 2006;111(1) 272-286.

[13] Hevner RF, Shi L, Justice N, Hsueh Y, Sheng M, Smiga S, Bulfone A, Goffinet AM, Campagnoni AT, Rubenstein JL. Tbr1 regulates differentiation of the preplate and layer 6. Neuron 2001;29(2) 353-366.

[14] Chen Y, Kundakovic M, Agis-Balboa RC, Pinna G, Grayson DR. Induction of the reelin promoter by retinoic acid is mediated by Sp1. Journal of Neurochemistry 2007;103(2) 650-665.

[15] Lambert de Rouvroit C, de Bergeyck V, Cortvrindt C, Bar I, Eeckhout Y, Goffinet AM. Reelin, the extracellular matrix protein deficient in reeler mutant mice, is processed by a metalloproteinase. Experimental Neurology 1999;156(1) 214-217.

[16] Hisanaga A, Morishita S, Suzuki K, Sasaki K, Koie M, Kohno T, Hattori M. A disintegrin and metalloproteinase with thrombospondin motifs 4 (ADAMTS-4) cleaves Reelin in an isoform-dependent manner. FEBS Letters 2012.

[17] Jossin Y, Gui L, Goffinet AM. Processing of Reelin by embryonic neurons is important for function in tissue but not in dissociated cultured neurons. Journal of Neuroscience 2007;27(16) 4243-4252.

[18] Jossin Y, Ignatova N, Hiesberger T, Herz J, Lambert de Rouvroit C, Goffinet AM. The central fragment of Reelin, generated by proteolytic processing in vivo, is critical to its function during cortical plate development. Journal of Neuroscience 2004;24(2) 514-521.

[19] D'Arcangelo G, Nakajima K, Miyata T, Ogawa M, Mikoshiba K, Curran T. Reelin is a secreted glycoprotein recognized by the CR-50 monoclonal antibody. Journal of Neuroscience 1997;17(1) 23-31.

[20] Utsunomiya-Tate N, Kubo K, Tate S, Kainosho M, Katayama E, Nakajima K, Mikoshiba K. Reelin molecules assemble together to form a large protein complex, which is inhibited by the function-blocking CR-50 antibody. Proceedings of the National Academy of Sciences of the United States of America 2000;97(17) 9729-9734.

[21] de Bergeyck V, Nakajima K, Lambert de Rouvroit C, Naerhuyzen B, Goffinet AM, Miyata T, Ogawa M, Mikoshiba K. A truncated Reelin protein is produced but not secreted in the 'Orleans' reeler mutation (Reln[rl-Orl]). Brain Research: Molecular Brain Research 1997;50(1-2) 85-90.

[22] D'Arcangelo G, Miao GG, Curran T. Detection of the reelin breakpoint in reeler mice. Brain Research: Molecular Brain Research 1996;39(1-2) 234-236.

[23] Gupta A, Tsai LH, Wynshaw-Boris A. Life is a journey: a genetic look at neocortical development. Nature Reviews Genetics 2002;3(5) 342-355.

[24] O'Rourke NA, Dailey ME, Smith SJ, McConnell SK. Diverse migratory pathways in the developing cerebral cortex. Science 1992;258(5080) 299-302.

[25] Caviness VS, Jr. Neocortical histogenesis in normal and reeler mice: a developmental study based upon [3H]thymidine autoradiography. Brain Research 1982;256(3) 293-302.

[26] Ogawa M, Miyata T, Nakajima K, Yagyu K, Seike M, Ikenaka K, Yamamoto H, Mikoshiba K. The reeler gene-associated antigen on Cajal-Retzius neurons is a crucial molecule for laminar organization of cortical neurons. Neuron 1995;14(5) 899-912.

[27] Frotscher M. Dual role of Cajal-Retzius cells and reelin in cortical development. Cell and Tissue Research 1997;290(2) 315-322.

[28] Curran T, D'Arcangelo G. Role of reelin in the control of brain development. Brain Research: Brain Research Reviews 1998;26(2-3) 285-294.

[29] Tissir F, Lambert de Rouvroit C, Goffinet AM. The role of reelin in the development and evolution of the cerebral cortex. Brazilian Journal of Medical and Biological Research 2002;35(12) 1473-1484.

[30] Goffinet AM, So KF, Yamamoto M, Edwards M, Caviness VS, Jr. Architectonic and hodological organization of the cerebellum in reeler mutant mice. Brain Research 1984;318(2) 263-276.

[31] Stanfield BB, Cowan WM. The development of the hippocampus and dentate gyrus in normal and reeler mice. Journal of Comparative Neurology 1979;185(3) 423-459.

[32] Badea A, Nicholls PJ, Johnson GA, Wetsel WC. Neuroanatomical phenotypes in the reeler mouse. NeuroImage 2007;34(4) 1363-1374.

[33] Chai X, Forster E, Zhao S, Bock HH, Frotscher M. Reelin stabilizes the actin cytoskeleton of neuronal processes by inducing n-cofilin phosphorylation at serine3. Journal of Neuroscience 2009;29(1) 288-299.

[34] Gonzalez-Billault C, Del Rio JA, Urena JM, Jimenez-Mateos EM, Barallobre MJ, Pascual M, Pujadas L, Simo S, Torre AL, Gavin R, Wandosell F, Soriano E, Avila J. A role of MAP1B in Reelin-dependent neuronal migration. Cerebral Cortex 2005;15(8) 1134-1145.

[35] Niu S, Renfro A, Quattrocchi CC, Sheldon M, D'Arcangelo G. Reelin promotes hippocampal dendrite development through the VLDLR/ApoER2-Dab1 pathway. Neuron 2004;41(1) 71-84.

[36] Niu S, Yabut O, D'Arcangelo G. The Reelin signaling pathway promotes dendritic spine development in hippocampal neurons. Journal of Neuroscience 2008;28(41) 10339-10348.

[37] Trommsdorff M, Gotthardt M, Hiesberger T, Shelton J, Stockinger W, Nimpf J, Hammer R, Richardson J, Herz J. Reeler/Disabled-like disruption of neuronal migration in knockout mice lacking the VLDL receptor and ApoE receptor 2. Cell 1999;97(6) 689-1390.

[38] Hiesberger T, Trommsdorff M, Howell BW, Goffinet A, Mumby MC, Cooper JA, Herz J. Direct binding of Reelin to VLDL receptor and ApoE receptor 2 induces tyrosine phosphorylation of disabled-1 and modulates tau phosphorylation. Neuron 1999;24(2) 481-489.

[39] Borrell V, Del Rio JA, Alcantara S, Derer M, Martinez A, D'Arcangelo G, Nakajima K, Mikoshiba K, Derer P, Curran T, Soriano E. Reelin regulates the development and synaptogenesis of the layer-specific entorhino-hippocampal connections. Journal of Neuroscience 1999;19(4) 1345-1358.

[40] Chen Y, Beffert U, Ertunc M, Tang TS, Kavalali ET, Bezprozvanny I, Herz J. Reelin modulates NMDA receptor activity in cortical neurons. Journal of Neuroscience 2005;25(36) 8209-8216.

[41] Herz J, Chen Y. Reelin, lipoprotein receptors and synaptic plasticity. Nature Reviews Neuroscience 2006;7(11) 850-859.

[42] Qiu S, Zhao LF, Korwek KM, Weeber EJ. Differential reelin-induced enhancement of NMDA and AMPA receptor activity in the adult hippocampus. Journal of Neuroscience 2006;26(50) 12943-12955.

[43] Ventruti A, Kazdoba TM, Niu S, D'Arcangelo G. Reelin deficiency causes specific defects in the molecular composition of the synapses in the adult brain. Neuroscience 2011;189 32-42.

[44] Hellwig S, Hack I, Kowalski J, Brunne B, Jarowyj J, Unger A, Bock HH, Junghans D, Frotscher M. Role for Reelin in neurotransmitter release. Journal of Neuroscience 2011;31(7) 2352-2360.

[45] Knuesel I. Reelin-mediated signaling in neuropsychiatric and neurodegenerative diseases. Progress in Neurobiology 2010;91(4) 257-274.

[46] Qiu S, Weeber EJ. Reelin signaling facilitates maturation of CA1 glutamatergic synapses. Journal of Neurophysiology 2007;97(3) 2312-2321.

[47] Guidotti A, Auta J, Davis JM, Di-Giorgi-Gerevini V, Dwivedi Y, Grayson DR, Impagnatiello F, Pandey G, Pesold C, Sharma R, Uzunov D, Costa E. Decrease in reelin and glutamic acid decarboxylase67 (GAD67) expression in schizophrenia and bipolar disorder: a postmortem brain study. Archives of General Psychiatry 2000;57(11) 1061-1069.

[48] Abdolmaleky HM, Cheng KH, Russo A, Smith CL, Faraone SV, Wilcox M, Shafa R, Glatt SJ, Nguyen G, Ponte JF, Thiagalingam S, Tsuang MT. Hypermethylation of the reelin (RELN) promoter in the brain of schizophrenic patients: a preliminary report. American Journal of Medical Genetics Part B, Neuropsychiatric Genetics 2005;134B(1) 60-66.

[49] Fatemi SH, Earle JA, McMenomy T. Reduction in Reelin immunoreactivity in hippocampus of subjects with schizophrenia, bipolar disorder and major depression. Molecular Psychiatry 2000;5(6) 654-663, 571.

[50] Chin J, Massaro CM, Palop JJ, Thwin MT, Yu GQ, Bien-Ly N, Bender A, Mucke L. Reelin depletion in the entorhinal cortex of human amyloid precursor protein transgenic mice and humans with Alzheimer's disease. Journal of Neuroscience 2007;27(11) 2727-2733.

[51] Maynard TM, Sikich L, Lieberman JA, LaMantia AS. Neural development, cell-cell signaling, and the "two-hit" hypothesis of schizophrenia. Schizophrenia Bulletin 2001;27(3) 457-476.

[52] Girirajan S, Rosenfeld JA, Cooper GM, Antonacci F, Siswara P, Itsara A, Vives L, Walsh T, McCarthy SE, Baker C, Mefford HC, Kidd JM, Browning SR, Browning BL, Dickel DE, Levy DL, Ballif BC, Platky K, Farber DM, Gowans GC, Wetherbee JJ, Asamoah A, Weaver DD, Mark PR, Dickerson J, Garg BP, Ellingwood SA, Smith R, Banks VC, Smith W, McDonald MT, Hoo JJ, French BN, Hudson C, Johnson JP, Ozmore JR, Moeschler JB, Surti U, Escobar LF, El-Khechen D, Gorski JL, Kussmann J, Salbert B, Lacassie Y, Biser A, McDonald-McGinn DM, Zackai EH, Deardorff MA, Shaikh TH, Haan E, Friend KL, Fichera M, Romano C, Gecz J, DeLisi LE, Sebat J, King MC, Shaffer LG, Eichler EE. A recurrent 16p12.1 microdeletion supports a two-hit model for severe developmental delay. Nature Genetics 2010;42(3) 203-209.

[53] Laviola G, Ognibene E, Romano E, Adriani W, Keller F. Gene-environment interaction during early development in the heterozygous reeler mouse: clues for modelling of major neurobehavioral syndromes. Neuroscience and Biobehavioral Reviews 2009;33(4) 560-572.

[54] Lussier AL, Romay-Tallon R, Kalynchuk LE, Caruncho HJ. Reelin as a putative vulnerability factor for depression: examining the depressogenic effects of repeated corticosterone in heterozygous reeler mice. Neuropharmacology 2011;60(7-8) 1064-1074.

[55] Teixeira CM, Martin ED, Sahun I, Masachs N, Pujadas L, Corvelo A, Bosch C, Rossi D, Martinez A, Maldonado R, Dierssen M, Soriano E. Overexpression of Reelin prevents the manifestation of behavioral phenotypes related to schizophrenia and bipolar disorder. Neuropsychopharmacology 2011;36(12) 2395-2405.

[56] Zhu X, Lee HG, Perry G, Smith MA. Alzheimer disease, the two-hit hypothesis: an update. Biochimica et Biophysica Acta 2007;1772(4) 494-502.

[57] Zhu X, Castellani RJ, Takeda A, Nunomura A, Atwood CS, Perry G, Smith MA. Differential activation of neuronal ERK, JNK/SAPK and p38 in Alzheimer disease: the 'two hit' hypothesis. Mechanisms of Ageing and Development 2001;123(1) 39-46.

[58] Stranahan AM, Haberman RP, Gallagher M. Cognitive decline is associated with reduced reelin expression in the entorhinal cortex of aged rats. Cerebral Cortex 2011;21(2) 392-400.

[59] Botella-Lopez A, Burgaya F, Gavin R, Garcia-Ayllon MS, Gomez-Tortosa E, Pena-Casanova J, Urena JM, Del Rio JA, Blesa R, Soriano E, Saez-Valero J. Reelin expression and glycosylation patterns are altered in Alzheimer's disease. Proceedings of the National Academy of Sciences of the United States of America 2006;103(14) 5573-5578.

[60] Hibi T, Hattori M. The N-terminal fragment of Reelin is generated after endocytosis and released through the pathway regulated by Rab11. FEBS Letters 2009;583(8) 1299-1303.

[61] Baloyannis SJ. Morphological and morphometric alterations of Cajal-Retzius cells in early cases of Alzheimer's disease: a Golgi and electron microscope study. International Journal of Neuroscience 2005;115(7) 965-980.

[62] Riedel A, Miettinen R, Stieler J, Mikkonen M, Alafuzoff I, Soininen H, Arendt T. Reelin-immunoreactive Cajal-Retzius cells: the entorhinal cortex in normal aging and Alzheimer's disease. Acta Neuropathologica 2003;106(4) 291-302.

[63] Seripa D, Matera MG, Franceschi M, Daniele A, Bizzarro A, Rinaldi M, Panza F, Fazio VM, Gravina C, D'Onofrio G, Solfrizzi V, Masullo C, Pilotto A. The RELN locus in Alzheimer's disease. Journal of Alzheimer's Disease 2008;14(3) 335-344.

[64] Wirths O, Multhaup G, Czech C, Blanchard V, Tremp G, Pradier L, Beyreuther K, Bayer TA Reelin in plaques of beta-amyloid precursor protein and presenilin-1 double-transgenic mice. Neuroscience Letters 2001;316(3) 145-148.

[65] Knuesel I, Nyffeler M, Mormede C, Muhia M, Meyer U, Pietropaolo S, Yee BK, Pryce CR, LaFerla FM, Marighetto A, Feldon J. Age-related accumulation of Reelin in amyloid-like deposits. Neurobiology of Aging 2009;30(5) 697-716.

[66] Doehner J, Madhusudan A, Konietzko U, Fritschy JM, Knuesel I. Co-localization of Reelin and proteolytic AbetaPP fragments in hippocampal plaques in aged wild-type mice. Journal of Alzheimer's Disease 2010;19(4) 1339-1357.

[67] Kocherhans S, Madhusudan A, Doehner J, Breu KS, Nitsch RM, Fritschy JM, Knuesel I. Reduced Reelin expression accelerates amyloid-beta plaque formation and tau pathology in transgenic Alzheimer's disease mice. Journal of Neuroscience 2010;30(27) 9228-9240.

[68] Botella-Lopez A, Cuchillo-Ibanez I, Cotrufo T, Mok SS, Li QX, Barquero MS, Dierssen M, Soriano E, Saez-Valero J. Beta-amyloid controls altered Reelin expression and processing in Alzheimer's disease. Neurobiology of Disease 2010;37(3) 682-691.

[69] Kosik KS, Joachim CL, Selkoe DJ. Microtubule-associated protein tau (tau) is a major antigenic component of paired helical filaments in Alzheimer disease. Proceedings of the National Academy of Sciences of the United States of America 1986;83(11) 4044-4048.

[70] Weingarten MD, Lockwood AH, Hwo SY, Kirschner MW. A protein factor essential for microtubule assembly. Proceedings of the National Academy of Sciences of the United States of America 1975;72(5) 1858-1862.

[71] Lee G, Cowan N, Kirschner M. The primary structure and heterogeneity of tau protein from mouse brain. Science 1988;239(4837) 285-288.

[72] Lee G, Neve RL, Kosik KS. The microtubule binding domain of tau protein. Neuron 1989;2(6) 1615-1624.

[73] Lindwall G, Cole RD. The purification of tau protein and the occurrence of two phosphorylation states of tau in brain. Journal of Biological Chemistry 1984;259(19) 12241-12245.

[74] Seubert P, Mawal-Dewan M, Barbour R, Jakes R, Goedert M, Johnson GV, Litersky JM, Schenk D, Lieberburg I, Trojanowski JQ, Lee VM. Detection of phosphorylated Ser262 in fetal tau, adult tau, and paired helical filament tau. Journal of Biological Chemistry 1995;270(32) 18917-18922.

[75] Iqbal K, Alonso Adel C, Grundke-Iqbal I. Cytosolic abnormally hyperphosphorylated tau but not paired helical filaments sequester normal MAPs and inhibit microtubule assembly. Journal of Alzheimer's Disease 2008;14(4) 365-370.

[76] Grundke-Iqbal I, Iqbal K, Tung YC, Quinlan M, Wisniewski HM, Binder LI. Abnormal phosphorylation of the microtubule-associated protein tau (tau) in Alzheimer cytoskeletal pathology. Proceedings of the National Academy of Sciences of the United States of America 1986;83(13) 4913-4917.

[77] Ihara Y, Nukina N, Miura R, Ogawara M. Phosphorylated tau protein is integrated into paired helical filaments in Alzheimer's disease. Journal of Biochemistry 1986;99(6) 1807-1810.

[78] Steiner B, Mandelkow EM, Biernat J, Gustke N, Meyer HE, Schmidt B, Mieskes G, Soling HD, Drechsel D, Kirschner MW, Goedert M, Mandelkow E. Phosphorylation of microtubule-associated protein tau: identification of the site for Ca2(+)-calmodulin dependent kinase and relationship with tau phosphorylation in Alzheimer tangles. EMBO Journal 1990;9(11) 3539-3544.

[79] Andorfer CA, Davies P. PKA phosphorylations on tau: developmental studies in the mouse. Developmental Neuroscience 2000;22(4) 303-309.

[80] Liu SJ, Zhang JY, Li HL, Fang ZY, Wang Q, Deng HM, Gong CX, Grundke-Iqbal I, Iqbal K, Wang JZ. Tau becomes a more favorable substrate for GSK-3 when it is prephosphorylated by PKA in rat brain. Journal of Biological Chemistry 2004;279(48) 50078-50088.

[81] Jensen PH, Hager H, Nielsen MS, Hojrup P, Gliemann J, Jakes R. alpha-synuclein binds to Tau and stimulates the protein kinase A-catalyzed tau phosphorylation of serine residues 262 and 356. Journal of Biological Chemistry 1999;274(36) 25481-25489.

[82] Hoshi M, Nishida E, Miyata Y, Sakai H, Miyoshi T, Ogawara H, Akiyama T. Protein kinase C phosphorylates tau and induces its functional alterations. FEBS Letters 1987;217(2) 237-241.

[83] Correas I, Diaz-Nido J, Avila J. Microtubule-associated protein tau is phosphorylated by protein kinase C on its tubulin binding domain. Journal of Biological Chemistry 1992;267(22) 15721-15728.

[84] Reynolds CH, Utton MA, Gibb GM, Yates A, Anderton BH. Stress-activated protein kinase/c-jun N-terminal kinase phosphorylates tau protein. Journal of Neurochemistry 1997;68(4) 1736-1744.

[85] Hanger DP, Hughes K, Woodgett JR, Brion JP, Anderton BH. Glycogen synthase kinase-3 induces Alzheimer's disease-like phosphorylation of tau: generation of paired helical filament epitopes and neuronal localisation of the kinase. Neuroscience Letters 1992;147(1) 58-62.

[86] Reynolds CH, Betts JC, Blackstock WP, Nebreda AR, Anderton BH. Phosphorylation sites on tau identified by nanoelectrospray mass spectrometry: differences in vitro between the mitogen-activated protein kinases ERK2, c-Jun N-terminal kinase and P38, and glycogen synthase kinase-3beta. Journal of Neurochemistry 2000;74(4) 1587-1595.

[87] Baumann K, Mandelkow EM, Biernat J, Piwnica-Worms H, Mandelkow E. Abnormal Alzheimer-like phosphorylation of tau-protein by cyclin-dependent kinases cdk2 and cdk5. FEBS Letters 1993;336(3) 417-424.

[88] Trojanowski JQ, Lee VM. Phosphorylation of paired helical filament tau in Alzheimer's disease neurofibrillary lesions: focusing on phosphatases. FASEB Journal 1995;9(15) 1570-1576.

[89] Minamide LS, Striegl AM, Boyle JA, Meberg PJ, Bamburg JR. Neurodegenerative stimuli induce persistent ADF/cofilin-actin rods that disrupt distal neurite function. Nature Cell Biology 2000;2(9) 628-636.

[90] Davis RC, Marsden IT, Maloney MT, Minamide LS, Podlisny M, Selkoe DJ, Bamburg JR. Amyloid beta dimers/trimers potently induce cofilin-actin rods that are inhibited by maintaining cofilin-phosphorylation. Molecular Neurodegeneration 2011;6(10).

[91] Bernard O Lim kinases, regulators of actin dynamics. International Journal of Biochemistry & Cell Biology 2007;39(6) 1071-1076.

[92] Zhao L, Ma QL, Calon F, Harris-White ME, Yang F, Lim GP, Morihara T, Ubeda OJ, Ambegaokar S, Hansen JE, Weisbart RH, Teter B, Frautschy SA, Cole GM. Role of p21-activated kinase pathway defects in the cognitive deficits of Alzheimer disease. Nature Neuroscience 2006;9(2) 234-242.

[93] Heredia L, Helguera P, de Olmos S, Kedikian G, Sola Vigo F, LaFerla F, Staufenbiel M, de Olmos J, Busciglio J, Caceres A, Lorenzo A. Phosphorylation of actin-depolymerizing factor/cofilin by LIM-kinase mediates amyloid beta-induced degeneration: a potential mechanism of neuronal dystrophy in Alzheimer's disease. Journal of Neuroscience 2006;26(24) 6533-6542.

[94] Mendoza-Naranjo A, Contreras-Vallejos E, Henriquez DR, Otth C, Bamburg JR, Maccioni RB, Gonzalez-Billault C. Fibrillar amyloid-beta1-42 modifies actin organization affecting the cofilin phosphorylation state: a role for Rac1/cdc42 effector proteins and the slingshot phosphatase. Journal of Alzheimer's Disease 2012;29(1) 63-77.

[95] Mendoza-Naranjo A, Gonzalez-Billault C, Maccioni RB. Abeta1-42 stimulates actin polymerization in hippocampal neurons through Rac1 and Cdc42 Rho GTPases. Journal of Cell Science 2007;120(Pt 2) 279-288.

[96] Davis RC, Maloney MT, Minamide LS, Flynn KC, Stonebraker MA, Bamburg JR. Mapping cofilin-actin rods in stressed hippocampal slices and the role of cdc42 in amyloid-beta-induced rods. Journal of Alzheimer's Disease 2009;18(1) 35-50.

[97] Huang TY, Minamide LS, Bamburg JR, Bokoch GM. Chronophin mediates an ATP-sensing mechanism for cofilin dephosphorylation and neuronal cofilin-actin rod formation. Developmental Cell 2008;15(5) 691-703.

[98] Herring A, Donath A, Steiner KM, Widera MP, Hamzehian S, Kanakis D, Kolble K, Elali A, Hermann DM, Paulus W, Keyvani K. Reelin Depletion is an Early Phenomenon of Alzheimer's Pathology. Journal of Alzheimer's Disease 2012;30(4) 963-979.

[99] Saez-Valero J, Costell M, Sjogren M, Andreasen N, Blennow K, Luque JM. Altered levels of cerebrospinal fluid reelin in frontotemporal dementia and Alzheimer's disease. Journal of Neuroscience Research 2003;72(1) 132-136.

[100] D'Arcangelo G, Homayouni R, Keshvara L, Rice DS, Sheldon M, Curran T. Reelin is a ligand for lipoprotein receptors. Neuron 1999;24(2) 471-479.

[101] Howell B, Hawkes R, Soriano P, Cooper J. Neuronal position in the developing brain is regulated by mouse disabled-1. Nature 1997;389(4c369df1-0b52-a4f8-d881-0c77f39fea11) 733-740.

[102] Howell B, Herrick T, Cooper J. Reelin-induced tyrosine [corrected] phosphorylation of disabled 1 during neuronal positioning. Genes & Development 1999;13(6) 643-651.

[103] Howell B, Herrick T, Hildebrand J, Zhang Y, Cooper J. Dab1 tyrosine phosphorylation sites relay positional signals during mouse brain development. Current Biology 2000;10(10) 877-962.

[104] Matsuki T, Zaka M, Guerreiro R, van der Brug MP, Cooper JA, Cookson MR, Hardy JA, Howell BW. Identification of Stk25 as a genetic modifier of Tau phosphorylation in Dab1-mutant mice. PLoS One 2012;7(2) e31152.

[105] Ohkubo N, Lee YD, Morishima A, Terashima T, Kikkawa S, Tohyama M, Sakanaka M, Tanaka J, Maeda N, Vitek MP, Mitsuda N. Apolipoprotein E and Reelin ligands modulate tau phosphorylation through an apolipoprotein E receptor/disabled-1/glycogen synthase kinase-3beta cascade. FASEB Journal 2003;17(2) 295-297.

[106] Brich J, Shie FS, Howell BW, Li R, Tus K, Wakeland EK, Jin LW, Mumby M, Churchill G, Herz J, Cooper JA. Genetic modulation of tau phosphorylation in the mouse. Journal of Neuroscience 2003;23(1) 187-192.

[107] Beffert U, Morfini G, Bock HH, Reyna H, Brady ST, Herz J. Reelin-mediated signaling locally regulates protein kinase B/Akt and glycogen synthase kinase 3beta. Journal of Biological Chemistry 2002;277(51) 49958-49964.

[108] Bock HH, Jossin Y, Liu P, Forster E, May P, Goffinet AM, Herz J. Phosphatidylinositol 3-kinase interacts with the adaptor protein Dab1 in response to Reelin signaling and is required for normal cortical lamination. Journal of Biological Chemistry 2003;278(40) 38772-38779.

[109] Patrick GN, Zukerberg L, Nikolic M, de la Monte S, Dikkes P, Tsai LH. Conversion of p35 to p25 deregulates Cdk5 activity and promotes neurodegeneration. Nature 1999;402(6762) 615-622.

[110] Beffert U, Weeber EJ, Morfini G, Ko J, Brady ST, Tsai LH, Sweatt JD, Herz J. Reelin and cyclin-dependent kinase 5-dependent signals cooperate in regulating neuronal migration and synaptic transmission. Journal of Neuroscience 2004;24(8) 1897-1906.

[111] Leemhuis J, Bouche E, Frotscher M, Henle F, Hein L, Herz J, Meyer DK, Pichler M, Roth G, Schwan C, Bock HH. Reelin signals through apolipoprotein E receptor 2 and Cdc42 to increase growth cone motility and filopodia formation. Journal of Neuroscience 2010;30(44) 14759-14772.

[112] Jimenez S, Torres M, Vizuete M, Sanchez-Varo R, Sanchez-Mejias E, Trujillo-Estrada L, Carmona-Cuenca I, Caballero C, Ruano D, Gutierrez A, Vitorica J. Age-dependent

accumulation of soluble amyloid beta (Abeta) oligomers reverses the neuroprotective effect of soluble amyloid precursor protein-alpha (sAPP(alpha)) by modulating phosphatidylinositol 3-kinase (PI3K)/Akt-GSK-3beta pathway in Alzheimer mouse model. Journal of Biological Chemistry 2011;286(21) 18414-18425.

Chapter 4

γ-Secretase — Regulated Signaling and Alzheimer's Disease

Kohzo Nakayama, Hisashi Nagase,
Chang-Sung Koh and Takeshi Ohkawara

Additional information is available at the end of the chapter

http://dx.doi.org/10.5772/54230

1. Introduction

Alzheimer's disease (AD) is an incurable and progressive neurodegenerative disorder and the most common form of dementia that occurs with aging. The main hallmarks of this disease are the extracellular deposition of amyloid plaques and the intracellular aggregation of tangles in the brain [1, 2]. Although the causes of both the onset and progression of AD are still uncertain, much evidence, including results of genetic analysis, indicates that amyloid precursor protein (APP) itself and its proteolytic processing are responsible for AD. Indeed, familial forms of AD (FAD) have mutations [3] or a duplication of the *APP* gene [4] or mutations in the presenilin1 or 2 (*PS1* or *PS2*) genes [5-7] that code for a catalytic component of the γ-secretase complex [8].

Although APP plays a central role in AD [1, 2], the physiological function of this membrane protein is not clear [9]. On the other hand, γ-secretase was first identified as a protease that cleaves APP within the transmembrane domain and produces amyloid-β (Aβ) peptides [10], which are the main constituent of amyloid plaques and are thought to be involved in AD pathogenesis. However, similar to the physiological functions of APP, those of γ-secretase are also still unclear [11, 12].

The signaling hypothesis suggests that the primary function of γ-secretase is to regulate signaling of type 1 membrane proteins (the amino terminus is extracellular, and the carboxy terminus is cytoplasmic); this was proposed by analogy of Notch signaling [13-15]. Notch is a family of evolutionarily conserved type 1 membrane proteins that mediate the fates of numerous cells in both invertebrates and vertebrates [16-18]. The molecular mechanism of the Notch signaling pathway is unique because it is controlled by proteolytic cleavage reactions [19, 20]. In the canonical Notch signaling pathway, ligands bind to the extracellular domain of Notch expressed on neighboring cells and trigger sequential proteolytic cleavage. Finally, the intracellular domain (ICD) of Notch (NICD) is released from the cell membrane by γ-secretase; NICD then translocates into the nucleus where it modulates gene expression through binding to transcription factors. Therefore, γ-secretase plays a central regulatory role in Notch signaling.

Recently, more than five dozen type 1 transmembrane proteins, including Notch and APP, have been reported as substrates for γ-secretase [21]. The ICDs of these proteins are also released from the cell membrane [13-15, 22]. Furthermore, it has been shown that some of these ICDs exist in the nucleus. These processes are very similar to those involved in Notch signaling. Thus, the common enzyme γ-secretase modulates the proteolysis and turnover of putative signaling molecules; this suggests that mechanisms similar to the Notch signaling pathway may widely contribute to γ-secretase–regulated signaling [13-15, 23]. Indeed, it has been shown that the ICD of APP (AICD), which is released from the cell membrane by γ-secretase, also translocates to the nucleus [24-26] and may function as a transcriptional regulator [27, 28]. These observations suggest the existence of APP signaling.

To test the hypothesis that APP has a signaling mechanism similar to that of Notch, we established embryonic carcinoma P19 cell lines that overexpressed AICD [29], which may mimic signaling mechanisms. Although neurons differentiated from these cell lines, AICD expression induced dynamic changes in gene expression profile and neuron-specific apoptosis [30]. These results suggest that APP also has a signaling mechanism, which may be closely related to AD.

In this chapter, we first summarize current research progress regarding Notch, APP, and γ-secretase. We also focus on the signaling hypothesis; γ-secretase–regulated mechanisms similar to Notch signaling may widely play roles in signaling events involving type 1 transmembrane proteins, including APP. Next, we review recent evidence supporting the existence of APP signaling. Furthermore, we discuss the possibility that APP signaling is involved in the onset and progression of AD.

2. γ-Secretase controls Notch signaling

Notch is a family of evolutionarily conserved type 1 membrane proteins with a mass of about 300 kDa [31] that mediates fates of numerous cells in both invertebrates and vertebrates [16, 17]. For example, cells expressing the major ligand Delta inhibit the neural differentiation of neighboring Notch-expressing cells during neurogenesis. Disruption of or disorder in Notch signaling leads to developmental defects or cancer in mammals [18].

While *Drosophila* has only one Notch gene, four Notch isoforms (Notch1 to 4) have been identified in mammals. The typical Notch protein contains 36 tandem epidermal growth factor (EGF)-like repeats in its extracellular domain, and six tandem ankyrin-like (CDC10) repeats, a nuclear localization signal, and a PEST sequence in its intracellular domain [31]. The 11th and 12th EGF-like repeats are essential for binding to its ligands [32]. Notch is cleaved in the trans-Golgi network, apparently by furin-like covertase, and is expressed on the cell surface as a heterodimer [33].

http://dx.doi.org/10.5772/54230

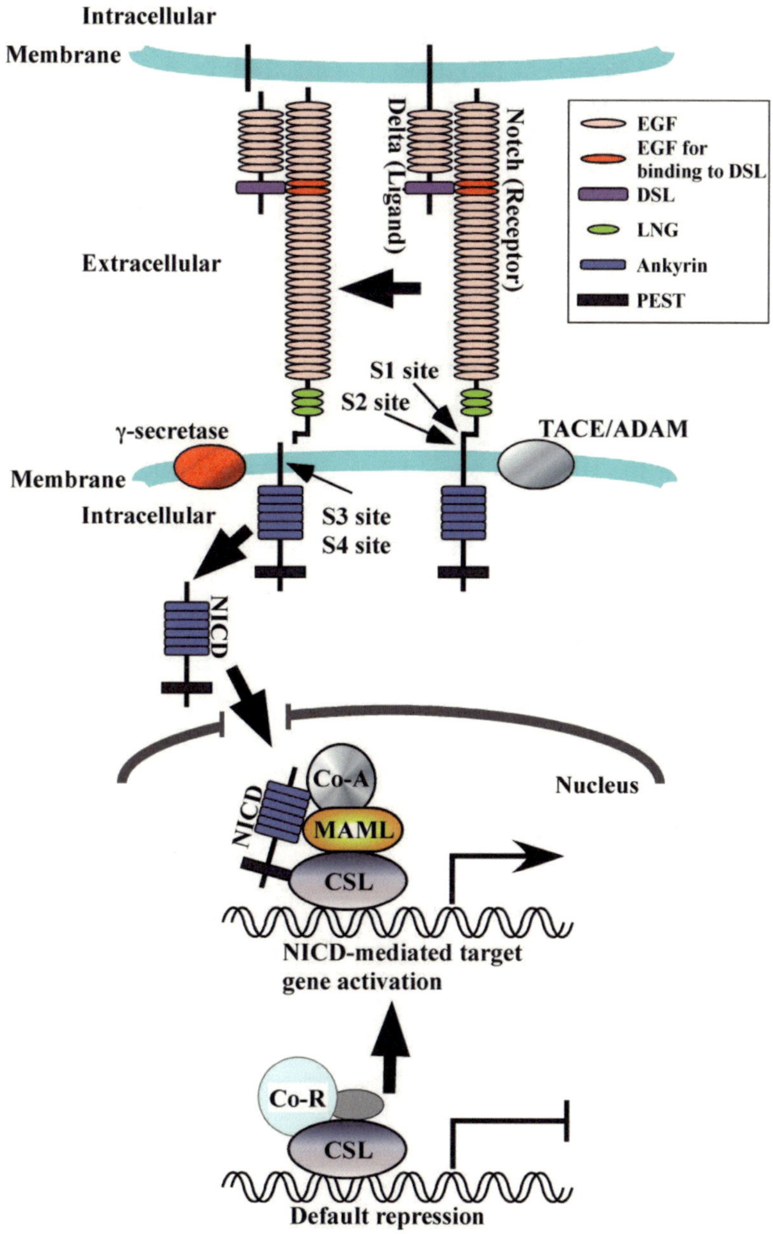

Figure 1. Notch signaling pathway. Notch proteins are expressed on the cell surface as heterodimers after cleavage at the S1 site by furin. The binding of Notch to the ligand triggers sequential proteolytic cleavage of the regulated intramembrane proteolysis (RIP). When Notch binds to the ligand, Notch is cleaved at the S2 site in the juxtamembrane region by TACE or ADAM protease. Next, the remaining protein stub is further cleaved by γ-secretase at the S3 and S4 sites within the transmembrane domain and NICD is released from the membrane. Then, NICD translocates into the nucleus and binds to the CSL together with MAML. The resultant CSL–NICD–MAML complex removes co-repressors (Co-R) from CSL transcription factor and recruits a co-activator (Co-A), resulting in conversion from repressor to activator. Finally, the complexes of CSL-NICD-MAML-Co-activators promote transcription of the target genes.

Drosophila has two different Notch ligands, Delta [34] and Serrate [35]. In mammals, two families of Notch ligands, Delta-like protein family (Dll1, 3, and 4) [36-38] and Jagged family (Jagged 1 and 2) [39, 40], have been identified. The extracellular domains of all these ligands also contain variable number of EGF-like repeats, e.g., *Drosophila* Delta has nine, while most vertebrate Deltas have eight, and *Caenorhabditis elegans* Lag-2 has two repeats. All these ligands share a single copy of a 2nd cysteine-rich conservative motif called the DSL (**D**elta: **S**errate: **L**ag-2) domain [41], which is essential for binding to Notch [42].

As shown in Fig.1, in the canonical Notch signaling pathway, ligands bind to the extracellular domain of Notch proteins on neighboring cells and trigger sequential proteolytic cleavage reactions; this is called the regulated intramembrane proteolysis (RIP) mechanism [43]. Precise steps of Notch processing are mentioned in section 4.2 of this chapter. In brief, first, Notch is cleaved within the juxtamembrane (JM) domain by metalloproteases to remove most of the extracellular region [44, 45]. Next, the remaining protein stub is further cleaved by γ-secretase within the transmembrane (TM) domain and NICD is released from the membrane [46-48]. The released NICD translocates to the nucleus and controls the expression of certain genes through binding to transcription factors. Thus, γ-secretase plays a central regulatory role in Notch signaling.

Members of the CSL transcription factor family (CBF1/RBP-jκ in mammals, Su(H) in *Drosophila*, and Lag-1 in *C. elegans*) are major downstream targets of Notch signaling [19]. NICD binds to CSL transcription factors, and six tandem ankyrin-like repeats in NICD are essential for binding to CSL transcription factors [49]. NICD also binds to Mastermind-like proteins (MAML family in mammals) [50], thus forming the CSL-NICD-MAML complex. The formation of these complexes results in removal of co-repressors from CSL and recruitment of co-activators, such as P/CAF and P300 [50, 51]. Through this process, the CSL complex is converted from a transcriptional repressor to an activator. Finally, these complexes bind to the *cis*-acting DNA sequences of target genes, such as Hes (Hairy/Enhancer of split in *Drosophila*), which encode the basic helix-loop-helix (bHLH) transcription factors, and promote their transcription [52].

3. Amyloid Precursor Protein (APP)

3.1. Overview of APP

APP was identified as a cDNA cloned using a partial amino acid sequence of the Aβ fragment isolated from the amyloid plaque of AD brains [53]. This cDNA coded for an evolutionarily conserved type 1 transmembrane protein. Fig. 2 shows schematic diagram of APP protein. Although APP is expressed in many tissues, this protein especially accumulates in the synapses of neurons. The human *APP* gene is about 240 kb in length containing at least 18 exons [54] and is localized on the long arm of chromosome 21 [53], an extra copy of which is present in patients with Down's syndrome (trisomy 21). Several alternative splicing isoforms of APP have been found, which differ mainly in the absence (APP-695, predominantly expressed in neurons) or presence (APP-751 and APP-770) of the Kunitz protease inhibitor (KPI) domain toward the N-terminus of the protein [55].

As described below, APP undergoes sequential proteolytic cleavage reactions to generate the extracellular fragment, intracellular fragment (AICD), and Aβ fragment that is located in the membrane-spanning region. Note that both the extracellular fragment and AICD are generated at the same time as Aβ. Extensive post-translational modifications of APP, such as glycosylation, phosphorylation, and tyrosine sulfation, have been observed.

Mammals have two other members of APP family called APP-like protein 1 (APLP1) and 2 (APLP2) [56]. APLP1 expression is restricted to neurons. On the other hand, expression of APLP2 is detected in many tissues, although it is highly enriched in the brain. These APP family proteins share conserved domains, such as the E1 and E2, in the extracellular region. The E1 domain contains several subdomains, such as a growth factor-like domain and a metal-binding motif [57]. The E2 domain has a coiled coil dimerization motif and may bind proteoglycans in the extracellular matrix [58].

Interestingly, the amino acid sequence of the Aβ fragment is not highly conserved and is unique to APP; on the other hand, the highest degree of sequence conservation is found in the ICD not only within the APP homologues [29] but also within the APP family [9]. This strong sequence conservation most likely reflects functional importance of the ICDs in the APP family proteins.

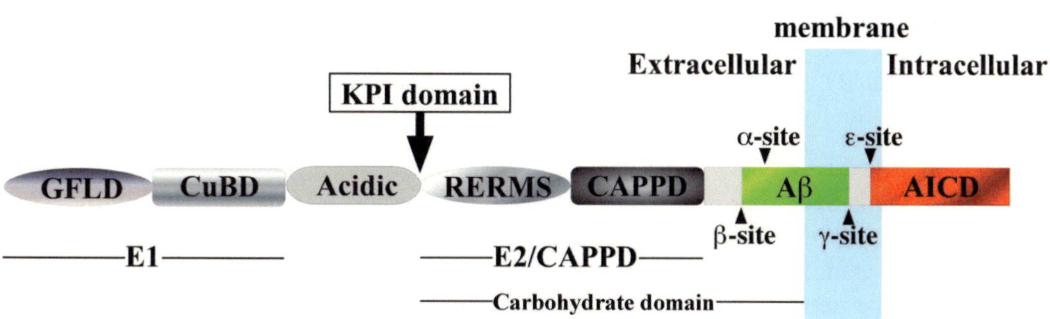

Figure 2. Schematic domain structure of APP. APP protein family shares the conserved E1 and E2 domains in their extracellular region. The E1 domain contains N-terminal growth factor-like domain (GFLD) and copper-binding domain (CuBD). The E1 domain is linked via acidic domain to the carbohydrate domain including E2 domain, which consists of RERMS sequence and central APP domain (CAPPD). E2 domain is followed by the Aβ region, and the intracellular domain (AICD) which is the most conserved region. Although the Kunitz protease inhibitor (KPI) domain is present at the indicated site in APP-751 and APP-770, APP-695 lacks this domain.

3.2. Proposed APP functions

Although the physiological functions of APP are not clear, several possibilities have been proposed. The most considerable functions are synapse formation and repair [59, 60]. Indeed, APP expression is upregulated after neural injury as well as during neuronal differentiation [59, 60]. After translation in the soma, APP is transported in an anterograde manner to the synaptic region, where the amount of APP is correlated with synaptogenesis. APP knockout mice show impaired long-term potentiation and declined memory without remarkable neuronal loss [61]. This evidence also supports this idea.

It has also been suggested that APP acts as a cell adhesion molecule and plays a role in cell–cell interaction. Indeed, the E1 and E2 domains can interact with extracellular matrix proteins and heparan sulfate proteoglycans [57, 58]. In addition, it has also been shown that extracellular domains of APP family proteins can interact with each other *in trans*. Therefore, APP family proteins may bind to each other in a homophilic or heterophilic manner to enhance cell–cell adhesion [62].

As APP may have a signaling mechanism, as described in detail below, the idea that APP is a cell-surface receptor is interesting. Indeed, several candidates of ligand for APP have been proposed. For example, F-spondin [63] and Nogo-66 [64] receptor bind to the extracellular domain of APP and regulate the production of Aβ. In addition, Aβ itself can also bind to the extracellular domain of APP [65].

3.3. Aβ amyloid

Aβ is the main constituent of an amyloid plaque, which is thought to be the hallmark and a major cause of AD pathogenesis in the brain. Thus, the amyloid hypothesis is generally accepted as the mechanism of the onset and progression of AD. The traditional amyloid hypothesis is that overproduced Aβ forms insoluble amyloid plaques, which are commonly observed in the AD brain and are believed to be the toxic form of APP and responsible for neurodegeneration [66].

As detailed in section 4.2., Aβ is generated after sequential cleavage of APP by β- and γ-secretases. Although these fragments range from 36 to 43 amino acid residues in length, Aβ40 and Aβ42 are the most common isoforms. Aβ40 is predominant over Aβ42, but Aβ42 is more amyloidogenic [67] and is, therefore, thought to be closely associated with AD. Furthermore, similar amyloid plaques are found in particular variants of Lewy body dementia [68] and in the muscle disease inclusion body myositis [69]. Aβ also forms aggregates that coat cerebral blood vessels in cerebral amyloid angiopathy (CAA), which is observed in over 90% of AD patients [70].

Deposition of Aβ in the AD brain is thought to be formed due to imbalances between the production of Aβ and its removal from the brain through various clearance mechanisms, including enzyme-mediated degradation [71]. Therefore, mechanisms of not only production but also degradation of Aβ have been studied extensively. As a result, several candidates for Aβ degradation enzymes are proposed. Neprilysin (NEP) and insulin-

http://dx.doi.org/10.5772/54230

degrading enzyme (IDE) are expressed in neurons as well as within the vasculature and the levels of both these enzymes are reduced in AD [71]; therefore, these enzymes have been well studied in relation to AD. Interestingly, it has been reported that *APOE* e4, which is the most-established genetic risk factor for the onset of AD and CAA, is associated with reduced levels of both enzymes [72, 73]. Furthermore, other candidates for Aβ degradation enzymes have been proposed, including endothelin-converting enzymes 1 and 2 (ECE-1 and ECE-2) [74] and angiotensin-converting enzyme (ACE) [75]. The levels of plasmin and plasminogen activators (uPA and tPA) and ECE-2 have also been shown to be reduced in the AD brain [71].

4. γ-Secretase

4.1. Overview of γ-secretase

γ-Secretase was first identified as a protease that cleaves APP within the TM domain and produces Aβ peptides [10], which is thought to be a major cause of the pathogenesis in the AD brain.

γ-Secretase is a complicated complex composed of PS, nicastrin (NCT), anterior pharynx defective-1 (Aph-1), and PS enhancer-2 protein (Pen-2) [8, 11, 12]. Two PS genes, *PS1* located on chromosome 14 [5] and *PS2* located on chromosome 1 [6, 7], have been identified by genetic linkage analyses as the genes responsible for early-onset FAD. The *PS1* and *PS2* genes encode proteins with eight or nine transmembrane domains of 467 and 448 amino acids, respectively, with about 65% sequence identity between the two proteins. Both proteins are the catalytic components of the γ-secretase complex. Although both PS1 and PS2 are expressed ubiquitously in the brain and peripheral tissues of adult mammals, PS1 expression level is significantly higher than that of PS2 [76]. NCT is a single-pass membrane protein and may recognize the substrate proteins of γ-secretase [77]. Indeed, the extracellular domain of NCT resembles an aminopeptidase, but lacks catalytic residues. Thus, this domain can interact with the free N-terminal of stubs of γ-secretase substrates generated by ectodomain shedding [78]; hence, shedding of γ-secretase substrates may be essential for the production of free N-termini of these proteins retained in the membrane to be recognized by NCT. Aph-1 may act as a scaffold during the process of γ-secretase complex assembly, and Pen-2 may act as a trigger for the proteolytic cleavage of PS in order to activate it [11, 12].

The physiological functions of γ-secretase have not been clarified. However, this protease can cleave a surprisingly large number of transmembrane proteins [79]. Indeed, more than five dozen proteins, most of which are type 1 membrane proteins, have been reported as γ-secretase substrates [21]. Interestingly, these substrates have a wide range of biological functions. Representative γ-secretase substrates are shown in Table 1.

Substrate	Function	PS or ICD function
ApoER2	Lipoprotein receptor, neuronal migration	Activates nuclear reporter
APP	Precursor to Aβ, adhesion, trophic properties, axonal transport?	Ab generation, release of ICD, Complex with Fe65/Tip60, Cell death?
APLP1/2	Cell adhesion?	Forms complex with Fe65 and Tip60
β-Catenin	Transduce Wnt signals stabilize adherens junctions	Facilitates phosphorylation
CD43	Signal transduction	Signaling molecule?
CD44	Cell adhesion	Activates TRE-mediated nuclear transcription
CSF1-R	Protein tyrosine kinase	Unknown
CXCL16 & CX3CL1	Membrane chemokine ligands	Unknown
DCC	Axon guidance, tumor suppressor	Activates nuclear reporter
Delta	Notch ligand	Transcriptional regulation
E-cadherin	Cell adhesion	Promotes disassembly of adhesion complex
ERBB4	Receptor tyrosine kinase	Regulates heregulin-induced growth inhibition
HLA-A2	MHC class I molecule	Unknown
IFN-αR2	Subunit of type I IFN-α receptor	Transcriptional regulation
Insulin receptor	Receptor tyrosine kinase	Accumulates in nucleus
IGIF-R	Receptor tyrosine kinase	Unknown
IL-1RI	Cytokine receptor	Unknown
IL-1RII	Cytokine receptor	Unknown
Jagged	Notch ligand	Modulates AP-1-mediated transcription
LAR	Receptor tyrosine phosphatase	Accumulates in nucleus
LDLR	Lipoprotein receptor	Unknown
LRP	Scavenger and signaling receptor	Activates nuclear reporter
Na channel β-subunit	Cell adhesion, an auxiliary subunit of voltage-gated Na channel	Alters cell adhesion and migration
N-cadherin	Cell adhesion	Promotes CBP degradation
Nectin-1α	Adherens junction, synapse receptor	Remodeling of cell junctions?
Notch1-4	Signaling receptor	Transcriptional regulation
NRADD	Apoptosis in neuronal cells	Modulates glycosylation/maturation of NRADD
P75NTR	Neurotrophin co-receptor, dependence receptor	Modulates p75-TrkA complex? Nuclear signaling?
γ-Protocadherin	Cell adhesion, neuronal differentiation	Regulation of gene transcription?
Syndecan-3	Cell surface proteoglycan co-receptor	Regulation of membrane-targeting of CASK
Telencephalin	Cell adhesion	Turnover of telencephalin
Tyrosinase,Tyrosinase-related protein 1/2	Pigment synthesis	Intracellular transport of Post-Golgi Tyr-containing vesicles
Vasorin	TGF-β inhibitor	Unknown

Table 1. Substrates for γ-secretase

4.2. Some γ-secretase substrates share a common proteolytic process

Fig.3 shows the proteolytic processes of Notch, APP, and CD44. There are surprising similarities between these processes and all of these processes follow the RIP mechanism. For example, in the canonical Notch signaling pathway, ligands bind to the extracellular domain of Notch on neighboring cells and trigger sequential proteolytic cleavage reactions (the RIP mechanism) and shedding at the S2 site by TACE or ADAM protease making the truncated Notch [44, 45]. Truncated Notch is further cleaved by γ-secretase in at least two sites within the TM domain [46-48], i.e., at the S3 site to release NICD and at the S4 site to release the remaining small peptide (Nβ). As mentioned above, NICD, which is released from the cell membrane to the cytoplasm by γ-secretase, translocates to the nucleus where its activity is expressed through binding to transcription factors.

The proteolytic process of APP is very similar to that of Notch and also follows the RIP mechanism. Cleavage of APP by α- secretase [80] or β-secretase [81] at the α- or β-site, respectively, within the JM region results in shedding of almost the entire extracellular domain and generates membrane-tethered α- or β-carboxy terminal fragments (CTFs). Several zinc metalloproteinases, such as TACE and ADAM [82, 83], and the aspartyl protease BACE2 [84] can cleave APP at the α-site, while BACE1 (β-site APP cleaving enzyme) cleaves APP at the β-site [81]. Once the extracellular domain has been shed, the remaining stub is further cleaved at least twice by γ-secretase within the TM domain at γ- and ε-sites resulting in production of either non-amyloidogenic p3 peptide (in combination with α-secretase) or amyloidogenic Aβ (in combination with BACE1), respectively, and AICD [11, 12]. As discussed in the next paragraph, although a large proportion of AICD is rapidly degraded in the cytoplasm, a small amount of the remaining AICD may translocate to the nucleus.

It has been reported that several other type 1 membrane proteins also follow the RIP mechanism and their ICDs are released from the cell membrane [13, 14, 22]. For example, as shown in Fig.3, the process of sequential proteolytic cleavage of CD44, which is important for immune system function, is very similar to those of Notch and APP [22]. In addition, the ICD of this protein (CD44ICD) also translocates to the nucleus (Fig.3).

As discussed here, several γ-secretase substrates follow the RIP mechanism. The ICDs of these substrates are released from the cell membrane by γ-secretase, and these ICDs translocate to the nucleus. These processes are very similar to those involved in Notch signaling. Therefore, the observations that the common enzyme, γ-secretase, modulates proteolysis and the turnover of possible signaling molecules led to the attractive idea, the signaling hypothesis, which suggests that mechanisms similar to those occurring in the Notch signaling pathway may contribute widely to γ-secretase–regulated signaling mechanisms.

Actually, Dll1, a major ligand of Notch, is cleaved sequentially by metalloproteases and γ-secretase, and ICD of Dll1 (Dll1IC) is released from the cell membrane and then translocates to the nucleus [85, 86]. Furthermore, we have shown that Dll1IC then binds to Smad 2 and 3, which are transcription factors involved in the TGF-β/activin signaling pathway, and may alter transcription of specific genes that are involved in neuronal differentiation [87]. These results suggest that Dll1 also has a signaling mechanism similar to that of Notch.

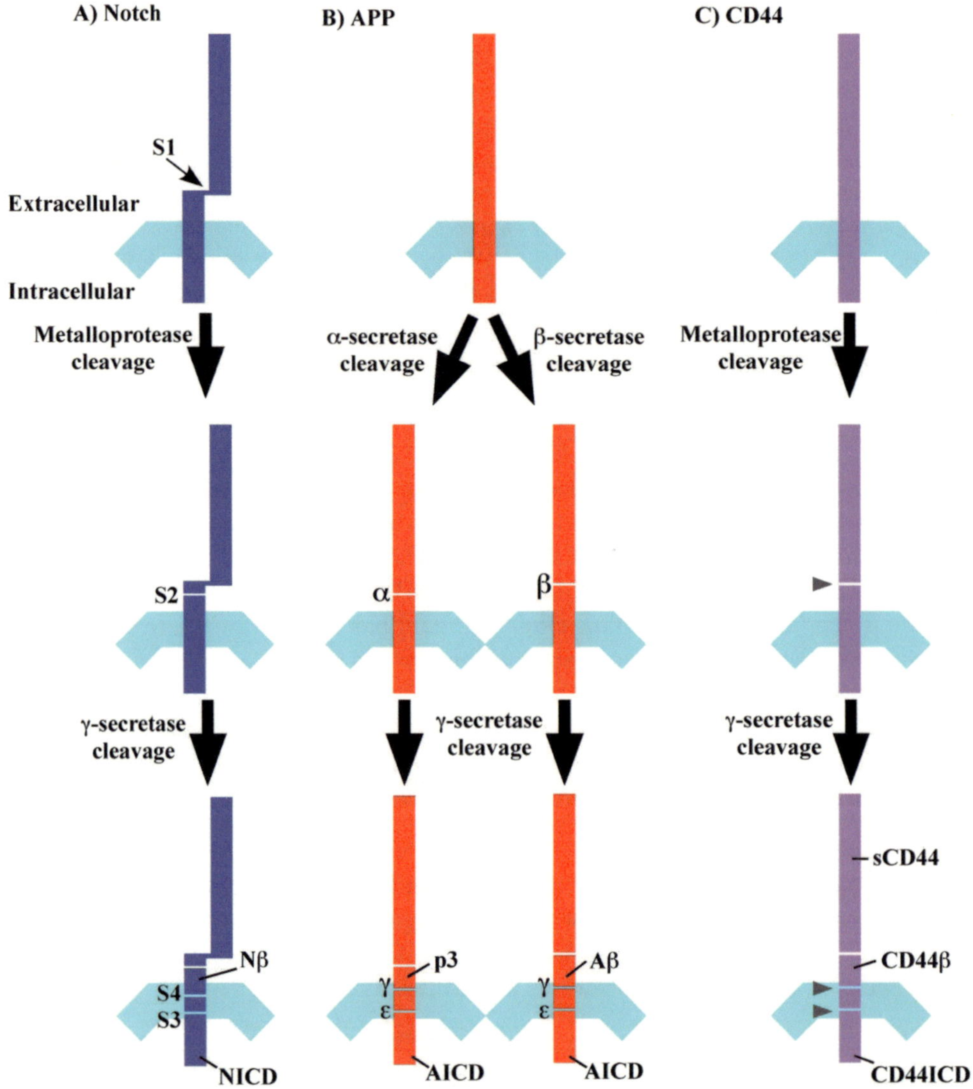

Figure 3. Similarities in the proteolytic processes among Notch, APP, and CD44. (A) In response to ligand binding, Notch undergoes shedding due to metalloprotease cleavage at the S2 site within the juxtamembrane domain. After shedding the extracellular domain, the remaining Notch stub is further cleaved by γ-secretase at S3 and S4 sites within the transmembrane domain. This sequential proteolysis produces NICD and Nβ fragment. (B) Cleavage of APP by α-secretase or β-secretase at the α-site or β-site, respectively, within the juxtamembrane domain results in shedding of almost the entire extracellular domain and generates membrane-tethered α- or β-carboxy terminal fragments (CTFs). Several zinc metalloproteinases and BACE2 can cleave APP at the α-site, while BACE1 cleaves APP at the β-site. After shedding the extracellular domain, the remaining stub is further cleaved at least twice within the transmembrane domain at γ- and ε-sites by γ-secretase, producing either p3 peptide (in combination with α-secretase) or Aβ (in combination with BACE1), respectively, and AICD. (C) Several stimuli, such as PKC activation and Ca^{2+} influx, trigger ectodomain cleavage of CD44 by a metalloprotease at the site within the juxtamembrane domain, resulting in the secretion of soluble CD44 (sCD44). After shedding the extracellular domain, the remaining CD44 stub is further cleaved by γ-secretase at two sites within the transmembrane domain. This sequential proteolysis produces the CD44ICD and CD44β, an Aβ-like peptide.

4.3. Is γ-secretase a proteasome of the membrane?

As mentioned above, more than five dozen γ-secretase substrates, most of which are type 1 membrane proteins, have been reported. This raises the simple question against the signaling hypothesis, why so many membrane proteins can transmit signals to the nucleus. In reply to this question, another possibility that γ-secretase acts as a proteasome of the membrane has been proposed [11, 12]. Indeed, as the ICDs of these substrates including AICD, which are released by γ-secretase, are rapidly degraded [24, 88], it is usually difficult to detect their ICDs by western blotting. Furthermore, ectodomain shedding seems to be constitutive for some substrates, and ligand binding has been reported to enhance only cleavage of Notch [47], Delta [87], Syndecan-3 [89], and ERBB4 [90]. In addition, much evidence supporting the signaling hypothesis was obtained in overexpression assays that differ somewhat from normal physiological conditions. Based on these observations, the proteasome hypothesis suggesting that the primary function of γ-secretase is to facilitate the selective disposal of type 1 membrane proteins has been proposed [11, 12].

Although the proteasome hypothesis for γ-secretase is reasonable and potent, there is no doubt that the certain signaling mechanisms regulated by γ-secretase, such as Notch signaling, exist. Therefore, it is likely that different functions of γ-secretases reflect their variant complexes in different combinations with multiple components, such as Aph-1, Pen2, and/or PS isoforms, with different cellular functions, such as roles in signaling or degradation.

In addition, it seems that a small proportion of ICDs of these substrates that are released by γ-secretase are sufficient for signaling mechanisms. Generally, γ-secretase substrates like APP are considerably more abundant than transcription factors, which are usually rare molecules. Although a large proportion of ICDs of these substrates are rapidly degraded, a small amount of the remaining ICDs may be sufficient for their signaling functions with small quantities of transcription factors. Thus, the majority of ICDs of these substrates may be degraded, and only a small proportion may play roles in signaling.

In relation to this issue, an attractive idea has been proposed in which a certain stimulus controls APP signaling through phosphorylation and dephosphorylation of AICD. Since AICD is stabilized [91] and translocated into the nucleus by Fe65 [26], it is thought that Fe65 is essential for the signaling function of AICD. Non-phosphorylated AICD can bind to Fe65 and form a complex; thus, this complex is stabilized and immediately translocates to the nucleus, where it mediates the expression of target genes in association with Tip60. On the other hand, phosphorylated AICD cannot bind to Fe65. Therefore, phosphorylated AICD without Fe65 cannot translocate to the nucleus. Phosphorylated AICD that remains in the cytosol is rapidly degraded by degradation enzymes such as the proteasome and/or IDE. Indeed, it has been reported that phosphorylation at Thr^{668} in the APP-695 isoform strongly inhibited binding to Fe65 [92, 93].

5. The role of AICD

5.1. Signaling functions of AICD

As mentioned above, the observations that the common enzyme, γ-secretase, modulates proteolysis and the turnover of possible signaling molecules led to the signaling hypothesis. This suggests that mechanisms similar to the Notch signaling pathway may contribute widely to γ-secretase–regulated signaling mechanisms, including APP signaling. If APP signaling exists, it may be closely related to AD.

Actually, there is accumulating evidence for the existence of APP signaling and its contribution to the onset and progression of AD. As mentioned above, the highest degree of sequence conservation within the APP homologues is found in the ICD [9, 29]. This sequence conservation suggests the functional importance of AICD, which may reflect the existence of APP signaling. In addition, several AICD-interacting proteins, which may regulate AICD stability, cellular localization, and transcriptional activity, have been identified. Based on this, several models of APP signaling have also been proposed. As mentioned above, it has been suggested that AICD recruits Fe65 proteins and translocates into the nucleus where the AICD-Fe65-Tip60 ternary complex may control transcription of target genes [27]. Furthermore, *NEP* gene expression requires binding of the AICD to its promoter [94].

Transgenic mice overexpressing both AICD and Fe65 showed abnormal activity of glycogen synthase kinase 3 beta (Gsk3b protein) [95], leading to hyperphosphorylation and aggregation of tau. This results in microtubule destabilization and the reduction of nuclear β-catenin levels causing a loss of cell-cell contact that may contribute to neurotoxicity in AD. Subsequent neurodegeneration and working memory deficits were also observed in these transgenic mice [96]. In other experiments, similar transgenic mice exhibited abnormal spiking events in their electroencephalograms and susceptibility to kainic acid-induced seizures independent of Aβ [97]. Furthermore, the function of c-Abl kinase in the transcriptional regulation of AICD was reported and c-Abl was shown to modulate AICD-dependent cellular responses, transcriptional induction, as well as apoptotic responses [98]. Interestingly, elevated AICD levels have also been reported in AD brains [96]. In addition, AICD was detected in the nucleus in injured brains [99]. Taken together, it is likely that APP signaling changes the expression of certain genes, which may cause AD pathology.

To explore APP signaling, we established several AICD-overexpressing embryonic carcinoma P19 cell lines [29]. Undifferentiated AICD-overexpressing cells retained epithelial cell-like morphology and healthy as well as control cells. Although neurons were differentiated from these cell lines after aggregation culture with all-*trans*-retinoic acid (RA) treatment, AICD expression induced neuron-specific cell death. Indeed, as shown in Fig.4, while neurons from control cells that carried the vector alone were healthy, almost all neurons differentiated from AICD-overexpressing P19 cells showed severe degeneration, becoming spherical with numerous vacuoles and detaching from the culture dishes 4 days after the induction of differentiation.

Since DNA fragmentation was detected, these cells died by apoptosis. In addition, all terminal deoxynucleotidyl transferase (TdT)-mediated deoxyuridine triphosphate (dUTP)-biotin nick end-labeling (TUNEL)-positive cells were also Tuj1-positive neurons. Taken together, we concluded that AICD could induce neuron-specific apoptosis [29]. The effects of AICD were restricted to neurons, with no effects observed in non-neural cells.

Thus, although further studies are required, these results strongly suggest that AICD plays a role in APP signaling and induces neuronal cell death, which may closely relate to the onset and progression of AD.

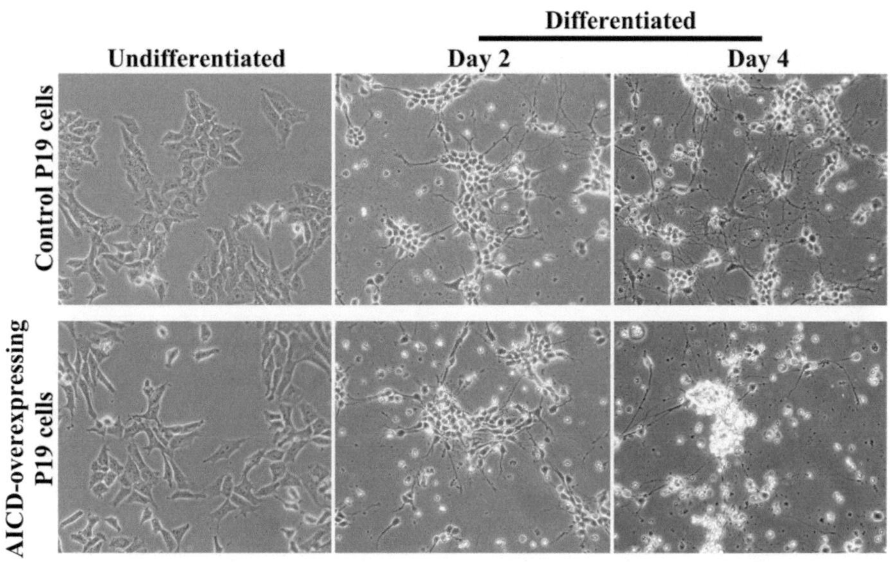

Figure 4. Expression of AICD in P19 cells induced neuronal cell death. After aggregation culture with RA, AICD-expressing P19 and control P19 cells carrying vector alone were replated and cultured for the indicated periods on dishes and allowed to differentiate. Undifferentiated AICD-expressing P19 cells retained epithelial cell-like morphology similar to control cells, while the differentiated cells became round and showed a bipolar morphology with neurite extension. Two days after replating (Day 2), all cell lines grew well and neurons with long neurites appeared. Four days after replating (Day 4), control cells still grew well as clusters and many neurons had differentiated from these cells. However, many AICD-expressing P19 cells showed severe degeneration, becoming spherical with numerous vacuoles and detached from the culture dishes.

5.2. AICD changes the gene expression profile

If APP signaling exists, AICD should change the expression of certain genes. To examine this possibility and identify the genes involved in this neuron-specific apoptosis, we performed DNA microarray analyses to evaluate the changes in the expression of more than 20,000 independent genes induced by AICD through the process of neuron-specific apoptosis [30]. Gene expression levels were deduced by hybridization signal intensity on the DNA microarrays, and the data from AICD-overexpressing cells were compared to data from control cells at the same 3 points during culture: 1) the undifferentiated state; 2) after 4 days of aggregation with RA (aggregated state); and 3) 2 days after replating (differentiated state). According to our expectations, AICD was shown to alter the expression of a great many genes; in the presence of AICD, the expression levels of 277 genes were upregulated by more than 10-fold, while those of 341 genes were downregulated to less than 10% of the original level [30].

Gene Symbol	Gene Name	Function	Relative Expression Levels (fold)		
			Undifferentiated	Aggregated	Differentiated
Non-regulated genes (housekeeping genes)					
Actb	β-actin	cytoskeleton protein	-1.2	1.2	1
Sdha	succinate dehydrogenase subunit A	electron transporter in the TCA cycle and respiratory chain	-1.1	-1.6	-1.2
Eef1a1	eukaryotic translation elongation factor-1 alpha 1	essential component for the elongation phase during protein translation	1	-1.1	1.2
Upregulated genes					
Ptprt	protein tyrosine phosphatase receptor T	protein tyrosine phosphatase that regulates STAT3 activity	906	204	116
Cpb1	carboxypeptidase B1	hydrolysis of C-terminal end of basic amino acid peptide bond	16	296	222
Nr2e1	tailless homolog	transcription factor that is essential for neural stem cell proliferation and self-renewal	5.8	244	54
Myh1	myosin heavy chain 1	one of the components of the motor protein myosin	-4.2	259	-1.1
Dnahc7c	axonemal dynein heavy chain	essential for motility of cilia and flagellae	133	41	43
Alkbh3	alkylation repair homolog 3	AlkB enzyme that repairs methylation damage in DNA and RNA	69	80	43
Ctgf	connective tissue growth factor	skeletogenesis/vasculogenesis by modulating BMP, Wnt, and IGF-I signals	90	54	40
Downregulated genes					
Hes5	hairy and enhancer of split 5	transcription factor that inhibits neurogenesis	-8.7	-3039	-2515
Slc10a6	sodium-dependent organic anion transporter	transport of sulfoconjugated steroid hormones and bile acids	-145	-785	-1212
Nid1	nidogen-1	extracellular matrix linker protein	-304	-165	-507
LOC213332	analog of Na^+-dependent glucose transporter 1	putative glucose transporter	-232	-325	-306
Dtx1	Deltex1	regulator of Notch signaling pathway	-30	-85	-691
Rbp4	retinol-binding protein 4	retinol transporter from the liver to extrahepatic tissues	-525	-100	-24
Col3a1	collagen type III alpha 1	extracellular matrix protein	4.1	-29	-234

Relative expression levels (fold) were estimated from the intensities of hybridization signals. Housekeeping gene expression was unaltered in AICD-overexpressing P19 and control P19 cells in all states, suggesting that these genes are not affected by AICD. These results also indicated that the observed differences in expression were not due to technical problems, such as uneven hybridization or poor RNA quality.

Table 2. Expression levels of 7 upregulated and 7 downregulated genes, as well as 3 housekeeping genes

http://dx.doi.org/10.5772/54230

AICD strongly induced expression of several genes, representative examples of which are listed in Table 2. For example, AICD-overexpressing P19 cells showed strong expression of the protein tyrosine phosphatase receptor T (*Ptprt*) gene at all sampling points: 906-fold, 204-fold, and 116-fold upregulation, in undifferentiated, aggregated, and differentiated states, respectively, compared with control cells. In contrast to these upregulated genes, the expression of several genes was strongly inhibited by AICD. Although *Hes5* expression was markedly increased through the process of neural differentiation, with an increase of almost 300-fold in control cells, AICD inhibited this induction. As shown in Fig.5, these results were confirmed by RT-PCR. Thus, AICD may induce both upregulation and downregulation of certain genes, suggesting that AICD plays an important role in APP signaling.

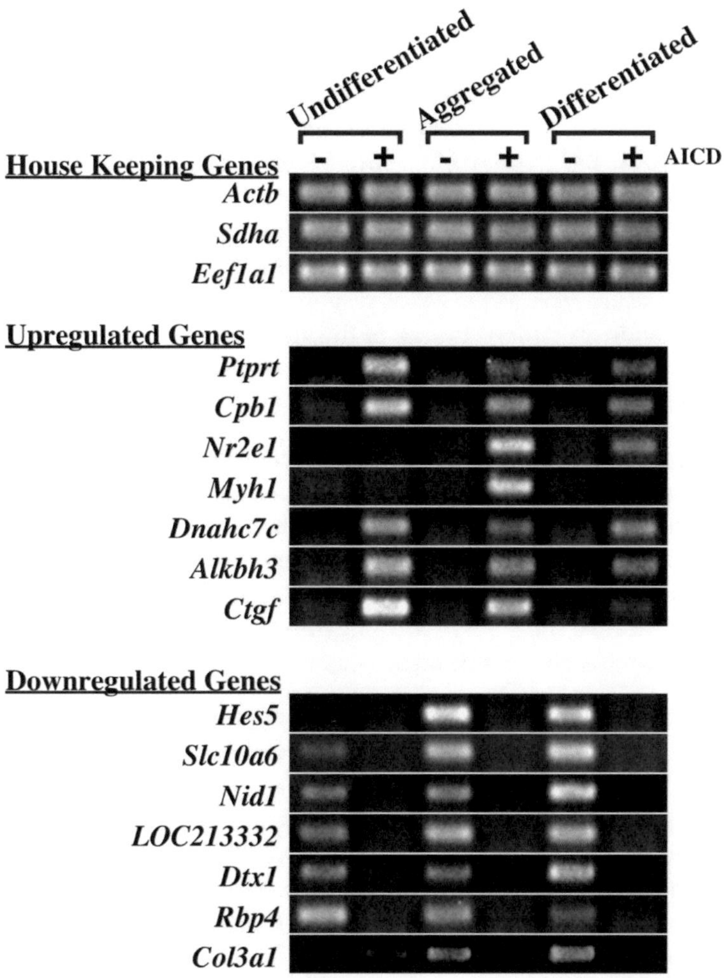

Figure 5. RT-PCR analysis of representative 7 upregulated genes and 7 downregulated genes, as well as 3 housekeeping genes, in P19 cells overexpressing AICD. The RNA samples same as applied to DNA microarray analysis was used in this RT-PCR analysis.

We performed Gene Ontology (GO) analysis and classified these upregulated and downregulated genes according to the GO terms [30]; however, we did not find genes that were significantly related to cell death among those with altered expression. Furthermore, we evaluated AICD-induced changes in the expression of genes thought to be involved in cell death in AD [30]; however, we found no significant changes in expression of these genes. Thus, it is likely that AICD does not directly induce the expression of genes involved in cell death, but the extreme dynamic changes in gene expression disrupt the homeostasis of certain neurons and thus give rise to neuron-specific cell death. Taken together, these results strongly suggest the existence of APP signaling.

6. Can Aβ clarify all aspects of the onset and progression of AD?

Autosomal dominant mutations in and around the Aβ region of the *APP* gene, which accelerate proteolytic processing, are responsible for hereditary early-onset AD [3]. The human *APP* gene is located on the long arm of chromosome 21 [53], an extra copy of which is present in individuals with Down's syndrome (trisomy 21). Patients with Down's syndrome develop AD by 40 years of age, most likely due to this gene dosage effect [4]. In addition, both PS1 and PS2, which are catalytic components of the γ-secretase complex, were identified by genetic linkage analyses as the genes responsible for FAD [5-7]. In many cases, familial diseases can provide an understanding of the sporadic ones. Therefore, both APP itself and its proteolytic processing may be responsible for the onset and progression of not only FAD but also sporadic AD.

As mentioned above, Aβ is the main constituent of amyloid plaque, which is thought to play a major role in the pathogenesis of AD; its presence is a hallmark of the AD brain. Thus, the amyloid hypothesis is generally accepted as the mechanism of the onset and progression of AD. Although an alternative hypothesis has also been proposed, which suggests that soluble Aβ oligomers rather than insoluble amyloid plaques are responsible for the onset and progression of AD because the soluble form of the Aβ oligomer is toxic for neurons [100, 101], Aβ still plays a central role in this idea.

However, several doubts have recently been raised regarding the amyloid hypothesis that Aβ plays a central role in the onset and progression of AD. One of the most critical arguments against this hypothesis is the presence of high levels of Aβ deposition in many nondemented elderly people [102], suggesting that Aβ amyloid plaques are not toxic. Indeed, transgenic mice overproducing Aβ show amyloid deposition mimicking that seen in the AD brain but do not show neurodegeneration [61]. Furthermore, several anti-Aβ drugs and vaccines have failed to show efficacy in phase III clinical trials [103]. Surprisingly, long-term follow-up studies showed unexpected problems [104]. Immunization of AD patients with the anti-Aβ vaccine, AN-1792, cleared Aβ amyloid plaques. Actually, patients with high titers of antibody against Aβ showed virtually complete plaque removal. However, there was no evidence of improvement in survival and/or cognitive function, even in patients with high titers of anti-Aβ antibody [104]. Although several interpretation for this lack of improvement have been proposed, these results lead to the idea that both soluble and insoluble forms of Aβ may not be involved in the onset and progression of AD.

Based on these observations, it has been suggested that AD may be caused by an APP-derived fragment, just not necessarily Aβ [105]. As both extracellular fragments and AICD are generated at the same time as Aβ, acceleration of proteolytic processing leads to overproduction of not only Aβ but also of both the extracellular fragments and AICD. Therefore, it is likely that the extracellular fragments and/or AICD are responsible for the onset and progression of AD. Indeed, AICD has been shown to induce neuron-specific apoptosis, which leads to AD pathology, as mentioned above.

In addition, it has also been proposed that APP is a ligand of Death receptor 6 (DR6) [106], which mediates cell death and is expressed at high levels in the human brain regions most affected by AD. APP is cleaved by β-secretase, releasing the extracellular domain (sAPPβ), which is further cleaved by an as yet unknown mechanism to release a 35 kDa N-terminal fragment (N-APP). This N-APP fragment binds DR6 to trigger neurodegeneration through caspase 6 in axons and caspase 3 in cell bodies [106]. These results suggest that N-APP may also be involved in the onset and progression of AD.

7. The model of APP signaling

Through this chapter, we discussed the possibility of the existence of APP signaling. It is likely that disorders of this signaling mechanism are involved in the onset and progression of AD. As AICD is generated at the same time as Aβ, acceleration of proteolytic processing leads to overproduction of not only Aβ but also AICD in AD brain as discussed above. Furthermore, we showed that AICD alters the expression of certain genes and induces neuron-specific apoptosis [29, 30].

If the APP signaling hypothesis is correct, certain molecules involved in APP signaling may be attractive candidates for the targets of drug discovery for treating AD. Fig.6 is a schematic model of APP signaling. As mentioned above, after cleavage within the JM domain by α- or β-secretase, AICD is released from the membrane by γ-secretase. Inhibiters for these proteases are being studied extensively.

As mentioned in section 4.3, non-phosphorylated AICD can bind to the nuclear adaptor protein Fe65 [92, 93], which is essential for translocation of AICD to the nucleus. However, phosphorylated AICD cannot bind to Fe65. These results suggest the possibility that a certain stimulus controls APP signaling through phosphorylation and dephosphorylation of AICD. It has also been shown that the majority of cell membrane-associated APP is phosphorylated specifically at Thr^{668} in neurons [107]. Therefore, phosphorylated AICD, which is released from the cell membrane to the cytoplasm by γ-secretase, cannot bind to Fe65 and thus cannot translocate to the nucleus. Phosphorylated AICD left in the cytosol is rapidly degraded, probably by the proteasome and/or IDE [88]. However, if AICD is dephosphorylated by certain phosphatase, AICD can binds to Fe65. Thus, AICD/Fe65 complexes may immediately translocate to the nucleus, where they mediate expressions of certain target genes in association with histone acetyltransferase Tip60 [27]. Besides dephosphorylation of AICD, if phosphorylation of membrane-associated APP is inhibited, non-phosphorylated AICD may also increase. Therefore, it is likely that non-phosphorylated AICD is involved in the onset and progression of AD.

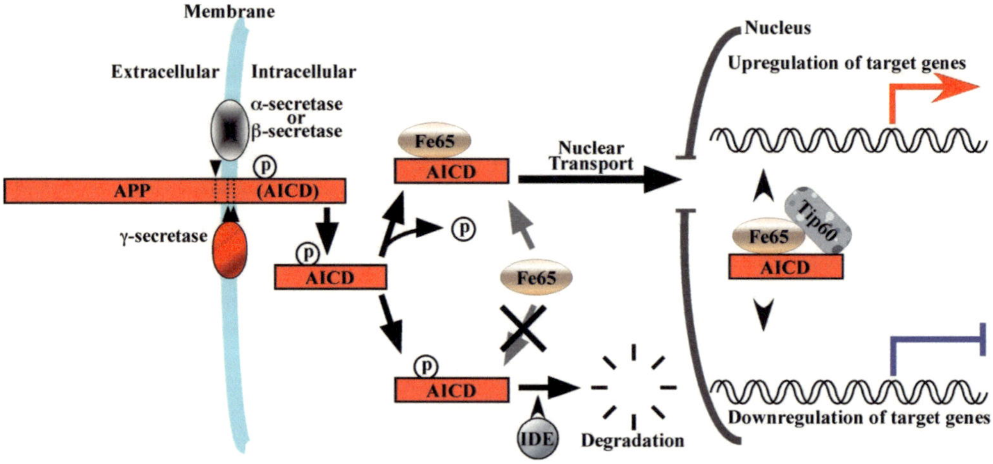

Figure 6. Model of APP signaling pathway. The majority of cell membrane-associated APP is phosphorylated within its ICD in neurons. After cleavage of JM domain by α- or β-secretase, AICD is released from the membrane by γ-secretase. Phosphorylated AICD cannot bind to the nuclear adaptor protein Fe65, which is thought to be essential for translocation of AICD to the nucleus, and thus cannot translocate to the nucleus. Phosphorylated AICD left in the cytosol is rapidly degraded, probably by the proteasome and/or insulin-degrading enzyme (IDE). On the other hand, dephosphorylated AICD binds to Fe65. Therefore, dephosphorylated AICD/Fe65 complexes immediately translocate to the nucleus, where they meidate up- and downregulation of certain target genes in association with Tip60.

In addition to these possibilities, it is also likely that AICD is ineffective in the normal brain, because almost all AICD is degraded rapidly, and APP signaling cannot be transmitted. However, both AICD and Aβ are overproduced in the AD brain compared to normal brain. Thus, although the majority of AICD is degraded, a small amount of the remaining AICD may play a role in signaling and cause neuron-specific cell death in the AD brain. In addition, if the degrading activity of AICD is reduced or lost in the AD brain, APP signaling, which leads to neuron-specific cell death, may be enhanced. Thus, compounds that inhibit translocation of AICD to the nucleus will be good candidates for AD therapy. From this point of view, protein phosphatase inhibitors and chemicals that impair the interaction between AICD and Fe65 may be potential ones.

8. Conclusion

γ-Secretase was first identified as a protease that cleaves APP within the transmembrane domain and produces Aβ peptides, which are the main hallmark of AD and are thought to be involved in the pathogenesis in the AD brains. However, the physiological functions of this protease remain to be clarified.

The signaling hypothesis for γ-secretase suggesting that its primary function is to regulate the signaling of type 1 membrane proteins was proposed by analogy of Notch signaling. In the canonical Notch signaling pathway, ligands bind to the extracellular domain of Notch expressed on neighboring cells, and trigger sequential proteolytic cleavage. Finally, NICD is released from the cell membrane by γ-secretase and translocates into the nucleus where it modulates gene expression through binding to transcription factors. Thus, γ-secretase plays a central regulatory role in Notch signaling.

While APP is thought to play central roles in the onset and progression of AD, the physiological functions of this protein also have not yet been fully elucidated. However, it has been shown that AICD, which is released from the cell membrane by γ-secretase, also translocates to the nucleus and may function as a transcriptional regulator. These observations suggest the existence of a signaling mechanism similar to that of Notch.

In this chapter, we focused on the signaling aspects of APP and its pathological roles in AD. Indeed, we showed that AICD alters gene expression and induces neuron-specific apoptosis. Thus, it is likely that APP has a signaling mechanism similar to that of Notch and that APP signaling is at least partially responsible for the onset and progression of AD. If the APP signaling hypothesis is correct, several molecules involved in APP signaling may be attractive candidates for the targets of drug discovery for treating AD. Thus, extensive studies about this issue are expected.

Abbreviations

AD, Alzheimer's disease;

Aβ, amyloid-β;

APP, amyloid precursor protein;

AICD, the intracellular domain of APP;

Aph-1, anterior pharynx defective-1;

CAA, cerebral amyloid angiopathy;

Dll, Delta-like protein

Dll1IC, the intracellular domain of Dll1;

EGF, epidermal growth factor;

FAD, familial AD;

Hes, Hairy/Enhancer of split;

ICD, intracellular domain;

IDE, insulin-degrading enzyme;

JM, juxtamembrane;

KPI, Kunitz inhibitor domain;

NICD, the intracellular domain of Notch;

NCT, nicastrin;

NEP, neprilysin;

PS, presenilin;

Pen-2, PS enhancer-2 protein;

RIP, regulated intramembrane proteolysis;

RA, all-trans-retinoic acid;

TM, transmembrane;

Acknowledgments

Our works described here were supported by the grants-in-aid from the Ministry of Education, Culture, Sports, Science, and Technology of Japan. Some parts of this manuscript have been taken from our publications in Cellular and Molecular Neurobiology Volume 31, Number 6, 887-900 (2011) and in Current Psychopharmacology, Volume 1, Number 2, 155-166 (2012).

Author details

Kohzo Nakayama[1,4*], Hisashi Nagase[2], Chang-Sung Koh[3] and Takeshi Ohkawara[1]

*Address all correspondence to: kohzona@shinshu-u.ac.jp

1 Department of Anatomy, Shinshu University, School of Medicine, Matsumoto, Nagano, Japan

2 Department of Immunology and Infectious Diseases, Shinshu University, School of Medicine, Japan

3 Department of Biomedical Sciences, Shinshu University, School of Health Sciences, Matsumoto, Nagano, Japan

4 Department of Developmental and Regenerative Medicine, Mie University, Graduate School of Medicine, Tsu, Mie, Japan

References

[1] Hardy J. Amyloid, the presenilins and Alzheimer's disease. Trends Neurosci. 1997;20:154-9.

[2] Selkoe DJ. Alzheimer's disease: genes, proteins, and therapy. Physiol Rev. 2001;81:741-66.

[3] Goate A, Chartier-Harlin MC, Mullan M, Brown J, Crawford F, Fidani L, et al. Segregation of a missense mutation in the amyloid precursor protein gene with familial Alzheimer's disease. Nature. 1991;349:704-6.

[4] Lott IT, Head E. Alzheimer disease and Down syndrome: factors in pathogenesis. Neurobiol Aging. 2005;26:383-9.

[5] Sherrington R, Rogaev EI, Liang Y, Rogaeva EA, Levesque G, Ikeda M, et al. Cloning of a gene bearing missense mutations in early-onset familial Alzheimer's disease. Nature. 1995;375:754-60.

[6] Levy-Lahad E, Wasco W, Poorkaj P, Romano DM, Oshima J, Pettingell WH, et al. Candidate gene for the chromosome 1 familial Alzheimer's disease locus. Science. 1995;269:973-7.

[7] Rogaev EI, Sherrington R, Rogaeva EA, Levesque G, Ikeda M, Liang Y, et al. Familial Alzheimer's disease in kindreds with missense mutations in a gene on chromosome 1 related to the Alzheimer's disease type 3 gene. Nature. 1995;376:775-8.

[8] Iwatsubo T. The gamma-secretase complex: machinery for intramembrane proteolysis. Curr Opin Neurobiol. 2004;14:379-83.

[9] Zheng H, Koo EH. The amyloid precursor protein: beyond amyloid. Mol Neurodegener. 2006;1:5.

[10] Haass C, Selkoe DJ. Cellular processing of beta-amyloid precursor protein and the genesis of amyloid beta-peptide. Cell. 1993;75:1039-42.

[11] Kopan R, Ilagan MX. Gamma-secretase: proteasome of the membrane? Nat Rev Mol Cell Biol. 2004;5:499-504.

[12] Selkoe DJ, Wolfe MS. Presenilin: running with scissors in the membrane. Cell. 2007;131:215-21.

[13] Nakayama K, Nagase H, Hiratochi M, Koh CS, Ohkawara T. Similar mechanisms regulated by gamma-secretase are involved in both directions of the bi-directional Notch-Delta signaling pathway as well as play a potential role in signaling events involving type 1 transmembrane proteins. Curr Stem Cell Res Ther. 2008;3:288-302.

[14] Nakayama K, Nagase H, Koh CS, Ohkawara T. gamma-Secretase-Regulated Mechanisms Similar to Notch Signaling May Play a Role in Signaling Events, Including

APP Signaling, Which Leads to Alzheimer's Disease. Cell Mol Neurobiol. 2011;31:887-900.

[15] Nakayama K, Nagase H, Koh C-S, Ohkawara T. Gamma-Secretase-Regulated Signaling: Notch, APP, and Alzheimer's Disease. Current Psychopharmacology. 2012;1:155-66.

[16] Artavanis-Tsakonas S, Matsuno K, Fortini ME. Notch signaling. Science. 1995;268:225-32.

[17] Lewis J. Notch signalling and the control of cell fate choices in vertebrates. Semin Cell Dev Biol. 1998;9:583-9.

[18] Bolos V, Grego-Bessa J, de la Pompa JL. Notch signaling in development and cancer. Endocr Rev. 2007;28:339-63.

[19] Artavanis-Tsakonas S, Rand MD, Lake RJ. Notch signaling: cell fate control and signal integration in development. Science. 1999;284:770-6.

[20] Justice NJ, Jan YN. Variations on the Notch pathway in neural development. Curr Opin Neurobiol. 2002;12:64-70.

[21] McCarthy JV, Twomey C, Wujek P. Presenilin-dependent regulated intramembrane proteolysis and gamma-secretase activity. Cell Mol Life Sci. 2009;66:1534-55.

[22] Nagase H, Koh CS, Nakayama K. gamma-Secretase-regulated signaling pathways, such as notch signaling, mediate the differentiation of hematopoietic stem cells, development of the immune system, and peripheral immune responses. Curr Stem Cell Res Ther. 2011;6:131-41.

[23] Koo EH, Kopan R. Potential role of presenilin-regulated signaling pathways in sporadic neurodegeneration. Nat Med. 2004;10 Suppl:S26-33.

[24] Cupers P, Orlans I, Craessaerts K, Annaert W, De Strooper B. The amyloid precursor protein (APP)-cytoplasmic fragment generated by gamma-secretase is rapidly degraded but distributes partially in a nuclear fraction of neurones in culture. Journal of neurochemistry. 2001;78:1168-78.

[25] Gao Y, Pimplikar SW. The gamma -secretase-cleaved C-terminal fragment of amyloid precursor protein mediates signaling to the nucleus. Proc Natl Acad Sci U S A. 2001;98:14979-84.

[26] Kimberly WT, Zheng JB, Guenette SY, Selkoe DJ. The intracellular domain of the beta-amyloid precursor protein is stabilized by Fe65 and translocates to the nucleus in a notch-like manner. The Journal of biological chemistry. 2001;276:40288-92.

[27] Cao X, Sudhof TC. A transcriptionally [correction of transcriptively] active complex of APP with Fe65 and histone acetyltransferase Tip60. Science. 2001;293:115-20.

[28] Guenette SY. A role for APP in motility and transcription? Trends in pharmacological sciences. 2002;23:203-5; discussion 5-6.

[29] Nakayama K, Ohkawara T, Hiratochi M, Koh CS, Nagase H. The intracellular domain of amyloid precursor protein induces neuron-specific apoptosis. Neurosci Lett. 2008;444:127-31.

[30] Ohkawara T, Nagase H, Koh CS, Nakayama K. The amyloid precursor protein intracellular domain alters gene expression and induces neuron-specific apoptosis. Gene. 2011;475:1-9.

[31] Wharton KA, Johansen KM, Xu T, Artavanis-Tsakonas S. Nucleotide sequence from the neurogenic locus notch implies a gene product that shares homology with proteins containing EGF-like repeats. Cell. 1985;43:567-81.

[32] Rebay I, Fleming RJ, Fehon RG, Cherbas L, Cherbas P, Artavanis-Tsakonas S. Specific EGF repeats of Notch mediate interactions with Delta and Serrate: implications for Notch as a multifunctional receptor. Cell. 1991;67:687-99.

[33] Logeat F, Bessia C, Brou C, LeBail O, Jarriault S, Seidah NG, et al. The Notch1 receptor is cleaved constitutively by a furin-like convertase. Proc Natl Acad Sci U S A. 1998;95:8108-12.

[34] Kopczynski CC, Alton AK, Fechtel K, Kooh PJ, Muskavitch MA. Delta, a Drosophila neurogenic gene, is transcriptionally complex and encodes a protein related to blood coagulation factors and epidermal growth factor of vertebrates. Genes Dev. 1988;2:1723-35.

[35] Fleming RJ, Scottgale TN, Diederich RJ, Artavanis-Tsakonas S. The gene Serrate encodes a putative EGF-like transmembrane protein essential for proper ectodermal development in Drosophila melanogaster. Genes Dev. 1990;4:2188-201.

[36] Bettenhausen B, Hrabe de Angelis M, Simon D, Guenet JL, Gossler A. Transient and restricted expression during mouse embryogenesis of Dll1, a murine gene closely related to Drosophila Delta. Development. 1995;121:2407-18.

[37] Dunwoodie SL, Henrique D, Harrison SM, Beddington RS. Mouse Dll3: a novel divergent Delta gene which may complement the function of other Delta homologues during early pattern formation in the mouse embryo. Development. 1997;124:3065-76.

[38] Shutter JR, Scully S, Fan W, Richards WG, Kitajewski J, Deblandre GA, et al. Dll4, a novel Notch ligand expressed in arterial endothelium. Genes Dev. 2000;14:1313-8.

[39] Lindsell CE, Shawber CJ, Boulter J, Weinmaster G. Jagged: a mammalian ligand that activates Notch1. Cell. 1995;80:909-17.

[40] Shawber C, Boulter J, Lindsell CE, Weinmaster G. Jagged2: a serrate-like gene expressed during rat embryogenesis. Dev Biol. 1996;180:370-6.

[41] Tax FE, Yeargers JJ, Thomas JH. Sequence of C. elegans lag-2 reveals a cell-signalling domain shared with Delta and Serrate of Drosophila. Nature. 1994;368:150-4.

[42] Henderson ST, Gao D, Christensen S, Kimble J. Functional domains of LAG-2, a putative signaling ligand for LIN-12 and GLP-1 receptors in Caenorhabditis elegans. Mol Biol Cell. 1997;8:1751-62.

[43] Brown MS, Ye J, Rawson RB, Goldstein JL. Regulated intramembrane proteolysis: a control mechanism conserved from bacteria to humans. Cell. 2000;100:391-8.

[44] Pan D, Rubin GM. Kuzbanian controls proteolytic processing of Notch and mediates lateral inhibition during Drosophila and vertebrate neurogenesis. Cell. 1997;90:271-80.

[45] Brou C, Logeat F, Gupta N, Bessia C, LeBail O, Doedens JR, et al. A novel proteolytic cleavage involved in Notch signaling: the role of the disintegrin-metalloprotease TACE. Mol Cell. 2000;5:207-16.

[46] Kopan R, Schroeter EH, Weintraub H, Nye JS. Signal transduction by activated mNotch: importance of proteolytic processing and its regulation by the extracellular domain. Proc Natl Acad Sci U S A. 1996;93:1683-8.

[47] Schroeter EH, Kisslinger JA, Kopan R. Notch-1 signalling requires ligand-induced proteolytic release of intracellular domain. Nature. 1998;393:382-6.

[48] Okochi M, Steiner H, Fukumori A, Tanii H, Tomita T, Tanaka T, et al. Presenilins mediate a dual intramembranous gamma-secretase cleavage of Notch-1. EMBO J. 2002;21:5408-16.

[49] Roehl H, Bosenberg M, Blelloch R, Kimble J. Roles of the RAM and ANK domains in signaling by the C. elegans GLP-1 receptor. EMBO J. 1996;15:7002-12.

[50] Wu L, Aster JC, Blacklow SC, Lake R, Artavanis-Tsakonas S, Griffin JD. MAML1, a human homologue of Drosophila mastermind, is a transcriptional co-activator for NOTCH receptors. Nat Genet. 2000;26:484-9.

[51] Wallberg AE, Pedersen K, Lendahl U, Roeder RG. p300 and PCAF act cooperatively to mediate transcriptional activation from chromatin templates by notch intracellular domains in vitro. Mol Cell Biol. 2002;22:7812-9.

[52] Kageyama R, Ohtsuka T, Kobayashi T. The Hes gene family: repressors and oscillators that orchestrate embryogenesis. Development. 2007;134:1243-51.

[53] Kang J, Lemaire HG, Unterbeck A, Salbaum JM, Masters CL, Grzeschik KH, et al. The precursor of Alzheimer's disease amyloid A4 protein resembles a cell-surface receptor. Nature. 1987;325:733-6.

[54] Yoshikai S, Sasaki H, Doh-ura K, Furuya H, Sakaki Y. Genomic organization of the human amyloid beta-protein precursor gene. Gene. 1990;87:257-63.

[55] Sisodia SS, Koo EH, Hoffman PN, Perry G, Price DL. Identification and transport of full-length amyloid precursor proteins in rat peripheral nervous system. J Neurosci. 1993;13:3136-42.

[56] Coulson EJ, Paliga K, Beyreuther K, Masters CL. What the evolution of the amyloid protein precursor supergene family tells us about its function. Neurochem Int. 2000;36:175-84.

[57] Dahms SO, Hoefgen S, Roeser D, Schlott B, Guhrs KH, Than ME. Structure and biochemical analysis of the heparin-induced E1 dimer of the amyloid precursor protein. Proc Natl Acad Sci U S A.107:5381-6.

[58] Wang Y, Ha Y. The X-ray structure of an antiparallel dimer of the human amyloid precursor protein E2 domain. Mol Cell. 2004;15:343-53.

[59] Hung AY, Koo EH, Haass C, Selkoe DJ. Increased expression of beta-amyloid precursor protein during neuronal differentiation is not accompanied by secretory cleavage. Proc Natl Acad Sci U S A. 1992;89:9439-43.

[60] Leyssen M, Ayaz D, Hebert SS, Reeve S, De Strooper B, Hassan BA. Amyloid precursor protein promotes post-developmental neurite arborization in the Drosophila brain. EMBO J. 2005;24:2944-55.

[61] McGowan E, editor. Alzheimer animal models: models of Abeta deposition in transgenic mice. Basel: ISN Neuropath Press; 2003.

[62] Soba P, Eggert S, Wagner K, Zentgraf H, Siehl K, Kreger S, et al. Homo- and heterodimerization of APP family members promotes intercellular adhesion. EMBO J. 2005;24:3624-34.

[63] Ho A, Sudhof TC. Binding of F-spondin to amyloid-beta precursor protein: a candidate amyloid-beta precursor protein ligand that modulates amyloid-beta precursor protein cleavage. Proc Natl Acad Sci U S A. 2004;101:2548-53.

[64] Park JH, Gimbel DA, GrandPre T, Lee JK, Kim JE, Li W, et al. Alzheimer precursor protein interaction with the Nogo-66 receptor reduces amyloid-beta plaque deposition. J Neurosci. 2006;26:1386-95.

[65] Lorenzo A, Yuan M, Zhang Z, Paganetti PA, Sturchler-Pierrat C, Staufenbiel M, et al. Amyloid beta interacts with the amyloid precursor protein: a potential toxic mechanism in Alzheimer's disease. Nat Neurosci. 2000;3:460-4.

[66] Hardy J, Selkoe DJ. The amyloid hypothesis of Alzheimer's disease: progress and problems on the road to therapeutics. Science. 2002;297:353-6.

[67] Jarrett JT, Berger EP, Lansbury PT, Jr. The carboxy terminus of the beta amyloid protein is critical for the seeding of amyloid formation: implications for the pathogenesis of Alzheimer's disease. Biochemistry. 1993;32:4693-7.

[68] Lippa CF, Smith TW, Swearer JM. Alzheimer's disease and Lewy body disease: a comparative clinicopathological study. Ann Neurol. 1994;35:81-8.

[69] Askanas V, Engel WK, Alvarez RB. Light and electron microscopic localization of beta-amyloid protein in muscle biopsies of patients with inclusion-body myositis. Am J Pathol. 1992;141:31-6.

[70] Haan J, Roos RA. Amyloid in central nervous system disease. Clin Neurol Neurosurg. 1990;92:305-10.

[71] Miners JS, Baig S, Palmer J, Palmer LE, Kehoe PG, Love S. Abeta-degrading enzymes in Alzheimer's disease. Brain Pathol. 2008;18:240-52.

[72] Miners JS, Van Helmond Z, Chalmers K, Wilcock G, Love S, Kehoe PG. Decreased expression and activity of neprilysin in Alzheimer disease are associated with cerebral amyloid angiopathy. J Neuropathol Exp Neurol. 2006;65:1012-21.

[73] Cook DG, Leverenz JB, McMillan PJ, Kulstad JJ, Ericksen S, Roth RA, et al. Reduced hippocampal insulin-degrading enzyme in late-onset Alzheimer's disease is associated with the apolipoprotein E-epsilon4 allele. Am J Pathol. 2003;162:313-9.

[74] Turner AJ, Murphy LJ. Molecular pharmacology of endothelin converting enzymes. Biochem Pharmacol. 1996;51:91-102.

[75] Erdos EG, Skidgel RA. The angiotensin I-converting enzyme. Lab Invest. 1987;56:345-8.

[76] Lee MK, Slunt HH, Martin LJ, Thinakaran G, Kim G, Gandy SE, et al. Expression of presenilin 1 and 2 (PS1 and PS2) in human and murine tissues. J Neurosci. 1996;16:7513-25.

[77] Yu G, Nishimura M, Arawaka S, Levitan D, Zhang L, Tandon A, et al. Nicastrin modulates presenilin-mediated notch/glp-1 signal transduction and betaAPP processing. Nature. 2000;407:48-54.

[78] Shah S, Lee SF, Tabuchi K, Hao YH, Yu C, LaPlant Q, et al. Nicastrin functions as a gamma-secretase-substrate receptor. Cell. 2005;122:435-47.

[79] Struhl G, Adachi A. Requirements for presenilin-dependent cleavage of notch and other transmembrane proteins. Mol Cell. 2000;6:625-36.

[80] Esch FS, Keim PS, Beattie EC, Blacher RW, Culwell AR, Oltersdorf T, et al. Cleavage of amyloid beta peptide during constitutive processing of its precursor. Science. 1990;248:1122-4.

[81] Vassar R, Bennett BD, Babu-Khan S, Kahn S, Mendiaz EA, Denis P, et al. Beta-secretase cleavage of Alzheimer's amyloid precursor protein by the transmembrane aspartic protease BACE. Science. 1999;286:735-41.

[82] Buxbaum JD, Liu KN, Luo Y, Slack JL, Stocking KL, Peschon JJ, et al. Evidence that tumor necrosis factor alpha converting enzyme is involved in regulated alpha-secretase cleavage of the Alzheimer amyloid protein precursor. The Journal of biological chemistry. 1998;273:27765-7.

[83] Lammich S, Kojro E, Postina R, Gilbert S, Pfeiffer R, Jasionowski M, et al. Constitutive and regulated alpha-secretase cleavage of Alzheimer's amyloid precursor protein by a disintegrin metalloprotease. Proc Natl Acad Sci U S A. 1999;96:3922-7.

[84] Farzan M, Schnitzler CE, Vasilieva N, Leung D, Choe H. BACE2, a beta -secretase homolog, cleaves at the beta site and within the amyloid-beta region of the amyloid-beta precursor protein. Proc Natl Acad Sci U S A. 2000;97:9712-7.

[85] Ikeuchi T, Sisodia SS. The Notch ligands, Delta1 and Jagged2, are substrates for presenilin-dependent "gamma-secretase" cleavage. The Journal of biological chemistry. 2003;278:7751-4.

[86] LaVoie MJ, Selkoe DJ. The Notch ligands, Jagged and Delta, are sequentially processed by alpha-secretase and presenilin/gamma-secretase and release signaling fragments. The Journal of biological chemistry. 2003;278:34427-37.

[87] Hiratochi M, Nagase H, Kuramochi Y, Koh CS, Ohkawara T, Nakayama K. The Delta intracellular domain mediates TGF-beta/Activin signaling through binding to Smads and has an important bi-directional function in the Notch-Delta signaling pathway. Nucleic Acids Res. 2007;35:912-22.

[88] Edbauer D, Willem M, Lammich S, Steiner H, Haass C. Insulin-degrading enzyme rapidly removes the beta-amyloid precursor protein intracellular domain (AICD). The Journal of biological chemistry. 2002;277:13389-93.

[89] Schulz JG, Annaert W, Vandekerckhove J, Zimmermann P, De Strooper B, David G. Syndecan 3 intramembrane proteolysis is presenilin/gamma-secretase-dependent and modulates cytosolic signaling. The Journal of biological chemistry. 2003;278:48651-7.

[90] Ni CY, Murphy MP, Golde TE, Carpenter G. gamma -Secretase cleavage and nuclear localization of ErbB-4 receptor tyrosine kinase. Science. 2001;294:2179-81.

[91] Buoso E, Lanni C, Schettini G, Govoni S, Racchi M. beta-Amyloid precursor protein metabolism: focus on the functions and degradation of its intracellular domain. Pharmacol Res. 2011;62:308-17.

[92] Ando K, Iijima KI, Elliott JI, Kirino Y, Suzuki T. Phosphorylation-dependent regulation of the interaction of amyloid precursor protein with Fe65 affects the production of beta-amyloid. The Journal of biological chemistry. [Research Support, Non-U.S. Gov't]. 2001;276:40353-61.

[93] Kimberly WT, Zheng JB, Town T, Flavell RA, Selkoe DJ. Physiological regulation of the beta-amyloid precursor protein signaling domain by c-Jun N-terminal kinase JNK3 during neuronal differentiation. J Neurosci. 2005;25:5533-43.

[94] Belyaev ND, Nalivaeva NN, Makova NZ, Turner AJ. Neprilysin gene expression requires binding of the amyloid precursor protein intracellular domain to its promoter: implications for Alzheimer disease. EMBO reports. [Research Support, Non-U.S. Gov't]. 2009;10:94-100.

[95] Ryan KA, Pimplikar SW. Activation of GSK-3 and phosphorylation of CRMP2 in transgenic mice expressing APP intracellular domain. J Cell Biol. 2005;171:327-35.

[96] Ghosal K, Vogt DL, Liang M, Shen Y, Lamb BT, Pimplikar SW. Alzheimer's disease-like pathological features in transgenic mice expressing the APP intracellular domain. Proc Natl Acad Sci U S A. 2009;106:18367-72.

[97] Vogt DL, Thomas D, Galvan V, Bredesen DE, Lamb BT, Pimplikar SW. Abnormal neuronal networks and seizure susceptibility in mice overexpressing the APP intracellular domain. Neurobiol Aging. 2009.

[98] Vazquez MC, Vargas LM, Inestrosa NC, Alvarez AR. c-Abl modulates AICD dependent cellular responses: transcriptional induction and apoptosis. J Cell Physiol. 2009;220:136-43.

[99] DeGiorgio LA, DeGiorgio N, Milner TA, Conti B, Volpe BT. Neurotoxic APP C-terminal and beta-amyloid domains colocalize in the nuclei of substantia nigra pars reticulata neurons undergoing delayed degeneration. Brain research. [Research Support, Non-U.S. Gov't Research Support, U.S. Gov't, P.H.S.]. 2000;874:137-46.

[100] Klein WL, Krafft GA, Finch CE. Targeting small Abeta oligomers: the solution to an Alzheimer's disease conundrum? Trends Neurosci. 2001;24:219-24.

[101] Selkoe DJ. Alzheimer's disease is a synaptic failure. Science. 2002;298:789-91.

[102] Terry RD KR, Bick KL, Sisodia SS. Alzheimer's disease. Philadelphia: Lippincott, Williams & Wilkins; 1999.

[103] Abbot A. The plaque plan. Nature. 2008;456:161-4.

[104] Holmes C, Boche D, Wilkinson D, Yadegarfar G, Hopkins V, Bayer A, et al. Long-term effects of Abeta42 immunisation in Alzheimer's disease: follow-up of a randomised, placebo-controlled phase I trial. Lancet. [Research Support, Non-U.S. Gov't]. 2008;372:216-23.

[105] Schnabel J. Alzheimer's theory makes a splash. Nature. 2009;459:310.

[106] Nikolaev A, McLaughlin T, O'Leary DD, Tessier-Lavigne M. APP binds DR6 to trigger axon pruning and neuron death via distinct caspases. Nature. 2009;457:981-9.

[107] Iijima K, Ando K, Takeda S, Satoh Y, Seki T, Itohara S, et al. Neuron-specific phosphorylation of Alzheimer's beta-amyloid precursor protein by cyclin-dependent kinase 5. Journal of neurochemistry. [Research Support, Non-U.S. Gov'tResearch Support, U.S. Gov't, P.H.S.]. 2000;75:1085-91.

Chapter 5

Phosphorylation of Tau Protein Associated as a Protective Mechanism in the Presence of Toxic, C-Terminally Truncated Tau in Alzheimer's Disease

José Luna-Muñoz, Charles R. Harrington,
Claude M. Wischik, Paola Flores-Rodríguez,
Jesús Avila, Sergio R. Zamudio, Fidel De la Cruz,
Raúl Mena, Marco A. Meraz-Ríos and
Benjamin Floran-Garduño

Additional information is available at the end of the chapter

http://dx.doi.org/10.5772/54228

1. Introduction

Alzheimer's disease (AD) is the most common cause of dementia in the elderly and is characterized by progressive memory loss leading to a gradual and irreversible deterioration of cognitive function. The neuropathology of AD is characterized by the accumulation of fibrillary lesions in the form of neuritic plaques (NPs, Fig. 1A), neurofibrillary tangles (NFTs, Fig. 1C,D; small arrow) and dystrophic neurites (DNs, Fig. 1; arrows) in neocortex, amygdala and hippocampus [1]. The density of the NPs and NFTs correlate with the degree of dementia in AD [2]. The accumulation of these lesions does not occur at random; the presence of NFTs is associated with vulnerability of the perforant pathway [3]. NPs are comprised of extracellular deposits of amyloid-β peptide fibrils that are associated with DNs of dendritic and axonal origin (Fig. 1A; arrows). Intracellular NFTs selectively kill neurons in specific brain areas. In AD, the distribution of NFTs follows a stereotypical profile arising first in layer II of the entorhinal cortex, hippocampal region and CA1/subicular layer IV of the entorhinal cortex and then neocortex (mainly in fronto-temporal and parietal areas). This pattern of distribution was first described by Braak and Braak in 1991 [4], and provides the most important neuropathological criteria for a definite diagnosis of AD (Fig. 2) [5]. Ultrastructurally, NFTs are composed of dense accumulations of structures known as paired helical filaments (PHFs) [6, 7], which are mainly distributed in the perinuclear area of the neuron and in proximal processes (Fig. 1C). Tau protein is the major structural constituent of the PHF subunits [7-9]. Normally, tau protein exists as a family of microtubule-associated protein (MAPs) that are found predominantly in axons. Through repeated domains located toward the carboxy-terminus of the protein, tau provides stability to the microtubule and this process can be regulated through a balance in the phosphorylation/dephosphorylation process of tau protein [10]. In AD, tau protein accumulates as PHFs in the somatodendritic compartment, with consequent destabilization of axonal microtubules. Tau is further post-translationally in AD, with modifications of ubiquitination [11, 12], glycation [13, 14], glycosylation [15], nitration [16], polyamination [17], hyperphosphorylation [18, 19] and proteolysis [7, 20-24]. The latter two changes occur throughout the tau molecule [25-27].

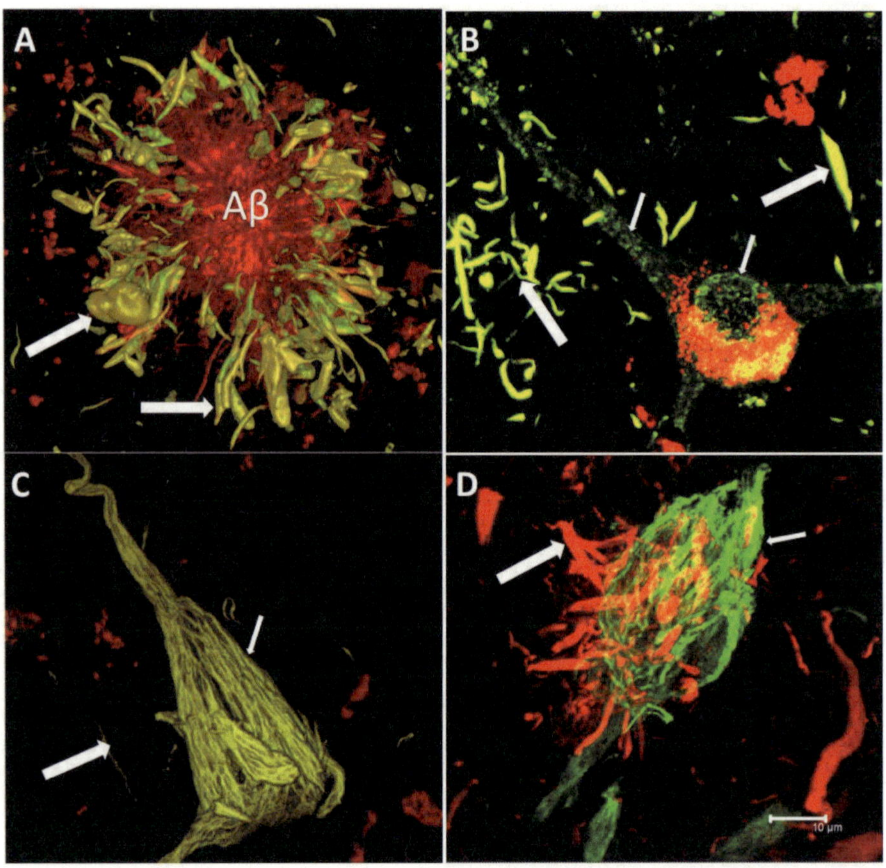

Figure 1. Neuropathological hallmarks of Alzheimer´s disease. Double labelling with tau antibody (green channel) counterstained with thiazine red (red channel). A) A classical neuritic plaquein which an amyloid fibrillar plaque (Aβ), recognized by thiazine red, is associated with dystrophic neurites (arrows). B). Pre-tangle cells are characterized by diffuse granular deposits throughout the perinuclear area (small arrow) and proximal processes. C) A neurofibrillary tangle that is strongly labeled by tau antibody and colocalized with tiazine red. (A,B) projection of 20 and 9 confocal microscopy sections, respectively, each of 1.0 μm thickness.

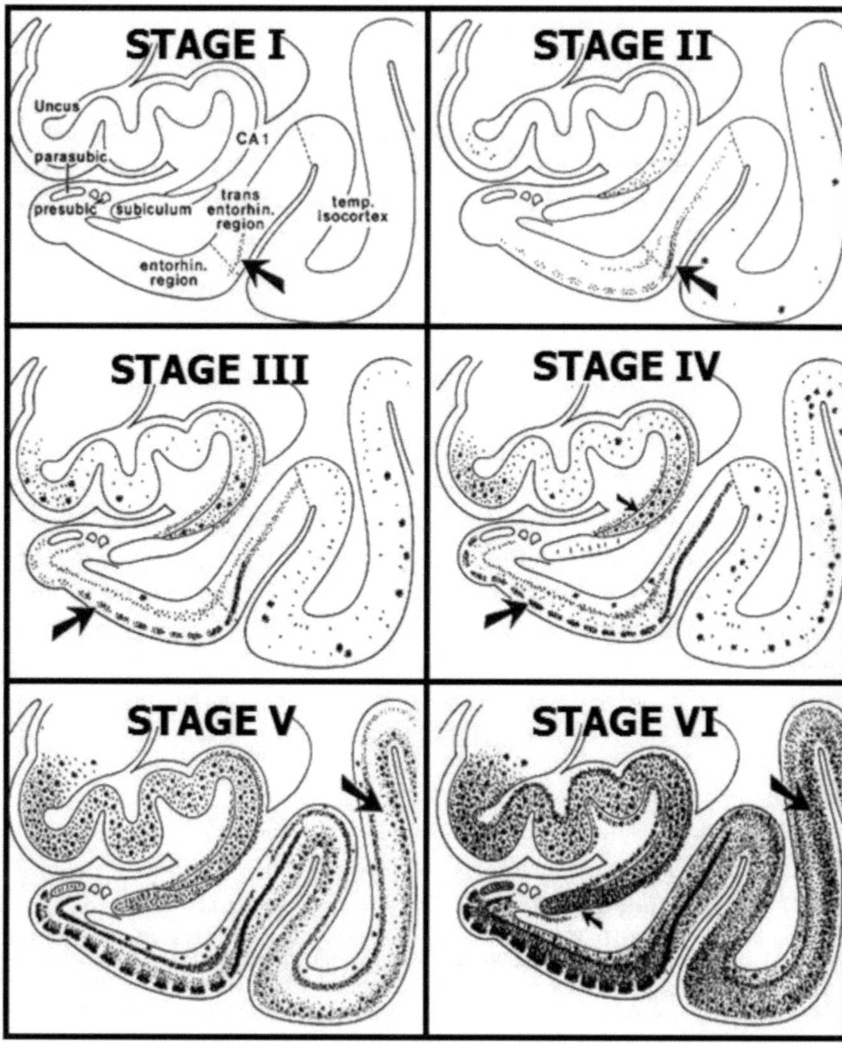

Figure 2. Braak stages of AD neuropathology base on the pattern of neurofibrillary change (NFT, Neuropil threads and plaques dystrofic neurites) [4], Although clinic-pathological correlations were not made, Braak and Braak did speculate that the entorhinal stage (I-II) represents clinically silent periods of the disease with NFT involvement confined to trans-entorhinal layer pre-alpha. Limbic stages (III/IV) correspond with clinically incipient AD, and NFT involvement of CA1, and neocortical stages (V/VI) represent fully developed AD, with NFT involvement of all areas of association cortex.

Tau protein can be phosphorylated at multiple sites. While there is evidence that phosphorylation of tau protein promotes its assembly into PHFs [18, 19, 28, 29], the role of phosphorylation in the genesis of PHFs has been limited to the analysis of "mature", intracellular NFTs (NFT-I). By this stage in the disease, tau protein will have been affected by many different pathological processes, several of which may be associated with the hyperphosphorylation process [25, 26, 30].

Another post-translational modification found in AD is the proteolytic truncation of the C-terminal portion of tau protein [7, 20, 21, 23, 31, 32]. It has been proposed that such truncation unlike hyperphosphorylation, favours polymerisation of tau [33, 34][35].

In recent years, evidence from both *in vitro* and *in vivo* studies[36, 37], suggests that hyperphosphorylation of tau protein has a protective role. In this review, we analyze the protective effects of hyperphosphorylated species of tau protein and their relationship to toxicity, and the participation of truncated species of tau in the formation of PHFs.

2. Tau protein

The cytoskeleton is formed by three types of filaments: microfilaments, intermediate filaments and microtubules [38]. The cytoskeleton provides a dynamic scaffold to proteins, vesicles and organelles, essential for proper cell function and changes in the state of its polymerization, play an important role in neuronal process such as polarization, axonal transport, maintenance of neuronal extensions, synaptic plasticity and protein sorting [39]. Tau protein functions as a regulator of microtubule assembly [40]. Tau protein participates in microtubule polymerization [41], regulation of axonal diameter [42], regulation of axonal transport [43], neurogenesis and the establishment of neuronal polarity in development [44]. Furthermore, tau participates in the regulation of signaling pathways by acting as a protein scaffold.

The gene that encodes for tau consists of 16 exons and is located at the chromosomal locus 17q21 [45]. Through alternative splicing, six tau isoforms are generated in the CNS, varying from 352-441 amino acids in length (Fig. 3). Tau protein can be divided into three domains: an acidic region in the N-terminal projection, a proline-rich domain and a microtubule-binding domain (Fig. 4) [46]. The alternative transcription of exons 2, 3 and 10 modifies the presence of repeats in the N-terminus of tau (0-2N) and the number of microtubule-binding repeat domains (3R or 4R), respectively.

3. Tau protein metabolism

The *MAPT* (tau) gene is transcribed mainly in neurons and a promoter that confers neuronal specificity has been described [47]. It has been reported that the presence of a tau promoter lacking neuronal specificity might account for the expression of tau in peripheral tissue [48]. In both cases, sequences containing binding sites for transcription factors AP2 and Sp1 were described. Whereas tau protein synthesis is unaffected by microtubule polymerization or depolymerization, degradation of tau is stimulated by microtubule depolymerization [49].

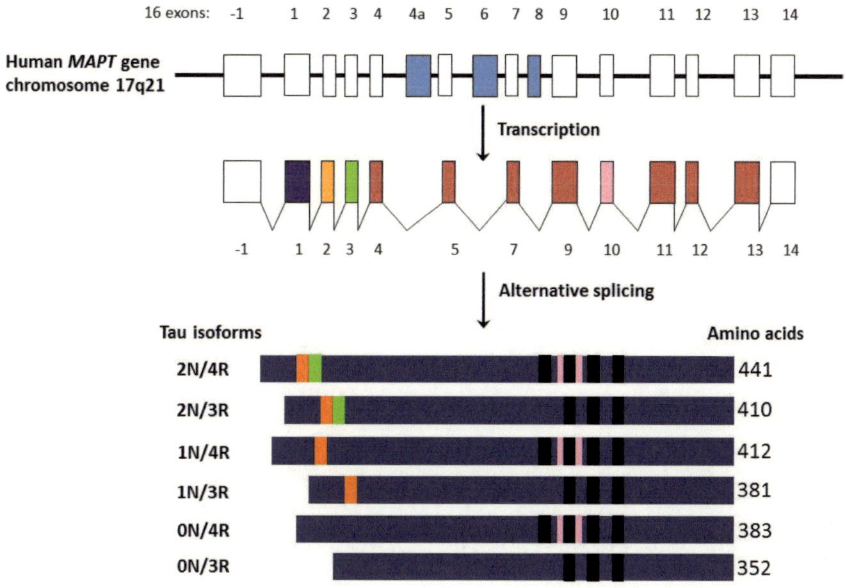

Figure 3. Schematic representation of the human *MAPT* (tau) gene, the primary tau transcript and the six CNS tau protein isoforms. The *MAPT* gene is located over 100kb of the long arm of chromosome 17 at position 17q21. It contains 16 exons, with exon −1 is a part of the promoter (upper panel). The tau primary transcript contains 13 exons. Exons −1 and 14 are transcribed but not translated. Exons 1, 4, 5, 7, 9, 11, 12, 13 are constitutive, and exons 2, 3, and 10 are alternatively spliced, giving rise to six different mRNAs, translated in six different CNS tau isoforms (lower panel). These isoforms differ by the absence or presence of one or two N-terminal inserts of 29 amino acids encoded by exon 2 (yellow box) and 3 (green box), in combination with either three (R1, R3 and R4) or four (R1–R4) C-terminal repeat-regions (black boxes). The additional microtubule-binding domain is encoded by exon 10 (pink box) (lower panel). Adult tau includes all six tau isoforms, including the largest isoform of 441-amino acids containing all inserts and other isoforms as indicated. The shortest 352-amino acids isoform is the only one found only in fetal brain.

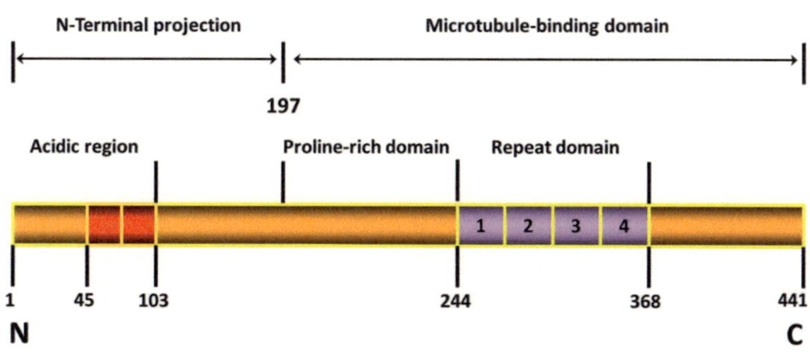

Figure 4. Schematic representation of the functional domains of the largest tau isoform (441 amino acids). The projection domain, including an acidic and a proline-rich region, interacts with cytoskeletal elements to determine the spacing between microtubules in axons. The N-terminal part is also involved in signal transduction pathways by interacting with proteins such as PLC-γ and Src-kinases. The C-terminal part, referred to as the microtubule-binding domain, regulates the rate of microtubules polymerization and is involved in binding with functional proteins such as protein phosphatase 2A (PP2A) or presenilin 1(PS1).

It is technically difficult to determine the half life of the different tau isoforms and several factors may regulate tau degradation such as, for example, the extent of phosphorylation and acetylation of tau (see below). The half life of tau decreases in rats by neonatal period P20 and there is less demand for tau in non-dividing, mature neurons [50].

Two main mechanisms for tau protein degradation have been documented: 1) the proteasomal ubiquitin pathway and 2) the lysosomal autophagic pathway. Proteasomal degradation of tau protein has been described by 20S proteasomal processing [51], although there have also been reports suggesting that tau is not normally degraded by the proteasome [52]. Tau, modified by phosphorylation, can be ubiquitinated by the CHIP-hsc70 complex and degraded by the proteasome [53]. Furthermore, acetylation of tau can regulate its proteasomal degradation by modifying those lysine residues needed for ubiquitination. In this way, acetylation of tau inhibits its degradation through a competition between ubiquitination and acetylation [54].

On the other hand, tau may get processed through a lysosomal autophagic mechanism. It has been reported that tau can be degraded by lysosomal proteases [55] and, more recently, it was shown that tau fragmentation and clearance can occur by lysosomal processing [56].

Tau protein is a microtubule-associated protein. It's mostly abundant in neurons in the Central Nervous System (CNS). The main function of Tau protein is to interact with tubulin to stabilize microtubules and promote tubulin assembly into microtubules. Tau protein controls microtubule stability in two different ways : isoforms and phosphorylation.

Normally, the tau protein is very important, as it manages the transport of materials within soma and other cellular regions through the myelin sheaths. Once it spotted something suspicious or irrelevant, it stops the information sending process automatically. However, in Alzheimer's disease, the tau proteins started to perform uncommon reaction, where it transmitting the information to the brain simultaneously, regardless of its validity.

Once the above problem happening, it causes the brain overloading with information and might lead to inflammation, clumps or tangles, which kill most of the brain cells (Fig. 5).

4. Phosphporylation of tau protein

Protein phosphorylation is the addition of a phosphate group, by esterification, to one of three different amino acids: serine, threonine and tyrosine. Phosphorylation is the most common post-translational modification of tau described and increased tau phosphorylation reduces its affinity for microtubules leading to cytoskeletal destabilization. Eighty-five putative phosphorylation sites on tau protein have been described in AD brain tissue (Fig. 6). The formation of fibrillar aggregates of post-translationally modified tau protein in the brain are characteristic of AD and other tauopathies. The phosphorylation of tau protein affects its solubility, localization, function, interaction with partners and susceptibility to other post-translational modifications. However, the role of specific sites of tau phosphorylation in early neurodegenerative mechanisms is unknown. The molecular mechanisms of aggregation of tau into insoluble forms may help to account for the different dementias in which both clinical symptoms and age of onset differ.

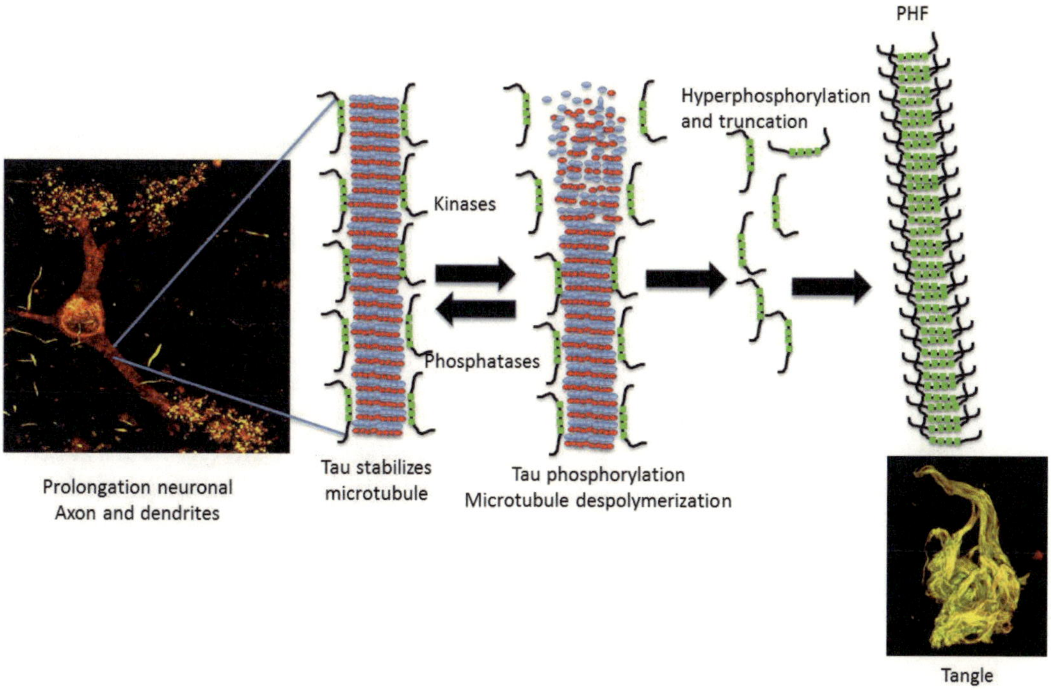

Figure 5. tau protein, which forms part of a microtubule. The microtubule helps transpot nutrients and other important substances from one part of the nerve cells to another. Axon are long threadlike extensions that conduct nerve impulses away from the nerve cells; dendrites are short branched threadlike extensions that conduct nerve impulses toward the verve cell body. In Alzheimer´s disease the tau protein is abnormal and the microtubule structures collapse.

5. C-terminal truncation of tau protein in AD

5.1. PHF-core concept

In 1988, Wischik et al, [7, 22] identified tau protein as the major constituent of Pronase-resistant PHFs and tau was characterized by a specific C-terminal truncation of the protein at Glu-391. This truncation is identified by the monoclonal antibody (mAb) 423 [23, 31], and the acid-reversible occlusion of the intact core tau domain. PHFs are labeled by the fluorescent dye, thiazin-red, a dye which can be used to differentiate between amorphous and fibrillar states of tau and amyloid proteins in AD. The minimum tau fragment in the PHF [20, 24] corresponds to the tandem repeat region in the C-terminal domain of tau protein, a species having a molecular weight of 12.5 kDa. Characteristically, this fragment is highly stable to proteolysis, insoluble and toxic and is referred to as PHF-core tau [22, 57, 58]. PHF-core tau and mAb 423 immunoreactivity of NFTs, have a close clinical-pathological relationship; the density of NFTs immunolabelled with mAb 423 is correlated with the progression of neurofibrilary pathology, as determined by Braak staging criteria (Fig. 2). Most significantly, there is a correlation between mAb 423 immunoreactivity and both clinical severity and progression to dementia [3]. On the other hand, over-expression of PHF-core tau, in cell culture, favors a programmed cell death or apoptosis, which shows that it is highly toxic[59]. Recombinant tau protein truncated at Glu-391 also shows increased rates of polymerization compared with recombinant full-length tau. From confocal microscopy studies, it has been shown that this fragment of tau is hidden within the PHF-core and exposed by formic acid treatment [57]. In the cytoplasm of susceptible neurons, this truncated tau triggers an autocatalytic process in which the fragment has a high affinity for full length tau and, once bound, leads to cycles of proteolysis and further tau binding to form a proto-filament [60]. In this scenario, the initiating tau species that gave rise to the filament is hidden within a large number of covering tau molecules, some of which become hyperphosphorylated. This would correspond to the early aggregation of tau protein associated with PHF in small NFT. Tau molecules of the NFT would become exposed on death of the neuron to reveal the extracellular NFT, or "ghost tangle" (Fig. 1D, small arrow) which shares the properties of being stable, insoluble and immunoreactive with mAb 423 [57, 61]. The proteases responsible for truncation at Glu-391 are not known.

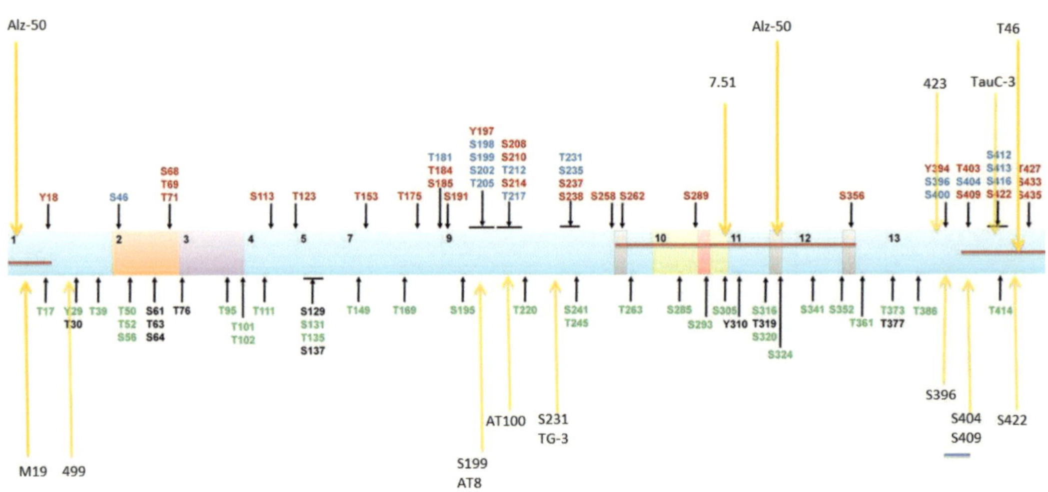

Figure 6. Location of tau phosphorylation sites and epitopes for tau antibodies. Multiple amino acids are phosphorylated with some those observed in AD brain [5], normal brain (green) and both normal and AD brains (blue). Putative phosphorylation sites that have not yet been demonstrated *in vitro* or *in vivo* (black). Localization of antibody epitopes are indicated arrows. Residues are numbered according to the longest tau isoform.

6. Truncation of tau protein at Asp-421

In 2003, a second truncation of tau protein was found to be associated with PHFs [62-65]. This truncation is found at position Asp-421 in the C-terminus of the tau molecule and its presence can be detected specifically by using mAb TauC-3[25, 63]. Unlike truncation at Glu-391, for which the protease responsible is unknown, caspase-3 (an enzyme involved in the apoptotic pathway) is responsible for the truncation at Asp-421 *in vitro* [59, 62, 63]. This suggests that cleavage of the carboxyl terminus of tau protein, could result as a neuronal response to prevent or control the polymerization of tau in PHF [58]. In 2005, Binder and colleagues discovered a truncation at the amino terminus of the tau protein associated with PHFs. This cut corresponds to Asp-13, which is produced by caspase-6, another enzyme involved in the apoptotic pathway [66]. An antibody to detect this cleavage site of the amino terminus of tau protein has not yet been generated.

Tau-C3 has an affinity for NFTs, NDs and neuropil threads in AD brains. Immunohistochemical studies indicated that truncation at Asp-421 occurs after conformational change; the antibody binds with greatest affinity when the amino terminus of tau molecule contacts the third microtubule binding repeat (MTBR), as recognized by mAb Alz-50 [26]. However, other studies have shown Tau-C3 immunoreactivity in pre-tangle cells before they become Alz-50 immunoreactive and in the absence of PHFs [64, 67].

7. Impact of phosphorylation and truncation on the abnormal processing of tau protein in AD

7.1. A neuroprotective mechanism for the phosphorylation of tau protein in the AD brain

During neurodegeneration in AD, tau protein is abnormally phosphorylated in the proline-rich region at Ser and Thr residues [68], and such phosphorylation sites can be identified using highly specific antibodies such as: AT8 (Ser-202/Thr-205) AT100 (Ser-212 and Ser-214), TG3 (Thr-231/Ser-235) and PHF-1 (Ser-396/Ser-404), among others (Fig. 6). However, NFTs are found in viable neurons at late stages of the disease, and they persist in neuronal cells for decades with a significant number of NFTs being found in the cognitively intact elderly [69, 70]. Such NFT-bearing neurons contain normal content and structure of microtubules [68]. The findings from studies in transgenic mice and human data, suggest that tau accumulation in the somatodendritic compartment may represent the manifestation of a protective mechanism or a cellular adaptation that arises with advancing age. An increase in tau phosphorylation in AD brain has been associated with a protective mechanism against oxidative stress [71]. In another study, intact microtubules were found in NFT-bearing neurons [8], calling into question whether accumulation of phosphorylated tau and destabilization of microtubules are necessarily linked. Although microtubules are depolymerized in neurons with fibrillary degeneration, one study found evidence that the reduction of microtubules in AD is marked and specifically limited to vulnerable pyramidal neurons, and that even these alterations were observed in the absence of PHF [72]. This finding is also consistent with previous work by one of the authors noting a microtubule decrease of nearly 50% in dendrites that did not correlate with either PHFs or age [73], suggesting that a proportion of phosphorylated tau protein is associated with microtubules [71]. In animal models, it has been confirmed that axonal transport is not affected by either over-expression or reduction of tau protein *in vivo* [42, 74]. Another study found evidence that axonopathy precedes the formation of NFTs in a transgenic mouse [75]. A transgenic mouse expressing a human tau isoform developed NFTs, neuronal loss and behavioral impairments [58]. After suppression of tau expression, the behavioral deficits stabilized yet NFTs continued to accumulate, suggesting that NFTs are not sufficient to cause cognitive decline or neuronal death.

Within NFTs, different species of tau protein associated with phosphorylation are observed, but the neurodegenerating neurons still appear to be functional [75]. These observations suggest that the cytoplasmic accumulation of hyperphosphorylated tau protein is non-toxic, similar to the accumulation of lipofuscin that does not alter cellular metabolism[68]. It is generally assumed that disintegration of microtubules is associated with an imbalance between kinase and phosphatase activities, which lead to an alteration in the stability of microtubules, disruption of cell function and culminate in neuronal death. The data, however, suggest that, at least, a subpopulation of hyperphosphorylated NFTs may be not toxic. This is controversial, given the fact that the hyperphosphorylation of tau and NFTs are considered to be toxic. However, the ability of tau protein fractions, purified from AD brains, to alter microtubule assembly, *in vitro,* has been attributed to sequestration of normal tau molecules [18]. Alonso and colleagues [28] demonstrated that recombinant hyperphosphorylated tau, *in vitro*, decreases the breakdown of the recombinant microtubule when assembled into small aggregates [19, 28]. On this basis, the authors suggested that hyperphosphorylated tau protein plays a protective role against the disintegration of the microtubule.

Tau that has been hyperphosphorylated with GSK3-β kinase becomes immunoreactive with mAbs AT8, PHF1 and TG-3, antibodies whose epitopes are very closely related to AD [29, 76]. The fact that GSK3-β is capable of creating epitopes considered pathological in AD suggests that there are other participants that require to be considered. These data suggest the possible existence of a toxic species of non-phosphorylated tau protein, which would be responsible for capturing further molecules of tau in PHFs, yet would not be exposed on the filament [7, 57, 61]. It is possible that, by hiding the toxic form in PHFs could protect the neuron [77]. It is important to note that the presumed "intermediaries" are present in the cytoplasm of the neuron when it is still viable. Another study showed that NFTs (and presumably tau oligomers) could remain in the cytoplasm of the neuron for decades [78], an observation that would further argue against a primary toxicity of phosphorylated tau protein in AD.

7.2. Hyperphosphorylation of tau protein protecting neurons from apoptosis

It is also proposed that apoptosis plays an important role in neuronal damage in AD. This proposal is based on the detection of fragmented DNA and expression of apoptosis signaling proteins such as caspases 3, 6, 8 and 9, Bax, Fas and Fas-L, in the cortex and hippocampus, in postmortem brain tissue [79, 80] and observations that amyloid-β can induce neuronal apoptosis [81]. Apoptosis is a process that usually occurs over a period of hours, whereas the accumulation of tangles found in AD brains occurs over a period of years or decades [78]. It has been suggested that hyperphosphorylation of tau protein is a mechanism used to evade cell death by apoptosis. Cells over-expressing hyperphosphorylated tau appear to avoid the apoptotic process [82].

8. Participation of hyperphosphorylated and truncated tau species in the early formation of PHFs

8.1. Model for the mechanism of assembly

Despite suggestions of a neuroprotective role for tau protein in AD, links between phosphorylated species (that are presumed to be protective) and the complex assembly of toxic, truncated tau into insoluble PHFs is not clear. In recent years, we have characterized the early stages of tau protein processing in neurons (pre-tangle state) (Fig. 1B, small arrows) and have described accumulations of tau that possess pathological species present in NFT, yet which do not show the presence of assembled structures in PHFs [67, 83]. The pre-tangle (Fig. 1B) is the first step in non-fibrillar aggregation of tau protein in AD and one in which at least 5 different changes take place (Fig 1 C,D). These events include: a) the presence of a C-terminally truncated and toxic tau species (Glu-391); b) a cascade of specific phosphorylation of tau protein in the N-terminus; c) C-terminal truncation via the action of caspase-3; d) oligomerization and aggregation of tau species and e) assembly of tau into PHFs.

A model to accommodate the observations are represented schematically in Fig. 7. In this model, the first event to occur would be the emergence of tau oligomers or a PHF subunit (Fig. 7 A,B). The mechanism whereby this is initiated is unknown, but its toxicity and high affinity for binding to intact tau molecules would trigger an immediate need for the cell to protect itself. That would be reflected by hyperphosphorylation of the molecule in a failed attempt to hide the PHF and prevent the capture of further intact tau molecules (Fig. 7 B,C). In AD, this protective function of the phosphorylated species favors more molecules becoming available for sequestration and formation into PHFs (Fig. 7D). Gradually, phosphorylated tau will be affected by exogenous proteolysis to re-expose the PHF-core (Fig. 7E). These steps follow as a molecular consequence of the catastrophic fragmentation of the microtubule, synaptic dysfunction, oxidative stress and post-translational modifications of tau. This model emphasizes that polymerization and neuroprotective mechanisms are both involved in the development of PHFs. The phosphorylated species of tau protein play a role in the initial protective response of the neuron to prevent the assembly of these filaments [35]. Thus NFTs, in which externally available tau is hyperphosphorylated, represents a mechanism whereby the neuron may try to protect itself from neurofibrillary degeneration and further studies to confirm this hypothesis are warranted.

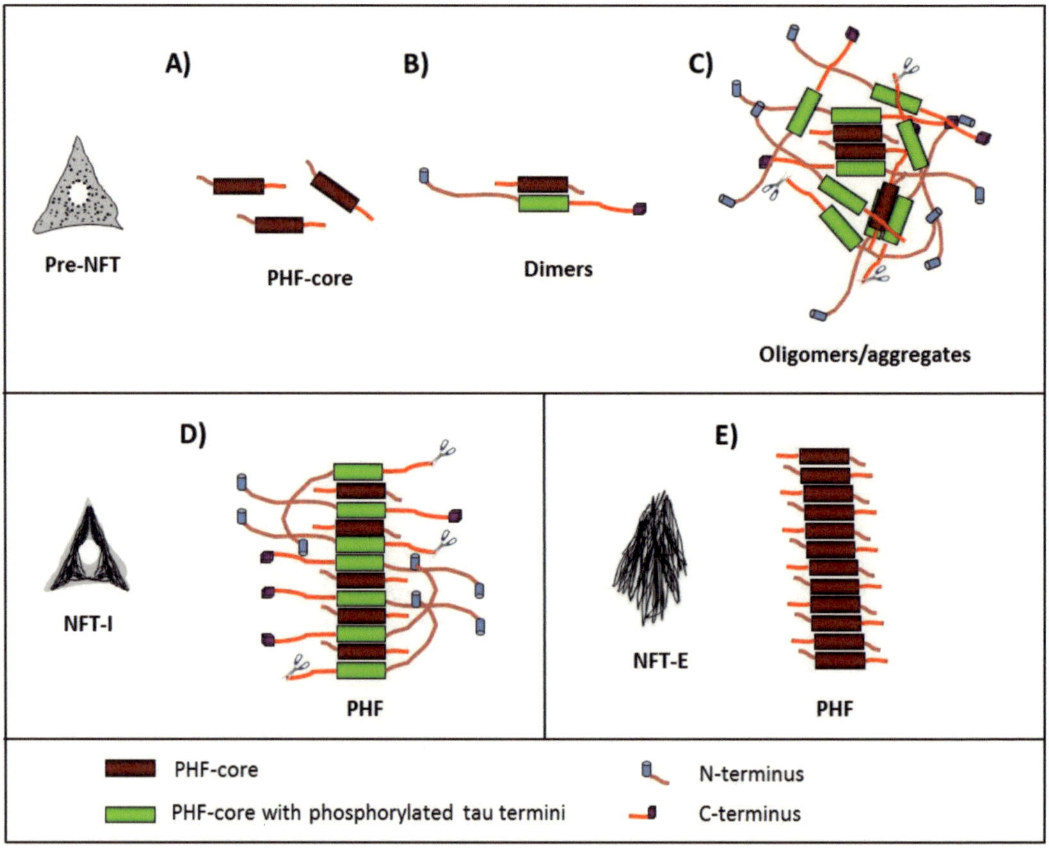

Figure 7. Scheme illustrating the early steps of aggregation and polymerization of tau protein in Alzheimer´s disease. (A) The model starts with the appearance of PHF-core tau in cytoplasm of susceptible neurons. (B) The high binding capacity of PHF-tau results in the assembly of dimers of PHF-core and intact tau molecules in the cytoplasm. (C) The phosphorylation of intact tau would be an early event to hide the toxic soluble aggregates of molecules. (D). The high affinity and stability of the proto-filaments that make up the mature intracellular NFT allows tau molecules to form PHFs. (E) With the death of the neuron, the PHF-core subunit becomes exposed again in the extracellular space following proteolysis. Further details are described in the text.

Acknowledgements

Authors express their gratitude to the Mexican families for the donation of brain tissue from their beloved and without which these studies would not be possible. Amparo Viramontes Pintos for the handling of brain tissue.This work was financially supported by CONACyT grants, No. 142293 (to B.F.).

Author details

José Luna-Muñoz[1], Charles R. Harrington[2], Claude M. Wischik[2], Paola Flores-Rodríguez[1], Jesús Avila[3], Sergio R. Zamudio[4], Fidel De la Cruz[4], Raúl Mena[1], Marco A. Meraz-Ríos[5] and Benjamin Floran-Garduño[1]

1 Departments of Physiology, Biophysics and Neurosciences, National Laboratory of experimental services (LaNSE), CINVESTAV-IPN, Mexico

2 Division of Applied Health Sciences, School of Medicine and Dentistry, University of Aberdeen, USA

3 Centro de Biología Molecular "Severo Ochoa", CSIC/UAM, Universidad Autónoma de Madrid, Madrid, Spain

4 Department of Physiology, ENCB-IPN, Mexico

5 Molecular Biomedicine, CINVESTAV-IPN, Mexico

References

[1] Arnold, S.E., et al., The topographical and neuroanatomical distribution of neurofibrillary tangles and neuritic plaques in the cerebral cortex of patients with Alzheimer's disease. Cerebral cortex, 1991. 1(1): p. 103-16.

[2] Arriagada, P.V., et al., Neurofibrillary tangles but not senile plaques parallel duration and severity of Alzheimer's disease. Neurology, 1992. 42(3 Pt 1): p. 631-9.

[3] Garcia-Sierra, F., et al., The extent of neurofibrillary pathology in perforant pathway neurons is the key determinant of dementia in the very old. Acta Neuropathol, 2000. 100(1): p. 29-35.

[4] Braak, H. and E. Braak, Neuropathological stageing of Alzheimer-related changes. Acta Neuropathol, 1991. 82(4): p. 239-59.

[5] Braak, H., et al., Staging of Alzheimer disease-associated neurofibrillary pathology using paraffin sections and immunocytochemistry. Acta Neuropathol, 2006. 112(4): p. 389-404.

[6] Kidd, M., Paired helical filaments in electron microscopy of Alzheimer's disease. Nature, 1963. 197: p. 192-3.

[7] Wischik, C.M., et al., Structural characterization of the core of the paired helical filament of Alzheimer disease. Proc Natl Acad Sci U S A, 1988. 85(13): p. 4884-8.

[8] Crowther, R.A. and C.M. Wischik, Image reconstruction of the Alzheimer paired helical filament. Embo J, 1985. 4(13B): p. 3661-5.

[9] Kondo, J., et al., The carboxyl third of tau is tightly bound to paired helical filaments. Neuron, 1988. 1(9): p. 827-34.

[10] Lee, G., R.L. Neve, and K.S. Kosik, The microtubule binding domain of tau protein. Neuron, 1989. 2(6): p. 1615-24.

[11] Perry, G., et al., Ubiquitin is detected in neurofibrillary tangles and senile plaque neurites of Alzheimer disease brains. Proc Natl Acad Sci U S A, 1987. 84(9): p. 3033-6.

[12] Mori, H., J. Kondo, and Y. Ihara, Ubiquitin is a component of paired helical filaments in Alzheimer's disease. Science, 1987. 235(4796): p. 1641-4.

[13] Ledesma, M.D., P. Bonay, and J. Avila, Tau protein from Alzheimer's disease patients is glycated at its tubulin-binding domain. J Neurochem, 1995. 65(4): p. 1658-64.

[14] Ledesma, M.D., et al., Analysis of microtubule-associated protein tau glycation in paired helical filaments. J Biol Chem, 1994. 269(34): p. 21614-9.

[15] Wang, J.Z., I. Grundke-Iqbal, and K. Iqbal, Glycosylation of microtubule-associated protein tau: an abnormal posttranslational modification in Alzheimer's disease. Nat Med, 1996. 2(8): p. 871-5.

[16] Horiguchi, T., et al., Nitration of tau protein is linked to neurodegeneration in tauopathies. Am J Pathol, 2003. 163(3): p. 1021-31.

[17] Tucholski, J., J. Kuret, and G.V. Johnson, Tau is modified by tissue transglutaminase in situ: possible functional and metabolic effects of polyamination. J Neurochem, 1999. 73(5): p. 1871-80.

[18] Alonso, A.C., I. Grundke-Iqbal, and K. Iqbal, Alzheimer's disease hyperphosphorylated tau sequesters normal tau into tangles of filaments and disassembles microtubules. Nat Med, 1996. 2(7): p. 783-7.

[19] Alonso Adel, C., et al., Polymerization of hyperphosphorylated tau into filaments eliminates its inhibitory activity. Proc Natl Acad Sci U S A, 2006. 103(23): p. 8864-9.

[20] Novak, M., J. Kabat, and C.M. Wischik, Molecular characterization of the minimal protease resistant tau unit of the Alzheimer's disease paired helical filament. Embo J, 1993. 12(1): p. 365-70.

[21] Wischik, C.M., et al., Quantitative analysis of tau protein in paired helical filament preparations: implications for the role of tau protein phosphorylation in PHF assembly in Alzheimer's disease. Neurobiol Aging, 1995. 16(3): p. 409-17; discussion 418-31.

[22] Wischik, C.M., et al., Isolation of a fragment of tau derived from the core of the paired helical filament of Alzheimer disease. Proc Natl Acad Sci U S A, 1988. 85(12): p. 4506-10.

[23] Novak, M., Truncated tau protein as a new marker for Alzheimer's disease. Acta Virol, 1994. 38(3): p. 173-89.

[24] Novak, M., et al., Difference between the tau protein of Alzheimer paired helical filament core and normal tau revealed by epitope analysis of monoclonal antibodies 423 and 7.51. Proc Natl Acad Sci U S A, 1991. 88(13): p. 5837-41.

[25] Guillozet-Bongaarts, A.L., et al., Tau truncation during neurofibrillary tangle evolution in Alzheimer's disease. Neurobiol Aging, 2005. 26(7): p. 1015-22.

[26] Garcia-Sierra, F., et al., Conformational changes and truncation of tau protein during tangle evolution in Alzheimer's disease. J Alzheimers Dis, 2003. 5(2): p. 65-77.

[27] Garcia-Sierra, F., S. Mondragon-Rodriguez, and G. Basurto-Islas, Truncation of tau protein and its pathological significance in Alzheimer's disease. J Alzheimers Dis, 2008. 14(4): p. 401-9.

[28] Alonso, A., et al., Hyperphosphorylation induces self-assembly of tau into tangles of paired helical filaments/straight filaments. Proc Natl Acad Sci U S A, 2001. 98(12): p. 6923-8.

[29] Iqbal, K. and I. Grundke-Iqbal, Discoveries of tau, abnormally hyperphosphorylated tau and others of neurofibrillary degeneration: a personal historical perspective. J Alzheimers Dis, 2006. 9(3 Suppl): p. 219-42.

[30] Augustinack, J.C., et al., Specific tau phosphorylation sites correlate with severity of neuronal cytopathology in Alzheimer's disease. Acta Neuropathol, 2002. 103(1): p. 26-35.

[31] Novak, M., et al., Characterisation of the first monoclonal antibody against the pronase resistant core of the Alzheimer PHF. Prog Clin Biol Res, 1989. 317: p. 755-61.

[32] Garcia-Sierra, F., et al., Accumulation of C-terminally truncated tau protein associated with vulnerability of the perforant pathway in early stages of neurofibrillary pathology in Alzheimer's disease. J Chem Neuroanat, 2001. 22(1-2): p. 65-77.

[33] Wischik, C.M., Lay R.Y., Harrington C.R. , Modelling prion-like processing of tau protein in Alzheimer´s disease for pharmaceutical development., in Modifications in Alzheimer´s disease, B.R. Avila J., Kosik K.S., Editor 1997, Harwood Academic: Amsterdam. p. 185-241.

[34] Guillozet-Bongaarts, A.L., et al., Pseudophosphorylation of tau at serine 422 inhibits caspase cleavage: in vitro evidence and implications for tangle formation in vivo. J Neurochem, 2006. 97(4): p. 1005-14.

[35] Schneider, A., et al., Phosphorylation that detaches tau protein from microtubules (Ser262, Ser214) also protects it against aggregation into Alzheimer paired helical filaments. Biochemistry, 1999. 38(12): p. 3549-58.

[36] Arendt, T., et al., Reversible paired helical filament-like phosphorylation of tau is an adaptive process associated with neuronal plasticity in hibernating animals. J Neurosci, 2003. 23(18): p. 6972-81.

[37] Su, B., et al., Physiological regulation of tau phosphorylation during hibernation. J Neurochem, 2008. 105(6): p. 2098-108.

[38] Doherty, G.J. and H.T. McMahon, Mediation, modulation, and consequences of membrane-cytoskeleton interactions. Annu Rev Biophys, 2008. 37: p. 65-95.

[39] Morris, M., et al., The many faces of tau. Neuron, 2011. 70(3): p. 410-26.

[40] Weingarten, M.D., et al., A protein factor essential for microtubule assembly. Proc Natl Acad Sci U S A, 1975. 72(5): p. 1858-62.

[41] Witman, G.B., et al., Tubulin requires tau for growth onto microtubule initiating sites. Proc Natl Acad Sci U S A, 1976. 73(11): p. 4070-4.

[42] Harada, A., et al., Altered microtubule organization in small-calibre axons of mice lacking tau protein. Nature, 1994. 369(6480): p. 488-91.

[43] Dixit, R., et al., Differential regulation of dynein and kinesin motor proteins by tau. Science, 2008. 319(5866): p. 1086-9.

[44] Caceres, A. and K.S. Kosik, Inhibition of neurite polarity by tau antisense oligonucleotides in primary cerebellar neurons. Nature, 1990. 343(6257): p. 461-3.

[45] Neve, R.L., et al., Identification of cDNA clones for the human microtubule-associated protein tau and chromosomal localization of the genes for tau and microtubule-associated protein 2. Brain Res, 1986. 387(3): p. 271-80.

[46] Mandelkow, E.M., et al., Structure, microtubule interactions, and phosphorylation of tau protein. Ann N Y Acad Sci, 1996. 777: p. 96-106.

[47] Heicklen-Klein, A. and I. Ginzburg, Tau promoter confers neuronal specificity and binds Sp1 and AP-2. J Neurochem, 2000. 75(4): p. 1408-18.

[48] Andreadis, A., et al., A tau promoter region without neuronal specificity. J Neurochem, 1996. 66(6): p. 2257-63.

[49] Drubin, D., et al., Regulation of microtubule protein levels during cellular morphogenesis in nerve growth factor-treated PC12 cells. J Cell Biol, 1988. 106(5): p. 1583-91.

[50] Vila-Ortiz, G.J., et al., The rate of Tau synthesis is differentially regulated during postnatal development in mouse cerebellum. Cell Mol Neurobiol, 2001. 21(5): p. 535-43.

[51] David, D.C., et al., Proteasomal degradation of tau protein. J Neurochem, 2002. 83(1): p. 176-85.

[52] Delobel, P., et al., Proteasome inhibition and Tau proteolysis: an unexpected regulation. FEBS Lett, 2005. 579(1): p. 1-5.

[53] Dickey, C.A., et al., The high-affinity HSP90-CHIP complex recognizes and selectively degrades phosphorylated tau client proteins. J Clin Invest, 2007. 117(3): p. 648-58.

[54] Min, S.W., et al., Acetylation of tau inhibits its degradation and contributes to tauopathy. Neuron, 2010. 67(6): p. 953-66.

[55] Kenessey, A., et al., Degradation of tau by lysosomal enzyme cathepsin D: implication for Alzheimer neurofibrillary degeneration. J Neurochem, 1997. 69(5): p. 2026-38.

[56] Wang, Y., et al., Tau fragmentation, aggregation and clearance: the dual role of lysosomal processing. Hum Mol Genet, 2009. 18(21): p. 4153-70.

[57] Mena, R., et al., Staging the pathological assembly of truncated tau protein into paired helical filaments in Alzheimer's disease. Acta Neuropathol, 1996. 91(6): p. 633-41.

[58] Mena R., L.-M.J., Stages of pathological tau-protein processing in Alzheimer´s disease: From soluble aggregation to polymetization into insoluble tau-PHFs, in Currents Hypotheses and Research Milestones, R.B.M.a.G. Perry, Editor 2009. p. 79-91.

[59] Fasulo, L., Visintin M., Novak M., Cattaneo A., Tau truncation in Alzheimer´s disease: encompassing PHF core tau induces apoptosis ina COS cells. Alzheimes´s reports, 1998. 1: p. 25-32.

[60] Wischik, C.M., et al., Selective inhibition of Alzheimer disease-like tau aggregation by phenothiazines. Proceedings of the National Academy of Sciences of the United States of America, 1996. 93(20): p. 11213-8.

[61] Mena, R., et al., Monitoring pathological assembly of tau and beta-amyloid proteins in Alzheimer's disease. Acta Neuropathol, 1995. 89(1): p. 50-6.

[62] Fasulo, L., et al., The neuronal microtubule-associated protein tau is a substrate for caspase-3 and an effector of apoptosis. J Neurochem, 2000. 75(2): p. 624-33.

[63] Gamblin, T.C., et al., Caspase cleavage of tau: linking amyloid and neurofibrillary tangles in Alzheimer's disease. Proc Natl Acad Sci U S A, 2003. 100(17): p. 10032-7.

[64] Rissman, R.A., et al., Caspase-cleavage of tau is an early event in Alzheimer disease tangle pathology. J Clin Invest, 2004. 114(1): p. 121-30.

[65] Gamblin, T.C., et al., In vitro polymerization of tau protein monitored by laser light scattering: method and application to the study of FTDP-17 mutants. Biochemistry, 2000. 39(20): p. 6136-44.

[66] Horowitz, P.M., et al., N-terminal fragments of tau inhibit full-length tau polymerization in vitro. Biochemistry, 2006. 45(42): p. 12859-66.

[67] Luna-Munoz, J., et al., Earliest stages of tau conformational changes are related to the appearance of a sequence of specific phospho-dependent tau epitopes in Alzheimer's disease. J Alzheimers Dis, 2007. 12(4): p. 365-75.

[68] Castellani, R.J., et al., Phosphorylated tau: toxic, protective, or none of the above. J Alzheimers Dis, 2008. 14(4): p. 377-83.

[69] Nelson, P.T., H. Braak, and W.R. Markesbery, Neuropathology and cognitive impairment in Alzheimer disease: a complex but coherent relationship. Journal of neuropathology and experimental neurology, 2009. 68(1): p. 1-14.

[70] Abner, E.L., et al., "End-stage" neurofibrillary tangle pathology in preclinical Alzheimer's disease: fact or fiction? Journal of Alzheimer's disease : JAD, 2011. 25(3): p. 445-53.

[71] Lee, H.G., et al., Tau phosphorylation in Alzheimer's disease: pathogen or protector? Trends Mol Med, 2005. 11(4): p. 164-9.

[72] Cash, A.D., et al., Microtubule reduction in Alzheimer's disease and aging is independent of tau filament formation. Am J Pathol, 2003. 162(5): p. 1623-7.

[73] Paula-Barbosa, M., M.A. Tavares, and A. Cadete-Leite, A quantitative study of frontal cortex dendritic microtubules in patients with Alzheimer's disease. Brain research, 1987. 417(1): p. 139-42.

[74] Yuan, A., et al., Axonal transport rates in vivo are unaffected by tau deletion or overexpression in mice. J Neurosci, 2008. 28(7): p. 1682-7.

[75] Leroy, K., et al., Early axonopathy preceding neurofibrillary tangles in mutant tau transgenic mice. Am J Pathol, 2007. 171(3): p. 976-92.

[76] Jicha, G.A., et al., A conformation- and phosphorylation-dependent antibody recognizing the paired helical filaments of Alzheimer's disease. J Neurochem, 1997. 69(5): p. 2087-95.

[77] McMillan, P.J., et al., Truncation of tau at E391 promotes early pathologic changes in transgenic mice. Journal of neuropathology and experimental neurology, 2011. 70(11): p. 1006-19.

[78] Morsch, R., W. Simon, and P.D. Coleman, Neurons may live for decades with neurofibrillary tangles. J Neuropathol Exp Neurol, 1999. 58(2): p. 188-97.

[79] Guo, H., et al., Active caspase-6 and caspase-6-cleaved tau in neuropil threads, neuritic plaques, and neurofibrillary tangles of Alzheimer's disease. Am J Pathol, 2004. 165(2): p. 523-31.

[80] Lassmann, H., et al., Cell death in Alzheimer's disease evaluated by DNA fragmentation in situ. Acta Neuropathol, 1995. 89(1): p. 35-41.

[81] Kudo, W., et al., Inhibition of Bax protects neuronal cells from oligomeric Abeta neurotoxicity. Cell death & disease, 2012. 3: p. e309.

[82] Li, H.L., et al., Phosphorylation of tau antagonizes apoptosis by stabilizing beta-catenin, a mechanism involved in Alzheimer's neurodegeneration. Proc Natl Acad Sci U S A, 2007. 104(9): p. 3591-6.

[83] Luna-Munoz, J., et al., Regional conformational change involving phosphorylation of tau protein at the Thr231, precedes the structural change detected by Alz-50 antibody in Alzheimer's disease. J Alzheimers Dis, 2005. 8(1): p. 29-41.

Chapter 6

Pin1 Protects Against Alzheimer's Disease: One Goal, Multiple Mechanisms

Lucia Pastorino, Asami Kondo, Xiao Zhen Zhou and Kun Ping Lu

Additional information is available at the end of the chapter

http://dx.doi.org/10.5772/55085

1. Introduction

1.1. Plaque and tangle pathology in AD

Alzheimer's disease (AD] is the most common form of dementia, and it accounts for more than 60% of all cases of dementia. Although many factors may increase the risk for AD, the only cause so far known is aging [1]. Most of the cases are sporadic, as only less than 0.1% of the cases occur because of inherited mutations on genes directly involved in the disease (familial AD, FAD] [2].

AD is caused by progressive and irreversible neurodegeneration. At the moment, there is no cure for AD. Therapies available are only aimed at lessening the progression of the cognitive decline and neurodegeneration and do not target pathways directly causative of the disease [3]. These include the acetylcholinesterase inhibitors (Aricept] [4] or inhibitors of the glutamatergic NMDA receptor (Namenda] [5] and were shown to be mostly effective when administered at early stages [6-8]. However, a proper diagnostic approach able to identify AD early in the development is still missing, and this reduces the efficacy of the treatments available. Therefore, there is the need to develop both diagnostic tools able to detect early stages of the disease, and to generate effective treatments targeting the early pathogenic events in AD. This is becoming increasingly important also considering that the population affected by AD will dramatically increase in the years to come. Numbers are in fact dramatic: 10 million baby boomers may develop AD within the next 10-20 years [9]. Currently, in the United States alone there are more than 5 million AD patients, and the costs to the US government exceeds the 200 billion/year.These numbers are expected to quadruple in the next 40 years, causing unsustainable costs for the care of these patients and their caregivers, who could not receive support and care and would then have to face undignified life conditions.

Studying the molecular mechanisms responsible for the neurodegeneration in AD can help identify new effective therapeutic targets. Two main pathways are identified in AD. They involve two proteins, the amyloid precursor protein APP and the microtubule-associated protein tau, as they are responsible for the formation of the two characteristic lesions, the extracellular plaques and the intracellular neurofibrillary tangles (NFTs], respectively [10, 11]. Both plaques and tangles are considered causative of the disease; they deposit following the progression of the disease, and they could contribute to alter neuronal morphology leading to neuronal death [12-16].

The origin and composition of plaques and tangles are quite different. Plaques are forms of aggregated, fibrillar material called amyloid, insoluble fibrous protein aggregations organized in β-sheet strands that deposits in the outer part of the brain [17-19]. Their core is mainly composed of Abeta (beta-amyloid], a peptide of small molecular weight deriving from APP, which tends to form small size aggregates called oligomers with known toxic properties [20]. Oligomers are found intracellularly, but can be secreted to the extracellular space, where they will aggregate into larger structures called fibrils, forming the core of the plaque [18, 21, 22].

Similarly, tangles are formed by insoluble structures organized into fibrils, the pair helical filaments (PHFs], which eventually organize and aggregate into larger structures, the tangles [19]. The main component is hyperphosphorylated protein tau, which in this form becomes insoluble and tends to form aggregates [13, 23].

The biological functions of APP and tau are very different [13, 24], but during the disease both the beta amyloid product and the hyperphosphorylated tau become toxic to the neuron, causing neurodegeneration. However, the mechanisms by which tau and Abeta may be toxic differ. In fact, as a microtubule stabilizing protein, tau can become toxic to the cytoskeleton when hyperphosphorylated, as in this form it would detach from the microtubules destabilizing them. Hyperphosphorylated tau would also tend to aggregate into NFTs, impairing cellular functions [23]. As to the plaques, their mechanism of toxicity is still under debate. Although they cause the formation of dystrophic neuritis [18], it is still unclear whether they are really toxic or rather protecting, by sequestering Abeta oligomers from the environment. In facts, Abeta is sequestered from the extracellular space to form the plaque [25]. Indeed, oligomers are considered toxic: they form early in the pathology [26], associate with impaired cognitive functions in mice [27] and in AD patients [28], and impair neurotransmission [29-33]. Therefore, identifying the pathways that lead to both increased Abeta production and/or tau hyperphosphorylation and also regulate their aggregation into organized insoluble structure may dramatically help find a cure to treat AD.

1.2. Pin1–regulated protein isomerization as a mechanism to control tangle and plaque pathologies

Protein phosphorylation seems to be a common feature of both plaque and tangle pathologies. In fact, changes in the levels of phosphorylated APP seems to influence APP function and toxicity in the pathology, as increased phosphorylation of APP at specific domains positively regulates Abeta production [34-36]. Of note, both APP and tau can be phosphorylated by the same kinases, such as cdc2, CDK5 and GSK3, and such kinases seem to be particularly active

http://dx.doi.org/10.5772/55085

during the disease [23, 37-40]. Hence, the identification of molecular pathways that can control non physiologic phosphorylation of both tau and APP in the disease could help identify targets to tackle at the same time both tangle and plaque pathologies.

We found that the enzyme Pin1 protects from both tangle and Abeta pathology, since a genetically modified animal model lacking Pin1 (Pin1KO] developed age-dependent tauopathy and was characterized by increased production of Abeta, deposited in form of intracellular aggregates [41, 42]. This seems to be due to the capability of Pin1 to regulate the conformation of cis and trans isomers of both phosphorylated tau and APP, as shown using conformation specific antibodies for tau, and by means of NMR.

Pin1 (Protein interacting with NIMA (never in mitosis A]-1] is a prolyl isomerase, which regulates the function of phosphorylated protein substrates by regulating their cis/trans isomerization [43, 44]. Pin1 belongs to the family of PPIase (peptidyl prolyl cis trans isomerase], enzymes that are evolutionary conserved. Unlike other PPIases, Pin1 specifically regulates the conformation of substrates phosphorylated at specific serine or threonine residues preceding a proline (S/T-P motifs] [45-47]. The stereochemistry of Proline allows the protein to undergo two different conformations (cis and trans], which could be determined by the presence of a phospho group on the S or T residue [43, 48]. Since Proline-directed phosphorylation regulates key cellular mechanisms, by maintaining the equilibrium between the two conformations, Pin1 may dramatically contribute to the maintenance of vital cellular functions.

The structure of Pin1 consists of two domains, an N-terminal WW domain comprised of the first 40 aminoacids which is responsible for Pin1 binding to its substrates, and a larger PPIase domain that spans the remaining part of the protein and catalyzes the substrate's isomerization [49]. Of note, although mostly in the nucleus, Pin1 subcellular localization is driven by the presence of its substrates [50], to extranuclear compartments, with obvious expression in the plasma membrane, cytosol and cytosolic organelles involved in endocytosis [41, 51]. The ubiquitous expression of Pin1 allows the protein to control the isomerization of multiple substrates in different cellular compartments, including cytosolic proteins like NF-KappaB [52], p53 [53], beta-catenin [54], IRAK1 [55] and others [46], or protein that localize at different compartments like APP [41, 51] and tau [42, 56]. This determines a crucial role for Pin1 in controlling the physiological activity of proteins involved in diverse functions, such as protein transcription and stability, and protein interaction, by regulating the aforementioned substrates [43].

Notably, Pin1 function is highly regulated and its aberration affects Pin1's ability to isomerize its substrates with consequences on their function, contributing to an increasing number of pathological conditions, including Alzheimer's disease, cancer and immunologic disorders and aging. Lack of Pin1 function was found to impair immune responses in Pin1KO animal models [55], due to lack of activation of IRAK1, which is involved in the regulation of the TLR signaling [57]. In cancer, Pin1 levels are increased due to transcriptional activation and loss of inhibitory phosphorylation and other mechanisms [45, 58]. This leads to up-regulated isomerization of substrates involved in hyperproliferative processes, activating two dozens of oncogenes and inactivating a dozen of tumor suppressors [46, 59, 60]. On the contrary, in AD brain Pin1 activity is reduced due to decreased protein level and to oxidation [56, 61, 62]. Some genetic polymorphisms on the Pin1 gene were found to associate with forms of late onset AD [63-65]. Interestingly, a polymorphism that associated with increased Pin1 levels by regulating AP-4 mediated transcription, was found to be protective as it correlates with delayed disease onset in a Chinese cohort [66]. In AD, the changes in Pin1 levels and activity prevent from an effective isomerization of the phosphorylated APP and tau [41, 56]. As a consequence, the equilibrium between the cis and trans conformation is not maintained and the proteins exist in the pathogenic cis conformation: APP will generate more Abeta and tau will lose normal microtubule function and become toxic, leading to both plaque and tangle pathologies.

In this book chapter we will discuss findings from our and other labs that point to a crucial role of Pin1 in protecting against AD by regulating diverse cellular pathways using multiple mechanisms. We will specifically highlight how Pin1 regulates protein conformation of APP and tau to control APP trafficking, APP stability and Abeta production as well as tau phosphorylation, microtubule function, stabilization and aggregation in vivo and in vitro. We will also emphasize the importance of Pin1-mediated regulation of APP and tau conformation as a modulator of pathogenic mechanisms that might occur early in the development of the disease. Finally, we will also discuss how Pin1 is emerging as a novel diagnostic and therapeutic tool for early intervention to tackle both tau and Abeta pathologies in AD.

2. Pin1 as a crucial regulator of APP trafficking and stabilization to protect from Abeta pathology in AD

Although both tau and Abeta pathologies define AD, only Abeta is the characteristic feature that distinguishes AD from other forms of dementia. In fact, only the presence of plaques containing Abeta peptide allows a definite AD diagnosis [10,67-69], whereas the presence of PHF alone could be related also to other forms of tauopathies, like FTPD, Pick disease and others [13]. The specificity of Abeta pathology to AD makes of Abeta and its precursor APP ideal therapeutic targets. Here we will review the role of APP in AD, the molecular mechanisms that regulate Abeta formation, focusing on the role of Pin1 as a post-phosphorylative event to regulate both APP intracellular localization and trafficking, and also turnover, preventing Abeta formation. These topics are of particular relevance for the understanding of the mechanisms underlying Abeta production in AD. In fact, the intracellular localization of APP will determine whether APP will be toxic influencing the production of beta-amyloid peptides. Moreover, impaired APP turnover will cause APP stabilization, which will lead to increased levels of both APP and beta-amyloid peptides. Thisphenomenon is particularly consistent with pathologies associated with higher levels of APP and development of AD, such as Down syndrome.

2.1. APP trafficking and processing pathways

APP is a type 1 transmembrane protein that is ubiquitously expressed. APP is characterized by a long extracellular domain, a short transmembrane domain and a small intracellular domain that regulates APP phosphorylation and trafficking [68, 70]. The domain that contains the sequence for Abeta spans a region of approximately 40 aminoacids across the N-terminal portion of the trasmembrane domain [71]. Three isoforms of APP exists characterized by different molecular weight, the result of alternative RNA splicing, APP751, APP750 and APP695 [72]. Since the splicing occurs in the most N-terminal region of the protein, all the three isoforms express the domains for both Abeta and the intracellular domain [72]. APP isoforms may be differently expressed in the various organs. AP770 is for example mostly present in the heart and in peripheral cells, whereas APP695 is the only form expressed in the brain and therefore linked to Abeta generation in AD [72]. For this reason, the APP isoform considered in AD studies is APP695, and the numbering of the aminoacids follows this sequence.

Within the cell, APP localization is not limited to a single part, as it undergoes trafficking through different compartments. Upon synthesis in the ER, APP travels through the Golgi compartment where it undergoes glycosylation, to finally reach the plasma membrane. It eventually will recycle to the Golgi, following internalization from the plasma membrane and trafficking through the endosomal pathway [70, 73, 74]. Of note, the significance of APP physiological function may depend on the compartment where APP localizes during the life of the cell. In fact, depending on whether APP is retained at the plasma membrane or it is internalized to the endosomes, it will generate different metabolites with diverse function, either neurotrophic and therefore protective from AD, or toxic. More in details, at the plasma membrane APP will undergo a processing pathway called non-amyloidogenic [75, 76], in which metalloproteases of the ADAMs family and others (ADAM10, ADAM17 and TACE [77-81]], called alpha secretase, will cleave APP in the middle of the sequence for Abeta, generating the extracellular stub alphaAPPs with known neurotrophic properties [82], and a C-terminal stub called C83. C83 will be further cleaved in the late endosomes by a complex of four proteins called gamma-secretase, to generate a small fragment called p3 with no amyloidogenic properties. This pathway is called non-amyloidogenic, as it prevents the formation of intact Abeta peptides. The amount of APP at the plasma membrane that does not undergo alpha-secretase cleavage will internalize in the cell through the endocytic pathway [70, 73, 74]. This occurs thanks to the binding of proteins such as Fe65 to the 682YNPTY687 motif at the intracellular, C-terminal domain of APP [83-85]. Once in the early endosomes, full length APP is cleaved by BACE or beta secretase [86, 87], an aspartyl protease that cuts APP at the beginning of the sequence for Abeta. Such cleavage generates a soluble stub called betaAPPs with known apoptotic properties in the neuron [88], and a C-terminal stub called C99 which still contains the intact sequence for Abeta. C99 will traffic to the late endosomes, where it will be cleaved by gamma-secretase to generate intact Abeta [17, 89]. This pathway is called amyloidogenic as it produces Abeta peptides, and is increased in AD [90, 91].

It is clear that the intracellular localization of APP will determine whether APP will be amyloidogenic or not. Therefore, any mechanism that may help APP stay retained at the plasma membrane will protect from Abeta production and AD, whereas those that help APP internalize to the endosomes will favor the amyloidogenic processing and Abeta formation.

2.2. APP phosphorylation and conformation to regulate APP processing

One such mechanism is APP phosphorylation. In fact, it was shown that the Y682 residue can be phosphorylated by different kinases such as abl and TrkA [92, 93]. Phosphorylation at this level can regulate the association of APP to binding partners such as Fe65, X11/MINTs and Shc [94-97], ultimately controlling APP trafficking, processing and function also associated with cell movement and axonal branching [98, 99], and with NGF activity [100]. Tyr phosphorylation at Y682 motif has also been associated with increased Abeta production and amyloidogenic processing in vitro [101], in vivo [102] and in AD [103].

Interestingly, APP can be phosphorylated at a further N-terminal part of the intracellular domain, the 668Thr-669Pro residue [104], and phosphorylation at this domain has been associated with increased amyloidogenic processing of APP, both in vivo [39, 40] and in vitro [34]. The kinases involved in such phosphorylation are GSK3beta, CDK5, cdc2, known to be overactive in AD and responsible also for tau phosphorylation [23, 38, 39, 104, 105]. Of note, T668 phosphorylation was found to be elevated in AD brain [34], suggesting that it might induce toxic mechanisms linked to Abeta production. Such mechanisms seemed to relate to conformational changes affecting the 682YNPTY687 motif and therefore its ability to interact with binding partners [106, 107]. In support of this hypothesis, T668 has been linked to specific isomer formation. In fact, by means of NMR studies, it was observed that phosphorylation at the Thr668 residue causes an isomerization of APP from trans to cis. In fact, non-phosphorylated APP retains 100% trans conformation, and upon phosphorylation at T668 approximately 10% of the population turns to cis [108, 109].

Altogether, these findings draw attention to the role of T668 phosphorylation as an initiator of molecular pathways that lead to Abeta production by regulating APP conformation, trafficking and processing. They also suggest that different cis and trans APP isomers may contribute to shift the processing of APP towards either the amyloidogenic or the non-amyloidogenic processing, and therefore T668 phosphorylation may emerge as a potential target to halt amyloidogenic pathways in AD.

2.3. Pin1 to protect from Abeta pathology in animal models

Based on these findings and on the capability of Pin1 to protect from tau pathology by regulating tau conformation [42, 56], we hypothesized that Pin1 might regulate also the conformation of APP protecting from Abeta pathology. We found that Pin1 can bind to phosphorylated APP at T668, maintains the equilibrium between cis and trans conformation, ultimately shifting the processing of APP from the toxic amyloidogenic to the protective non-amyloidogenic [41].

More in detail, by means of pull down experiments, we observed that Pin1 can bind to APP only if phosphorylated at T668 [41]. Such interaction regulates APP isomerization. In fact, using a pentapetide containing part of the C-terminal domain and the T668-P motif, we observed that Pin1 isomerizes the conformation of this peptide from cis to trans 1000 times faster than the reversed equilibrium, suggesting that shifting the isomerization towards the trans conformation may be crucial for APP function, and that Pin1 might be key to regulate APP physiologic activity. We then tested whether altering the equilibrium between cis and trans conformation might result in changes of APP functions. For this purpose, we manipulated Pin1 cellular levels either by knocking Pin1 out in genetically modified animals (Pin1KO], or by overexpressing Pin1 in cultured cells. Our in vitro experiments showed that when levels of

Pin1 were elevated beyond physiologic, APP amyloidogenic processing would be reduced, as Abeta levels were decreased in the media of the cultured cells. On the contrary, lack of Pin1 expression in cultured Pin1KO breast cancer cells resulted in decreased alphaAPPs secretion and increased Abeta production. Similarly, in the brain of Pin1KO mice we could observe age-dependent increase of Abeta production, since levels of aggregated insoluble Abeta were elevated in 18 months old mice when compared to 5 months old mice.

We then crossed PinKO animals to APPtg2576 and studied the processing of APP. We observed an age-dependent shift in the processing of APP that would result in an increase of the amyloidogenic versus the non-amyloidogenic, paralleled by the accumulation of Abeta42 deposits in multivesicular bodies, a form of deposited Abeta associated with early stages of AD [32, 33]. This led us to hypothesize a model in which Pin1 would protect against neurodegeneration possibly by maintaining the equilibrium between the cis and the trans conformation of APP. In particular, in physiological conditions, Pin1 would favor the trans conformation of APP, increasing the non-amylodogenic processing. Vice versa in the absence of Pin1, the cis form would accumulate as the isomerization between the two forms would be lost, ultimately favoring the amyloidogenic processing.

2.4. Pin1 inhibits APP trafficking and internalization

Because Pin1 was found to localize with full length APP at the plasma membrane, we speculated that Pin1 may be involved in APP trafficking and internalization, regulating the amount of APP that undergoes amyloidogenic processing. We therefore tested the hypothesis whether Pin1 protects from Abeta formation by inhibiting APP internalization to amyloidogenic compartments [51]. For this purpose we used brain derived human H4 neuroglioma cells expressing APP either at endogenous level or stably overexpressing it, and Pin1 expression was knocked down by RNAi. We found that lower Pin1 levels associated with i) decreased levels of APP at the plasma membrane, ii) increased levels of betaAPPs and decreased alphaAPPs and iii) increased kinetic of internalization, as evidenced by means of immunocytochemistry in both fixed and living cells [51]. Levels of APP phosphoryated at T668 seemed to be elevated too. These data are in agreement with data from other groups that propose a toxic role of T688 phosphorylated APP [34], and may suggest that reduced Pin1 levels could be toxic in the same pathways. Interestingly, Ando and colleagues suggested that phosphorylation at T668 may affect APP conformation to ultimately alter the capability of APP to bind to partners such as Fe65 regulating APP trafficking, even if such interaction occurs at the 682YNPTY687 domain, further C-terminal than T668 [106]. This effect could be related to Pin1-mediated changes in APP conformation that could change the 682YNPTY687 stereochemistry. Of note, in Pin1 KD treated cells that were also overexpressing Fe65, we found that higher amounts of Fe65 associated with APP and that C99 accumulated, as compared to wild type cells. This was probably due to stabilization of Fe65 under these conditions, since Fe65 levels were elevated at the steady state in Pin1KD cells. Together with our immunocytochemistry data, under conditions that promote Fe65/APP interaction, these results suggest that reduced Pin1 expression may be linked to fastened internalization of APP to amyloidogenic compartments, where C99 is produced and accumulates (Fig. 1).

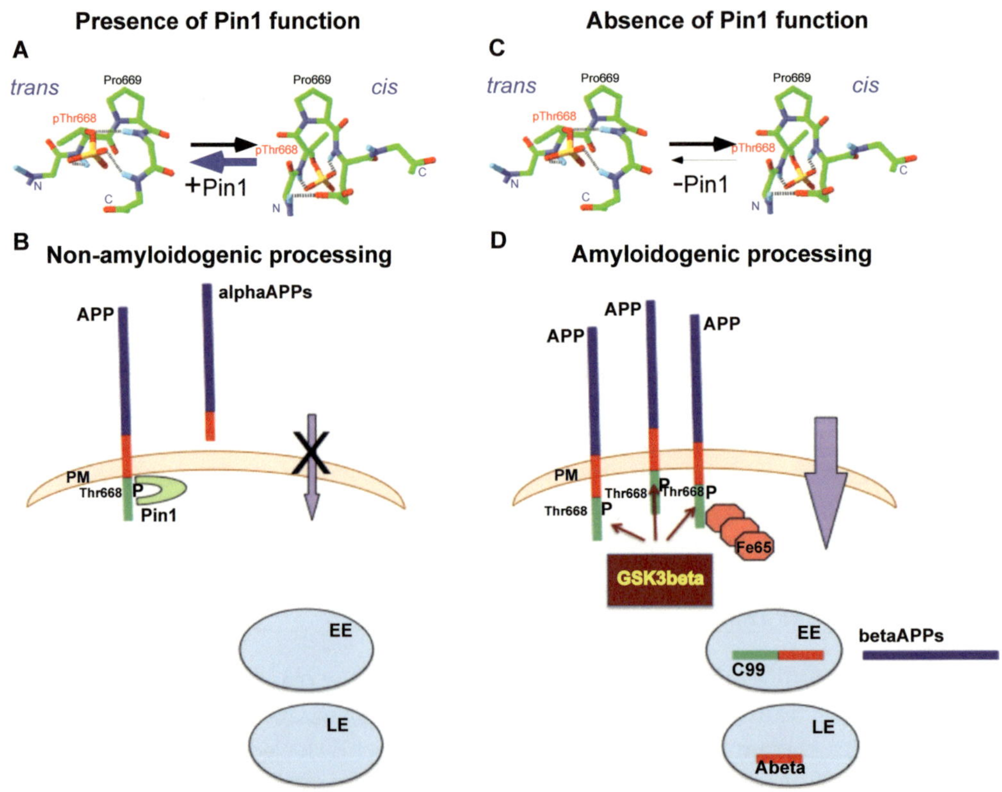

Our hypothesis is that Pin1 binds to and isomerizes the phosphorylated T668-Pro motif in full length APP, resulting in protein conformational changes that ultimately affect APP intracellular trafficking. (A, B]. In the presence of proper Pin1 function, the equilibrium between the cis and the trans form of phosphorylated APP is maintained [41] (A], and this may help APP stay anchored at the plasma membrane where it will undergo the non-amyloidogenic processing (B]. On the contrary, when Pin1 function is reduced, as in AD, the equilibrium between the cis and the trans form of phosphorylated APP will be disrupted, as the cis form of phosphorylated APP would not be isomerized to trans in a timely manner (C], and the levels of Fe65 will be stabilized. Moreover, reduced Pin1 function will enhance GSK3beta activity, leading to overall increase of phosphorylated APP at T668 and inhibiting APP turnover. These effects may lead to overall increased levels of APP undergoing internalization, trafficking and amyloidogenic processing (D]. PM: Plasma membrane. EE: Early Endosomes. LE: Late Endosomes.

Figure 1. A model for the role of Pin1 in inhibiting APP accumulation and amyloidogenic processing.

We had previously observed that reduced Pin1 expression is linked to Abeta production [41], and we found that Pin1KD may increase gamma-secretase cleavage of APP to generate AICD [51]. Hence, we could assume that AD-associated reduced Pin1 expression is linked to increased amyloidogenic processing, promoting both internalization and gamma-secretase dependent cleavage of APP.

2.5. Pin1 increases APP protein turnover

Recent findings from our lab link Pin1 deficit and amyloidogenic processing in AD to increased APP stabilization [110]. This is particularly relevant to a role of increased APP in the disease, as it is known that higher APP levels correlate with AD. In fact, genetic modifications causing either duplication of the APP gene [111] or increased expression [112] were found to cause familial early onset AD. In addition, in Down syndrome patients, the triplication of the APP gene associates with the development of AD after age 40 [113], with the exception of those individuals affected by partial trisomy excluding the APP region [114]. In our experimental paradigm, such APP stabilization is caused by the lack of GSK3beta inhibition under conditions of impaired Pin1 activity. This may suggest that lack of Pin1 in AD impacts Abeta pathology by targeting multiple pathways, from APP trafficking to APP stabilization via GSK3beta activation.

More in details, we found that GSK3beta inhibitory mechanism was decreased in Pin1KO mice [110], since phoshorylation at S9, a mechanism that inhibits the kinase's activity, was decreased in these mice. We speculated that GSK3beta, which contains several Ser-Pro motifs, might serve as a substrate of Pin1 and that, by regulating GSK3beta conformation, Pin1 could control GSK3beta activity. This mechanism would contribute to the understanding of a link between loss of Pin1 activity and APP and tau pathologies in AD. GSK3beta in fact is responsible for the phosphorylation of both T668 in APP and T231 in tau, crucial in determining toxic conformations of both proteins in the disease. We found that Pin1 binds to GSK3beta at the T330 residue, and that lack of phosphorylation at this site using a T330A mutant would prevent such interaction. Of note, changes in Pin1 levels would affect GSK3beta activity, in vivo and in vitro. In fact, in crude brain lysates from Pin1Tg mice, GSK3beta activity was decreased, whereas it increased in Pin1KO mice. Similarly, overexpression of a wild type form of Pin1 reduced GSK3beta activity in H4 cells, whereas overexpression of mutants in regulatory regions of Pin1 such as the WW (W34A) or at the PPIase (K63A) domains, or at the Pin1 binding site (T330A) would not induce any change in the kinase activity, suggesting that by binding to T330, Pin1 is a crucial negative regulator of GSK3beta activity.

We then tested the hypothesis whether the Pin1-mediated control of GSK3beta activity could help prevent APP from entering the amyloidogenic processing. We found that lack of Pin1-mediated regulation of GSK3beta activity in T330A mutant expressing H4 cells reduced the levels of the non-amyloidogenic alphaAPPs, whereas it increased overall T668 APP phosphorylation. Of note, under these conditions, levels of APP were elevated at the steady state in cells, as well as in mice Pin1 concentration regulated APP levels. In fact, APP was reduced in Pin1Tg mice, whereas it accumulated in the brain of Pin1KO mice, similarly to what we had previously observed [41]. We found that APP accumulation in Pin1KO mice or in Pin1KD cells is the result of a failed physiologic degradation of APP, which is stabilized under these conditions. In fact, by means of cycloheximide treatment, we tested APP turnover under conditions of either reduced Pin1 expression (Pin1KD cells) or in absence of Pin1-mediated regulation of GSK3beta activity, in cells overexpressing the T330A mutant. We found not only that APP was stabilized in Pin1 KD cells as compared to wild type cells, also such stabilization seemed to depend on Pin1-mediated regulation of GSK3beta activity, since APP was stabilized in cells overexpressing the GSK3beta mutant T330A as compared to cells GSK3beta wild type.

Altogether, these data suggest that Pin1 regulates APP turnover by inhibiting GSK3beta activation and therefore contributes to lower T668 phosphorylation, which is responsible for toxic conformations of APP, as previously discussed in this chapter. These evidences suggest that in the pathology, mechanisms that favor the accumulation of APP will be toxic by increasing the amount of APP that will undergo amyloidogenic processing, and lack of Pin1 function could be one of these (Fig.1). Therefore, Pin1-mediated GSK3beta activity is an additional mechanism that Pin1 uses to protect from Abeta pathology, and strengthen the possibility to consider Pin1 as a valid tool to target Abeta pathologies in AD.

3. Role of T668 phosphorylation and APP conformation in AD: Pin1 as a molecular switch to regulate APP function

The question how increased APP phosphorylation at T668 is linked to AD has raised a real debate in the field. Many evidences point to a role in the disease. In fact, not only phospho-T668 levels were increased in AD brains [34], also many studies in vitro and in vivo point to a role of T668 phosphorylation by different kinases in altered protein transport in neurons [115, 116], also associated with increased amyloidogenic processing and Abeta production in cellular and animal models [34, 36, 39, 117]. In these studies, a non-phosphorylatable mutant T668A was used as an experimental paradigm to compare the effects of phosphorylated endogenous APP to the non-phosphorylated T668A form. Interestingly, a knock-in T668A animal model did not show any age-dependent alteration in APP processing [118], since in this study levels of Abeta, alphaAPPs and betaAPPs were comparable in both T668A and wild type mice during aging. Although at a first glance these data seem to challenge the hypothesis that regulation of T668 phosphorylation might be involved in AD, from these data it cannot be concluded that such phosphorylation is irrelevant to AD progression. It is not by abolishing APP phosphorylation at T668 by either knocking out APP or knocking in a non-phosphorylatable version of it that we can exclude a role for such pathway in the disease. APP KO mice are viable and their development and aging does not rely on alterations of APP processing [119, 120], and yet a role for APP in the development of AD is not disputed. Similarly, tau KO mice develop properly, reach adulthood and age normally [121-123], however a role for hyperphosphorylated tau in AD is quite clear.

It is possible that the controversy around the role of T668 phosphorylation in AD lies in the fact that physiologic phosphorylation at this domain is low, and it is only elevated in AD. This would explain why the T668A knock in mice did not show any difference from the wild type [118], because basal levels of phosphorylated T668 APP are very low, and phosphorylation-mediated regulation of APP activity in wild type mice was therefore comparable to the T668A mutant mice in this study.

Based on our data in vivo in Pin1KO mice and in vitro in Pin1KD cells [41, 51], we could hypothesize that the relevance of physiological T668 phosphorylation could be to maintain allow the equilibrium between cis and trans conformation. We could also assume that reduced Pin1 levels or increased T668 phosphorylation, both conditions associated with AD [34, 56],

http://dx.doi.org/10.5772/55085

may disturb such equilibrium leading to increased Abeta production. Of note, the overexpression in Pin1KO breast cancer cells of a T668A APP mutant, which retains 100% trans conformation, rescued the amount of APP anchored at the plasma membrane, and also the levels of alphaAPPs [51]. These data may suggest that the protective non-amyloidogenic processing of APP is maintained only if APP is in the trans conformation, a conditions that associates with physiologic low levels of phosphorylated T668 and to physiologic levels of Pin1. This poses attention on protein isomerization and Pin1 as a fine post-phosphorylative tool to regulate a protein function, bypassing the regulation of the kinases. Targeting abnormal protein isomerization and Pin1 function may therefore offer a preferred approach in AD to halt the toxic effects of hyperphosphorylated proteins, such as phosphorylated T668 APP and T231 tau, instead of the pharmacological inhibition of the many kinases responsible for their phosphorylation.

Altogether, the data discussed here emphasize a role for Pin1-mediated isomerization of APP and GSK3beta as a mechanism to control APP physiologic function, shifting APP processing toward the non-amyloidogenic pathway (Fig.1). Such regulation prevents the formation of toxic species produced downstream the amyloidogenic pathway, such as Abeta and betaAPPs, by regulating both APP trafficking and stabilization, and occurs as a post-phosphorylative event to maintain the equilibrium between cis and trans conformations. Therefore, Pin1 and regulation of APP conformation emerge as ideal candidates in the search of therapeutic targets for AD.

4. Pin1 and tau pathology in animal models and in AD

Tau-mediated neurodegeneration may result from the combination of toxic gains-of-function acquired by the aggregates or their precursors and the detrimental effects that arise from the loss of the normal function(s) of tau in the disease state [15]. The toxic gains-of-function includes sequestration of normal tau function by NFTs made of hyperphosphorylated tau. NFTs also become physical obstacles to the transport of vesicles and other cargos[15]. The loss of the normal function of tau includes detachment of tau from microtubules that causes loss of microtubule-stabilizing function [124]. Although dynamic tau phosphorylation occurs during embryonic development [125], aberrant tau phosphorylation in mature neurons is harmful to the neuron [126]. Tau hyperphosphorylation is a key regulatory mechanism that leads to both such toxic gains-of-function and the loss of the normal function(s) of tau [15].

4.1. Prolyl isomerization of tau

A high proportion of prolines residues are common to intrinsically disordered proteins, and tau is no exception [127]. Nearly 10% of full-length tau is composed of proline residues and around 20% of the residues between I151 and Q244 are proline. Many functions of tau are mediated through microtubule (MT) binding domains distal to this proline-rich domain. Interestingly, many disease-associated phosphorylation events that seed tau tangle formation occur at proline-directed serine (S) and threonine (T) residues in this proline-rich region. This indicates that important structural changes in the proline-rich region of tau are regulating tangle formation. In particular, cis-trans isomerization around these prolines modulates protein phosphatase binding and activity at specific S/T sites. We discovered that Pin1 regulates tau phosphorylation in concert with protein phosphatase 2A (PP2A) especially at T231 [42, 56, 128-130]. Findings by Dickey's group suggest that FKBP51 has a similar activity to Pin1; but unlike Pin1, FKBP51 coordinates with Hsp90 to isomerize tau [131].

4.2. Deletion of Pin1 causes tauopathy in mice

Pin1 knockout (KO) mice [42] serve as a good model to investigate the effect of Pin1 on endogenous tau *in vivo*. Pin1-deficient mice showed progressive age-dependent motor and behavioral deficits including abnormal limb-clasping reflexes, hunched postures and reduced mobility [42] similar to tau transgenic mice [132, 133]. These phenotypes in Pin1 mutant mice are significant because the total level of NFTs correlates with the degree of cognitive impairment [134, 135]. Pioneering studies that used immunohistochemical techniques to determine the level of both NFTs and senile plaques in different brain regions of AD patients, as well as non-demented elderly individuals, demonstrated that the number of NFTs, but not the numbers of senile plaques, correlates with the degree of cognitive impairment [134, 135].

4.3. Pin1 acts on the pT231–P motif in p–tau to protect against tauopathy in AD

It is increasingly evident that tauopathy in AD may result from the combination of toxic gains-of function acquired by phosphorylated tau (p-tau) aggregates, and the malignant effects from loss of tau normal function, including the failure of p-tau to bind and promote microtubule (MT) assembly [15]. Interestingly, a common characteristic event that disrupts tau MT function and precedes tangle formation is increased phosphorylation of tau especially on S/T-P motifs [11, 126, 136-141]. Indeed, tau kinases, such as mitogen-activated protein (MAP) kinases, cyclin-dependent protein kinase 5 (CDK5) and glycogen synthase 3 (GSK3) [142-144] or phosphatases, such as protein phosphatase 2A (PP2A) [145, 146] are deregulated in AD and modulating these enzymes can affect tauopathy [23, 39, 147-155]. Moreover, recent GWAS studies identify several new AD genes that might modulate tau phosphorylation and/or cytoskeleton, including MARK4 (pro-directed tau kinase) and BIN1 [156], and CD2AP [157, 158]. Notably, T231 phosphorylation in tau is reported to be the first of a number of tau phosphoepitopes appearing sequentially during early stages in pretangle AD neurons: pT231 → TG3 → AT8 → AT100 → Alz50 →→ NFTs. However, it is still unclear how this phosphorylation leads to tau misfolding, aggregation and tangle formation [130, 159-161]. The results from our group and others support a critical role for Pin1 in protecting against tauopathy in AD by acting on the phosphorylated T231-P (pT231-P)motif (Fig.2). We discovered that pT231-P motif in tau exists in distinct cis and trans conformations, and that the cis to trans conversion is accelerated by a unique isomerase, Pin1 [44, 56, 128, 162], thereby protecting against tangle formation in AD [42, 48, 56, 163, 164]. pT231 is the first of sequential tau phosphoepitopes appearing in pretangle neurons in prodromal AD [159, 160] and its cerebrospinal fluid (CSF) level is an early biomarker that tracks MCI (mild cognitive impairment) conversion to AD, albeit with wide interindividual variations [165, 166]. Pin1 acts on the pT231-P motif in tau (i) to restore the ability of p-tau to promote MT assembly [56], (ii) to facilitate p-

http://dx.doi.org/10.5772/55085

tau dephosphorylation because PP2A is trans-specific [42, 128], and (iii) to promote p-tau degradation [164] (Fig.2). Indeed, Pin1 overexpression promotes tau dephosphorylation selectively on pT231 in neurons and mouse brains [167, 168]. Pin1 has no effect on T231A mutant tau in vitro or vivo [56, 128, 139, 164]. Furthermore, Pin1 deficiency (Pin1-KO) mice display age-dependent tauopathy [42], whereas Pin1 overexpression in postnatal neurons effectively suppresses tauopathy induced by human wild-type (WT) tau in mice, albeit it enhances tauopathy induced by the P301L mutant tau [164].

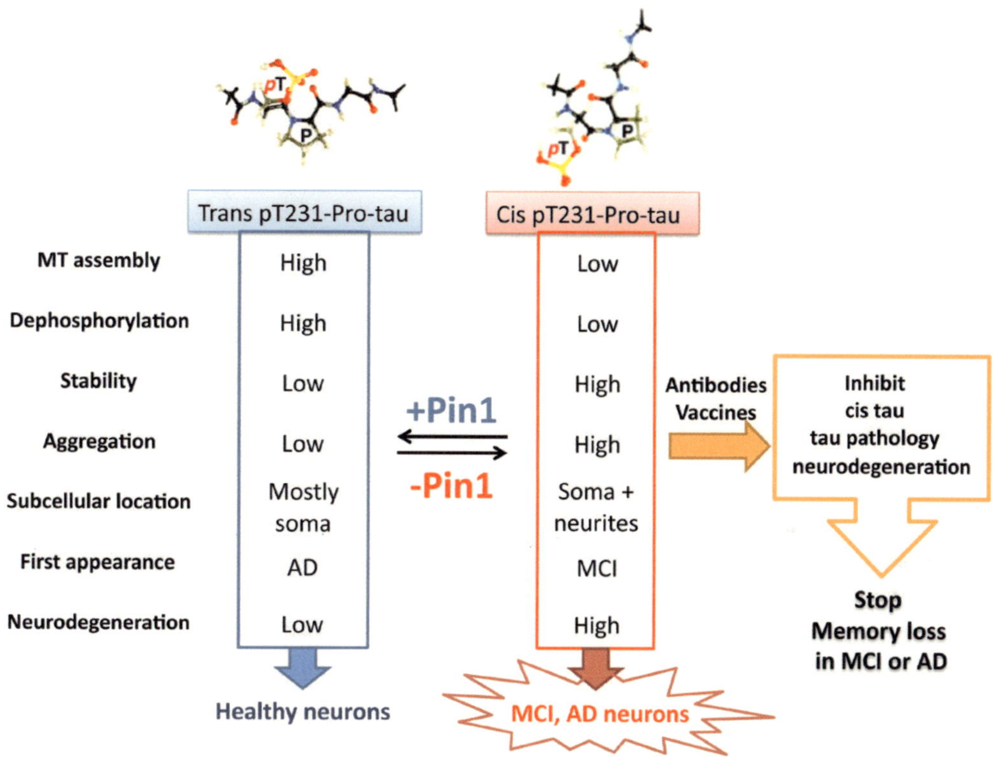

pT231-tau protein exists in the two completely different cis and trans conformations, as depicted in cartoons of the primary backbone structures. Cis, but not trans, pT231-tau loses normal function and also gains toxic function. Pin1 inhibits the accumulation of the pathogenic cis pT231-tau conformation in AD by converting it to the nonpathogenic trans form. Conformation-specific antibody and/or vaccines against the pathogenic cis pT231-tau might be developed for the diagnosis and treatment of AD, especially during its early stages.

Figure 2. Pin1 inhibits the accumulation of the pathogenic cis pT231-tau conformation in AD by converting it to the nonpathogenic trans form

These findings are highly relevant to human AD. We found that Pin1 localize to tangle and is depleted in AD brains [56], which has been confirmed and expanded to other tauopathies including FTD [61, 62, 169-172]. Furthermore, Pin1 is induced by neuron differentiation and highly expressed in most normal neurons, but inhibited by various mechanisms in AD neurons [44, 54, 56, 59, 62, 167, 169, 171-175]. For example, Pin1 expression is especially low in AD vulnerable neurons or actual degenerated neurons in AD [42]. Pin1 can be inactivated by oxidation in mild cognitive impairment (MCI) and AD neurons [61, 169, 170]. Pin1 is sequestered into tangles [56] or tangle or Ab-free granulovacuolar bodies with increasing tauopaty [176]. The human Pin1 gene is located at 19p13.2, a new late onset AD locus distinct from ApoE4 [173] and Pin1 promoter SNPs that reduce Pin1 expression [177] are associated with increased risk for AD in some cohorts [174], although not in others [65, 178]. A different Pin1 promoter SNP that prevents its suppression by AP4 is associated with delayed onset of AD [178]. Our findings of the opposite effects of Pin1 on cancer and AD [43, 45] have been supported by genetic association studies [174, 177, 179] and epidemiological studies [180-182]. Our analysis of the Framingham Study has further shown that cancer patients have decreased risk of AD, that AD patients have reduced cancer risk, and importantly, that this inverse relationship in not due to selective mortality or underdiagnosis [183]. Thus, we recently proposed that lack of sufficient Pin1 to catalyze cis to trans isomerization of pT231-tau might be a pathogenic mechanism leading to tauopathy in AD [48, 163].

5. Regulation of tau conformation as an early change in AD pathology: Implications for Pin1–catalyzed protein conformational regulation as a therapeutic and diagnostic tool

5.1. Cis pT231–tau is extremely early pathogenic conformation that is accumulated in MCI and AD

To analysis Pin1-catalyzed cis/trans protein conformational regulation and conformation-specific function or regulation, we have developed a novel technology to generate the first cis and trans-specific antibodies. We discovered that cis, but not trans, pT231-tau is extremely early pathogenic conformation in AD due to lack of Pin1 convert it to the physiological trans [129].

We found that replacing the five membered ring of Pro232 with the six membered ring homoproline (Pip) increases cis to 74%, since ~90% of pT231-P motif in a synthetic peptide in trans. Polyclonal antibodies raised against a pT231-Pip tau peptide recognize human and mouse p-tau. Resulting cis-specific antibody recognize regular pT231-Pro tau and cis pT231-5,5-demethylproline (Dmp) tau peptide, whereas trans-specific antibody recognizes regular pT231-Pro and trans pT231-Ala tau peptide. Neither antibody recognizes the non-phosphopeptide. Furthermore, both antibodies recognize tau, but not its T231A mutant expressed in SY5Y cells. Thus, cis- or trans- antibodies are highly specific [129]. Antibodies against cis pT231-tau might provide opportunity for efficient immunotherapy and diagnostic tools against early pathogenic tau conformation, raising the possibility of preventing tauopathy in AD patients at early stages.

5.2. Cis pT231–tau not only loses normal MT functions, but also gains toxic functions

As we and other groups had been shown [56, 184-186], phosphorylation of tau on T231 by Ccd2 abolishes its ability to promote MT assembly, which can be restored after dephosphor-

http://dx.doi.org/10.5772/55085

ylation by PP2A or Pin1 [129]. Importantly, the ability of Pin1 to restore p-tau MT function is fully blocked by incubation of Pin1-treated p-tau with trans antibodies, but not cis antibodies. Furthermore, trans pT231-tau peptide is readily dephosphorylated by the tau phosphatase PP2A, which dephosphorylate on trans pS/T-P motifs [128]. Moreover, cis pT231-tau is much more stable than the trans both in cells and in Tau-transgenic (Tg) mouse brain slice cultures. Finally cis pT231-tau is much more prone to aggregation than the trans in Tau-Tg mouse brains and human MCI brains, as detected by sarcosyl fractionation experiments [42, 164, 187]. Thus, cis, but not trans, p-tau loses normal MT functions, and gains toxic functions.

5.3. Pin1 overexpression increases cis to trans pT231–P conversion in WT tau–Tg mice

To detect the ability of Pin1 to increase cis to trans isomerization, we showed that Pin1 reduces cis, but increases trans pT231-tau in vitro [129]. Moreover, Pin1 overexpression in Tau-Tg mice (Tau+Pin1) reduces the cis content, but increases the trans content, whereas Pin1 deficiency in Tau-Tg mice (Tau+Pin1-KO) has the opposite effects, as shown by immunoblots and immunostains [129]. In contrast to Wt tau-Tg mice, Pin1 overexpression increased cis, but decreased trans pT231-tau in P301L tau Tau-Tg mice because the P301L tau mutation greatly reduced cis, but not trans, pT231-tau, as we hypothesized [164]. These results explain why Pin1 has the opposite effects on WT tau and P301L tau [164] and are consistent with that CSF pT231-tau can differentiate AD form frontotemporal dementia[165, 166].

5.4. Cis, but not trans, pT231–tau is significantly elevated and localized to dystrophic neurites in MCI and further accumulated in AD

To examine p-tau conformational changes during the development of AD, we analyzed different Braak brain tissues with *cis* or *trans*-specific tau antibodies. There is little *cis* or *trans* pT231-tau in normal brains [129]. In AD cortex, *trans* pT231-tau is very low, but the *cis* is readily detected, even at Braak stages III and IV (MCI), and further accumulates as the Braak stage increases [129]. Notably, *cis*, but not *trans*, is localized to the dystrophic neurites [129], an early hallmark change highly correlating with synaptic and cognitive loss in AD [188-194]. Given Pin1 inhibition by oxidation in MCI brains [169, 170, 195], Pin1 might act at a very early step to inhibit tauopathy in AD.

5.5. Cis pT231–tau fully overlaps with neurofibrillary degeneration and correlates with reduced Pin1 levels in the AD hippocampus

As shown [42, 134, 196, 197], Pin1 is highly expressed in the CA2 region of the hippocampus, but dramatically reduced in the CA1 region, whereas PHF-1, a solid neurofibrillary neurodegeneration marker [161], is prevalent in the CA1, but not in CA2 region [129]. Importantly, trans-positive neurons are dominant in the CA2 region. However, in the CA region, cis-positive neurons are greatly increased. All cis-positive neurons are also positive for PHF-1 in both CA2 and CA1 regions. However, 74% of trans-positive cells in the CA2 region are negative for PHF-1. Thus, cis, but not trans, pT231-tau is fully overlapped with neurofibrillary degeneration.

5.6. Potential novel cis and trans conformation–specific disease diagnoses and therapies

Our exciting new insight into the role and regulation of p-tau conformations in AD might have important and novel therapeutic implications. For example, it has been shown that Thr231 phosphorylation is the earliest detectable tau phosphorylation event in human AD [130, 159, 160, 198] and its levels are elevated in cerebrospinal fluids and tracks AD progression, but with large individual variations [199, 200], making it difficult to become a standardized test. Our findings that the *cis* conformation appears earlier in MCI and is pathologically more relevant suggest that *cis* pThr231-tau and especially its ratio with *trans* might be a better and easier standardized diagnostic marker, especially for early diagnosis and patient comparison. Furthermore, the findings that Pin1 overexpression converts *cis* to *trans*, promotes tau degradation and inhibits tau pathology and neurodegeneration in AD mouse models [201] and that Pin1 SNPs preventing its inhibition by brain-specific transcription factor AP-4 is associated with delayed onset of AD [202] suggest that overexpressing Pin1 or preventing Pin1 inhibition might be a new approach to reduce the *cis* to *trans* pThr231-tau ratio to block tau pathology at early stages. Finally, active or passive immunization against some pSer/Thr-Pro motifs in tau including the pThr231-Pro motif has been shown to reduce tau aggregates and improve memory deficits in mouse models [203-209]. However, we have here shown that only ~10% of regular synthetic pThr231-tau peptides is in the pathologically relevant *cis* conformation and the remaining 90% is in *trans*, which can still promote MT assembly and is not related to neurofibrillary degeneration. Therefore, immunotherapies either using conformation-specific vaccines or antibodies specifically against the pathologically relevant *cis* pT231-tau conformation might be more specific and effective and safer in treating AD. Given the critical role of Pin1 and other isomerases in controlling the function of many other key regulators in the pathogenesis of human disease, notable Alzheimer's disease, cancer, viral infection, inflammation and autoimmune disorders [210-213], it would be interesting to determine whether prolyl isomerization regulates the cellular function of these proteins and whether these conformational switches might be explored for developing novel diagnoses and therapies.

6. Finding a proper animal model to study AD: A lesson from the pin1KO mice

One of the biggest challenges when studying a disease is to develop the proper animal model that would reproduce the main features of that disease within the animal's biological environment. In the case of AD, this is not an easy goal, since mice do not spontaneously develop the features characteristic of this disease.

The only way to induce AD-like pathology with plaques and/or tangles in mice is by generating genetically altered animals. These may either overexpress aggressive mutants of APP linked to familial forms of AD (FAD) [214-218] and hence produce higher amounts of Abeta peptide, or express either wild type or aggressive mutants of tau [217, 218], leading to sustained tau hyperphosphorylation and tangle formation or may express both [217, 218]. These models may recapitulate plaque (APPTg) or tangle (tauTg) pathologies, or both (APPtg crossed to tauTg) [217, 218], and are extremely useful to understand the molecular pathways involved in AD, however they may [216] or may not [219] undergo neurodegeneration, which is a feature of AD. Moreover, they may not be representative of the way the disease progresses in sporadic AD, which affects the vast majority of AD patients, as they may represent only those familial cases of AD caused by those same mutations. Furthermore, these models may not be all specific for AD, since tau hyperphosphorylation and tangle formation occur also in other neurodegenerative diseases, and some of the tau mutations used to generate animal models for AD do not associate with AD, but with other neurodegenerative diseases, such as frontotemporal dementia associated with parkinsonism FTDP [17, 220, 221].

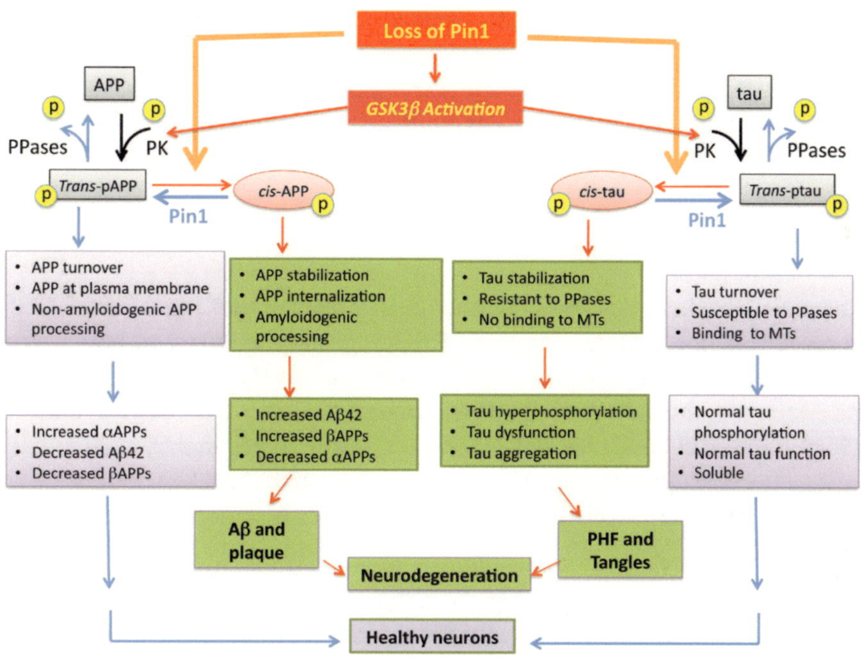

Both APP and tau are phosphorylated by protein kinase (PKs) as part of their normal function. The trans-conformation of phosphorylated APP and tau may present the physiological conformation that promotes their normal function (green boxes). Pin1 expression is induced during neuron differentiation and necessary to maintain normal neuronal function by preventing the unscheduled activation of mitotic events and/or controlling the function of phosphoproteins in the event that they become abnormally phosphorylated. For example, by catalyzing isomerization of the cis to trans conformation, Pin1 might promote non-amyloidogenic APP processing reducing Abeta production, as well as promote tau dephosphorylation and restore tau function. However in AD, a loss of Pin1 function, either through downregulation of Pin1 function, oxidative inactivation, phosphorylation or possible genetic alterations, can lead to build-up of cis-pS/T –P motifs. Cis-p-tau and cis-p-APP are proposed to represent pathological conformations (red ovals). Cis-p-APP is processed by the amyloidogenic pathway, which lead to a build-up of amyloid beta-42 (Abeta42), decreased levels of neurotropic alphaAPPs and the resultant formation of amyloid plaques. Cis-p-tau is resistant to protein phosphatases, which leads to a loss of MT binding, hyperphosphorylated tau an the formation of neurofibrillary tangles. The formation of tangles and plaques might further reduce Pin1 function by sequestering Pin1 and inducing oxidative modifications, respectively, in a positive feedback loop. In addition, a lack of proper Pin1 function leads to activation of kinases such as GSK3beta, which further increases both phosphorylation of tau and APP and also inhibits APP turnover, contributing to both tau and Abeta pathologies and causing neuronal death. Therefore, Pin1 deregulation might act on multiple pathways to contribute to AD development.

Figure 3. The regulation of APP processing and tau function by Pin1 in healthy and Alzheimer's neuron.

In addition, also animal models developed to understand a specific pathway even in absence of plaques [118], show limitations in the interpretation of the results.

In contrast, the model offered by knocking out the Pin1 gene in our Pin1KO model may recapitulate some of the features characteristic of both tau and Abeta pathology in sporadic AD, and therefore could serve as a valid tool to investigate the pathways that can be targeted to prevent or halt the disease progression. In fact, Pin1KO mice 1) develop age-dependent Abeta pathology associated with early neuronal deficit that leads to neurodegeneration (elevated Abeta levels associated with increased intracellular deposition) [41], 2) are characterized by age-dependent tau hyperphosphorylation, stabilization and PHF formation [42], and 3) show age-dependent neurodegeneration in selected areas [42]. Because genetic and proteomic findings link decreased Pin1 levels and/or activity to AD [56,61], we could speculate that the Pin1KO animal model be very close to recapitulating the features that characterize AD in humans, and therefore may serve as a valid model to study the molecular pathways involved in AD.

7. Conclusion

We have here reviewed studies showing how Pin1 is an essential regulator of APP, tau and GSK3beta conformations, maintaining their physiological functions, and how loss of Pin1 in AD contributes to the accumulation of toxic conformations that turn the proteins' function pathologic. Moreover, the data here discussed present Pin1 as a link between both Abeta and tau pathology that could be exploited to tackle both pathologies in AD, even at early stages. The emerging new concept is that protein conformation might be a key regulatory element in toxic pathways in AD, and that Pin1 regulation of protein conformations might be a promising avenue to fight AD.

The debate about Abeta and tau pathology, which occurs first, which causes the other, is still unsolved, and clarifying it would help identify the correct therapeutic target to successfully prevent AD progression. Although studies in animal models in vivo showed that Abeta pathology occurs first and may be causative of tau pathology [222, 223], they were performed in animal models genetically modified to develop both tau and Abeta pathologies, and therefore may not be representative of the molecular mechanisms underlying sporadic forms of AD. In fact, it is still unclear which pathology occurs first in human AD, and only fine diagnostic tools able to identify early modification on both APP and tau that may render the proteins toxic would be of help.

As appropriate early diagnostic tools are still missing, the evidences here presented highlight Pin1 as an ideal therapeutic target to block the toxicity of both APP and tau in AD. In fact, the data here discussed show that equilibrium between cis and trans conformation of APP and tau is crucial to maintain their physiological function, and that this is disrupted either by hyperphosphorylation at S/T-P or by lower Pin1 levels or both in AD. In addition, we show here evidences that, in tau, alteration in the equilibrium between cis and trans conformation is an event that precedes massive cognitive decline, since the cis form of phosphorylated tau accumulates in MCI patients [129]. These results directly link conformational changes to

http://dx.doi.org/10.5772/55085

pathologic protein functions, and highlight Pin1 as a successful regulator of such toxic conformations, opening new avenues in the medical field of AD. In fact, if a therapeutic target, Pin1 could block both tau and Abeta pathologies early in the disease, also resolving the eternal and unsolvable conflict: What happens first?

Author details

Lucia Pastorino, Asami Kondo, Xiao Zhen Zhou and Kun Ping Lu

*Address all correspondence to: lpastori@bidmc.harvard.edu

*Address all correspondence to: klu@bidmc.harvard.edu

Department of Medicine, Beth Israel Deaconess Medical Center, Harvard Medical School, Boston, USA

References

[1] Holtzman DM, Morris JC, Goate AM. Alzheimer's disease: the challenge of the second century. Sci Transl Med. 2011 Apr 6;3(77):77sr1.

[2] Bateman RJ, Aisen PS, De Strooper B, Fox NC, Lemere CA, Ringman JM, et al. Autosomal-dominant Alzheimer's disease: a review and proposal for the prevention of Alzheimer's disease. Alzheimers Res Ther. 2011;3(1):1.

[3] Aisen PS, Cummings J, Schneider LS. Symptomatic and nonamyloid/tau based pharmacologic treatment for Alzheimer disease. Cold Spring Harb Perspect Med. 2012 Mar;2(3):a006395.

[4] Winblad B, Engedal K, Soininen H, Verhey F, Waldemar G, Wimo A, et al. A 1-year, randomized, placebo-controlled study of donepezil in patients with mild to moderate AD. Neurology. 2001 Aug 14;57(3):489-95.

[5] Winblad B, Poritis N. Memantine in severe dementia: results of the 9M-Best Study (Benefit and efficacy in severely demented patients during treatment with memantine). Int J Geriatr Psychiatry. 1999 Feb;14(2):135-46.

[6] Tariot PN, Farlow MR, Grossberg GT, Graham SM, McDonald S, Gergel I. Memantine treatment in patients with moderate to severe Alzheimer disease already receiving donepezil: a randomized controlled trial. JAMA. 2004 Jan 21;291(3):317-24.

[7] Schneider LS, Insel PS, Weiner MW. Treatment with cholinesterase inhibitors and memantine of patients in the Alzheimer's Disease Neuroimaging Initiative. Arch Neurol. 2011 Jan;68(1):58-66.

[8] Whitehead A, Perdomo C, Pratt RD, Birks J, Wilcock GK, Evans JG. Donepezil for the symptomatic treatment of patients with mild to moderate Alzheimer's disease: a meta-analysis of individual patient data from randomised controlled trials. Int J Geriatr Psychiatry. 2004 Jul;19(7):624-33.

[9] Holtzman DM, Goate A, Kelly J, Sperling R. Mapping the road forward in Alzheimer's disease. Sci Transl Med. 2011 Dec 21;3(114):114ps48.

[10] Glenner GG, Wong CW, Quaranta V, Eanes ED. The amyloid deposits in Alzheimer's disease: their nature and pathogenesis. Appl Pathol. 1984;2(6):357-69.

[11] Goedert M, Spillantini MG, Cairns NJ, Crowther RA. Tau proteins of Alzheimer paired helical filaments: abnormal phosphorylation of all six brain isoforms. Neuron. 1992 Jan;8(1):159-68.

[12] Meyer-Luehmann M, Spires-Jones TL, Prada C, Garcia-Alloza M, de Calignon A, Rozkalne A, et al. Rapid appearance and local toxicity of amyloid-beta plaques in a mouse model of Alzheimer's disease. Nature. 2008 Feb 7;451(7179):720-4.

[13] Buee L, Bussiere T, Buee-Scherrer V, Delacourte A, Hof PR. Tau protein isoforms, phosphorylation and role in neurodegenerative disorders. Brain Res Brain Res Rev. 2000 Aug;33(1):95-130.

[14] Gomez-Isla T, Hollister R, West H, Mui S, Growdon JH, Petersen RC, et al. Neuronal loss correlates with but exceeds neurofibrillary tangles in Alzheimer's disease. Ann Neurol. 1997 Jan;41(1):17-24.

[15] Ballatore C, Lee VM, Trojanowski JQ. Tau-mediated neurodegeneration in Alzheimer's disease and related disorders. Nat Rev Neurosci. 2007 Sep;8(9):663-72.

[16] Parvathy S, Davies P, Haroutunian V, Purohit DP, Davis KL, Mohs RC, et al. Correlation between Abetax-40-, Abetax-42-, and Abetax-43-containing amyloid plaques and cognitive decline. Arch Neurol. 2001 Dec;58(12):2025-32.

[17] De Strooper B. Proteases and proteolysis in Alzheimer disease: a multifactorial view on the disease process. Physiol Rev. 2010 Apr;90(2):465-94.

[18] Masters CL, Selkoe DJ. Biochemistry of Amyloid beta-Protein and Amyloid Deposits in Alzheimer Disease. Cold Spring Harb Perspect Med. 2012 Jun;2(6):a006262.

[19] Jucker M, Walker LC. Pathogenic protein seeding in Alzheimer disease and other neurodegenerative disorders. Ann Neurol. 2011 Oct;70(4):532-40.

[20] Benilova I, Karran E, De Strooper B. The toxic Abeta oligomer and Alzheimer's disease: an emperor in need of clothes. Nat Neurosci. 2012 Mar;15(3):349-57.

[21] Larson ME, Lesne SE. Soluble Abeta oligomer production and toxicity. J Neurochem. 2012 Jan;120 Suppl 1:125-39.

[22] Haass C, Selkoe DJ. Soluble protein oligomers in neurodegeneration: lessons from the Alzheimer's amyloid beta-peptide. Nat Rev Mol Cell Biol. 2007 Feb;8(2):101-12.

[23] Noble W, Olm V, Takata K, Casey E, Mary O, Meyerson J, et al. Cdk5 is a key factor in tau aggregation and tangle formation in vivo. Neuron. 2003 May 22;38(4):555-65.

[24] Reinhard C, Hebert SS, De Strooper B. The amyloid-beta precursor protein: integrating structure with biological function. EMBO J. 2005 Dec 7;24(23):3996-4006.

[25] Hong S, Quintero-Monzon O, Ostaszewski BL, Podlisny DR, Cavanaugh WT, Yang T, et al. Dynamic analysis of amyloid beta-protein in behaving mice reveals opposing changes in ISF versus parenchymal Abeta during age-related plaque formation. J Neurosci. 2011 Nov 2;31(44):15861-9.

[26] Walsh DM, Selkoe DJ. Deciphering the molecular basis of memory failure in Alzheimer's disease. Neuron. 2004 Sep 30;44(1):181-93.

[27] Cleary JP, Walsh DM, Hofmeister JJ, Shankar GM, Kuskowski MA, Selkoe DJ, et al. Natural oligomers of the amyloid-beta protein specifically disrupt cognitive function. Nat Neurosci. 2005 Jan;8(1):79-84.

[28] Santos AN, Ewers M, Minthon L, Simm A, Silber RE, Blennow K, et al. Amyloid-beta oligomers in cerebrospinal fluid are associated with cognitive decline in patients with Alzheimer's disease. J Alzheimers Dis. 2012 Jan 1;29(1):171-6.

[29] Walsh DM, Klyubin I, Fadeeva JV, Cullen WK, Anwyl R, Wolfe MS, et al. Naturally secreted oligomers of amyloid beta protein potently inhibit hippocampal long-term potentiation in vivo. Nature. 2002 Apr 4;416(6880):535-9.

[30] Wang Q, Walsh DM, Rowan MJ, Selkoe DJ, Anwyl R. Block of long-term potentiation by naturally secreted and synthetic amyloid beta-peptide in hippocampal slices is mediated via activation of the kinases c-Jun N-terminal kinase, cyclin-dependent kinase 5, and p38 mitogen-activated protein kinase as well as metabotropic glutamate receptor type 5. J Neurosci. 2004 Mar 31;24(13):3370-8.

[31] Shankar GM, Li S, Mehta TH, Garcia-Munoz A, Shepardson NE, Smith I, et al. Amyloid-beta protein dimers isolated directly from Alzheimer's brains impair synaptic plasticity and memory. Nat Med. 2008 Aug;14(8):837-42.

[32] Takahashi RH, Milner TA, Li F, Nam EE, Edgar MA, Yamaguchi H, et al. Intraneuronal Alzheimer abeta42 accumulates in multivesicular bodies and is associated with synaptic pathology. Am J Pathol. 2002 Nov;161(5):1869-79.

[33] Takahashi RH, Almeida CG, Kearney PF, Yu F, Lin MT, Milner TA, et al. Oligomerization of Alzheimer's beta-amyloid within processes and synapses of cultured neurons and brain. J Neurosci. 2004 Apr 7;24(14):3592-9.

[34] Lee MS, Kao SC, Lemere CA, Xia W, Tseng HC, Zhou Y, et al. APP processing is regulated by cytoplasmic phosphorylation. J Cell Biol. 2003 Oct 13;163(1):83-95.

[35] Suzuki T, Nakaya T. Regulation of amyloid beta-protein precursor by phosphorylation and protein interactions. J Biol Chem. 2008 Oct 31;283(44):29633-7.

[36] Phiel CJ, Wilson CA, Lee VM, Klein PS. GSK-3alpha regulates production of Alzheimer's disease amyloid-beta peptides. Nature. 2003 May 22;423(6938):435-9.

[37] Lee MS, Tsai LH. Cdk5: one of the links between senile plaques and neurofibrillary tangles? J Alzheimers Dis. 2003;5(2):127-37.

[38] Mandelkow EM, Drewes G, Biernat J, Gustke N, Van Lint J, Vandenheede JR, et al. Glycogen synthase kinase-3 and the Alzheimer-like state of microtubule-associated protein tau. FEBS Lett. 1992 Dec 21;314(3):315-21.

[39] Cruz JC, Kim D, Moy LY, Dobbin MM, Sun X, Bronson RT, et al. p25/cyclin-dependent kinase 5 induces production and intraneuronal accumulation of amyloid beta in vivo. J Neurosci. 2006 Oct 11;26(41):10536-41.

[40] Cruz JC, Tsai LH. Cdk5 deregulation in the pathogenesis of Alzheimer's disease. Trends Mol Med. 2004 Sep;10(9):452-8.

[41] 41. Pastorino L, Sun A, Lu PJ, Zhou XZ, Balastik M, Finn G, et al. The prolyl isomerase Pin1 regulates amyloid precursor protein processing and amyloid-beta production. . Nature. 2006;440:528-34.

[42] Liou YC, Sun A, Ryo A, Zhou XZ, Yu ZX, Huang HK, et al. Role of the prolyl isomerase Pin1 in protecting against age-dependent neurodegeneration. Nature. 2003 Jul 31;424(6948):556-61.

[43] Lu KP, Zhou XZ. The prolyl isomerase PIN1: a pivotal new twist in phosphorylation signalling and disease. Nat Rev Mol Cell Biol. 2007 Nov;8(11):904-16.

[44] Lu KP, Hanes SD, Hunter T. A human peptidyl-prolyl isomerase essential for regulation of mitosis. Nature. 1996;380(6574):544-7.

[45] Lu KP. Pinning down cell signaling, cancer and Alzheimer's disease. Trends Biochem Sci. 2004;29:200-9.

[46] Wulf G, Finn G, Suizu F, Lu KP. Phosphorylation-specific prolyl isomerization: is there an underlying theme? Nat Cell Biol. 2005 May;7(5):435-41.

[47] Yaffe MB, Schutkowski M, Shen M, Zhou XZ, Stukenberg PT, Rahfeld J, et al. Sequence-specific and phosphorylation-dependent proline isomerization: A potential mitotic regulatory mechanism. Science. 1997;278:1957-60.

[48] Lu KP, Finn G, Lee TH, Nicholson LK. Prolyl cis-trans isomerization as a molecular timer. Nat Chem Biol. 2007 Oct;3(10):619-29.

[49] Lu KP, Liou YC, Zhou XZ. Pinning down proline-directed phosphorylation signaling. Trends Cell Biol. 2002 Apr;12(4):164-72.

[50] Lu PJ, Zhou XZ, Liou YC, Noel JP, Lu KP. Critical role of WW domain phosphorylation in regulating phosphoserine binding activity and Pin1 function. J Biol Chem. 2002 Jan 25;277(4):2381-4.

[51] Pastorino L, Ma SL, Balastik M, Huang P, Pandya D, Nicholson L, et al. Alzheimer's disease-related loss of Pin1 function influences the intracellular localization and the processing of AbetaPP. J Alzheimers Dis. 2012 Jan 1;30(2):277-97.

[52] Ryo A, Suizu F, Yoshida Y, Perrem K, Liou YC, Wulf G, et al. Regulation of NF-kappaB signaling by Pin1-dependent prolyl isomerization and ubiquitin-mediated proteolysis of p65/RelA. Mol Cell. 2003;12:1413-26.

[53] Wulf GM, Liou YC, Ryo A, Lee SW, Lu KP. Role of Pin1 in the regulation of p53 stability and p21 transactivation,and cell cycle checkpoints in response to DNA damage. J Biol Chem. 2002;277:47976-9.

[54] Ryo A, Nakamura M, Wulf G, Liou YC, Lu KP. Pin1 regulates turnover and subcellular localization of beta-catenin by inhibiting its interaction with APC. Nat Cell Biol. 2001 Sep;3(9):793-801.

[55] Tun-Kyi A, Finn G, Greenwood A, Nowak M, Lee TH, Asara JM, et al. Essential role for the prolyl isomerase Pin1 in Toll-like receptor signaling and type I interferon-mediated immunity. Nat Immunol. 2011 Aug;12(8):733-41.

[56] Lu PJ, Wulf G, Zhou XZ, Davies P, Lu KP. The prolyl isomerase Pin1 restores the function of Alzheimer-associated phosphorylated tau protein. Nature. 1999 Jun 24;399(6738):784-8.

[57] Cook DN, Pisetsky DS, Schwartz DA. Toll-like receptors in the pathogenesis of human disease. Nat Immunol. 2004 Oct;5(10):975-9.

[58] Ryo A, Liou YC, Lu KP, Wulf G. Prolyl isomerase Pin1: a catalyst for oncogenesis and a potential therapeutic target in cancer. J Cell Sci. 2003 Mar 1;116(Pt 5):773-83.

[59] Wulf GM, Ryo A, Wulf GG, Lee SW, Niu T, Petkova V, et al. Pin1 is overexpressed in breast cancer and cooperates with Ras signaling in increasing the transcriptional activity of c-Jun towards cyclin D1. EMBO J. 2001 Jul 2;20(13):3459-72.

[60] Wulf G, Ryo A, Liou YC, Lu KP. The prolyl isomerase Pin1 in breast development and cancer. Breast Cancer Res. 2003;5(2):76-82.

[61] Sultana R, Boyd-Kimball D, Poon HF, Cai J, Pierce WM, Klein JB, et al. Oxidative modification and down-regulation of Pin1 in Alzheimer's disease hippocampus: A redox proteomics analysis. Neurobiol Aging. 2006 Jul;27(7):918-25.

[62] Wang S, Simon BP, Bennett DA, Schneider JA, Malter JS, Wang DS. The significance of Pin1 in the development of Alzheimer's disease. J Alzheimers Dis. 2007 Mar;11(1): 13-23.

[63] Lambert JC, Bensemain F, Chapuis J, Cottel D, Amouyel P. Association study of the PIN1 gene with Alzheimer's disease. Neurosci Lett. 2006 Jul 24;402(3):259-61.

[64] Poli M, Gatta LB, Dominici R, Lovati C, Mariani C, Albertini A, et al. DNA sequence variations in the prolyl isomerase Pin1 gene and Alzheimer's disease. Neurosci Lett. 2005 Dec 2;389(2):66-70.

[65] Nowotny P, Bertelsen S, Hinrichs AL, Kauwe JS, Mayo K, Jacquart S, et al. Association studies between common variants in prolyl isomerase Pin1 and the risk for late-onset Alzheimer's disease. Neurosci Lett. 2007 May 23;419(1):15-7.

[66] Ma SL, Tang NL, Tam CW, Cheong Lui VW, Lam LC, Chiu HF, et al. A PIN1 polymorphism that prevents its suppression by AP4 associates with delayed onset of Alzheimer's disease. Neurobiol Aging.Jun 24.

[67] Hardy J. A hundred years of Alzheimer's disease research. Neuron. 2006 Oct 5;52(1): 3-13.

[68] Hardy J, Selkoe DJ. The amyloid hypothesis of Alzheimer's disease: progress and problems on the road to therapeutics. Science. 2002 Jul 19;297(5580):353-6.

[69] Wong CW, Quaranta V, Glenner GG. Neuritic plaques and cerebrovascular amyloid in Alzheimer disease are antigenically related. Proc Natl Acad Sci U S A. 1985 Dec; 82(24):8729-32.

[70] Thinakaran G, Koo EH. Amyloid precursor protein trafficking, processing, and function. J Biol Chem. 2008 Oct 31;283(44):29615-9.

[71] Goldgaber D, Lerman MI, McBride OW, Saffiotti U, Gajdusek DC. Characterization and chromosomal localization of a cDNA encoding brain amyloid of Alzheimer's disease. Science. 1987 Feb 20;235(4791):877-80.

[72] Golde TE, Estus S, Usiak M, Younkin LH, Younkin SG. Expression of beta amyloid protein precursor mRNAs: recognition of a novel alternatively spliced form and quantitation in Alzheimer's disease using PCR. Neuron. 1990 Feb;4(2):253-67.

[73] Haass C, Kaether C, Thinakaran G, Sisodia S. Trafficking and Proteolytic Processing of APP. Cold Spring Harb Perspect Med. 2012 May;2(5):a006270.

[74] Rajendran L, Annaert W. Membrane trafficking pathways in Alzheimer's disease. Traffic. 2012 Jun;13(6):759-70.

[75] Parvathy S, Hussain I, Karran EH, Turner AJ, Hooper NM. The amyloid precursor protein (APP) and the angiotensin converting enzyme (ACE) secretase are inhibited by hydroxamic acid-based inhibitors. Biochem Soc Trans. 1998 Aug;26(3):S242.

[76] Parvathy S, Hussain I, Karran EH, Turner AJ, Hooper NM. Cleavage of Alzheimer's amyloid precursor protein by alpha-secretase occurs at the surface of neuronal cells. Biochemistry. 1999 Jul 27;38(30):9728-34.

[77] Lammich S, Kojro E, Postina R, Gilbert S, Pfeiffer R, Jasionowski M, et al. Constitutive and regulated alpha-secretase cleavage of Alzheimer's amyloid precursor protein by a disintegrin metalloprotease. Proc Natl Acad Sci U S A. 1999 Mar 30;96(7): 3922-7.

[78] Postina R. Activation of alpha-secretase cleavage. J Neurochem. 2012 Jan;120 Suppl 1:46-54.

[79] Postina R, Schroeder A, Dewachter I, Bohl J, Schmitt U, Kojro E, et al. A disintegrin-metalloproteinase prevents amyloid plaque formation and hippocampal defects in an Alzheimer disease mouse model. J Clin Invest. 2004 May;113(10):1456-64.

[80] Buxbaum JD, Liu KN, Luo Y, Slack JL, Stocking KL, Peschon JJ, et al. Evidence that tumor necrosis factor alpha converting enzyme is involved in regulated alpha-secretase cleavage of the Alzheimer amyloid protein precursor. J Biol Chem. 1998 Oct 23;273(43):27765-7.

[81] Asai M, Hattori C, Szabo B, Sasagawa N, Maruyama K, Tanuma S, et al. Putative function of ADAM9, ADAM10, and ADAM17 as APP alpha-secretase. Biochem Biophys Res Commun. 2003 Jan 31;301(1):231-5.

[82] Young-Pearse TL, Chen AC, Chang R, Marquez C, Selkoe DJ. Secreted APP regulates the function of full-length APP in neurite outgrowth through interaction with integrin beta1. Neural Dev. 2008;3:15.

[83] Cao X, Sudhof TC. A transcriptionally [correction of transcriptively) active complex of APP with Fe65 and histone acetyltransferase Tip60. Science. 2001 Jul 6;293(5527): 115-20.

[84] Cao X, Sudhof TC. Dissection of amyloid-beta precursor protein-dependent transcriptional transactivation. J Biol Chem. 2004 Jun 4;279(23):24601-11.

[85] Sabo SL, Lanier LM, Ikin AF, Khorkova O, Sahasrabudhe S, Greengard P, et al. Regulation of beta-amyloid secretion by FE65, an amyloid protein precursor-binding protein. J Biol Chem. 1999 Mar 19;274(12):7952-7.

[86] Vassar R, Bennett BD, Babu-Khan S, Kahn S, Mendiaz EA, Denis P, et al. Beta-secretase cleavage of Alzheimer's amyloid precursor protein by the transmembrane aspartic protease BACE. Science. 1999 Oct 22;286(5440):735-41.

[87] Hussain I, Powell D, Howlett DR, Tew DG, Meek TD, Chapman C, et al. Identification of a novel aspartic protease (Asp 2) as beta-secretase. Mol Cell Neurosci. 1999 Dec;14(6):419-27.

[88] Nikolaev A, McLaughlin T, O'Leary DD, Tessier-Lavigne M. APP binds DR6 to trigger axon pruning and neuron death via distinct caspases. Nature. 2009 Feb 19;457(7232):981-9.

[89] De Strooper B, Vassar R, Golde T. The secretases: enzymes with therapeutic potential in Alzheimer disease. Nat Rev Neurol.Feb;6(2):99-107.

[90] De Strooper B, Vassar R, Golde T. The secretases: enzymes with therapeutic potential in Alzheimer disease. Nat Rev Neurol. 2010 Feb;6(2):99-107.

[91] O'Brien RJ, Wong PC. Amyloid precursor protein processing and Alzheimer's disease. Annu Rev Neurosci. 2011;34:185-204.

[92] Zambrano N, Bruni P, Minopoli G, Mosca R, Molino D, Russo C, et al. The beta-amyloid precursor protein APP is tyrosine-phosphorylated in cells expressing a constitutively active form of the Abl protoncogene. J Biol Chem. 2001 Jun 8;276(23):19787-92.

[93] Tarr PE, Contursi C, Roncarati R, Noviello C, Ghersi E, Scheinfeld MH, et al. Evidence for a role of the nerve growth factor receptor TrkA in tyrosine phosphorylation and processing of beta-APP. Biochem Biophys Res Commun. 2002 Jul 12;295(2):324-9.

[94] Rogelj B, Mitchell JC, Miller CC, McLoughlin DM. The X11/Mint family of adaptor proteins. Brain Res Rev. 2006 Sep;52(2):305-15.

[95] Schettini G, Govoni S, Racchi M, Rodriguez G. Phosphorylation of APP-CTF-AICD domains and interaction with adaptor proteins: signal transduction and/or transcriptional role--relevance for Alzheimer pathology. J Neurochem. 2010 Dec;115(6): 1299-308.

[96] McLoughlin DM, Miller CC. The FE65 proteins and Alzheimer's disease. J Neurosci Res. 2008 Mar;86(4):744-54.

[97] Tarr PE, Roncarati R, Pelicci G, Pelicci PG, D'Adamio L. Tyrosine phosphorylation of the beta-amyloid precursor protein cytoplasmic tail promotes interaction with Shc. J Biol Chem. 2002 May 10;277(19):16798-804.

[98] Sabo SL, Ikin AF, Buxbaum JD, Greengard P. The Alzheimer amyloid precursor protein (APP) and FE65, an APP-binding protein, regulate cell movement. J Cell Biol. 2001 Jun 25;153(7):1403-14.

[99] Sabo SL, Ikin AF, Buxbaum JD, Greengard P. The amyloid precursor protein and its regulatory protein, FE65, in growth cones and synapses in vitro and in vivo. J Neurosci. 2003 Jul 2;23(13):5407-15.

[100] Matrone C, Barbagallo AP, La Rosa LR, Florenzano F, Ciotti MT, Mercanti D, et al. APP is phosphorylated by TrkA and regulates NGF/TrkA signaling. J Neurosci. 2011 Aug 17;31(33):11756-61.

[101] Perez RG, Soriano S, Hayes JD, Ostaszewski B, Xia W, Selkoe DJ, et al. Mutagenesis identifies new signals for beta-amyloid precursor protein endocytosis, turnover, and the generation of secreted fragments, including Abeta42. J Biol Chem. 1999 Jul 2;274(27):18851-6.

[102] Barbagallo AP, Weldon R, Tamayev R, Zhou D, Giliberto L, Foreman O, et al. Tyr(682) in the intracellular domain of APP regulates amyloidogenic APP processing in vivo. PLoS One. 2010;5(11):e15503.

[103] Russo C, Salis S, Dolcini V, Venezia V, Song XH, Teller JK, et al. Amino-terminal modification and tyrosine phosphorylation of [corrected) carboxy-terminal fragments of the amyloid precursor protein in Alzheimer's disease and Down's syndrome brain. Neurobiol Dis. 2001 Feb;8(1):173-80.

[104] Suzuki T, Oishi M, Marshak DR, Czernik AJ, Nairn AC, Greengard P. Cell cycle-dependent regulation of the phosphorylation and metabolism of the Alzheimer amyloid precursor protein. EMBO J. 1994 Mar 1;13(5):1114-22.

[105] Vincent IJ, Davies P. A protein kinase associated with paired helical filaments in Alzheimer disease. Proc Natl Acad Sci U S A. 1992 Apr 1;89(7):2878-82.

[106] Ando K, Iijima KI, Elliott JI, Kirino Y, Suzuki T. Phosphorylation-dependent regulation of the interaction of amyloid precursor protein with Fe65 affects the production of beta-amyloid. J Biol Chem. 2001 Oct 26;276(43):40353-61.

[107] Tamayev R, Zhou D, D'Adamio L. The interactome of the amyloid beta precursor protein family members is shaped by phosphorylation of their intracellular domains. Mol Neurodegener. 2009;4:28.

[108] Ramelot TA, Gentile LN, Nicholson LK. Transient structure of the amyloid precursor protein cytoplasmic tail indicates preordering of structure for binding to cytosolic factors. Biochemistry. 2000 Mar 14;39(10):2714-25.

[109] Ramelot TA, Nicholson LK. Phosphorylation-induced structural changes in the amyloid precursor protein cytoplasmic tail detected by NMR. J Mol Biol. 2001 Mar 30;307(3):871-84.

[110] Ma SL, Pastorino L, Zhou XZ, Lu KP. Prolyl isomerase Pin1 promotes amyloid precursor protein (APP) turnover by inhibiting glycogen synthase kinase-3beta (GSK3beta) activity: novel mechanism for Pin1 to protect against Alzheimer disease. J Biol Chem. 2012 Mar 2;287(10):6969-73.

[111] Sleegers K, Brouwers N, Gijselinck I, Theuns J, Goossens D, Wauters J, et al. APP duplication is sufficient to cause early onset Alzheimer's dementia with cerebral amyloid angiopathy. Brain. 2006 Nov;129(Pt 11):2977-83.

[112] Theuns J, Brouwers N, Engelborghs S, Sleegers K, Bogaerts V, Corsmit E, et al. Promoter mutations that increase amyloid precursor-protein expression are associated with Alzheimer disease. American journal of human genetics. 2006 Jun;78(6):936-46.

[113] Mann DM. Alzheimer's disease and Down's syndrome. Histopathology. 1988 Aug; 13(2):125-37.

[114] Prasher VP, Farrer MJ, Kessling AM, Fisher EM, West RJ, Barber PC, et al. Molecular mapping of Alzheimer-type dementia in Down's syndrome. Ann Neurol. 1998 Mar; 43(3):380-3.

[115] Muresan Z, Muresan V. c-Jun NH2-terminal kinase-interacting protein-3 facilitates phosphorylation and controls localization of amyloid-beta precursor protein. J Neurosci. 2005 Apr 13;25(15):3741-51.

[116] Muresan Z, Muresan V. Coordinated transport of phosphorylated amyloid-beta precursor protein and c-Jun NH2-terminal kinase-interacting protein-1. J Cell Biol. 2005 Nov 21;171(4):615-25.

[117] Parr C, Carzaniga R, Gentleman S, Van Leuven F, Walter J, Sastre M. GSK3 inhibition promotes lysosomal biogenesis and the autophagic degradation of the Amyloid-beta Precursor Protein. Mol Cell Biol. 2012 Aug 27.

[118] Sano Y, Nakaya T, Pedrini S, Takeda S, Iijima-Ando K, Iijima K, et al. Physiological mouse brain Abeta levels are not related to the phosphorylation state of threonine-668 of Alzheimer's APP. PLoS One. 2006;1:e51.

[119] Zheng H, Jiang M, Trumbauer ME, Sirinathsinghji DJ, Hopkins R, Smith DW, et al. beta-Amyloid precursor protein-deficient mice show reactive gliosis and decreased locomotor activity. Cell. 1995 May 19;81(4):525-31.

[120] Heber S, Herms J, Gajic V, Hainfellner J, Aguzzi A, Rulicke T, et al. Mice with combined gene knock-outs reveal essential and partially redundant functions of amyloid precursor protein family members. J Neurosci. 2000 Nov 1;20(21):7951-63.

[121] Harada A, Oguchi K, Okabe S, Kuno J, Terada S, Ohshima T, et al. Altered microtubule organization in small-calibre axons of mice lacking tau protein. Nature. 1994 Jun 9;369(6480):488-91.

[122] Dawson HN, Ferreira A, Eyster MV, Ghoshal N, Binder LI, Vitek MP. Inhibition of neuronal maturation in primary hippocampal neurons from tau deficient mice. J Cell Sci. 2001 Mar;114(Pt 6):1179-87.

[123] Gomez de Barreda E, Perez M, Gomez Ramos P, de Cristobal J, Martin-Maestro P, Moran A, et al. Tau-knockout mice show reduced GSK3-induced hippocampal degeneration and learning deficits. Neurobiol Dis. 2010 Mar;37(3):622-9.

[124] Stoothoff WH, Johnson GV. Tau phosphorylation: physiological and pathological consequences. Biochim Biophys Acta. 2005 Jan 3;1739(2-3):280-97.

[125] Mawal-Dewan M, Henley J, Van de Voorde A, Trojanowski JQ, Lee VM. The phosphorylation state of tau in the developing rat brain is regulated by phosphoprotein phosphatases. J Biol Chem. 1994 Dec 9;269(49):30981-7.

[126] Matsuo ES, Shin RW, Billingsley ML, Van deVoorde A, O'Connor M, Trojanowski JQ, et al. Biopsy-derived adult human brain tau is phosphorylated at many of the

same sites as Alzheimer's disease paired helical filament tau. Neuron. 1994 Oct;13(4): 989-1002.

[127] Romero PR, Zaidi S, Fang YY, Uversky VN, Radivojac P, Oldfield CJ, et al. Alternative splicing in concert with protein intrinsic disorder enables increased functional diversity in multicellular organisms. Proc Natl Acad Sci U S A. 2006 May 30;103(22): 8390-5.

[128] Zhou XZ, Kops O, Werner A, Lu PJ, Shen M, Stoller G, et al. Pin1-dependent prolyl isomerization regulates dephosphorylation of Cdc25C and tau proteins. Mol Cell. 2000 Oct;6(4):873-83.

[129] Nakamura K, Greenwood A, Binder L, Bigio EH, Denial S, Nicholson L, et al. Proline isomer-specific antibodies reveal the early pathogenic tau conformation in Alzheimer's disease. Cell. 2012 Mar 30;149(1):232-44.

[130] Jicha GA, Lane E, Vincent I, Otvos L, Jr., Hoffmann R, Davies P. A conformation- and phosphorylation-dependent antibody recognizing the paired helical filaments of Alzheimer's disease. J Neurochem. 1997 Nov;69(5):2087-95.

[131] Pei H, Li L, Fridley BL, Jenkins GD, Kalari KR, Lingle W, et al. FKBP51 affects cancer cell response to chemotherapy by negatively regulating Akt. Cancer cell. 2009 Sep 8;16(3):259-66.

[132] Allen B, Ingram E, Takao M, Smith MJ, Jakes R, Virdee K, et al. Abundant tau filaments and nonapoptotic neurodegeneration in transgenic mice expressing human P301S tau protein. J Neurosci. 2002 Nov 1;22(21):9340-51.

[133] Lewis J, McGowan E, Rockwood J, Melrose H, Nacharaju P, Van Slegtenhorst M, et al. Neurofibrillary tangles, amyotrophy and progressive motor disturbance in mice expressing mutant (P301L) tau protein. Nat Genet. 2000 Aug;25(4):402-5.

[134] Arriagada PV, Growdon JH, Hedley-Whyte ET, Hyman BT. Neurofibrillary tangles but not senile plaques parallel duration and severity of Alzheimer's disease. Neurology. 1992 Mar;42(3 Pt 1):631-9.

[135] Arriagada PV, Marzloff K, Hyman BT. Distribution of Alzheimer-type pathologic changes in nondemented elderly individuals matches the pattern in Alzheimer's disease. Neurology. 1992 Sep;42(9):1681-8.

[136] Vincent I, Zheng JH, Dickson DW, Kress Y, Davies P. Mitotic phosphoepitopes precede paired helical filaments in Alzheimer's disease. Neurobiol Aging. 1998 Jul-Aug; 19(4):287-96.

[137] Preuss U, Mandelkow EM. Mitotic phosphorylation of tau protein in neuronal cell lines resembles phosphorylation in Alzheimer's disease. European journal of cell biology. 1998 Jul;76(3):176-84.

[138] Bancher C, Brunner C, Lassmann H, Budka H, Jellinger K, Wiche G, et al. Accumulation of abnormally phosphorylated tau precedes the formation of neurofibrillary tangles in Alzheimer's disease. Brain Res. 1989 Jan 16;477(1-2):90-9.

[139] Lu KP, Liou YC, Vincent I. Proline-directed phosphorylation and isomerization in mitotic regulation and in Alzheimer's Disease. Bioessays. 2003 Feb;25(2):174-81.

[140] Lee VM, Balin BJ, Otvos L, Jr., Trojanowski JQ. A68: a major subunit of paired helical filaments and derivatized forms of normal Tau. Science. 1991 Feb 8;251(4994):675-8.

[141] Greenberg SG, Davies P, Schein JD, Binder LI. Hydrofluoric acid-treated tau PHF proteins display the same biochemical properties as normal tau. J Biol Chem. 1992 Jan 5;267(1):564-9.

[142] Pelech SL. Networking with proline-directed protein kinases implicated in tau phosphorylation. Neurobiol Aging. 1995 May-Jun;16(3):247-56; discussion 57-61.

[143] Dolan PJ, Johnson GV. The role of tau kinases in Alzheimer's disease. Current opinion in drug discovery & development. 2010 Sep;13(5):595-603.

[144] Illenberger S, Zheng-Fischhofer Q, Preuss U, Stamer K, Baumann K, Trinczek B, et al. The endogenous and cell cycle-dependent phosphorylation of tau protein in living cells: implications for Alzheimer's disease. Mol Biol Cell. 1998 Jun;9(6):1495-512.

[145] Goedert M, Satumtira S, Jakes R, Smith MJ, Kamibayashi C, White CL, 3rd, et al. Reduced binding of protein phosphatase 2A to tau protein with frontotemporal dementia and parkinsonism linked to chromosome 17 mutations. J Neurochem. 2000 Nov; 75(5):2155-62.

[146] Sontag E, Nunbhakdi-Craig V, Lee G, Bloom GS, Mumby MC. Regulation of the phosphorylation state and microtubule-binding activity of Tau by protein phosphatase 2A. Neuron. 1996 Dec;17(6):1201-7.

[147] Ishiguro K, Shiratsuchi A, Sato S, Omori A, Arioka M, Kobayashi S, et al. Glycogen synthase kinase 3 beta is identical to tau protein kinase I generating several epitopes of paired helical filaments. FEBS Lett. 1993 Jul 5;325(3):167-72.

[148] Sperber BR, Leight S, Goedert M, Lee VM. Glycogen synthase kinase-3 beta phosphorylates tau protein at multiple sites in intact cells. Neurosci Lett. 1995 Sep 8;197(2):149-53.

[149] Patrick GN, Zukerberg L, Nikolic M, de la Monte S, Dikkes P, Tsai LH. Conversion of p35 to p25 deregulates Cdk5 activity and promotes neurodegeneration. Nature. 1999 Dec 9;402(6762):615-22.

[150] James ND, Davis DR, Sindon J, Hanger DP, Brion JP, Miller CC, et al. Neurodegenerative changes including altered tau phosphorylation and neurofilament immunoreactivity in mice transgenic for the serine/threonine kinase Mos. Neurobiol Aging. 1996 Mar-Apr;17(2):235-41.

[151] Brownlees J, Irving NG, Brion JP, Gibb BJ, Wagner U, Woodgett J, et al. Tau phosphorylation in transgenic mice expressing glycogen synthase kinase-3beta transgenes. Neuroreport. 1997 Oct 20;8(15):3251-5.

[152] Ahlijanian MK, Barrezueta NX, Williams RD, Jakowski A, Kowsz KP, McCarthy S, et al. Hyperphosphorylated tau and neurofilament and cytoskeletal disruptions in mice overexpressing human p25, an activator of cdk5. Proc Natl Acad Sci U S A. 2000 Mar 14;97(6):2910-5.

[153] Kins S, Crameri A, Evans DR, Hemmings BA, Nitsch RM, Gotz J. Reduced protein phosphatase 2A activity induces hyperphosphorylation and altered compartmentalization of tau in transgenic mice. J Biol Chem. 2001 Oct 12;276(41):38193-200.

[154] Bian F, Nath R, Sobocinski G, Booher RN, Lipinski WJ, Callahan MJ, et al. Axonopathy, tau abnormalities, and dyskinesia, but no neurofibrillary tangles in p25-transgenic mice. The Journal of comparative neurology. 2002 May 6;446(3):257-66.

[155] Plattner F, Angelo M, Giese KP. The roles of cyclin-dependent kinase 5 and glycogen synthase kinase 3 in tau hyperphosphorylation. J Biol Chem. 2006 Sep 1;281(35): 25457-65.

[156] Seshadri S, Fitzpatrick AL, Ikram MA, DeStefano AL, Gudnason V, Boada M, et al. Genome-wide analysis of genetic loci associated with Alzheimer disease. JAMA. 2010 May 12;303(18):1832-40.

[157] Hollingworth P, Harold D, Sims R, Gerrish A, Lambert JC, Carrasquillo MM, et al. Common variants at ABCA7, MS4A6A/MS4A4E, EPHA1, CD33 and CD2AP are associated with Alzheimer's disease. Nat Genet. 2011 May;43(5):429-35.

[158] Naj AC, Jun G, Beecham GW, Wang LS, Vardarajan BN, Buros J, et al. Common variants at MS4A4/MS4A6E, CD2AP, CD33 and EPHA1 are associated with late-onset Alzheimer's disease. Nat Genet. 2011 May;43(5):436-41.

[159] Luna-Munoz J, Chavez-Macias L, Garcia-Sierra F, Mena R. Earliest stages of tau conformational changes are related to the appearance of a sequence of specific phospho-dependent tau epitopes in Alzheimer's disease. J Alzheimers Dis. 2007 Dec;12(4): 365-75.

[160] Luna-Munoz J, Garcia-Sierra F, Falcon V, Menendez I, Chavez-Macias L, Mena R. Regional conformational change involving phosphorylation of tau protein at the Thr231, precedes the structural change detected by Alz-50 antibody in Alzheimer's disease. J Alzheimers Dis. 2005 Sep;8(1):29-41.

[161] Augustinack JC, Schneider A, Mandelkow EM, Hyman BT. Specific tau phosphorylation sites correlate with severity of neuronal cytopathology in Alzheimer's disease. Acta Neuropathol. 2002 Jan;103(1):26-35.

[162] Yaffe MB, Schutkowski M, Shen M, Zhou XZ, Stukenberg PT, Rahfeld JU, et al. Sequence-specific and phosphorylation-dependent proline isomerization: a potential mitotic regulatory mechanism. Science. 1997 Dec 12;278(5345):1957-60.

[163] Lee TH, Pastorino L, Lu KP. Peptidyl-prolyl cis-trans isomerase Pin1 in ageing, cancer and Alzheimer disease. Expert reviews in molecular medicine. 2011;13:e21.

[164] Lim J, Balastik M, Lee TH, Nakamura K, Liou YC, Sun A, et al. Pin1 has opposite effects on wild-type and P301L tau stability and tauopathy. J Clin Invest. 2008 May; 118(5):1877-89.

[165] Hampel H, Blennow K, Shaw LM, Hoessler YC, Zetterberg H, Trojanowski JQ. Total and phosphorylated tau protein as biological markers of Alzheimer's disease. Experimental gerontology. 2010 Jan;45(1):30-40.

[166] Blennow K, Hampel H, Weiner M, Zetterberg H. Cerebrospinal fluid and plasma biomarkers in Alzheimer disease. Nat Rev Neurol. 2010 Mar;6(3):131-44.

[167] Hamdane M, Dourlen P, Bretteville A, Sambo AV, Ferreira S, Ando K, et al. Pin1 allows for differential Tau dephosphorylation in neuronal cells. Mol Cell Neurosci. 2006 May-Jun;32(1-2):155-60.

[168] Galas MC, Dourlen P, Begard S, Ando K, Blum D, Hamdane M, et al. The peptidyl-prolyl cis/trans-isomerase Pin1 modulates stress-induced dephosphorylation of Tau in neurons. Implication in a pathological mechanism related to Alzheimer disease. J Biol Chem. 2006 Jul 14;281(28):19296-304.

[169] Butterfield DA, Poon HF, St Clair D, Keller JN, Pierce WM, Klein JB, et al. Redox proteomics identification of oxidatively modified hippocampal proteins in mild cognitive impairment: insights into the development of Alzheimer's disease. Neurobiol Dis. 2006 May;22(2):223-32.

[170] Butterfield DA, Abdul HM, Opii W, Newman SF, Joshi G, Ansari MA, et al. Pin1 in Alzheimer's disease. J Neurochem. 2006 Sep;98(6):1697-706.

[171] Thorpe JR, Morley SJ, Rulten SL. Utilizing the peptidyl-prolyl cis-trans isomerase pin1 as a probe of its phosphorylated target proteins. Examples of binding to nuclear proteins in a human kidney cell line and to tau in Alzheimer's diseased brain. The journal of histochemistry and cytochemistry : official journal of the Histochemistry Society. 2001 Jan;49(1):97-108.

[172] Thorpe JR, Mosaheb S, Hashemzadeh-Bonehi L, Cairns NJ, Kay JE, Morley SJ, et al. Shortfalls in the peptidyl-prolyl cis-trans isomerase protein Pin1 in neurons are associated with frontotemporal dementias. Neurobiol Dis. 2004 Nov;17(2):237-49.

[173] Wijsman EM, Daw EW, Yu CE, Payami H, Steinbart EJ, Nochlin D, et al. Evidence for a novel late-onset Alzheimer disease locus on chromosome 19p13.2. American journal of human genetics. 2004 Sep;75(3):398-409.

[174] Segat L, Milanese M, Crovella S. Pin1 promoter polymorphisms in hepatocellular carcinoma patients. Gastroenterology. 2007 Jun;132(7):2618-9; author reply 9-20.

[175] Ramakrishnan P, Dickson DW, Davies P. Pin1 colocalization with phosphorylated tau in Alzheimer's disease and other tauopathies. Neurobiol Dis. 2003 Nov;14(2): 251-64.

[176] Dakson A, Yokota O, Esiri M, Bigio EH, Horan M, Pendleton N, et al. Granular expression of prolyl-peptidyl isomerase PIN1 is a constant and specific feature of Alzheimer's disease pathology and is independent of tau, Abeta and TDP-43 pathology. Acta Neuropathol. 2011 May;121(5):635-49.

[177] Lu J, Hu Z, Wei S, Wang LE, Liu Z, El-Naggar AK, et al. A novel functional variant (-842G>C) in the PIN1 promoter contributes to decreased risk of squamous cell carcinoma of the head and neck by diminishing the promoter activity. Carcinogenesis. 2009 Oct;30(10):1717-21.

[178] Ma SL, Tang NL, Tam CW, Lui VW, Lam LC, Chiu HF, et al. A PIN1 polymorphism that prevents its suppression by AP4 associates with delayed onset of Alzheimer's disease. Neurobiol Aging. 2012 Apr;33(4):804-13.

[179] Han CH, Lu J, Wei Q, Bondy ML, Brewster AM, Yu TK, et al. The functional promoter polymorphism (-842G>C) in the PIN1 gene is associated with decreased risk of breast cancer in non-Hispanic white women 55 years and younger. Breast cancer research and treatment. 2010 Jul;122(1):243-9.

[180] Roe CM, Behrens MI, Xiong C, Miller JP, Morris JC. Alzheimer disease and cancer. Neurology. 2005 Mar 8;64(5):895-8.

[181] Roe CM, Fitzpatrick AL, Xiong C, Sieh W, Kuller L, Miller JP, et al. Cancer linked to Alzheimer disease but not vascular dementia. Neurology. 2010 Jan 12;74(2):106-12.

[182] Behrens MI, Lendon C, Roe CM. A common biological mechanism in cancer and Alzheimer's disease? Curr Alzheimer Res. 2009 Jun;6(3):196-204.

[183] Driver JA, Beiser A, Au R, Kreger BE, Splansky GL, Kurth T, et al. Inverse association between cancer and Alzheimer's disease: results from the Framingham Heart Study. Bmj. 2012;344:e1442.

[184] Bramblett GT, Goedert M, Jakes R, Merrick SE, Trojanowski JQ, Lee VM. Abnormal tau phosphorylation at Ser396 in Alzheimer's disease recapitulates development and contributes to reduced microtubule binding. Neuron. 1993 Jun;10(6):1089-99.

[185] Yoshida H, Ihara Y. Tau in paired helical filaments is functionally distinct from fetal tau: assembly incompetence of paired helical filament-tau. J Neurochem. 1993 Sep; 61(3):1183-6.

[186] Alonso AC, Zaidi T, Grundke-Iqbal I, Iqbal K. Role of abnormally phosphorylated tau in the breakdown of microtubules in Alzheimer disease. Proc Natl Acad Sci U S A. 1994 Jun 7;91(12):5562-6.

[187] Ishihara T, Hong M, Zhang B, Nakagawa Y, Lee MK, Trojanowski JQ, et al. Age-dependent emergence and progression of a tauopathy in transgenic mice overexpressing the shortest human tau isoform. Neuron. 1999 Nov;24(3):751-62.

[188] Davies CA, Mann DM, Sumpter PQ, Yates PO. A quantitative morphometric analysis of the neuronal and synaptic content of the frontal and temporal cortex in patients with Alzheimer's disease. Journal of the neurological sciences. 1987 Apr;78(2):151-64.

[189] Scheff SW, DeKosky ST, Price DA. Quantitative assessment of cortical synaptic density in Alzheimer's disease. Neurobiol Aging. 1990 Jan-Feb;11(1):29-37.

[190] DeKosky ST, Scheff SW. Synapse loss in frontal cortex biopsies in Alzheimer's disease: correlation with cognitive severity. Ann Neurol. 1990 May;27(5):457-64.

[191] Terry RD, Masliah E, Salmon DP, Butters N, DeTeresa R, Hill R, et al. Physical basis of cognitive alterations in Alzheimer's disease: synapse loss is the major correlate of cognitive impairment. Ann Neurol. 1991 Oct;30(4):572-80.

[192] Masliah E, Ellisman M, Carragher B, Mallory M, Young S, Hansen L, et al. Three-dimensional analysis of the relationship between synaptic pathology and neuropil threads in Alzheimer disease. J Neuropathol Exp Neurol. 1992 Jul;51(4):404-14.

[193] Coleman PD, Yao PJ. Synaptic slaughter in Alzheimer's disease. Neurobiol Aging. 2003 Dec;24(8):1023-7.

[194] Thies E, Mandelkow EM. Missorting of tau in neurons causes degeneration of synapses that can be rescued by the kinase MARK2/Par-1. J Neurosci. 2007 Mar 14;27(11): 2896-907.

[195] Sultana R, Boyd-Kimball D, Poon HF, Cai J, Pierce WM, Klein JB, et al. Oxidative modification and down-regulation of Pin1 in Alzheimer's disease hippocampus: A redox proteomics analysis. Neurobiol Aging. 2006;27:918-25.

[196] Davies DC, Horwood N, Isaacs SL, Mann DM. The effect of age and Alzheimer's disease on pyramidal neuron density in the individual fields of the hippocampal formation. Acta Neuropathol. 1992;83(5):510-7.

[197] Hof PR, Morrison JH. Neocortical neuronal subpopulations labeled by a monoclonal antibody to calbindin exhibit differential vulnerability in Alzheimer's disease. Exp Neurol. 1991 Mar;111(3):293-301.

[198] Augustinack JC, Schneider A, Mandelkow EM, Hyman BT. Specific tau phosphorylation sites correlate with severity of neuronal cytopathology in Alzheimer's disease. Acta Neuropathol (Berl). 2002 Jan;103(1):26-35.

http://dx.doi.org/10.5772/55085

[199] Ewers M, Buerger K, Teipel SJ, Scheltens P, Schroder J, Zinkowski RP, et al. Multicenter assessment of CSF-phosphorylated tau for the prediction of conversion of MCI. Neurology. 2007 Dec 11;69(24):2205-12.

[200] Hampel H, Buerger K, Kohnken R, Teipel SJ, Zinkowski R, Moeller HJ, et al. Tracking of Alzheimer's disease progression with cerebrospinal fluid tau protein phosphorylated at threonine 231. Ann Neurol. 2001 Apr;49(4):545-6.

[201] Lim J, Balastik M, Lee TH, Liou YC, Sun A, Finn G, et al. Pin1 has opposite effects on wild-type and P301L tau stability and tauopathy. J Clin Invest. 2008;118:1877-89.

[202] Ma SL, Tang NLS, Tam CWC, Lui VWC, Lam LCW, Chiu HFK, et al. A functional polymorphism in Pin1 thatprevents its suppression by AP4 Is associated with delayed onset of Alzheimer's disease. Neurobiol Aging. 2010:(in press).

[203] Asuni AA, Boutajangout A, Quartermain D, Sigurdsson EM. Immunotherapy targeting pathological tau conformers in a tangle mouse model reduces brain pathology with associated functional improvements. J Neurosci. 2007 Aug 22;27(34):9115-29.

[204] Boutajangout A, Quartermain D, Sigurdsson EM. Immunotherapy targeting pathological tau prevents cognitive decline in a new tangle mouse model. J Neurosci. 2010 Dec 8;30(49):16559-66.

[205] Boimel M, Grigoriadis N, Lourbopoulos A, Haber E, Abramsky O, Rosenmann H. Efficacy and safety of immunization with phosphorylated tau against neurofibrillary tangles in mice. Exp Neurol. 2010 Aug;224(2):472-85.

[206] Kayed R, Jackson GR. Prefilament tau species as potential targets for immunotherapy for Alzheimer disease and related disorders. Current opinion in immunology. 2009 Jun;21(3):359-63.

[207] Wisniewski T, Boutajangout A. Vaccination as a therapeutic approach to Alzheimer's disease. The Mount Sinai journal of medicine, New York. 2010 Jan-Feb;77(1):17-31.

[208] Ubhi K, Masliah E. Recent advances in the development of immunotherapies for tauopathies. Exp Neurol. 2011 Oct 21;230.

[209] Boutajangout A, Ingadottir J, Davies P, Sigurdsson EM. Passive immunization targeting pathological phospho-tau protein in a mouse model reduces functional decline and clears tau aggregates from the brain. J Neurochem. 2011 Jun 3;118:658-67.

[210] Lu KP, Zhou XZ. The prolyl isomerase Pin1: a pivotal new twist in phosphorylation signalling and human disease. Nat Rev Mol Cell Biol. 2007;8:904-16.

[211] Lu KP, Finn G, Lee TH, Nicholson LK. Prolyl cis-trans isomerization as a molecular timer. Nature Chem Biol. 2007;3:619-29.

[212] Liou YC, Zhou XZ, Lu KP. The prolyl isomerase Pin1 as a molecular switch to determine the fate of phosphoproteins. Trends Biochem Sci. 2011:(Accepted).

[213] Theuerkorn M, Fischer G, Schiene-Fischer C. Prolyl cis/trans isomerase signalling pathways in cancer. Curr Opin Pharmacol. 2011 Apr 13:Epub 2011/04/19.

[214] Hsiao K, Chapman P, Nilsen S, Eckman C, Harigaya Y, Younkin S, et al. Correlative memory deficits, Abeta elevation, and amyloid plaques in transgenic mice. Science. 1996 Oct 4;274(5284):99-102.

[215] Duff K, Eckman C, Zehr C, Yu X, Prada CM, Perez-tur J, et al. Increased amyloid-beta42(43) in brains of mice expressing mutant presenilin 1. Nature. 1996 Oct 24;383(6602):710-3.

[216] Games D, Adams D, Alessandrini R, Barbour R, Berthelette P, Blackwell C, et al. Alzheimer-type neuropathology in transgenic mice overexpressing V717F beta-amyloid precursor protein. Nature. 1995 Feb 9;373(6514):523-7.

[217] Hall AM, Roberson ED. Mouse models of Alzheimer's disease. Brain Res Bull. 2012 May 1;88(1):3-12.

[218] Gotz J, Ittner LM. Animal models of Alzheimer's disease and frontotemporal dementia. Nat Rev Neurosci. 2008 Jul;9(7):532-44.

[219] Irizarry MC, Soriano F, McNamara M, Page KJ, Schenk D, Games D, et al. Abeta deposition is associated with neuropil changes, but not with overt neuronal loss in the human amyloid precursor protein V717F (PDAPP) transgenic mouse. J Neurosci. 1997 Sep 15;17(18):7053-9.

[220] Poorkaj P, Bird TD, Wijsman E, Nemens E, Garruto RM, Anderson L, et al. Tau is a candidate gene for chromosome 17 frontotemporal dementia. Ann Neurol. 1998 Jun; 43(6):815-25.

[221] Spillantini MG, Murrell JR, Goedert M, Farlow MR, Klug A, Ghetti B. Mutation in the tau gene in familial multiple system tauopathy with presenile dementia. Proc Natl Acad Sci U S A. 1998 Jun 23;95(13):7737-41.

[222] Gotz J, Chen F, van Dorpe J, Nitsch RM. Formation of neurofibrillary tangles in P301l tau transgenic mice induced by Abeta 42 fibrils. Science. 2001 Aug 24;293(5534): 1491-5.

[223] Lewis J, Dickson DW, Lin WL, Chisholm L, Corral A, Jones G, et al. Enhanced neurofibrillary degeneration in transgenic mice expressing mutant tau and APP. Science. 2001 Aug 24;293(5534):1487-91.

Chapter 7

Alzheimer Disease and Metabolism: Role of Cholesterol and Membrane Fluidity

Genaro G. Ortiz, Fermín P. Pacheco-Moisés,
Luis J. Flores-Alvarado, Miguel A. Macías-Islas,
Irma E. Velázquez-Brizuela,
Ana C. Ramírez-Anguiano,
Erandis D. Tórres-Sánchez,
Eddic W. Moráles-Sánchez, José A. Cruz-Ramos,
Genaro E Ortiz-Velázquez and
Fernando Cortés-Enríquez

Additional information is available at the end of the chapter

http://dx.doi.org/10.5772/54091

1. Introduction

Alzheimer's disease (AD) is an age-related disorder characterized by deposition of amyloid β-peptide (Aβ) and degeneration of neurons in brain regions such as the hippocampus, resulting in progressive cognitive dysfunction. The causes of Alzheimer's disease (AD) have not been fully discovered, there are three main hypotheses to explain the phenomenon: a) The deficit of acetylcholine; b) The accumulation of beta-amyloid (Aβ and / or tau protein; and c) Metabolic disorders.

The clinical criteria for diagnosing AD were defined in 1984 by the NINCDS-ADRDA; (National Institute of Neurological and Communicative Disorders and Stroke; Alzheimer's Disease and Related Disorders). It states that for the diagnosis of disease is required to prove the existence of chronic and progressive cognitive impairment in adults or elderly patients, without other underlying causes that can explain this phenomenon. However, using this criterion, it is difficult to differentiate between AD and other causes of deterioration in early stages of the disease.

A number of recent research has been related AD with metabolic disorders, particularly hyperglycemia and insulin resistance. The expression of insulin receptors has been demonstrated in the central nervous system neurons, preferably in the hippocampus. In these neurons, when insulin binds to its cellular receptor, promotes the activation of intracellular signaling cascades that lead to change in the expression of genes related to synaptic plasticity processes and enzymes involved in clearing the same insulin and Aβ. These enzymes degrading of insulin promotes the reduction of toxicity due to amyloid in animal models.

People with neuritic plaques accumulate in brain regions that correspond to brain regions in healthy people that rise in a metabolic process called aerobic glycolysis. While some regions such as prefrontal and parietal cortex, which is thought to have a role in self-recognition and control tasks, showed high levels of aerobic glycolysis, others such as the cerebellum and the hippocampal formation, believed to affect the control motor and memory, showed low levels. Brain cells use aerobic glycolysis for energy derived quickly from small amounts of glucose while obtaining the mass of its energy through a biochemical process effective to burn glucose. Since aerobic glycolysis may help the brain generate cell constituents, toxic metabolic byproducts manage and regulate programmed cell death; the findings suggest a possible link between brain function that provides energy to aerobic glycolysis and the onset of AD.

The causes of the late AD appear to be multifactorial, and cell biology studies point to cholesterol as a key factor in protein precursor of beta Amyloid (APP) processing and Aβ production. An alteration in cholesterol metabolism is attractive hypotheses, thus the carriers of the Apolipoprotein E4 genes, which is involved in cholesterol metabolism, are at increased genetic risk for Alzheimer's disease. Cholesterol is a component of cell membranes and particularly is found in microdomains functionally linked to the proteolytic processing of APP. In sporadic AD, a marked diminution of both membrane phospholipids and cholesterol has been found.

Epidemiological studies indicate that mild hypercholesterolemia may increase the risk of AD and decreased synthesis of cholesterol through statin administration can reduce the development of AD. Moreover, high cellular cholesterol content has been shown to favor the production of Aβ. Genetic studies have suggested links between AD and cholesterol control several genes including cholesterol acceptor ApoE (ε4 polymorphism). Liver X receptors (LRXs) are ligand-activated transcription factors of the nuclear hormone receptor superfamily LXRs and also are expressed in the brain. LXRs stimulate the expression of genes involved in cellular cholesterol transport, regulation of lipid content of lipoproteins (apoE, lipoprotein lipase, cholesterol ester transfer protein, and phospholipid transfer protein), metabolism of fatty acids and triglycerides (sterol regulatory element binding protein 1-c, fatty acid synthase, stearoyl coenzyme A desaturase 1, and acyl coenzyme A carboxylase). Many questions remain, but as a master regulator of cholesterol homeostasis, LXR may be considered as a potential molecular target for the treatment of AD.

In summary, numerous studies on the role of cholesterol in AD suggest that high cholesterol is a risk factor for early and late AD development.

http://dx.doi.org/10.5772/54091

2. Dementia and pathological changes

Dementia is a syndrome that cause cognitive and memory alterations; problems of orientation, attention, language and solving problems. Dementia involves a progressive decline in cognition that goes above and beyond the normal changes that come with age due to injuries or brain diseases. The two most common causes of dementia are AD and vascular dementia. More than 33% of women and 20% of men aged 65 year or more will develop dementia during their lifetime, and many more develop a milder form of cognitive impairment. Worldwide, the adult population is rapidly growing; prospective epidemiological studies suggest that there will be an increase of 50% of the total number of people with cognitive disorders in the next 25 years. Dementia is associated with increased mortality and disability, health care costs they mean a huge expenditure on health systems as well as a significant increase in social and economic responsibilities for caregivers and their families. With a current affection about 10% of the population over the 65 year-old Alzheimer's disease (AD) is the most common cause of progressive dementia [1].

AD is a progressive neurological disorder resulting in irreversible loss of neurons, particularly in the cortex and hippocampus, accounting for about one third of dementia syndromes, with a range that varies from 42 to 81% of all dementias. The clinical findings are characterized by progressive loose of memory, loss of: judgment, decision making, physical orientation and language disorders. The diagnosis is based on neurological examination and differential diagnosis with other dementias, but the definitive diagnosis is made only by autopsy. The pathological findings at microscopic level are: neuronal loss, gliosis, neurofibrillary tangles, neuritic plaques, Hirano bodies, granulo-vacuolar degeneration of neurons and amyloid angiopathy [2, 3]. A very early change in AD brain is the reduced glucose metabolism [4], and a recent analysis suggests that diabetes plays a role in the acceleration of brain aging. But, although it is known that type 2-diabetes may be associated with an increased risk of dementia, the exact mechanisms and mitigating factors still are not completely understood. The public health implications of this phenomenon are enormous. Although initially the association between type 2 diabetes and vascular dementia appeared to be more consistent than the relationship between type 2 diabetes and AD, there are recent studies that have yielded more consistent evidence of the relationship between diabetes and AD [5,6].

Neuritic plaques, neurofibrillary tangles and other proteins in AD brain are glycosylated [7]. Since people with diabetes have an increased blood glucose level is plausible to suspect that they have a higher chance of having AD. Animal models of induced diabetes suggest a direct neurodegenerative effect of diabetes; most of these studies show damage in the hippocampus, an area associated with learning and memory, and first structure to be affected by the neurodegeneration of AD disease. A post-mortem study revealed that people with diabetes and ApoE 4 allele, had more neuritic plaques and neurofibrilar tangles in the hippocampus and cortex, also cerebral amyloid angiopathy, in which the associated protein AD disease is deposited on the walls of blood vessels in the brain. It has been shown that those with diabetes have a greater cortical atrophy, independent of hypertension, the blood concentration of total cholesterol, smoking, coronary heart disease and sociodemographic factors than people without the condition. Today we know that obesity increases the risk of dementia and brain atrophy. However, the molecular mechanisms that are behind metabolic disorders caused by excess body fat are not fully understood yet, especially regarding its role in neurodegenerative diseases (see Figure 1). Preliminary evidence suggests that some adipocytokines could cross the blood brain barrier, and have some function in learning and memory [8].

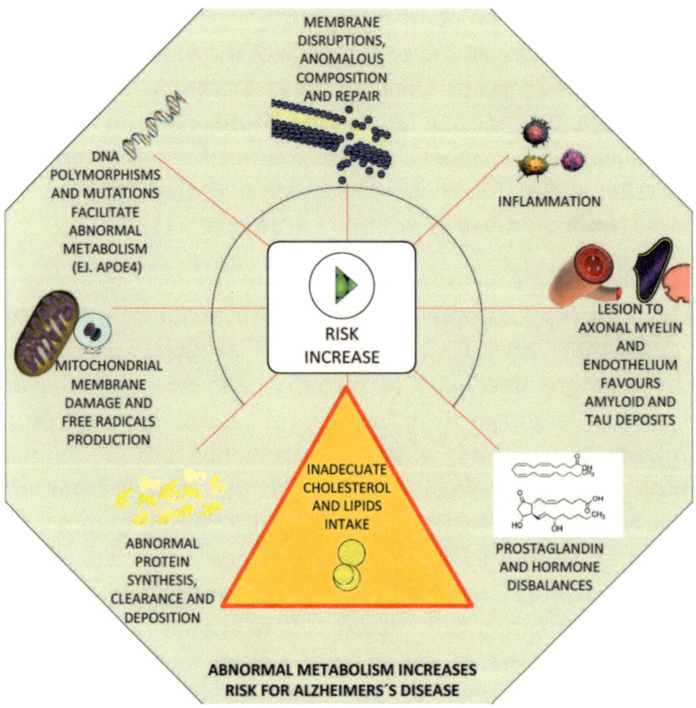

Figure 1. Abnormal metabolism increases risk for Alzheimer disease.

Recent findings from several longitudinal population studies have confirmed a link between obesity and risk of dementia. People with a body mass index (BMI) indicating obesity (≥ 30) have a greater probability of developing dementia (75%) compared with those with normal BMI (18.5 to 24.9). We must emphasize that abdominal obesity is more closely associated with dementia risk, that obesity spread throughout the body. Even for those with a healthy weight, abdominal obesity increases the risk of dementia [9].

3. Insulin-cholesterol-AD

Insulin signaling in the central nervous system has gained much interest for his participation in cognitive processes such as learning and memory and its possible relation to neurodegenerative diseases such as Alzheimer's disease. In peripheral tissues, mainly regulates insulin metabolism energetic and cell growth. The insulin receptor and several components of its signaling pathway are abundantly distributed in the mammalian brain and their activation modulates neuronal growth and synaptic plasticity [10].

It has been suggested that some alterations in the insulin signaling appear to be responsible for cognitive deficits and play an important role in the development of AD disease. Indeed, Type II diabetes is a risk factor for developing this type of dementia. Recently it has been observed that Aβ, which is overproduced in AD disease, causes alterations in the signaling pathway of insulin, supporting the causal relationships between this condition interesting and insulin [11]. In recent years the effects of insulin in the brain have drawn attention for his participation in mental processes such as memory and learning. Insulin in the brain plays an important role in the regulation of metabolism, and alterations in their activity are directly related to metabolic diseases such as obesity, diabetes or metabolic syndrome. In the mammalian brain, insulin anorexigenic effects, induces weight loss and regulates hypothalamic control of food intake. Also regulates glucose homeostasis by stimulating peripheral neurons producing pro-opiomelacortina (POMC) and agouti-related peptide (AgRP) through the IR and PI3K [12, 13].

Insulin can be generated in different brain sites. It is known that insulin is produced in the beta cells of the pancreas and can enter the brain through the blood brain barrier by active transport mediated by IR. Furthermore, the presence of messenger RNA in mammalian brain neurons, suggests that insulin can be produced locally. Likewise, there has been a strict regulation of the levels of insulin and its receptor (IR) in the brain, which may suggest that insulin level in the brain does not depend exclusively on the periphery [14]. However, if the source is local cerebral insulin, peripheral or shared has not been clarified yet. The IR is very abundant in the brains of rodents and humans with the highest concentration in the olfactory bulb, the hypothalamus, pituitary gland, hippocampus, cerebral cortex and cerebellum [15,16]. In addition, most of the proteins of the insulin signaling pathway have expression patterns that overlap with the IR in the brain. The IR is found abundantly in the hippocampus and its expression is increased after spatial learning tasks in rodents. The IR is widely found in the synapses of the dendritic trees which regulate the release of neurotransmitters and receptor recruitment [17] (see Figure 2).

Insulin regulates glutamatergic and GABAergic receptors, through the activation of the PI3K and MAPK. It is also known that the processes of long-term potentiation (LTP) and long-term depression (LTD), are associated with the molecular events underlying the establishment of memory and learning are regulated by the activation of PI3K through Complex formation with NMDA receptors, which regulates PI3K NMDA receptor translocation to the membrane. The response of the IR is reduced by the action of glutamate and depolarization, probably involving calcium influx of Ca2+ and activation of Ca2+-dependent kinases (Figure 3). This suggests a possible role of insulin in the synaptic plasticity and modulation of neuronal activity [18-20].

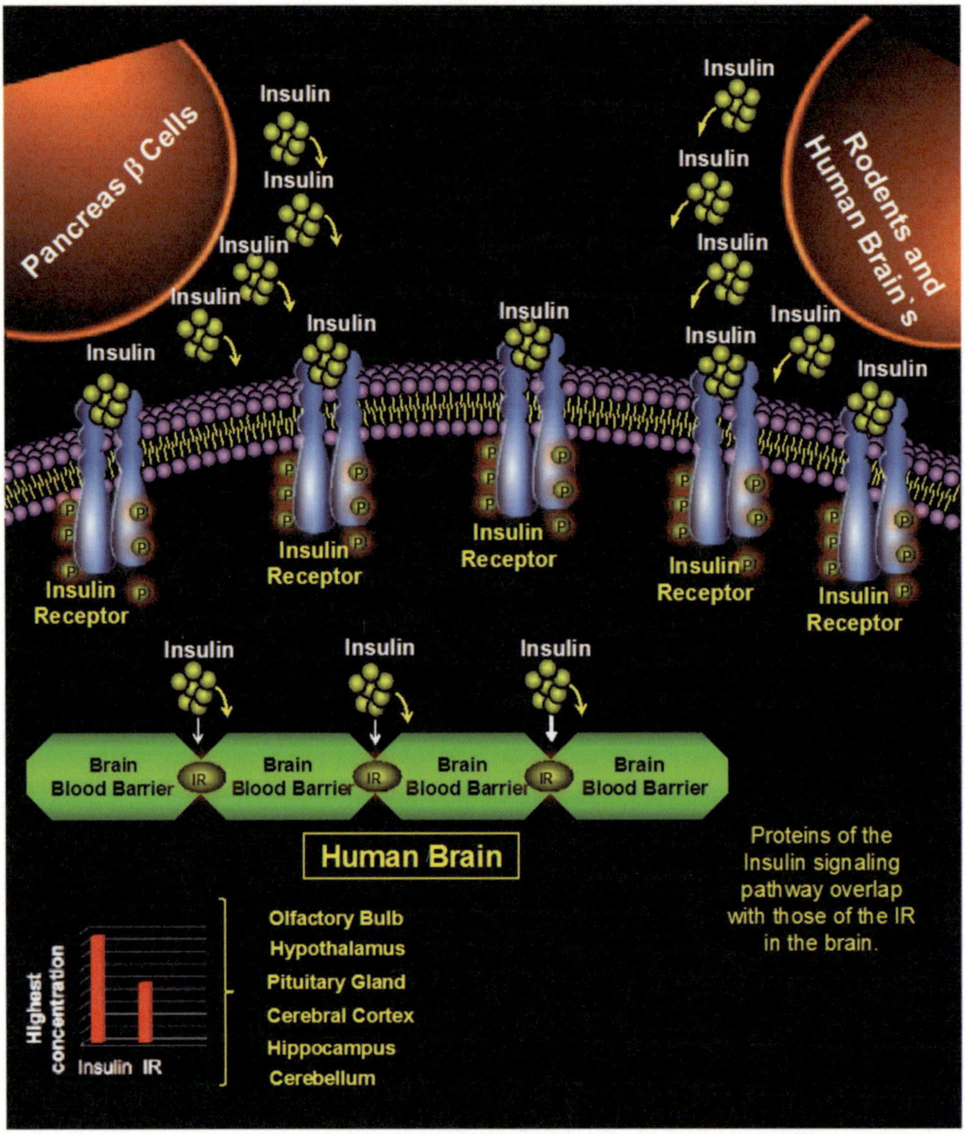

Figure 2. Insulin is produced in the Beta cells of the pancreasand enters the brain through the BBB (Brain Blood Barrier) via the IR (Insulin Receptor). Insulin levels on the brain do not depend exclusively on peripherical levels. The IR is very abundant in the brain of rodents and humans, showing its highest concentration in the following areas (in descending order): Olfactory bulb, hypothalamus, pituitary gland, cerebral cortex, hippocampus and the cerebellum. Most of the proteins involved in the insulin signaling pathway have expression patterns that overlap with the IR in the brain [125].

The presence of components via postsynaptic regions, such as mTOR, p70S6K, eIF-4E, 4E-BP1 and 4EBP2 suggest the existence of the regulation of protein synthesis at synapses. Insulin regulates the levels of the postsynaptic density protein PSD-95, which binds to the NMDA receptors in the synaptic membrane, through mTOR activation and modulation of protein translation at synapses. Furthermore, mTOR modulates synaptic plasticity Thus, insulin not only modulates neuronal synaptic activity [21]

Different strategies can be proposed to prevent the characteristics of AD-related dysfunction of the insulin signaling pathway. An important factor is the signal transduction through Akt. Akt activity can be improved with appropriate levels of omega-3 and DHA, which can help reduce βA levels and amyloid burden, as has been observed in transgenic mice Tg2576 regulating the activity of the enzyme IDE [22]. The loss of inhibition of GSK3 is involved in the production of neurofibrillary tangles and tau aggregation, which leads to oxidative stress, damage and toxicity in the neuronal synapses, so that GSK3 inhibitors could be used to prevent hyperphosphorylation of tau and the production of neurofibrillary tangles. Insulin has been used to improve memory and learning in healthy subjects and also in behavioral tasks in rats, suggesting a role in enhancing memory in humans, however, the actual effects of insulin on the CNS are just being elucidated [23,24].

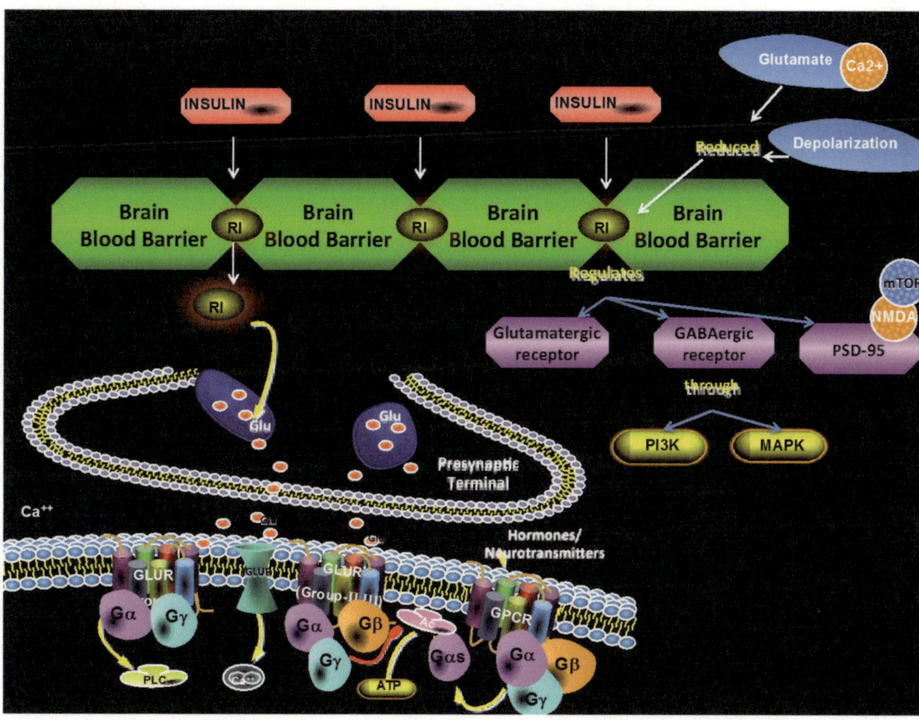

Figure 3. Insulin can enter the brain through the blood barrier by active transport mediated by IR. The IR is found abundantly in the hippocampus and synapses of dendritic trees, wich regulates the release of neurotransmitters and receptor recruitment. Insulin regulates glutamatergic and GABAergic receptors throug PI3K and MAPK [126].

Among the compounds which have been proposed as reducing agents include βA charging the statins, which lower cholesterol levels, some peptides that prevent Aβ fibril formation as PBT-531 and NC-1 (a chelating metals) and modulators of the activity of the secretases as

Bryostatin. Finally, the use of antioxidants such as vitamin E, have shown effectively to counter the effects of oxidative stress produced in the EA [25].

4. Proteins involved in cholesterol metabolism

Cholesterol, the most common steroid in humans, is a structural component of cell membranes and is a precursor of steroid hormones and bile salts. Since an excess of cholesterol is a major risk factor for the development of cardiovascular disease, it is essential a balance between cholesterol synthesis, uptake, and catabolism. Cholesterol is only synthesized in the liver and brain. The brain contains about 20% of total body cholesterol but only 2% of total body weight. The majority of this cholesterol is found in myelin membranes. Brain cholesterol is synthesized exclusively by *de novo* synthesis reaction from acetyl-CoA and acetoacetyl-CoA to form HMG-CoA. Then, is converted to mevalonate by HMG-CoA reductase, in the rate-limiting step of the process by oligodendrocytes, astrocytes and neurons [26].

After synthesis and secretion from glia via the ABCA1 transporter, cholesterol is packaged into lipoprotein particles resembling HDL. These HDL particles contain apoE. HDL is taken up into neurons through recognition of ApoE by a variety of lipoprotein receptors including the LDL receptor (LDLR); the LDL receptor related protein (LRP), the apoE receptor, as well as other lipoprotein receptors. Elimination of cholesterol from the brain occurs mainly via oxidation at the 24 and 27 positions to produce a class of compounds termed oxysterols. Water solubility of oxysterols is higher than cholesterol and diffuse across the BBB where they enter the peripheral circulation for excretion. *In vitro* studies showed a cholesterol shuttle from astrocytes to neurons that is mediated by apoE [27]. Virtually no cholesterol crosses the blood brain barrier from the peripheral circulation. Therefore, serum cholesterol levels have no effect on HMG-CoA reductase and its activity in the brain [28], and on total brain cholesterol levels [29]. The plasma half-life of cholesterol is several hours and fluctuates significantly according to intake. By contrast, cholesterol in the CNS is metabolized slowly, with a half life of 6 months in rats, and about 1 year in humans. In fact, changes in serum cholesterol have low impact on the CNS. Cholesterol metabolism in the brain is regulated by apoE4 and 24-hydroxylase. The rate-limiting enzyme 24-hydroxylase is uniquely expressed in the brain, and modulates the removal of cholesterol from the brain. The gene encoding this enzyme is called CYP46, and the CYP46 polymorphism was found to be associated with an increased Aβ deposition and tau phosphorylation, as well as with a higher risk of late-onset AD [30,31]. Cholesterol 24-hydroxylase (Cyp46) related to cytochrome P450, the ABC transporter (ABCA1), the receptor-associated protein to LDL (LRP) and the -2-macroglobulin. LRP1 is expressed mainly in neurons and activated astrocytes [32], and directly binds free Aβ, and mediates its egress from the brain [33]. Furthermore, it has been suggested that γ-secretase-mediated processing of APP plays a regulatory role in brain cholesterol and apoE metabolism through LRP1 [34]. In addition, the LRP polymorphism is negatively associated with Alzheimer. The Cyp46 is a brain specific enzyme that oxidizes cholesterol to form 24 (S)-hydroxycholesterol and its function is to remove cholesterol from the brain. Moreover, statins have been linked with AD, because the subjects medicated with them have lower prevalence of the disease [35]. The LRP-associated protein binds to LDL receptor very prominent in neurons. The α 2-macroglobulin is a protein capable of binding Aβ with high specificity and preventing its fibrillization [36]. α2M is found in neuritic plaques in AD brain [37] and it may play a role in Aβ clearance via LRP, as it is known to be able to bind other ligands and target them for internalization and degradation [38]. However, the putative role of these molecules in AD is controversial because some studies have failed to show an association between polymorphisms of α 2-macroglobulin and AD [39,40].

Studies *in vitro* showed that cholesterol depletion after treatment with both statins and methyl-β-cyclodextrin, which physically extracts membrane cholesterol, inhibits the generation of Aβ in hippocampal cells [41,42]. In transgenic AD animal models, hypercholesterolemia accelerates the development of Alzheimer's amyloid pathology [43]. Cholesterol-fed rabbits also develop changes in their brain that are typical of AD pathology [44].

Clinic-epidemiological studies suggest that increased serum cholesterol levels did not correlate substantially with AD in older ages [45,46]. However, all epidemiological studies, genetic, metabolic and laboratory show that many factors regulation of cholesterol metabolism are involved in the physiopathology of AD. The most prevalent risk factor identified to date is the Apolipoprotein E4 (Apo-E4), which is a protein carrier of cholesterol, Apo-E exists in the brain and the periphery. Although the E4 genotype appears to confer a risk for AD independent of plasma levels of cholesterol, the data do not clearly discriminate whether the polymorphism of the Apo E4 contributes to Alzheimer through a direct effect on Aβ, or an indirect effect through involving the catabolism of cholesterol (Figure 4). The levels of 24-hydroxycholesterol (24-OHC) is increased with age in subjects with AD, and recent studies suggest that genetic factors related to this molecule contribute to the pathogenesis of the disease [47].

Cholesterol catabolites also regulate the processing of the APP. Pharmacological inhibition of acyl-CoA:cholesterol acyltransferase (ACAT), which produces cholesterol esters, decreases Aβ. This is significant because the ACAT inhibitors are in development for the pharmaceutical companies for the treatment of atherosclerosis and such drugs may become useful for testing in AD. On the other hand, synthetic oxysterol, 22-hydroxycholesterol and synthetic LXR agonist reduces Aβ generation in murine models of AD via elevated apoE protein levels and increased lipidation of apoE, rather than through suppression of Aβ generation [48]. Furthermore, LXR agonist preserves cognitive function at a dose far below required to observe decreased Aβ levels [49] and AD neuropathology was exacerbated in mice lacking LXRs, providing further support for the central role of LXR target genes in the pathogenesis of AD. The enzyme that catalyzes the cleavage of β APP β-secretase is the (BACE) and their activity is particularly dependent on cholesterol levels [50] (Figure 5).

Studies on the cholesterol use in the brain of AD patients are also significant and consistent; cholesterol is removed from the brain to become 24-OHC, which appears in the plasma. The 24-OHC levels are increased in patients with AD or any other degenerative disease. The increase is probably, because cholesterol from degenerating neurons is captured and removed to maintain homeostasis. It has been shown that neurons with degenerative tangles showed increased levels of cholesterol. However, there is a striking difference between serum and brain levels of 24-OHC in AD, because the first increase; while the latter decrease. This perhaps reflects the decline in the number of neurons and synapses in the brains of subjects who died with AD [47]. Cholesterol is synthesized through a complex route that is blocked by a class of enzymes generically called statins. The clinical utility of statins has been demonstrated across multiple epidemiological studies, some of which have suggested that these drugs might be effective in treating AD disease. Advances in understanding the relationship between the biology of cholesterol and the production of Aβ peptide, crucial in the development of amyloid plaque, will lead to new therapeutic approaches for AD disease.

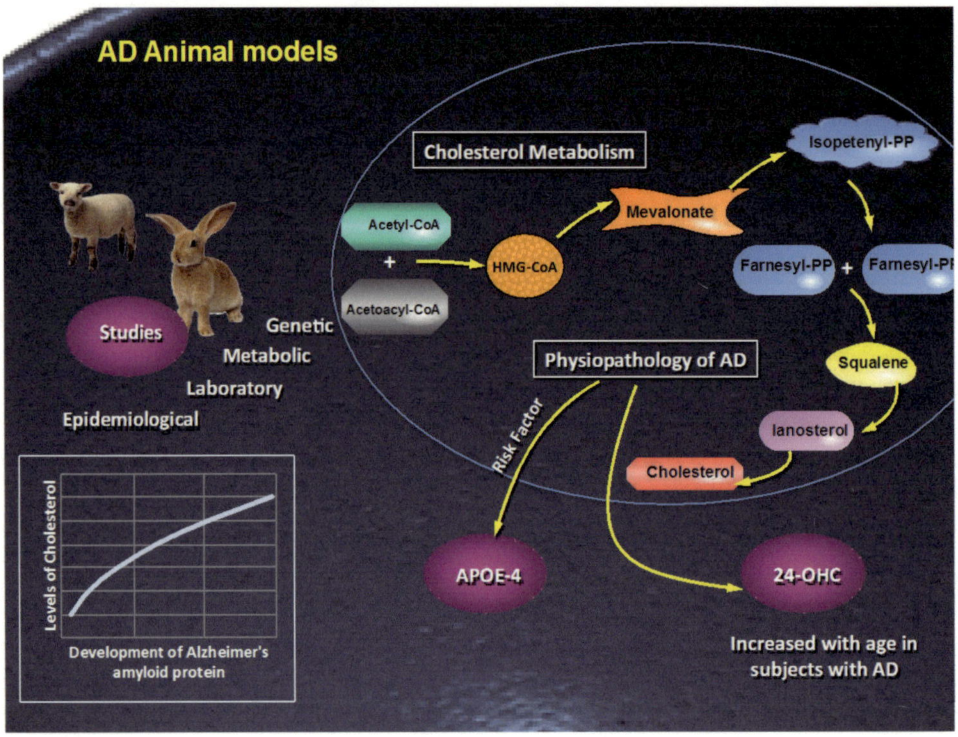

Figure 4. In Alzheimer's Disease (AD) animal models, hypercholesterolemia accelerates the development of Alzheimer's amyloid protein. Genetic, metabolic, clinical and epidemiological studies have shown that many factors involved in cholesterol's metabolism are involved in the pathophysiology of AD. The most prevalent risk factor is the APOE-4 (Apolipoprotein E4) genotype.

Statins are inhibitors of the enzyme 3-hydroxy-3-methylglutaryl coenzyme A (HMG-CoA) reductase, which converts HMG-CoA into mevalonate; this is the rate-limiting step in cholesterol biosynthesis [51]. These drugs decrease cholesterol levels about 30% and with few adverse effects. The first statin was lovastatin was synthesized, and since then have appeared fluvastatin, pravastatin, simvastatin and atorvastatin. Simvastatin and lovastatin are administered as pro-drugs and must be activated. These drugs differ in their lipid solubility; lipophilic statins, such as pravastatin, enter cells via an ATP-dependent anion transport system [52]. Pravastatin was not previously thought to cross the blood-brain barrier, however, it was recently demonstrated in mice that oral pravastatin treatment results in measurable pravastatin levels in the brain [53]. Pravastatin use is associated with a reduced risk of AD [54,55]. Statins inhibit cholesterol synthesis but also seem to affect other processes, because they can increase apoptosis and alter neuronal proliferation. Also decrease the immune response, anti-inflammatory property that has made recently has made the proposal to treat multiple sclerosis. Also appear to inhibit bone turnover and thereby reduce osteoporosis. The probable protective effects of statins in AD seem stronger than any association between plasma cholesterol and disease.

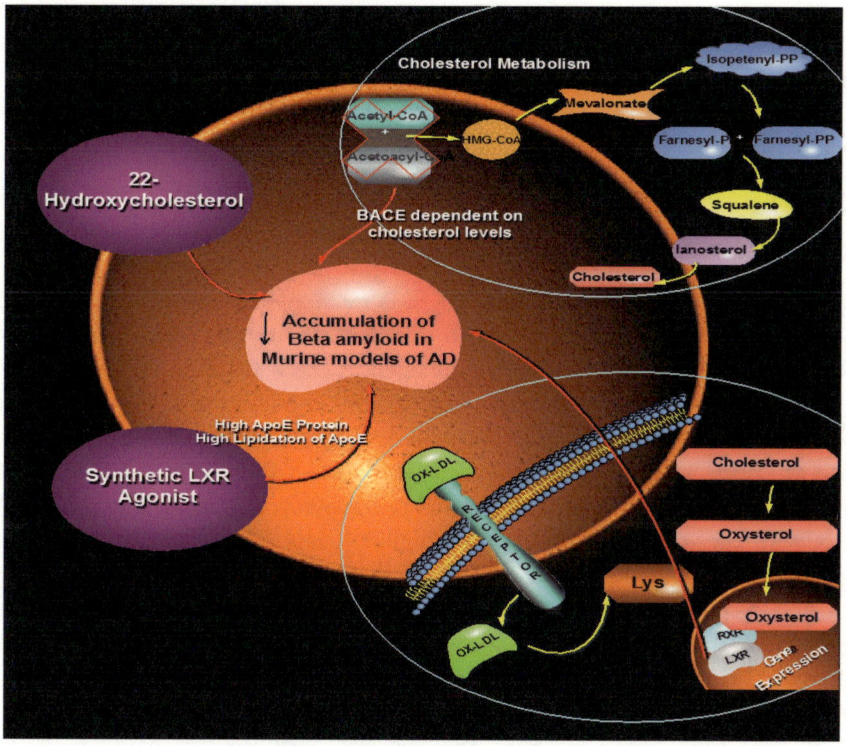

Figure 5. The inhibition of Acetyl-CoA and Acetoacyl-CoA (ACAT) produces cholesterol esters and decreases Amyloid Beta (AB). Synthetic oxysterol, 22-hydroxychoresterol and synthetic LXR agonists reduce AB generation in murine models of AD via elevated ApoE protein levels and increased lipidation of ApoE [124].

Oral administration of statins, in addition to inhibiting cholesterol synthesis, also affects gene expression the mouse brain [53]. Therefore, statins may protect the brain from AD by a mechanism independent of their effect on cholesterol. In addition to inhibition of cholesterol synthesis, statins block mevalonate formation and subsequently prevent formation of isoprenoids such as famesylpyrophosphate and geranylpyrophosphate. Statins inhibit isoprenylation of proteins, including the Rho family of small GTPases, in neuronal cells [56] and cultured microglia [57,58]. RhoA is a monomeric G-protein that is negatively coupled to cell growth; prevention of RhoA isoprenylation increases neurite extension [59]. At this regard, treatment of neurons with pravastatin enhanced neurite number, length and branching, and that this effect is mediated by inhibition of mevalonate synthesis and subsequent inhibition of isoprenylation of Rho GTPases and subsequent prevention of neuritic dystrophy and deterioration [60].

Epidemiological studies have found an inverse relationship between usage of the cholesterol-lowering drugs and risk of developing AD [54,55,61]. Statins are inhibitors of the enzyme HMG-CoA reductase, which converts HMG-CoA into mevalonate; this is the rate-limiting step in cholesterol biosynthesis [51]. However, reduction of cholesterol levels may or may not correlate with reduced risk of AD in patients taking statin drugs [62-64]. Furthermore, statin usage is associated with a decreased risk of depression and anxiety, which is not correlated with plasma cholesterol levels [65]. Oral administration of statins, in addition to inhibiting cholesterol synthesis, also affects gene expression in the mouse brain [53]. Thus, statins might prevent onset of AD by a mechanism independent of their effect on cholesterol.

Apolipoprotein E (apoE) is the major apolipoprotein in the brain and is a structural component of triglyceride-rich lipoproteins, chylomicrons, very-low-density lipoproteins (VLDL), and high-density-lipoproteins (HDL). ApoE is synthesized and secreted from astrocytes and microglia. Variation in the APOE gene sequence results in the 3 common alleles (ε2, ε3 and ε4), which can produce 6 different genotypes (ε2/ε2, ε2/ε3, ε2/ε4, ε3/ε3, ε3/ε4 and ε4/ε4). The ε2, ε3 and ε4 alleles encode three distinct forms of apoE (E2, E3 and E4) that differ in their amino acid composition at positions 112 and 158 [66]. ApoE3 seems to be the normal isoform, while apoE4 and apoE2 can each be dysfunctional [67]. Inheritance of apoE4 is associated with a greater risk of developing AD at an earlier age [68], whereas inheritance of apoE2 correlates with lower risk and later onset of AD [69]. individuals with the APOE ε4 allele show higher levels of plasma cholesterol, especially LDL cholesterol [70]. Subjects with APOE ε3/ε4 and ε4/ε4 genotypes absorb cholesterol effectively and have higher non-fasting serum triglyceride values than ε4 negative individuals [71,72]. A ApoE gene mutation (allele 4), the main risk factor for AD, may influence the risk of dementia more strongly among those with diabetes, in fact, findings from population studies show that people with diabetes and ApoE 4 are at greatest risk of AD compared with those without diabetes and without the ApoE 4. Although we know that people with diabetes are at increased risk of stroke, little is known about the effect of diabetes on the pathophysiology of neurodegeneration.

5. Membrane fluidity in Alzheimer disease

The role of the physical–chemical properties of intracellular membranous structures such as membrane fluidity in AD pathogenesis has been extensively studied. Membrane fluidity is a complex parameter, influenced both through some biophysical (temperature, electrical charges, pH) and biochemical factors (protein/phospholipids ratio, phospholipids/cholester-

http://dx.doi.org/10.5772/54091

ol ratio, degree of fatty acids unsaturation). It is a parameter that reflects the main membrane characteristic organization (gel or liquid crystal structure). Experiments provide consistent data about membrane fluidity relations to various cellular processes, especially membrane processes. Changes in the membrane composition and structure could alter the conformation and function of transmembranal ion channels, as well as affect the interaction of receptors and effectors, leading to altered signal transduction, handling of Ca", and response to exogenous stimuli [73].

Cholesterol distribution within the plasma membrane is not homogeneous: the highest level of free cholesterol inside the plasma membrane is found in cytofacial bilayer leaflet [74]. The exofacial leaflet contains substantially less cholesterol, and it is mostly condensed in lipid rafts, which are more tightly packed than nonlipid raft domains due to intermolecular hydrogen bonding involving sphingolipid and cholesterol [75]. This asymmetric distribution of cholesterol is altered by aging: it is significantly increased in exofacial leaflet with increasing age [76,77]. It has been reported that membrane fluidity of lipid membranes in the brain cortex of AD samples were significantly thinner (that is, had less microviscosity) than corresponding age-matched controls. This change in membrane width correlated with a 30% decrease in the ratio cholesterol/ phospholipid [78].

In our group of research we assessed the membrane fluidity in platelet submitochondrial particles and erythrocyte membranes from Mexican patients with Alzheimer disease. Submitochondrial particles are mainly constituted of inner mitochondrial membrane and are the site of oxidative phosphorylation and other enzymatic systems involved in the transport and utilization of metabolites. Membrane fluidity was estimated measuring the intramolecular excimer formation of the fluorescent probe 1,3 dipyrenylpropane incorporated in membranes. Similarly to the data reported from mitochondria in AD brains fluidity [79]., a reduced fluidity in the platelet inner mitochondrial membrane was found. It can partially be due to increased levels of lipid peroxidation [80]. Reduced membrane fluidity can diminish the activities of the enzymes of oxidative phosphorylation and other transport and receptor proteins, in as much as these enzymes are regulated by the physicochemical state of the lipid environment of the membrane. It may diminish significantly the ATP generation from the mitochondria. Interestingly, dysfunctional mitochondria and oxidative damage has been involved in Alzheimer's disease [81]. In agreement with previous reports, membrane fluidity from erythrocyte was not altered in AD [82], regardless of increased lipid oxidation in erythrocyte AD patients. This suggests that, in AD, mitochondrial membranes are more sensitive to oxidative stress than erythrocytes. In contrast to platelet inner mitochondrial membrane, it has been reported an increase in fluidity in whole membranes from platelets of AD patients [83]. This increase results from the elaboration of an internal membrane compartment resembling endoplasmic reticulum that is functionally abnormal [84]. At this regard, it is worth noting that the contribution of mitochondrial membranes to the whole cell membranes in platelets could be minimized since platelets contain few mitochondria [85].

On the other hand, it has been reported that using diphenil-hexatriene (DPH) and trimethylammonium-diphenyl-hexatriene (TMA-DPH) as fluorescent probes, the membrane fluidity in mitocondrial membranes was similar in platelets from AD patients and controls [86]. That discrepancy with our data may be due to intrinsic differences in the populations tested, the purity of the used mitochondrial fraction and the nature of the probes used. Additionally, it's clear that the lipophilic probes are sensitive to slightly different membrane properties. For instance, DPH and TMA-DPH are rotational probes [87] and dipyrenylpropane is a lateral diffusion sensitive probe [88]. In addition, DPH partitions into the interior of the bilayer and its average location has been shown to be about 8 Å from the center of the bilayer. TMA-DPH is oriented in the membrane bilayer with its positive charge localized at the lipid-water interface. Its DPH moiety is localized at about 11 Å from the center of the bilayer and reports the interfacial region of the membrane [89]. Whereas dipyrenylpropane is a highly hydrophobic probe which partitions into the membrane lipid bilayer [88].

As shown in figure 1, we found a significant decrease of membrane fluidity in hippocampal neurons from AD patients compared with membranes from elderly non demented controls (Figure 6). Lower membrane fluidity in AD patients was correlated with abnormal APP processing and cognitive decline [90].

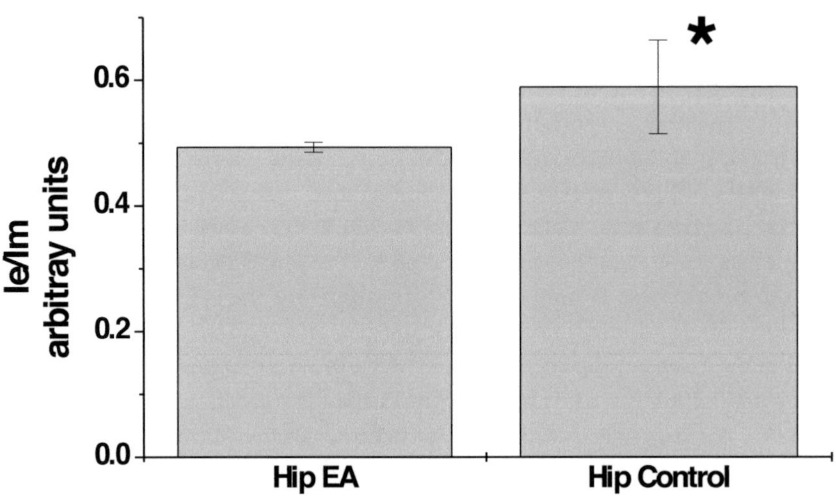

Figure 6. Excimer to monomer fluorescent ratio of dipirenylpropane on plasma membrane of hippocampus fom AD patients and aged-matched controls. The fluorescent probe was excited at 329 nm and emission of monomer (Ie) and excimer (Im) was read at 379 and 480 nm, respectively. Intramolecular excimer formation of this probe is related with the membrane fluidity. Therefore the ratio (Ie/Im) is directly proportional to membrane fluidity, which is reciprocal to membrane viscosity. The data shown are mean ± S.E.M. $*p < 0.01$.

Some strategies for the preservation of membrane fluidity include the use of polyunsaturated fatty acid (PUFAs). The brain is particularly rich in PUFAs such as eicosapentaenoic (EPA) and docosahexaenoic acids (DHA). PUFAs play an essential role in the normal development and functioning of brain [91]. Diets enriched in n-3 PUFA increased membrane fluidity, affect signal transduction and modulate gene expression for brain function [92]. Furthermore, DHA have the following effects: maintains membrane fluidity, improved synaptic and neurotransmitter functioning, enhanced learning and memory performances and displayed neuroprotective properties [93], decreased the amount of vascular Aβ deposition [94] and reduced Aβ burden [22]. In AD mouse model, DHA modulated APP processing by decreasing both α- and β-APP C-terminal fragment products and full-length APP [22]. However, caution should be taken when PUFAs are used for dietary supplementation, since DHA could be increasing oxidative stress, resulting in lipid peroxidation [95,96].

Addition of cholesterol restored the membrane width to that of the age-matched control samples. Alterations in other membrane components of AD brains have also been reported. The cholesterol content in lipid rafts has been shown to contribute to the integrity of the raft structure and the functions of the rafts in signaling and membrane trafficking [97]. At this regard, it has been shown that cholesterol depletion leads to increased membrane fluidity [98] mainly in intracellular membranes [99] and reduced endocytosis, shifting sAPP shedding from β-cleavage towards α-cleavage [63]. In fact, the cleavage of APP by β-secretase [100], occurs mainly in highly ordered membrane microdomains dispersed at the cell surface. These microdomains known as lipid rafts are enriched in cholesterol, sphingolipids and saturated phospholipids. Lipid rafts appear to be a mechanism to compartmentalize various processes on the cell surface by bringing together various receptor-mediated and signal transduction processes. The cleavage of APP by α-secretase is done mostly in nonraft domains [101]. Furthermore, it has been shown *in vitro* that lowering cholesterol leads to decreased BACE-cleavage of APP [102,103] and increased α-cleavage of APP [102].

Increased membrane fluidity due to cholesterol depletion inhibits endocytosis which might explain the observed increase of sAPPα and shift towards α-secretase cleavage that happens on the cell surface. Cholesterol increase is associated with enhanced membrane stiffness possibly explaining the disrupted proximity of APP and BACE. Surprisingly this is associated with enhanced sAPPβ production, possibly explained by altered transport and endocytosis mechanisms [103]. Another explanation therefore is the direct impact of cholesterol environment upon BACE activity. In living cells, BACE seems to require intact rafts for activity, and BACE outside rafts seems to be inactive [104].

6. Role of dietary lipids in Alzheimer disease

Recent theories suggests that there would be an interaction between genetic predisposition and environmental factors that lead to cell death by amyloid toxicity or disruption of tau protein. Dietary lipids could be a determining factor in the difference in risk between developed and underdeveloped countries. Dietary lipids could be the primary risk factor in late-onset sporadic AD (LO-SAT). The critical factors seem to be the ratios of polyunsaturated fatty acids (PUFAs) to monounsaturated (MUFA), saturated fatty acids (SFA) to essential fatty acids (EFAs). These contents are modified by the APOE4 genotype [105].

Oxidation of neuronal lipid membranes could be the initiating event in the cascade of synergistic processes with subsequent expression of Aβ and helical filaments of hyper-phosphorylated tau protein. PUFAs are important in modulating the inflammatory balance/systemic anti-inflammatory eicosanoids and fluidity and membrane function. Proinflammatory eicosanoids are derived from arachidonic acid (AA). The anti-inflammatory eicosanoids are derived from the via the n-3 EFA through DHA) and EPA. EFAs cannot be synthesized by animals and must be obtained from food. A diet rich in linoleic acid promotes proinflammatory state, while a diet rich in linolenic acid promotes inflammatory components. When lipids are exposed to free radicals begin an autoperoxidative process. This process is perpetual and changes the composition and rate of membrane lipids with loss of PUFA compared with MUFA and SFA. This causes the membrane to become less fluid and affecting the function of components, as well as of intracellular organelles and the vascular endothelium [106]. This seems to be the initial process of the cascade that culminates in neuronal death and neuropathological sequelae associated with LO-SAT. Antioxidant vitamins and vegetables may reduce the risk of AD. High levels of blood lipids are associated with atherosclerosis and diabetes, both risk factors for EA indirect. Recently it was found that the increase in LDL cholesterol, along with APOE epsilon4 genotype is associated with increased risk of AD [107].

The oxidative state of lipid membranes can have effects on neurons, at three levels:a) vascular;b) endothelial cell membrane; and c) membrane organelles.At the level of cellular membranes lipid oxidation accelerates the aggregation of amyloid which consequently decreases membrane fluidity. This also is observed with decreases of the content of MUFA and PUFA esterified to phospholipid. Interestingly, these changes are seen in brain regions affected in AD, especially at the hippocampus. The decrease of the membrane fluidity affects the synaptic connections [108]. The EA may be preventable and treatable and possibly reversible to some extent, if the proposed hypothesis is correct. The changes in the fat composition of the diet are reflected in plasma lipids and phospholipids in the membrane of red blood cells, likewise in the neural cell membranes, especially in areas of rapid lipid turnover. A diet low of n-6 PUFA and MUFA, and an adequate amount of n-3 PUFA, but not too caloric, with antioxidants should protect neuronal damage, lipid oxidation and the inflammatory cascade and amyloid deposition.

Lipid lowering agents appear to have a protective effect, although studies are not conclusive. Statins decrease the oxidizability of LDL, with decreased levels of oxygen reactive species, anti-inflammatory effects and improve endothelial dysfunction, also increased alpha-secretase activity. Increase the synthesis of LDL receptors, with decreased circulating level and reduced production of PPA.

The histological changes seen in the initial stages of AD confirmed that membrane lipids and inflammation are involved in the disease (Figure 7). AGE n-3/n-6 rate has a major impact on the balance of eicosanoid metabolism inflammatory and anti-inflammatory, and the degree of saturation of membrane lipids and fluidity affects its function. The apoE4 genotype may influence the risk of AD, as it is unable to protect that transports lipids from oxidation [109].

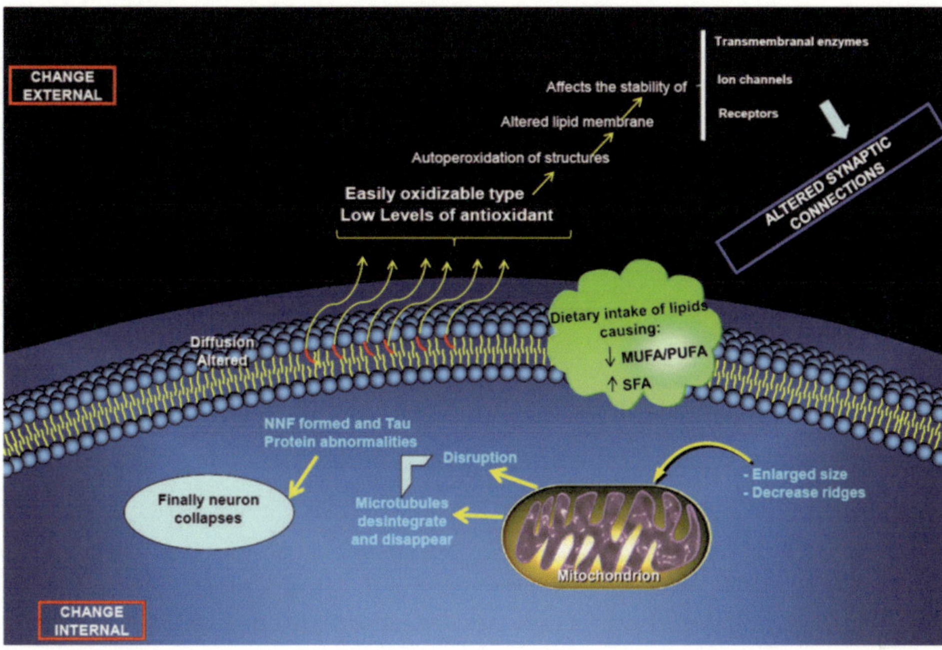

Figure 7. Cellular changes induced by lipid oxidation linked to dietary lipids. The change in dietary intake of lipids causing a low PUFA/MUFA (Polyunsaturated Fatty Acid/Monounsaturated Fatty Acids) ratio, which finally altered synaptic connections and neuron collapse [127].

7. Membrane phospholipid metabolism

The principal constituents of mammalian cell membranes are phospholipids, the most abundant of which is phosphatidylcholine (PC). PC biosynthesis is initiated by the phosphorylation of choline to form phosphocholine, which then combines with cytidine triphosphate (CTP) to form 5'-cytidine diphosphocholine (CDP-choline); this compound then reacts with diacylglycerol (DAG) to produce PC [110]. The rate at which cells form PC is affected by the availability of its precursors. Thus, uridine or cytidine increase CTP levels [111]; availability of CTP levels in turn can be rate-limiting in the syntheses of CDP-choline [112] and PC [113]; and DAG levels can control the conversion of CDP-choline to PC [114]. AD is also associated with abnormal metabolism of membrane phospholipids. Alterations in the metabolism of the phospholipids phosphatidylcholine (PC) have been detected in the cerebrospinal fluid of AD patients [115]. Neural membrane glycerophospholipids, particularly ethanolamine plasmalogens, are markedly decreased in autopsy samples from AD brain compared to age-matched control brain [116]. This decrease in glycerophospholipids is accompanied by a marked elevation in phospholipid degradation metabolites such as glycerophosphocholine, phosphocholine, and phosphoethanolamine [117]. Furthermore, marked increases have been reported in levels of prostaglandins and lipid peroxides in AD brain [118,119]. The marked changes observed in phospholipids and their catabolic products may be coupled to the elevated activities of lipolytic enzymes in AD brain [120]. Moreover, cortices of AD patients have decreased levels of PC and phosphatidylethanolamine, compared with age-matched controls [116]. PC synthesis is regulated by levels of its precursors [113,114]; therefore, stimulation of PC synthesis by increasing precursor levels prevents the disruption in normal phospholipid metabolism caused by AD. Furthermore, increasing cell membrane synthesis may have morphological consequences for the cell. For instance, dendritic atrophy and loss occur in mouse models of AD [121,122] and dystrophic neurites are observed in human cases of AD [123]

8. Concluding remarks

Data from a series of biochemical, genetic, epidemiological studies and others exhibited that cholesterol is a key factor in APP processing and Aβ production. For instance, high cholesterol levels are linked to increased Aβ generation and deposition. It appears that there are many different ways in which abnormalities in cholesterol metabolism can affect the development of AD. Some polymorphisms in genes involved in cholesterol catabolism and transport have been associated with an increased level of Aβ and are therefore potential risk factors for the disease. The best known of these genes is apoE4, which is the major genetic risk factor known for late-onset AD. Other genes implicated include cholesterol 24-hydroxylase (Cyp46), the LDL receptor related protein, the cholesterol transporter ABCA1, acyl-CoA:cholesterol acetyl transferase, and the LDL receptor. Then, we may conclude that what is bad for the heart is bad for the brain. We must pay attention to risk factors associated with heart disease to prevent Alzheimer's disease also. Considerable interest has also arisen regarding the effects of lifestyle interventions such as exercise and dietary/nutriceutical manipulations.

Acknowledgements

We dedicate this paper to Dr. Pedro Garzón de la Mora; who was for some of us a guide, and showed us to lose ourselves in the wonderful jungle of Biochemistry.

http://dx.doi.org/10.5772/54091

Author details

Genaro G. Ortiz[1*], Fermín P. Pacheco-Moisés[2], Luis J. Flores-Alvarado[3], Miguel A. Macías-Islas[4], Irma E. Velázquez-Brizuela[5], Ana C. Ramírez-Anguiano[2], Erandis D. Tórres-Sánchez[1], Eddic W. Moráles-Sánchez[1], José A. Cruz-Ramos[1], Genaro E Ortiz-Velázquez[1] and Fernando Cortés-Enríquez[1]

*Address all correspondence to: genarogabriel@yahoo.com

1 Lab. Estrés Oxidativo-Mitocondria & Enfermedad, Centro de Investigación Biomédica de Occidente. Instituto Mexicano del Seguro Social (IMSS). Guadalajara, Jalisco, México

2 Dpto. de Química. CUCEI, Universidad de Guadalajara. Guadalajara, Jalisco, México

3 Dpto. de Bioquímica. CUCS, Universidad de Guadalajara. Guadalajara, Jalisco, México

4 Depto. de Neurología. UMAE,HE- IMSS. Guadalajara, Jalisco, México

5 OPD-IJC-SSA- Jalisco. Guadalajara, Jalisco, México

References

[1] Reitz C, Carol Brayne & Richard Mayeux Epidemiology of Alzheimer disease. Nature Reviews Neurology 7, 137-152.

[2] Brookmeyer R, Johnson E, Ziegler-Graham K, Arrighi HM: Forecasting the global burden of Alzheimer's disease. Alzheimers Dement 2007, 3:186-191.

[3] Tiraboschi P, Hansen LA, Thal LJ, Corey-Bloom J (June 2004). The importance of neuritic plaques and tangles to the development and evolution of AD. Neurology 62 (11): pp. 1984–9

[4] L. Mosconi, Brain glucose metabolism in the early and specific diagnosis of Alzheimer's disease. FDG-PET studies in MCI and AD. Eur J Nucl Med Mol Imaging 2005: (32) 486-510.

[5] R. Peila, B.L. Rodriguez, L.J. Launer, Type 2 diabetes, APOE gene, and the risk for dementia and related pathologies: The Honolulu-Asia Aging Study. Diabetes 2002: (51) 1256-1262.

[6] Han W, Li C Linking type 2 diabetes and Alzheimer's disease. Proc Natl Acad Sci U S A. 2010 Apr 13;107(15):6557-8.

[7] T. Dyrks, A. Weidemann, G. Multhaup, J.M. Salbaum, H.G. Lemaire, J. Kang, B. Muller-Hill, C.L. Masters, K. Beyreuther, Identification, transmembrane orientation and

biogenesis of the amyloid A4 precursor of Alzheimer's disease. EMBO J 1988:(7) 949-957.

[8] K. Kos, A.L. Harte, N.F. da Silva, A. Tonchev, G. Chaldakov, S. James, D.R. Snead, B. Hoggart, J.P. O'Hare, P.G. McTernan, S. Kumar, Adiponectin and resistin in human cerebrospinal fluid and expression of adiponectin receptors in the human hypothalamus. J Clin Endocrinol Metab 2007:(92) 1129-1136.

[9] R.A. Whitmer, E.P. Gunderson, C.P. Quesenberry, Jr., J. Zhou, K. Yaffe, Body mass index in midlife and risk of Alzheimer disease and vascular dementia. Curr Alzheimer Res 2007:(4) 103-109. J Neurochem. 2005 Aug;94(4):1158-66.

[10] van der Heide LP, Kamal A, Artola A, Gispen WH, Ramakers GM. Insulin modulates hippocampal activity-dependent synaptic plasticity in a N-methyl-d-aspartate receptor and phosphatidyl-inositol-3-kinase-dependent manner.

[11] Son SM, Song H, Byun J, Park KS, Jang HC, Park YJ, Mook-Jung I. Altered APP Processing in Insulin-Resistant Conditions Is Mediated by Autophagosome Accumulation via the Inhibition of Mammalian Target of Rapamycin Pathway. Diabetes. 2012 Jul 24.

[12] Plum L, Belgardt BF, Brüning JC. Central insulin action in energy and glucose homeostasis. J Clin Invest 2006; 116(7): 1761-1766

[13] Pardini AW, Nguyen HT, Figlewicz DP, Baskin DG, Williams DL, Kim F, Schwartz MW. Distribution of insulin receptor substrate-2 in brain areas involved in energy homeostasis. Brain Res 2006; 1112(1): 169-178.

[14] Abbott MA, Wells DG, Fallon JR. The insulin receptor tyrosine kinase substrate p58/53 and the insulin receptor are components of CNS synapses. J Neurosci 1999; 19(17): 7300-7308.

[15] Gerozissis K. Brain insulin, energy and glucose homeostasis; genes, environment and metabolic pathologies. Eur J Pharmacol 2008; 585(1): 38-49.

[16] Gasparini L, Netzer WJ, Greengard P, Xu H. Does insulin dysfunction play a role in Alzheimer's disease? Trends Pharmacol Sci 2002; 23(6): 288-293.

[17] Wei Y, Williams JM, Dipace C, Sung U, Javitch JA, Galli A, Saunders C. Dopamine transporter activity mediates amphetamine-induced inhibition of Akt through a Ca2+/calmodulin-dependent kinase II-dependent mechanism. Mol Pharmacol 2007; 71(3): 835-842

[18] Man HY, Wang Q, Lu WY, Ju W, Ahmadian G, Liu L, D'Souza S, Wong TP, Taghibiglou C, Lu J, Becker LE, Pei L, Liu F, Wymann MP, MacDonald JF, Wang YT. Activation of PI3-Kinase is required for AMPA receptor insertion during LTP of mEPSCs in cultured hippocampal neurons. Neuron 2003; 38(4): 611-624.

[19] Zhao WQ, De Felice FG, Fernández S, Chen H, Lambert MP, Quon MJ, Krafft GA, Klein WL. Amyloid beta oligomers induce impairment of neuronal insulin receptors. FASEB J 2008; 22(1): 246-260.

[20] Nelson T, Alkon D. Insulin and cholesterol pathways in neuronal function, memory and neurodegeneration. Biochem Soc Trans 2005; 33(Pt 5): 1033-1036.

[21] Tang SJ, Reis G, Kang H, Gingras AC, Sonenberg N, Schuman EM. A rapamycin-sensitive signaling pathway contributes to long-term synaptic plasticity in the hippocampus. Proc Natl Acad Sci USA 2002; 99(1): 467-472.

[22] Lim GP, Calon F, Morihara T, Yang F, Teter B, Ubeda O, Salem N Jr, Frautschy SA, Cole GM. A diet enriched with the omega-3 fatty acid docosahexaenoic acid reduces amyloid burden in an aged Alzheimer mouse model. J Neurosci 2005; 25(12): 3032-3040.

[23] 2002; 22(22): 9785-9793. 45. Kern W, Peters A, Fruehwald-Schultes B, Deininger E, Born J, Fehm HL. Improving influence of insulin on cognitive functions in humans. Neuroendocrinology 2001; 74(4): 270-280

[24] Park CR, Seeley RJ, Craft S, Woods SC. Intracerebroventricular insulin enhances memory in a passive-avoidance task. Physiol Behav 2000; 68(4): 509-514.

[25] Blennow K, de Leon MJ, Zetterberg H. Alzheimer's disease. Lancet 2006; 368(9533): 387-403.

[26] J.M. Dietschy, S.D. Turley, Cholesterol metabolism in the brain. Curr Opin Lipidol 2001:(12) 105-112.

[27] O. Levi, D. Lutjohann, A. Devir, K. von Bergmann, T. Hartmann, D.M. Michaelson, Regulation of hippocampal cholesterol metabolism by apoE and environmental stimulation. J Neurochem 2005:(95) 987-997.

[28] H. Jurevics, J. Hostettler, C. Barrett, P. Morell, A.D. Toews, Diurnal and dietary-induced changes in cholesterol synthesis correlate with levels of mRNA for HMG-CoA reductase. J Lipid Res 2000:(41) 1048-1054.

[29] C. Kirsch, G.P. Eckert, A.R. Koudinov, W.E. Muller, Brain cholesterol, statins and Alzheimer's Disease. Pharmacopsychiatry 2003:(36 Suppl 2) S113-119.

[30] I. Bjorkhem, D. Lutjohann, U. Diczfalusy, L. Stahle, G. Ahlborg, J. Wahren, Cholesterol homeostasis in human brain: turnover of 24S-hydroxycholesterol and evidence for a cerebral origin of most of this oxysterol in the circulation. J Lipid Res 1998:(39) 1594-1600.

[31] A. Papassotiropoulos, J.R. Streffer, M. Tsolaki, S. Schmid, D. Thal, F. Nicosia, V. Iakovidou, A. Maddalena, D. Lutjohann, E. Ghebremedhin, T. Hegi, T. Pasch, M. Traxler, A. Bruhl, L. Benussi, G. Binetti, H. Braak, R.M. Nitsch, C. Hock, Increased brain beta-amyloid load, phosphorylated tau, and risk of Alzheimer disease associated with an intronic CYP46 polymorphism. Arch Neurol 2003:(60) 29-35.

[32] G.W. Rebeck, S.D. Harr, D.K. Strickland, B.T. Hyman, Multiple, diverse senile plaque-associated proteins are ligands of an apolipoprotein E receptor, the alpha 2-macroglobulin receptor/low-density-lipoprotein receptor-related protein. Ann Neurol 1995:(37) 211-217.

[33] M. Shibata, S. Yamada, S.R. Kumar, M. Calero, J. Bading, B. Frangione, D.M. Holtzman, C.A. Miller, D.K. Strickland, J. Ghiso, B.V. Zlokovic, Clearance of Alzheimer's amyloid-ss(1-40) peptide from brain by LDL receptor-related protein-1 at the blood-brain barrier. J Clin Invest 2000:(106) 1489-1499.

[34] Q. Liu, C.V. Zerbinatti, J. Zhang, H.S. Hoe, B. Wang, S.L. Cole, J. Herz, L. Muglia, G. Bu, Amyloid precursor protein regulates brain apolipoprotein E and cholesterol metabolism through lipoprotein receptor LRP1. Neuron 2007:(56) 66-78.

[35] M.D. Haag, A. Hofman, P.J. Koudstaal, B.H. Stricker, M.M. Breteler, Statins are associated with a reduced risk of Alzheimer disease regardless of lipophilicity. The Rotterdam Study. J Neurol Neurosurg Psychiatry 2009:(80) 13-17.

[36] S.R. Hughes, O. Khorkova, S. Goyal, J. Knaeblein, J. Heroux, N.G. Riedel, S. Sahasrabudhe, Alpha2-macroglobulin associates with beta-amyloid peptide and prevents fibril formation. Proc Natl Acad Sci U S A 1998:(95) 3275-3280.

[37] J. Bauer, S. Strauss, U. Schreiter-Gasser, U. Ganter, P. Schlegel, I. Witt, B. Yolk, M. Berger, Interleukin-6 and alpha-2-macroglobulin indicate an acute-phase state in Alzheimer's disease cortices. FEBS Lett 1991:(285) 111-114.

[38] W. Borth, Alpha 2-macroglobulin, a multifunctional binding protein with targeting characteristics. FASEB J 1992:(6) 3345-3353.

[39] D. Blacker, M.A. Wilcox, N.M. Laird, L. Rodes, S.M. Horvath, R.C. Go, R. Perry, B. Watson, Jr., S.S. Bassett, M.G. McInnis, M.S. Albert, B.T. Hyman, R.E. Tanzi, Alpha-2 macroglobulin is genetically associated with Alzheimer disease. Nat Genet 1998:(19) 357-360.

[40] E.A. Rogaeva, S. Premkumar, J. Grubber, L. Serneels, W.K. Scott, T. Kawarai, Y. Song, D.L. Hill, S.M. Abou-Donia, E.R. Martin, J.J. Vance, G. Yu, A. Orlacchio, Y. Pei, M. Nishimura, A. Supala, B. Roberge, A.M. Saunders, A.D. Roses, D. Schmechel, A. Crane-Gatherum, S. Sorbi, A. Bruni, G.W. Small, P.M. Conneally, J.L. Haines, F. Van Leuven, P.H. St George-Hyslop, L.A. Farrer, M.A. Pericak-Vance, An alpha-2-macroglobulin insertion-deletion polymorphism in Alzheimer disease. Nat Genet 1999:(22) 19-22.

[41] M. Simons, P. Keller, B. De Strooper, K. Beyreuther, C.G. Dotti, K. Simons, Cholesterol depletion inhibits the generation of beta-amyloid in hippocampal neurons. Proc Natl Acad Sci U S A 1998:(95) 6460-6464.

[42] D.S. Howland, S.P. Trusko, M.J. Savage, A.G. Reaume, D.M. Lang, J.D. Hirsch, N. Maeda, R. Siman, B.D. Greenberg, R.W. Scott, D.G. Flood, Modulation of secreted be-

ta-amyloid precursor protein and amyloid beta-peptide in brain by cholesterol. J Biol Chem 1998:(273) 16576-16582.

[43] L.M. Refolo, B. Malester, J. LaFrancois, T. Bryant-Thomas, R. Wang, G.S. Tint, K. Sambamurti, K. Duff, M.A. Pappolla, Hypercholesterolemia accelerates the Alzheimer's amyloid pathology in a transgenic mouse model. Neurobiol Dis 2000:(7) 321-331.

[44] D.L. Sparks, Y.M. Kuo, A. Roher, T. Martin, R.J. Lukas, Alterations of Alzheimer's disease in the cholesterol-fed rabbit, including vascular inflammation. Preliminary observations. Ann N Y Acad Sci 2000:(903) 335-344.

[45] A.G. Mainous, 3rd, S.L. Eschenbach, B.J. Wells, C.J. Everett, J.M. Gill, Cholesterol, transferrin saturation, and the development of dementia and Alzheimer's disease: results from an 18-year population-based cohort. Fam Med 2005:(37) 36-42.

[46] M.M. Mielke, P.P. Zandi, M. Sjogren, D. Gustafson, S. Ostling, B. Steen, I. Skoog, High total cholesterol levels in late life associated with a reduced risk of dementia. Neurology 2005:(64) 1689-1695.

[47] V. Leoni, C. Caccia, Oxysterols as biomarkers in neurodegenerative diseases. Chem Phys Lipids 2011:(164) 515-524.

[48] R.P. Koldamova, I.M. Lefterov, M. Staufenbiel, D. Wolfe, S. Huang, J.C. Glorioso, M. Walter, M.G. Roth, J.S. Lazo, The liver X receptor ligand T0901317 decreases amyloid beta production in vitro and in a mouse model of Alzheimer's disease. J Biol Chem 2005:(280) 4079-4088.

[49] D.R. Riddell, H. Zhou, T.A. Comery, E. Kouranova, C.F. Lo, H.K. Warwick, R.H. Ring, Y. Kirksey, S. Aschmies, J. Xu, K. Kubek, W.D. Hirst, C. Gonzales, Y. Chen, E. Murphy, S. Leonard, D. Vasylyev, A. Oganesian, R.L. Martone, M.N. Pangalos, P.H. Reinhart, J.S. Jacobsen, The LXR agonist TO901317 selectively lowers hippocampal Abeta42 and improves memory in the Tg2576 mouse model of Alzheimer's disease. Mol Cell Neurosci 2007:(34) 621-628.

[50] N. Zelcer, P. Tontonoz, Liver X receptors as integrators of metabolic and inflammatory signaling. J Clin Invest 2006:(116) 607-614.

[51] B.A. Hamelin, J. Turgeon, Hydrophilicity/lipophilicity: relevance for the pharmacology and clinical effects of HMG-CoA reductase inhibitors. Trends Pharmacol Sci 1998: (19) 26-37.

[52] K. Nezasa, K. Higaki, M. Takeuchi, M. Nakano, M. Koike, Uptake of rosuvastatin by isolated rat hepatocytes: comparison with pravastatin. Xenobiotica 2003:(33) 379-388.

[53] L.N. Johnson-Anuna, G.P. Eckert, J.H. Keller, U. Igbavboa, C. Franke, T. Fechner, M. Schubert-Zsilavecz, M. Karas, W.E. Muller, W.G. Wood, Chronic administration of statins alters multiple gene expression patterns in mouse cerebral cortex. J Pharmacol Exp Ther 2005:(312) 786-793.

[54] B. Wolozin, W. Kellman, P. Ruosseau, G.G. Celesia, G. Siegel, Decreased prevalence of Alzheimer disease associated with 3-hydroxy-3-methyglutaryl coenzyme A reductase inhibitors. Arch Neurol 2000:(57) 1439-1443.

[55] K. Rockwood, S. Kirkland, D.B. Hogan, C. MacKnight, H. Merry, R. Verreault, C. Wolfson, I. McDowell, Use of lipid-lowering agents, indication bias, and the risk of dementia in community-dwelling elderly people. Arch Neurol 2002:(59) 223-227.

[56] S. Pedrini, T.L. Carter, G. Prendergast, S. Petanceska, M.E. Ehrlich, S. Gandy, Modulation of statin-activated shedding of Alzheimer APP ectodomain by ROCK. PLoS Med 2005:(2) e18.

[57] X. Bi, M. Baudry, J. Liu, Y. Yao, L. Fu, F. Brucher, G. Lynch, Inhibition of geranylgeranylation mediates the effects of 3-hydroxy-3-methylglutaryl (HMG)-CoA reductase inhibitors on microglia. J Biol Chem 2004:(279) 48238-48245.

[58] A. Cordle, G. Landreth, 3-Hydroxy-3-methylglutaryl-coenzyme A reductase inhibitors attenuate beta-amyloid-induced microglial inflammatory responses. J Neurosci 2005:(25) 299-307.

[59] A. Sebok, N. Nusser, B. Debreceni, Z. Guo, M.F. Santos, J. Szeberenyi, G. Tigyi, Different roles for RhoA during neurite initiation, elongation, and regeneration in PC12 cells. J Neurochem 1999:(73) 949-960.

[60] A.M. Pooler, S.C. Xi, R.J. Wurtman, The 3-hydroxy-3-methylglutaryl co-enzyme A reductase inhibitor pravastatin enhances neurite outgrowth in hippocampal neurons. J Neurochem 2006:(97) 716-723.

[61] E. Zamrini, G. McGwin, J.M. Roseman, Association between statin use and Alzheimer's disease. Neuroepidemiology 2004:(23) 94-98.

[62] G.P. Eckert, Manipulation of lipid rafts in neuronal cells. The Open Biology Journal 2010:(3) 1874–1967.

[63] B. Wolozin, Cholesterol and the biology of Alzheimer's disease. Neuron 2004:(41) 7-10.

[64] W.G. Wood, F. Schroeder, U. Igbavboa, N.A. Avdulov, S.V. Chochina, Brain membrane cholesterol domains, aging and amyloid beta-peptides. Neurobiol Aging 2002:(23) 685-694.

[65] Y. Young-Xu, K.A. Chan, J.K. Liao, S. Ravid, C.M. Blatt, Long-term statin use and psychological well-being. J Am Coll Cardiol 2003:(42) 690-697.

[66] V.I. Zannis, J.L. Breslow, Human very low density lipoprotein apolipoprotein E isoprotein polymorphism is explained by genetic variation and posttranslational modification. Biochemistry 1981:(20) 1033-1041.

[67] Mahley RW, Rall SC: APOLIPOPROTEIN E: Far More Than a Lipid Transport Protein. Annu Rev Genomics Hum Genet 2000, 1:507-537.

[68] W.J. Strittmatter, A.D. Roses, Apolipoprotein E and Alzheimer disease. Proc Natl Acad Sci U S A 1995:(92) 4725-4727.

[69] E.H. Corder, A.M. Saunders, N.J. Risch, W.J. Strittmatter, D.E. Schmechel, P.C. Gaskell, Jr., J.B. Rimmler, P.A. Locke, P.M. Conneally, K.E. Schmader, et al., Protective effect of apolipoprotein E type 2 allele for late onset Alzheimer disease. Nat Genet 1994:(7) 180-184.

[70] Y. Song, M.J. Stampfer, S. Liu, Meta-analysis: apolipoprotein E genotypes and risk for coronary heart disease. Ann Intern Med 2004:(141) 137-147.

[71] A. Tammi, T. Ronnemaa, L. Rask-Nissila, T.A. Miettinen, H. Gylling, L. Valsta, J. Viikari, I. Valimaki, O. Simell, Apolipoprotein E phenotype regulates cholesterol absorption in healthy 13-month-old children--The STRIP Study. Pediatr Res 2001:(50) 688-691.

[72] A. Tammi, T. Ronnemaa, J. Viikari, E. Jokinen, H. Lapinleimu, C. Ehnholm, O. Simell, Apolipoprotein E4 phenotype increases non-fasting serum triglyceride concentration in infants - the STRIP study. Atherosclerosis 2000:(152) 135-141.

[73] P.A. Janmey, P.K. Kinnunen, Biophysical properties of lipids and dynamic membranes. Trends Cell Biol 2006:(16) 538-546.

[74] Eckert GP, Wood WG, Muller WE (2005) Statins: drugs for Alzheimer's disease? J Neural Transm.

[75] Y. Barenholz, Sphingomyelin and cholesterol: from membrane biophysics and rafts to potential medical applications. Subcell Biochem 2004:(37) 167-215.

[76] U. Igbavboa, N.A. Avdulov, F. Schroeder, W.G. Wood, Increasing age alters transbilayer fluidity and cholesterol asymmetry in synaptic plasma membranes of mice. J Neurochem 1996:(66) 1717-1725.

[77] Wood W, Eckert GP, Igbavboa U, Muller WE (2003) Amyloid beta-protein interactions with membranes and cholesterol: causes or casualties of Alzheimer's disease. Biochim Biophys Acta 1610:281-290.

[78] R.P. Mason, W.J. Shoemaker, L. Shajenko, T.E. Chambers, L.G. Herbette, Evidence for changes in the Alzheimer's disease brain cortical membrane structure mediated by cholesterol. Neurobiol Aging 1992:(13) 413-419.

[79] P. Mecocci, A. Cherubini, M.F. Beal, R. Cecchetti, F. Chionne, M.C. Polidori, G. Romano, U. Senin, Altered mitochondrial membrane fluidity in AD brain. Neurosci Lett 1996:(207) 129-132.

[80] G.G. Ortiz, F. Pacheco-Moises, M. El Hafidi, A. Jimenez-Delgado, M.A. Macias-Islas, S.A. Rosales Corral, A.C. de la Rosa, V.J. Sanchez-Gonzalez, E.D. Arias-Merino, I.E. Velazquez-Brizuela, Detection of membrane fluidity in submitochondrial particles of platelets and erythrocyte membranes from Mexican patients with Alzheimer disease

by intramolecular excimer formation of 1,3 dipyrenylpropane. Dis Markers 2008:(24) 151-156.

[81] E. Bonilla, K. Tanji, M. Hirano, T.H. Vu, S. DiMauro, E.A. Schon, Mitochondrial involvement in Alzheimer's disease. Biochim Biophys Acta 1999:(1410) 171-182.

[82] I. Hajimohammadreza, M.J. Brammer, S. Eagger, A. Burns, R. Levy, Platelet and erythrocyte membrane changes in Alzheimer's disease. Biochim Biophys Acta 1990: (1025) 208-214.

[83] G.S. Zubenko, U. Kopp, T. Seto, L.L. Firestone, Platelet membrane fluidity individuals at risk for Alzheimer's disease: a comparison of results from fluorescence spectroscopy and electron spin resonance spectroscopy. Psychopharmacology (Berl) 1999: (145) 175-180.

[84] G.S. Zubenko, I. Malinakova, B. Chojnacki, Proliferation of internal membranes in platelets from patients with Alzheimer's disease. J Neuropathol Exp Neurol 1987:(46) 407-418.

[85] M.H. Fukami, L. Salganicoff, Isolation and properties of human platelet mitochondria. Blood 1973:(42) 913-918.

[86] S.M. Cardoso, M.T. Proenca, S. Santos, I. Santana, C.R. Oliveira, Cytochrome c oxidase is decreased in Alzheimer's disease platelets. Neurobiol Aging 2004:(25) 105-110.

[87] M. Ameloot, H. Hendrickx, W. Herreman, H. Pottel, F. Van Cauwelaert, W. van der Meer, Effect of orientational order on the decay of the fluorescence anisotropy in membrane suspensions. Experimental verification on unilamellar vesicles and lipid/alpha-lactalbumin complexes. Biophys J 1984:(46) 525-539.

[88] K.A. Zachariasse, W.L. Vaz, C. Sotomayor, W. Kuhnle, Investigation of human erythrocyte ghost membranes with intramolecular excimer probes. Biochim Biophys Acta 1982:(688) 323-332.

[89] R.D. Kaiser, E. London, Location of diphenylhexatriene (DPH) and its derivatives within membranes: comparison of different fluorescence quenching analyses of membrane depth. Biochemistry 1998:(37) 8180-8190.

[90] I.A. Zainaghi, O.V. Forlenza, W.F. Gattaz, Abnormal APP processing in platelets of patients with Alzheimer's disease: correlations with membrane fluidity and cognitive decline. Psychopharmacology (Berl) 2007:(192) 547-553.

[91] J.P. Schuchardt, M. Huss, M. Stauss-Grabo, A. Hahn, Significance of long-chain polyunsaturated fatty acids (PUFAs) for the development and behaviour of children. Eur J Pediatr 2010:(169) 149-164.

[92] L.A. Horrocks, A.A. Farooqui, Docosahexaenoic acid in the diet: its importance in maintenance and restoration of neural membrane function. Prostaglandins Leukot Essent Fatty Acids 2004:(70) 361-372.

[93] I. Carrie, G. Abellan Van Kan, Y. Rolland, S. Gillette-Guyonnet, B. Vellas, PUFA for prevention and treatment of dementia? Curr Pharm Des 2009:(15) 4173-4185.

[94] C.R. Hooijmans, A.J. Kiliaan, Fatty acids, lipid metabolism and Alzheimer pathology. Eur J Pharmacol 2008:(585) 176-196.

[95] J.H. Song, T. Miyazawa, Enhanced level of n-3 fatty acid in membrane phospholipids induces lipid peroxidation in rats fed dietary docosahexaenoic acid oil. Atherosclerosis 2001:(155) 9-18.

[96] H. Grundt, D.W. Nilsen, M.A. Mansoor, A. Nordoy, Increased lipid peroxidation during long-term intervention with high doses of n-3 fatty acids (PUFAs) following an acute myocardial infarction. Eur J Clin Nutr 2003:(57) 793-800.

[97] K. Simons, E. Ikonen, Functional rafts in cell membranes. Nature 1997:(387) 569-572.

[98] E. Kojro, G. Gimpl, S. Lammich, W. Marz, F. Fahrenholz, Low cholesterol stimulates the nonamyloidogenic pathway by its effect on the alpha -secretase ADAM 10. Proc Natl Acad Sci U S A 2001:(98) 5815-5820.

[99] P. Weber, M. Wagner, H. Schneckenburger, Microfluorometry of cell membrane dynamics. Cytometry A 2006:(69) 185-188.

[100] C. Haass, A.Y. Hung, M.G. Schlossmacher, D.B. Teplow, D.J. Selkoe, beta-Amyloid peptide and a 3-kDa fragment are derived by distinct cellular mechanisms. J Biol Chem 1993:(268) 3021-3024.

[101] P.C. Reid, Y. Urano, T. Kodama, T. Hamakubo, Alzheimer's disease: cholesterol, membrane rafts, isoprenoids and statins. J Cell Mol Med 2007:(11) 383-392.

[102] R. Ehehalt, P. Keller, C. Haass, C. Thiele, K. Simons, Amyloidogenic processing of the Alzheimer beta-amyloid precursor protein depends on lipid rafts. J Cell Biol 2003:(160) 113-123.

[103] K. Fassbender, M. Simons, C. Bergmann, M. Stroick, D. Lutjohann, P. Keller, H. Runz, S. Kuhl, T. Bertsch, K. von Bergmann, M. Hennerici, K. Beyreuther, T. Hartmann, Simvastatin strongly reduces levels of Alzheimer's disease beta -amyloid peptides Abeta 42 and Abeta 40 in vitro and in vivo. Proc Natl Acad Sci U S A 2001:(98) 5856-5861.

[104] C.A. von Arnim, B. von Einem, P. Weber, M. Wagner, D. Schwanzar, R. Spoelgen, W.L. Strauss, H. Schneckenburger, Impact of cholesterol level upon APP and BACE proximity and APP cleavage. Biochem Biophys Res Commun 2008:(370) 207-212.

[105] Paula RS, Souza VC, Benedet AL, Souza ER, Toledo JO, Moraes CF, Gomes L, Alho CS, Córdova C, Nóbrega OT. Dietary fat and apolipoprotein genotypes modulate plasma lipoprotein levels in Brazilian elderly women. Mol Cell Biochem. 2010 Apr; 337(1-2):307-15.

[106] Catalá A. Lipid peroxidation modifies the picture of membranes from the "Fluid Mosaic Model" to the "Lipid Whisker Model" Biochimie 94 (2012) 101e109.

[107] Hoshino T, Kamino K, Matsumoto M. Gene dose effect of the APOE-epsilon4 allele on plasma HDL cholesterol level in patients with Alzheimer's disease. Neurobiol Aging. 2002 Jan-Feb;23(1):41-5.

[108] Eckert GP, Wood WG, Müller WE. Effects of aging and beta-amyloid on the properties of brain synaptic and mitochondrial membranes. J Neural Transm. 2001;108(8-9): 1051-64.

[109] Axelsen PH, Komatsu H, Murray IV. Oxidative stress and cell membranes in the pathogenesis of Alzheimer's disease. Physiology (Bethesda). 2011 Feb;26(1):54-69.

[110] E.P. Kennedy, S.B. Weiss, The function of cytidine coenzymes in the biosynthesis of phospholipides. J Biol Chem 1956:(222) 193-214.

[111] U.I. Richardson, C.J. Watkins, C. Pierre, I.H. Ulus, R.J. Wurtman, Stimulation of CDP-choline synthesis by uridine or cytidine in PC12 rat pheochromocytoma cells. Brain Res 2003:(971) 161-167.

[112] P.C. Choy, H.B. Paddon, D.E. Vance, An increase in cytoplasmic CTP accelerates the reaction catalyzed by CTP:phosphocholine cytidylyltransferase in poliovirus-infected HeLa cells. J Biol Chem 1980:(255) 1070-1073.

[113] V. Savci, R.J. Wurtman, Effect of cytidine on membrane phospholipid synthesis in rat striatal slices. J Neurochem 1995:(64) 378-384.

[114] W. Araki, R.J. Wurtman, Control of membrane phosphatidylcholine biosynthesis by diacylglycerol levels in neuronal cells undergoing neurite outgrowth. Proc Natl Acad Sci U S A 1997:(94) 11946-11950.

[115] C. Mulder, L.O. Wahlund, T. Teerlink, M. Blomberg, R. Veerhuis, G.J. van Kamp, P. Scheltens, P.G. Scheffer, Decreased lysophosphatidylcholine/phosphatidylcholine ratio in cerebrospinal fluid in Alzheimer's disease. J Neural Transm 2003:(110) 949-955.

[116] R.M. Nitsch, B.E. Slack, R.J. Wurtman, J.H. Growdon, Release of Alzheimer amyloid precursor derivatives stimulated by activation of muscarinic acetylcholine receptors. Science 1992:(258) 304-307.

[117] Pettegrew, J. W. (1989). Molecular insights into Alzheimer disease. Ann. N. Y. Acad. Sci. 568:5–28.

[118] Subbarao, K. V., Richardson, J. S., and Ang, L. C. (1990). Autopsy samples of Alzheimer's cortex show increased peroxidation in vitro. J. Neurochem. 55:342–345.

[119] Palmer, A. M., and Burns, M. A. (1994). Selective increase in lipid peroxidation in the inferior temporal cortex in Alzheimer's disease. Brain Res. 645:338–342.

[120] Farooqui, A. A., and Horrocks, L. A. (1991). Excitatory amino acid receptors, neural membrane phospholipid metabolism and neurological disorders. Brain Res. Rev. 16:171–191.

[121] F. Calon, G.P. Lim, F. Yang, T. Morihara, B. Teter, O. Ubeda, P. Rostaing, A. Triller, N. Salem, Jr., K.H. Ashe, S.A. Frautschy, G.M. Cole, Docosahexaenoic acid protects

from dendritic pathology in an Alzheimer's disease mouse model. Neuron 2004:(43) 633-645.

[122] D.L. Moolman, O.V. Vitolo, J.P. Vonsattel, M.L. Shelanski, Dendrite and dendritic spine alterations in Alzheimer models. J Neurocytol 2004:(33) 377-387.

[123] A.C. McKee, K.S. Kosik, N.W. Kowall, Neuritic pathology and dementia in Alzheimer's disease. Ann Neurol 1991:(30) 156-165.

[124] Figure Modified Pathway central: CD40 Signaling (Fig 5), www.sabiosciences.com/pathway.php?sn=CD40_Signaling

[125] Figure Modified Pathway central: Insulin Receptor (Fig 2), www.sabiosciences.com/pathway.php?sn=Insulin_Receptor

[126] Figure Modified Pathway Central: CREB Pathway (Figure 3), www.sabiosciences.com/pathway.php?sn=CREB

[127] Figure Modified Pathway Central: Mito (Figure 7), www.sabiosciences.com/pathway.php?sn=Mitochondrial_Apoptosis

Section 2

Diagnosis

Chapter 8

Pre-Analytical and Analytical Critical Factors Influencing the High Variability of the Concentrations Levels of Alzheimer Disease Biomarkers in Cerebral Spinal Fluid

Armand Perret-Liaudet, Aline Dorey,
Yannick Tholance, Benoit Dumont and
Isabelle Quadrio

Additional information is available at the end of the chapter

http://dx.doi.org/10.5772/55512

1. Introduction

Alzheimer's disease (AD) is a fatal neurodegenerative disorder characterized by a progressive neuronal death and loss of cognitive functions. AD is the most common type of dementia and its incidence rise to 10% in people aged over 90 [1]. Due to Increased longevity, it has been estimated that the number of people suffering from this neurodegenerative disorder will rise from 26.6 million cases in 2006 to 106,8 million worldwide in 2050 [2].

Although clinical intervention to halt the disease is inefficient, the clinical and psychological cares are likely known to significantly improve the quality of life of the patient but also those of the family. At the prodromal stage of the disease (Mild cognitive Impairment linked to AD), there are no sufficient evidences that treating the patient improves the patient outcome. This lack of evidence poses in some cases an ethical problem that is to announce the diagnosis of AD at an autonomous patient who will shift irreversibly in the coming years to the dementia stages. However, as reported in new criteria established by the National Institute on Aging (NIA) and the Alzheimer's Association, core clinical criteria could be used by healthcare providers without access to advanced imaging techniques or cerebrospinal fluid analysis. Criteria including these last advanced tools still remain in the research field [3]. On the contrary, the diagnosis is highly aimed to be accurate at least at the clinical stage of mild dementia, to detect the AD pathology. Core clinical criteria seems to be enough to ensure the AD diagnosis and the use of biomarkers (imaging or CSF biomarkers) can only increase the certainty that the basis of the clinical dementia syndrome is the AD pathophysiological process in a patient presenting the core clinical diagnosis [4]. The CSF biomarker panel of AD is a picture of the neurodegeneration, the neuronal loss, the tangle formation and Aβ-amyloid$_{42}$ (Aβ$_{42}$) peptide accumulation in the brain. Indeed, the core CSF biomarkers for AD diagnosis are a decrease of Aβ$_{42}$ levels and more recently a decrease of the ratio of Aβ-amyloid$_{42}$ / Aβ-amyloid$_{40}$ (Aβ$_{42}$/Aβ$_{40}$) which reflect senile plaques pathology as well as an increase of total tau (T-tau) and phosphorylated tau (P-tau) which reflect axonal degeneration [5,6]. The use of AD biomarker tests for routine diagnostic purposes at the present time, is only proposed as optional for use in patients with dementia when deemed appropriate by the clinician. From the several reasons for this limitation, the workgroup with the task of revising the 1984 criteria for Alzheimer's disease (AD) dementia, highlighted the limited standardization of biomarkers from one locale to another [4]. Despite a decrease in the number of side effects associated with the puncture, lumbar puncture remains an invasive procedure that is clearly the main factor preventing the wide dissemination of these biomarkers in the routine. However, we cannot ignore that the significant variability in measured biomarkers levels found in various studies, resulting in a high variability of both the diagnostic accuracy [7] and of the clinical cut-off for the diagnostic of AD [8], is a hindrance to the spread of these markers and their integration in the diagnostic criteria [3]. The cut-offs obtained in Europe for CSF total tau and beta-amyloid measured by the ELISA assays from the same manufacturer, were reported highly diverse, with two to three fold differences between the highest and lowest reported values [8]. Three major explanations are proposed in this report: first, the inter-laboratory comparisons are very difficult, as some laboratories have adopted the cut-off values from the research literature whereas others have established their own controls, these last controls being likely different in neuropsychology evaluation, neuroimaging and the follow-up. Secondly, the lack of standardized material between the different assays but also the lack of standardized protocols, seem to be a major source of this variation. Finally, pre-analytical factors are those factors that contribute to the variation of the laboratory results before the analysis of the sample. One consensus report has already established the main pre-analytical factors that should be standardized for CSF AD biomarkers analysis [9]. However, the importance of some pre-analytical confounding factors highlighted in this report remained to be elucidated. The aim of this report is to discuss and focus on main critical points in the different preanalytical steps likely to be responsible of data variability. For analytical steps, the introduction since 2009 of an external quality control at a large scale gave an overview of the «desaster», in the same line that prior results. We will discuss rapidly the prior results reported in 2011 and we will underline the urgent need for standardization.

2. Influence of confounding factors in pre-analytical phases on the analysis of AD biomarkers

The confounding factors in pre-analytical phases have a great importance to biochemical analysis and can affect the reliability of the results. Specially in the context of biomarkers of AD in CSF, there are some experimental studies that support this proposition [10,11,12]. Those factors are classically dichotomized in two different groups, «in vivo» and «in vitro». The «in vivo» factors are those biological factors that are linked directly to the patient, the «in vitro» factors are linked to the procedure of sample handling and processing.

2.1. *In vivo* factors

2.1.1. *Is there a specific time of day needed to collect the CSF?*

Answering this issue needs to know if a nycthemeral cycle exists that could modify the concentrations levels of AD CSF biomarkers during the day. Although a lack of standardization in the diagnostic strategy of the patient still exists, in most cases, after a first examination including a clinical and a neuropsychological evaluation, if needed, the lumbar puncture is generally scheduled in a second visit with morphological brain imaging in the same time, with the aim to minimize the duration of the hospitalization. As the time of the lumbar puncture is highly dependent of the coordinated organization of the clinical memory centre, of the biological laboratory and of the imaging department associated with it (waiting homeostasis results, scheduling imaging...), this question is highly relevant.

Previous results have suggested the existence of a large diurnal variability in Aβ levels during a time period of 36 hours, but without significant differences between the hours all along the day period [13]. Following these amazing and unexplained data, recent studies were unable to demonstrate the existence of a temporal fluctuation in CSF biomarker levels, not only for Aβ, but also for T-tau and P-tau [10, 14, 15]. Therefore, there is no need to standardize a specific time interval during the day for CSF collection dedicated to the AD biomarkers assays.

2.1.2. *Is fasting able to modify the concentrations levels of AD biomarkers ?*

At our knowledge, there are no study that has analyzed the influence of fasting on AD CSF biomarkers. The comparison of patients with and without fasting would give a set of indirect and biased data without clear conclusion. Moreover, for ethical reasons, it seems to be impossible to start a research study focused on this topic, as this study would imply a protocol with the realization of successive lumbar punctures in a short delay. Therefore, it is not possible to answer scientifically this issue. Nevertheless, it has been shown that, independently of the patient food intake, Aβ levels in plasma are very stable [10]. As there is a lack of data concerning this topic, as those kind of data could probably never be obtained, and taking account of the large diversity in the locale organization, it is not logical to recommend fasting for the analysis of AD biomarkers in CSF.

2.2. *In vitro* factors

2.2.1. *Localization of the puncture*

Due to the possible decreased rostro-caudal concentration gradient, the site of CSF withdrawal must be also standardized. At our knowledge, there is no study reporting any difference between AD biomarkers concentrations obtained by a ventricular puncture and those obtained by lumbar puncture. Therefore, it is not recommended to analyse these markers in the ventricular punctures obtained during neurosurgical interventions. Nowadays, diagnostic CSF is usually obtained by LP between the L3/L4 and L4/L5 intervertebral space.

2.2.2. Does a CSF gradient of AD biomarkers exist ?

Most brain-derived proteins have a decreased rostro-caudal concentration gradient [16]. Therefore, the volume of CSF taken can influence protein concentration. Using unpublished data from Le Bastard et al., Vanderstichele et al reported the absence of a gradient effect in AD CSF biomarkers concentrations during [9]. It was confirmed by another experimental study analyzing the gradient effect in the spinal cord on $A\beta_{42}$ [10]. Therefore, there is no reason to recommend any specific fraction of CSF volume for the assay of AD biomarkers.

2.2.3. What kind of needle for the puncture ?

The type of needle is likely known to influence the percentage of side effects in patients and to be a factor leading to the presence of red cells [17, 18]. Therefore, the needle could influence the biomarkers concentrations. It has been shown that post-lumbar puncture headache (PLPH) severity was significantly decreased when a 22G needle was used instead of a 20G needle [18]. Moreover, using a 22G atraumatic needle it was also observed a remarkably decrease of PLPH in comparison with 22G traumatic needles [19]. Finally, as lumbar puncture is sometimes difficult with 25G needle in elderly people, a korean group has compared the prevalence of PLPH using 23G and 25G needles. They concluded that the choice of a 23 or 25 gauge Quincke needle has no significant influence on post-dural puncture headache for Korean patients greater than 60 years old. Therefore, the 23 gauge Quincke needle is an option for lumbar punctures in this patient population [20].

2.2.4. Types of sampling tubes

It was established that polypropylene (PP) tubes should be preferred to glass or polystyrene tubes for collection of the CSF since $A\beta$ peptides, but also T-tau and P-tau, bind in a non specifically manner to the polystyrene tubes and to the glass tubes [10, 21]. However, two independent studies reported significant differences on $A\beta_{42}$ levels (up to 50 % compared to basal values !) when CSF was collected in PP tubes from different suppliers [11, 22]. For $A\beta_{42}$, we found that adsorption was effective in a contact time less than 15 minutes, the loss of $A\beta_{42}$ levels being highly significant [11]. Moreover the adsorption intensity was highly dependent on the levels of total proteinorachia, since we abolished this phenomenon when we spiked the CSF with solutions of bovine serum albumin. Amazingly, we also shown that, whereas all the tubes that we studied were commercialized by the providers as tubes in PP, a calorimetry and a spectroscopy analysis revealed that just one out of 11 tubes was pure PP while the others were copolymers made of PP and polyethylene (PE) [11]. Moreover, we also shown that the pure PP causes more adsorption of amyloid peptides than tubes in copolymers of PE and PP, with or without treatment surface, and that some tubes in copolymers could be worst than classical polystyrene: these highly striking results were reproducible in the independent laboratories which have collaborated in this study [11]. Moreover, it was also observed that the tubes that performed better for $A\beta_{42}$ were the worst for P-tau suggesting that hydrophilic-hydrophobic balance is a important point in protein adsorption [11, 23]. The variability of adsorption intensity of proteins onto the plastic of the tube is the result of the incredible jungle of the manufacturing of different tubes called PP: difference in the nature and in the percentage of the copolymers in the plastic, presence of additives, surface treatments, modification of the surface by the sterilization process... The possibility of modifying the protein adsorption by additives or surface treatments was underlined by different reports. First, when Tween-20 was added in the tube containing the CSF, the adsorption of amyloid peptides was significantly reduced [22]. Secondly we recently reported similar results using various plasma treatments of the tube surface, able to modify the adsorption of different proteins like prion protein, Tau and alpha synuclein [23]. These data highlight the need to standardize also the type of test tube used since the great variability found could even lead to a possible AD misdiagnosis. In our laboratory, we shifted to the best tube that we found in this study. This shift has introduced an averaged increase of 25 % of $A\beta_{42}$ levels leading to a modification of our cut off diagnostic value from 500 ng/L to 700 ng/L (data submitted). Currently the members of the Joint Programming Neurodegenerative Disease research (JPND*)* are performing a study which includes the analysis of the most suitable type of tube for AD CSF biomarkers research. Therefore, it is not reasonable to follow the actual guidelines recommending the use of generic PP tubes. Since the data of the JPND collaboration will probably not be available before 2 or 3 years, the best compromise would be that each laboratory concerned by these markers, compares its local tube with the best tubes identified in our study, which are easily available in the commercial market.

2.2.5. Time delay between CSF collection and storage before assay

This is an issue difficult to standardize due the high variety of existing procedures and its probable dependance of confounding factors (hemorragic puncture, hemolyzed samples, high levels of total protein, one sampling tube for AD biomarkers and various markers of others pathologies...) which could modify the stability of the biomarkers during this critical period.

For that, we will discuss first the need to centrifuge and the protocol of centrifugation. This step is able to avoid the presumed influence of the blood cells introduced by the hemorragic puncture. These hemorragic punctures occur in 14-20% cases of lumbar puncture. Bjerke et al. were unable to detect any difference in $A\beta_{42}$ levels when up to 5000 erythrocytes/µl were spiked to the CSF. This value was found ten fold higher than those recommended in the regulation's document included in the Innogenetics kits. However, they found significant decreased $A\beta_{42}$ levels in CSF when plasma was added which was attributed to the binding of $A\beta_{42}$ to different plasma proteins [10]. We cannot also neglect the presence of plasmatic proteases able to digest the peptides since it has been shown that blood contamination of CSF can also lead to protein degradation [25]. The guidelines of Vanderstichele et al. pointed out the absence of difference on the levels of $A\beta_{42}$, T-tau and P-tau between centrifuged and non-centrifuged samples (N. Le Bastard, unpublished data) [9] which could be explained by the fact that they used clear CSF samples. In these guidelines, it was pointed out that spinning speed did not modify significantly the concentration levels of the biomarkers. More recently, it was reported that the sample temperature was always similar to the temperature set up in the centrifuge showing that temperature is not increased by spinning itself [26]. We can then recommend, that centrifugation should be performed at 2,000 g during 10 minutes at room temperature (RT) following the standardized protocol [26].

If several publications and recommendations are related to the delay between sampling and storage [27], it seems that there is a lack of conclusive data about the influence of the delay between sampling and centrifugation for AD biomarkers, mainly for hemorragic puncture. Nevertheless, it was reported significant changes of various metabolites, various amino acids and proteins in presence of white blood cells in the CSF, using a proteomics approach when the CSF were left at RT in the first 30 minutes [28].These data could explain the apparent discrepancy between the study of Kaiser et al, describing a significant increase of the levels of $A\beta_{42}$ after 24 hours [29] and those of Bjerke, describing that $A\beta_{42}$ concentrations remained stable up to 24 hours after the sampling (storage at RT) [10]. The lack of centrifugation prior incubation is likely the reason of the increase in $A\beta_{42}$ previously observed. Taken all together, all these data highlight the importance of centrifugation to be realized, as soon as possible after sampling, for CSF biomarker analysis.

Although the aspect of the CSF was not always indicated, we can imagine that the different studies which have reported a stability of the CSF levels of $A\beta_{42}$, $A\beta_{40}$, T-tau and P-tau over a period of 24 h at least, were done with clear CSF. Thus, the concentrations of $A\beta_{42}$ were found stable 24 h [10], 72 h when the sample was stored at 4°C [12] and up to 7 days after LP at RT [30]. It was the same for the concentrations of T-tau [10, 12, 29, 30]. Regarding the temperature during the time delay, no significant difference was found between the storage of the CSF samples at RT, 4°C or frozen in any of the studies performed [9, 10].

2.2.6. *Freezing process*

This process is complex since different factors could influence the biomarkers concentrations: although it seems clear that heterogeneity also exists for storage tubes, the temperature of freezing, the volume of the aliquots, the length of the storage and the possible effect of freezing / thawing cycles are potential factors to evaluate. Moreover, these factors can be synergistic: the adsorption of proteins onto the tube walls could be increased by the lower volume of the aliquot and mainly by the ratio volume / surface, or by the temperature of freezing (-20 versus -80°C).

The first step is to choose a storage tube. In parallel to the test realized with 11 sampling tubes [11], we selected 9 different commercially available polypropylene storage tubes (Table 1, tubes 13 to 21), some of them being used by different clinical teams in the AD field. The volume capacity was ranged from 0,5 to 1,5 mL. We performed an analysis of the surface polymer composition using differential scanning calorimetry and Fourier Transformed Infrared spectroscopy. This revealed the same surprising results than obtained with the sampling tubes [11]: only one tube was constituted by pure polypropylene, the others being copolymers with at least polyethylene, with or without surface treatment. Using the same protocol as described for the sampling tubes [11], biomarkers concentrations showed variations that were significantly different for $A\beta_{42}$ peptide. Median values for $A\beta_{42}$ peptide varied from 94 % to 127 %.

http://dx.doi.org/10.5772/55512

These data confirmed those obtained for sampling tubes, although the variability was lower than those found with these last tubes. The effect was present after 15 min, but increasing the incubation time to 24h at 2-8°C, the values did not significantly change compared to 15 minutes incubation.

The next step consists to standardize if needed the temperature, i.e. the speed, of freezing.

Freezing temperatures may affect CSF proteins concentrations as it has previously been reported for cystatin C, which undergoes a proteolysis at -20°C but not at -80°C [31]. Recently, the levels of T-tau and P-tau were reported significantly lower when CSF samples were immediately frozen at -20°C instead of -80°C (N. Le Bastard, unpublished data) [19]. However, this group did not find any difference for the $A\beta_{42}$ levels when the CSF were frozen at -20°C or -80°C, confirming previous results [10]. Therefore, freezing and storage at -80°C the CSF samples, seem to be logical.

Aliquoting the supernatant of CSF is absolutely necessary since it avoids different Freeze/thaw cycles (see below). Although we did not realize a study designed to evaluate the possible synergy between the ratio volume/surface and the speed of freezing onto the absorption phenomenon in these storage tubes (total volume less than 1.5 ml), some procedures issued from previous reported guidelines can be logically applied [27]. They pointed out the need to use small volumes (never more than 0.5 ml), which would allow: a/to realize at least the assay of the 3 classical AD biomarkers and if needed the assay of $A\beta_{40}$, b/ to prevent freeze/thaw cycles and c/ fill the tube up to 75% to minimize the adsorption and the evaporation effect, this last effect being negligible when the sample is stored frozen at -80°C [26].

As mentioned before, the guidelines recommend separating the supernatant in several fractions, that which will reduce the numbers of freeze/thaw cycles since freezing was shown able to affect protein stability [32]. Some studies have already analyzed the influence of freeze/thaw cycles on AD CSF biomarkers. Most studies using an ELISA format no have found any change on $A\beta_{42}$ and Tau CSF levels after one freeze/thaw cycle [10, 12, 30, 33], whereas a significant loss of $A\beta_{42}$ was found after one single cycle in one study using a semi-quantitative method [34]. Increasing the number of cycles was reported able to modify the stability of $A\beta_{42}$ CSF levels. However, about the exact numbers of cycles able to impact the levels, no real consensus was found between the different studies. If the Tau CSF levels seem to be unaffected by 3 or 6 freeze/thaw cycles [30, 12], the $A\beta_{42}$ CSF levels were found either stable after 3 cycles [30], either were significantly decreased after the third cycle [12]. In case of immunoassay analysis, it is logically recommended to limit the number of freeze/thaw cycles up to two as maximum [9].

Finally, the length of storage at -80°C does not seem to present a major influence on stability of CSF AD biomarkers, at least for 2 years [30] according to unpublished data from Blennow K. et al., referenced in the guideline published by Vanderstichele et al. [19]. Moreover, the levels of $A\beta_{42}$ and T-tau but not $A\beta_{40}$, remained stable up to 6 years [35]. In summary, we can conclude that CSF can be stored up to 2 years at -80°C as previously reported [19].

3. Variability introduced by the analytical step

There are several available assays for the determination of CSF Aβ_{42}, T-Tau and P-Tau, commercialized by different companies (Covance, Cusabio, IBL international, Innogenetics, Invitrogen, Millipore, Meso Scale Discovery, Wako... list not exhaustive). Large variation, in assay performance and outcomes of CSF Aβ_{42}, T-Tau and P-Tau levels was observed between laboratories also when the same assay format was used, reaching in some cases an inter-assay and inter-laboratory coefficient variations of 20 to 35% [7, 36]. As shown in conclusions of the first report of the external quality control (EQC) program started by the Alzheimer's association [37], ELISA techniques dominate the market while multiplex techniques are used less. In this program, for Aβ_{42}, T-Tau and P-Tau, most of laboratories [26 laboratories) used the INNOTEST enzyme-linked immunosorbent assays (ELISAs) (Innogenetics, Ghent, Belgium, www.innogenetics.com), whereas 14 laboratories used the bead-based Luminex xMAP platform with the INNO-BIA AlzBio3 (Innogenetics, Ghent, Belgium, www.innogenetics.com). Moreover, for Aβ_{42} and T-Tau, 5 laboratories used Meso Scale Discovery (MSD, Gaithersburg, MD, www.mesoscale.com) technology [37].

3.1. Principles of assays

INNOTEST enzyme-linked immunosorbent assays (ELISAs) (Innogenetics) are classical ELISAs with colorimetric detection.

INNO-BIA AlzBio3 allows the simultaneous quantification of Aβ_{42}, T-Tau and P-Tau in CSF using xMAP® technology (xMAP is a registered trademark of Luminex Corp). The microsphere-based Luminex xMAP technology involves covalent coupling of a capture antibody to spectrally specific fluorescent microspheres [38]. Each microsphere number has a unique spectral identity. The classification of each bead is made by excitation at 635 nm. Each bead number is linked with only one antibody and the signals from analytes in the mixture are identified unequivocally. The quantification of the molecular reaction that has occurred at the microsphere surface, is done using a fluorochrome, the phycoerythrin coupled to streptavidin. The intensity of the fluorescence, derived after excitation of PE at 532 nm, is reported.

MSD offers the possibility to measure in simplex or multiplex format, depending on the biomarker analysed. Whereas t-Tau is measured in simplex format by the participants of the external control program, Aβ_{42} can be measured in simplex or multiplex format in combination with Aβ_{38} and Aβ_{40}. Multi-array plate formats include 96- and 384-well plates. The multi-spot plates are available with up to 100 spots per well. MSD uses electrochemiluminescence to detect binding events on patterned arrays. Electrochemiluminescence detection uses labels that emit light at ~620 nm when electrochemically stimulated, the stimulation mechanism (electricity) being decoupled from the signal (light). The signals are treated by the SECTOR Imager Instrument, which is medium throughput imaging detection systems (charge-coupled device camera), capable of multiplexing in all spot formats and reads 96- and 384-well plates.

3.2. Extent of the variability highlighted by this EQC program [37]

3.2.1. Total variability

In this report, results were grouped according to analytical techniques and samples [37]. The total CVs among centers were 16% to 28% for ELISA, 13% to 36% for xMAP, and 16% to 36% for MSD. CVs for MSD must be interpreted with caution, because they included 2 different Monoclonal antibodies (Mab) for $A\beta_{42}$ assays, binding to different epitopes on the amyloid peptide. These data were totally conformed to those reported earlier [7, 36]. There was no major modification of the CV in the longitudinal evaluation, except a decrease in variation for T-tau measured by ELISA. This was expected, since there was no active intervention between the 2 rounds [37].

3.2.2. Within-laboratory precision

Within-laboratory CVs were examined at the reference laboratories for ELISA and xMAP in two consecutive rounds. CVs were 3.2% to 24% for ELISA and 2.3% to 26% for xMAP, but differed between analytes within individual laboratories, indicating assay-dependent variations [37].

3.2.3. Differences in absolute values

The analytical techniques reported different absolute values for the biomarkers. ELISA values for $A\beta_{42}$, were about 2 fold higher than xMAP values. MSD values for $A\beta_{42}$, were dependent of the Mab used. ELISA values for T-Tau were about 3 fold higher than xMAP values. Finally for P-Tau, the differences inter techniques were clearly decreased in comparison to $A\beta_{42}$, and T-Tau. Considerable variability exists among the same manufacturer between mono and multiplex technology. For example, the decision threshold of clinical disease was reported to be at 86 pg / mL and 350 pg / mL for T-TAU measured by xMAP technology of Innogenetics on the platform Luminex and the conventional ELISA, respectively [39]. Factors of correction between values obtained by xMAP and ELISA, were used for global comparison of groups of patients, i.e. controls, Mild Cognitive Impairment and AD patients to predict incipient AD by CSF biomarkers [40]. In an other side, it was clearly shown that the use of factors of correction did not resolve the discrepancy in values observed between xMAP and ELISAs [41]. Although the observed biomarker concentrations may vary significantly between platforms, including MSD, xMAP and ELISA, these techniques seem to have similar diagnostic accuracy for patients with AD versus controls [39] or for detecting early AD [41, 42].

3.3. Possible sources of variability

In this study analysing the variability of results from only two rounds of an EQC program and from many different assay lots used, the authors limited their interpretation of the relative contributions from between-laboratory, within-laboratory, and between-lot components to the total variability [37]. Differences in within-laboratory CVs among the biomarkers within individual reference laboratories suggest that assay-related factors are important. Moreover, the high variability of the results of biomarkers measured by different commercial kits can be explained, by the use of different antibodies, the nature of the calibrator, the calibration method and many others factors as for example the nature of standard. Increasing data during years and by incorporation of new centers (since this first report concerning 40 laboratories, in summer of 2012, 64 laboratories were participating at this program) will permit to better identify the major sources of variability in analytical steps. Thus, we can just list the different points to be further investigated.

In the laboratory, the biologist will take care for:

a. Pipetting

The pipetting mode (inverse pipetting...) is not specified by the manufacturer. Using a single tip can influence the standard curve accuracy. However, the magnitude of this effect, if any, should be tested, to provide a better basis for recommendation [43].

b. Calibration

For lyophilised standard, accurate solubilization and accurate pipetting is critical. Moreover, since for INNOTEST Ab42, the first point of the curve calibration must be adjusted depending of the set value, accurate pipeting is absolutely needed. The type of curve fitting used and the software for data calculation were shown as possible factors of variability [43].

c. Reagent handling and adhesion of biologists to the manufacturer standard operating procedure (SOP)

The adhesion of routine laboratories to the manufacturer SOP is absolutely needed to reduce the part of the variability found in CSF biomarkers analysis. For that, a great effort must be done by the different manufacturers to limit individual interpretation of the technical instructions. The best example consists in the definition of the «room temperature» which can mainly vary from the north to the south of Europe. The maintenance of laboratory equipment is a crucial point to ensure the accuracy of pipeting volumes, the accuracy of temperatures, the accuracy of detection signals and the quality and reproducibility of washing steps.

d. Familiarization with the method and Competency Train

Implementing these techniques in the laboratory needs a training program ensured by the manufacturer. Moreover, habilitation and qualification of the laboratory staff must be done.

e. Validation criteria of runs for rejecting data

Different means are used to ensure validation of results. The definition of the criteria of acceptance of results must be strict. They include the calibration curve parameters, the CV of the duplicate samples and the use of an internal quality control program. For the CV criteria acceptance, in our experience, it seems that they are to be adequately defined since, the recommendation of CV < 20% done in the INNOTEST documentation, is not acceptable all along the dynamical range of the assay, in particular when the concentration level is near the clinical cut-off. Moreover, in the absence of QC samples in the kit, the biologist needs to implement its own QC program with different crucial points to resolve: the nature of the

http://dx.doi.org/10.5772/55512

sample (native CSF pools, spiked CSF with standards, peptides...) how many QC samples, range of concentrations to cover, absence of reference material. This point is crucial for laboratories concerned by accreditation scheme based on the application of ISO15189 standard.

3.3.1. Issues to be solved by manufacturers

Many crucial points need to be solved as the poor quality of the test procedure instructions to decrease variability induced by misunderstanding of the protocols. This lacking information is often an indicator of minimal method optimization of the protocol (for example incubation steps, handling the reagents...). The reagents must be proposed in a manner that permits to decrease variability, for instance the «ready to use» calibrators. The absence of quality control included in the kit is a major problem. In fact, part of the discrepancy observed in the concentrations levels between the analytical techniques ELISA, xMAP, and MSD is caused by the lack of certified reference materials (CRMs). This could mainly impact the interlot variability and is at least, a brake to standardization. Antibody purification, coating of plates and beads are also factors of lot-lot variability.

4. Conclusion

The present chapter highlights two main issues responsible for the lack of harmonization of CSF AD biomarkers cut-offs values: the lack of standardization of the pre-analytical steps and the high variability of results linked to the analytical step. This latter issue can be explained by the absence of transferability of results between the different platforms but also by the high inter laboratory dispersion within the same assays. Previous consensus guidelines for pre-analytical factor standardization gave the way to resolve this issue, evidencing the need to standardize sampling and storage tubes, the type of the needle for the CSF puncture and the long term storage. Establishing SOPs for sample processing would allow to compare diagnostic conclusions between different laboratories. The implementation of those SOPs in the clinical community may reduce part of the variability found in the analysis of AD CSF biomarkers. Antibody purification, coating surfaces, preparation of standards, manufacturers instructions are also sources of variation, which need to be decreased and requires increased efforts by kit manufacturers. The optimal approach is a collaborative effort between commercial kit and instrument platform manufacturers, laboratories concerned by those methods, and reference standardization programs.

Acknowledgements

We wish to thank all our collaborators of the JPND BIOMARKPD program, those of the French Society of Clinical Biology (SFBC) and those of the NEUROSCREEN European project for their valuable assistance.

Author details

Armand Perret-Liaudet[1,2*], Aline Dorey[1], Yannick Tholance[1,3], Benoit Dumont[1,2] and Isabelle Quadrio[1,2]

*Address all correspondence to: armand.perret-liaudet@chu-lyon.fr

1 Hospices Civils de Lyon, Neurobiologie, Centre Mémoire de Recherche et de Ressources; Hôpitaux de Lyon, Lyon, France

2 Université Lyon 1, CNRS UMR5292, INSERM U1028, Equipe BioRan, Lyon, France

3 Université Lyon 1, CNRS UMR5292, INSERM U1028, Equipe WAKING, Lyon, France

References

[1] Qiu C, Kivipelto M (2009) Epidemiology of Alzheimer's disease: occurrence, determinants, and strategies toward intervention. *Dialogues in Clinical Neuroscience* 111-128.

[2] Brookmeyer R, Johnson E, Ziegler-Graham K, Arrighi HM (2007) Forecasting the global burden of Alzheimer's disease. *Alzheimer's & dementia: the journal of the Alzheimer's Association* 3, 186-91.

[3] Albert M.A. DeKosky S.T., Dickson D., Dubois B., Feldman H., Fox N.C., Gamst A., Holtzman D.M., Jagust W.J., Petersen R.C., Snyder P, Carrillo M.C., Thies B., Phelps C. (2011) "The diagnosis of mild cognitive impairment due to Alzheimer's disease: Recommendations from the National Institute on Aging – Alzheimer's Association workgroups on diagnostic guidelines for Alzheimer's disease" Alzheimer's & *Dementia: The Journal of the Alzheimer's Association*, 7(3), 270 – 279.

[4] McKhann G.M., Knopman D.C., Chertkow H., Hyman T.H., Jack C.R.Jr., Kawash C.J., Klunkk W.E., Koroshetzl W.J., Manlym, J.J., Mayeux R., Mohs R.M.,. Morris J.C., Rossorr M.N, Scheltens P., Carrillo M.C., Weintraub S., Thies B., Phelps C. (2011) The diagnosis of dementia due to Alzheimer's disease: Recommendations from the National Institute on Aging-Alzheimer's Association workgroups on diagnostic guidelines for Alzheimer's disease : *The Journal of the Alzheimer's Association*, 7(3), 263 – 269.

[5] Teunissen C (2002) Biochemical markers related to Alzheimer's dementia in serum and cerebrospinal fluid. *Neurobiology of Aging* 23, 485-508.

[6] Blennow K, Hampel H, Weiner M, Zetterberg H (2010) Cerebrospinal fluid and plasma biomarkers in Alzheimer disease. *Nature reviews. Neurology* 6, 131-44.

[7] Verwey NA, van der Flier WM, Blennow K, Clark C, Sokolow S, De Deyn PP, Galasko D, Hampel H, Hartmann T, Kapaki E, Lannfelt L, Mehta PD, Parnetti L, Petzold A, Pirttila T, Saleh L, Skinningsrud A, Swieten JCV, Verbeek MM, Wiltfang J, Youn-

kin S, Scheltens P, Blankenstein MA (2009) A worldwide multicentre comparison of assays for cerebrospinal fluid biomarkers in Alzheimer's disease. *Annals of clinical biochemistry* 46, 235-40.

[8] Hort J., Bartos A., Pirttila T. and Scheltens P. (2010) Use of cerebrospinal fluid biomarkers in diagnosis of dementia across Europe. *European Journal of Neurology*, 17, 90–96

[9] Vanderstichele H, Bibl M, Engelborghs S, Le Bastard N, Lewczuk P, Molinuevo JL, Parnetti L, Perret-Liaudet A, Shaw LM, Teunissen C, Wouters D, Blennow K (2012) Standardization of preanalytical aspects of cerebrospinal fluid biomarker testing for Alzheimer's disease diagnosis: A consensus paper from the Alzheimer's Biomarkers Standardization Initiative. *Alzheimer's & dementia: the journal of the Alzheimer's Association* 8, 65-73.

[10] Bjerke M, Portelius E, Minthon L, Wallin A, Anckarsäter H, Anckarsäter R, Andreasen N, Zetterberg H, Andreasson U, Blennow K (2010) Confounding factors influencing amyloid Beta concentration in cerebrospinal fluid. *International journal of Alzheimer's disease*, 2010, Article ID 986310, 11 pages.

[11] Perret-Liaudet A, Pelpel M, Tholance Y, Dumont B, Vanderstichele H, Zorzi W, Elmoualij B, Schraen S, Moreaud O, Gabelle A, Thouvenot E, Thomas-Anterion C, Touchon J, Krolak-Salmon P, Kovacs GG, Coudreuse A, Quadrio I, Lehmann S (2012) Risk of Alzheimer's Disease Biological Misdiagnosis Linked to Cerebrospinal Collection Tubes. *Journal of Alzheimer's disease: JAD* 30, 1-8.

[12] Schoonenboom NSM, Mulder C, Vanderstichele H, Van Elk E-J, Kok A, Van Kamp GJ, Scheltens P, Blankenstein M a (2005) Effects of processing and storage conditions on amyloid beta (1-42) and tau concentrations in cerebrospinal fluid: implications for use in clinical practice. *Clinical chemistry* 51, 189-95.

[13] Bateman RJ, Wen G, Morris JC, Holtzman DM (2007) Fluctuations of CSF amyloid-beta levels: implications for a diagnostic and therapeutic biomarker. *Neurology* 68, 666-9.

[14] Moghekar A, Goh J, Li M, Albert M, O'Brien RJ (2012) Cerebrospinal fluid aβ and tau level fluctuation in an older clinical cohort. *Archives of neurology* 69, 246-50.

[15] Slats D, Claassen JAHR, Spies PE, Borm G, Besse KTC, van Aalst W, Tseng J, Sjögren MJC, Olde Rikkert MGM, Verbeek MM (2012) Hourly variability of cerebrospinal fluid biomarkers in Alzheimer's disease subjects and healthy older volunteers. *Neurobiology of aging* 33, 831.e1-9.

[16] Reiber H (2001) Dynamics of brain-derived proteins in cerebrospinal fluid. *Clinica Chimica Acta* 310, 173-186.

[17] Chevallier S, Monti M, Michel P, Vollenweider P. (2008) Lumbar puncture. *Rev Med Suisse* 177, 2312-4, 2316-8.

[18] Dietrich M. Post-lumbar puncture headache syndrome. (1996) In : Neurologic disorders : Course and treatment, Brandt T, Caplan LR, Dichgans J (Eds). San Diego : Elsevier Academic Press,;59.

[19] Lavi R, Yarnitsky D, Rowe JM, Weissman A, Segal D, Avivi I. Standard vs atraumatic Whitacre needle for diagnostic lumbar puncture: a randomized trial (2006) *Neurology.* 67(8), 1492-4.

[20] Kim M, Yoon H. (2011) Comparison of post-dural puncture headache and low back pain between 23 and 25 gauge Quincke spinal needles in patients over 60 years: randomized, double-blind controlled trial. *Int J Nurs Stud.* 48(11), 1315-22.

[21] Lewczuk P, Beck G, Esselmann H, Bruckmoser R, Zimmermann R, Fiszer M, Bibl M, Maler JM, Kornhuber J, Wiltfang J (2006) Effect of sample collection tubes on cerebrospinal fluid concentrations of tau proteins and amyloid beta peptides. *Clinical chemistry* 52, 332-4.

[22] Pica-Mendez AM, Tanen M, Dallob A, Tanaka W, Laterza OF (2010) Nonspecific binding of Aβ42 to polypropylene tubes and the effect of Tween-20. *Clinica chimica acta; international journal of clinical chemistry* 411, 1833.

[23] Poncin-Epaillard F, Mille C, Debarnot D, Zorzi W, Moualij BE, Coudreuse A, Legeay G, Quadrio I, Perret-Liaudet A. Study of the adhesion of neurodegenerative proteins on plasma-modified and coated polypropylene surfaces. *J Biomater Sci Polym Ed* 2011 Sep 22.

[24] Petzold A, Sharpe LT, Keir G (2006) Spectrophotometry for cerebrospinal fluid pigment analysis. *Neurocritical care* 4, 153-62.

[25] You J-S, Gelfanova V, Knierman MD, Witzmann FA, Wang M, Hale JE (2005) The impact of blood contamination on the proteome of cerebrospinal fluid. *Proteomics* 5, 290-6.

[26] Del Campo M, Mollenhauer B, Bertolotto A, Engelborghs S, Hampel H, Simonsen AH, Kapaki E, Kruse N, Le Bastard N, Lehmann S, Molinuevo JL, Parnetti L, Perret-Liaudet A, Sáez-Valero J, Saka E, Urbani A, Vanmechelen E, Verbeek M, Visser PJ, Teunissen C. (2012) Recommendations to standardize preanalytical confounding factors in Alzheimer's and Parkinson's disease cerebrospinal fluid biomarkers: an update. *Biomark Med.* 6, 419-30.

[27] Teunissen CE, Petzold a, Bennett JL, Berven FS, Brundin L, Comabella M, Franciotta D, Frederiksen JL, Fleming JO, Furlan R, Hintzen RQ, Hughes SG, Johnson MH, Krasulova E, Kuhle J, Magnone MC, Rajda C, Rejdak K, Schmidt HK, van Pesch V, Waubant E, Wolf C, Giovannoni G, Hemmer B, Tumani H, Deisenhammer F (2009) A consensus protocol for the standardization of cerebrospinal fluid collection and biobanking. *Neurology* 73, 1914-22.

[28] Rosenling T, Slim CL, Christin C, Coulier L, Shi S, Stoop MP, Bosman J, Suits F, Horvatovich PL, Stockhofe-Zurwieden N, Vreeken R, Hankemeier T, van Gool AJ, Luid-

er TM, Bischoff R (2009) The effect of preanalytical factors on stability of the proteome and selected metabolites in cerebrospinal fluid (CSF). *Journal of proteome research* 8, 5511-22.

[29] Kaiser E, Schönknecht P, Thomann P a, Hunt A, Schröder J (2007) Influence of delayed CSF storage on concentrations of phospho-tau protein (181), total tau protein and beta-amyloid (1-42). *Neuroscience letters* 417, 193-5.

[30] Zimmermann R, Lelental N, Ganslandt O, Maler JM, Kornhuber J, Lewczuk P (2011) Preanalytical sample handling and sample stability testing for the neurochemical dementia diagnostics. *Journal of Alzheimer's disease: JAD* 25, 739-45.

[31] Carrette O, Burkhard PR, Hughes S, Hochstrasser DF, Sanchez J-C (2005) Truncated cystatin C in cerebrospiral fluid: Technical artefact or biological process? *Proteomics* 5, 3060-5.

[32] Bhatnagar BS, Bogner RH, Pikal MJ (2007) Protein stability during freezing: separation of stresses and mechanisms of protein stabilization. Pharmaceutical development and technology 12, 505-23.

[33] Sjögren M, Vanderstichele H, Agren H, Zachrisson O, Edsbagge M, Wikkelsø C, Skoog I, Wallin A, Wahlund LO, Marcusson J, Nägga K, Andreasen N, Davidsson P, Vanmechelen E, Blennow K (2001) Tau and Abeta42 in cerebrospinal fluid from healthy adults 21-93 years of age: establishment of reference values. Clinical chemistry 47, 1776-81.

[34] Bibl M, Esselmann H, Otto M, Lewczuk P, Cepek L, Rüther E, Kornhuber J, Wiltfang J (2004) Cerebrospinal fluid amyloid beta peptide patterns in Alzheimer's disease patients and nondemented controls depend on sample pretreatment: indication of carrier-mediated epitope masking of amyloid beta peptides. Electrophoresis 25, 2912-8.

[35] Schipke CG, Jessen F, Teipel S, Luckhaus C, Wiltfang J, Esselmann H, Frölich L, Maier W, Rüther E, Heppner FL, Prokop S, Heuser I, Peters O (2011) Long-term stability of Alzheimer's disease biomarker proteins in cerebrospinal fluid. *Journal of Alzheimer's disease: JAD* 26, 255-62.

[36] Lewczuk P, Beck G, Ganslandt O, Esselmann H, Deisenhammer F, Regeniter A, Petereit H-F, Tumani H, Gerritzen A, Oschmann P, Schröder J, Schönknecht P, Zimmermann K, Hampel H, Bürger K, Otto M, Haustein S, Herzog K, Dannenberg R, Wurster U, Bibl M, Maler JM, Reubach U, Kornhuber J, Wiltfang J. International quality control survey of neurochemical dementia diagnostics. *Neurosci Lett.* 2006;409:1–4

[37] Mattsson N, Andreasson U, Persson S, Arai H, Batish SD, Bernardini S, Bocchio-Chiavetto L, Blankenstein M a, Carrillo MC, Chalbot S, Coart E, Chiasserini D, Cutler N, Dahlfors G, Duller S, Fagan AM, Forlenza O, Frisoni GB, Galasko D, Galimberti D, Hampel H, Handberg A, Heneka MT, Herskovits AZ, Herukka S-K, Holtzman DM, Humpel C, Hyman BT, Iqbal K, Jucker M, Kaeser S a, Kaiser E, Kapaki E, Kidd D,

Klivenyi P, Knudsen CS, Kummer MP, Lui J, Lladó A, Lewczuk P, Li Q-X, Martins R, Masters C, McAuliffe J, Mercken M, Moghekar A, Molinuevo JL, Montine TJ, Nowatzke W, O'Brien R, Otto M, Paraskevas GP, Parnetti L, Petersen RC, Prvulovic D, de Reus HPM, Rissman R a, Scarpini E, Stefani A, Soininen H, Schröder J, Shaw LM, Skinningsrud A, Skrogstad B, Spreer A, Talib L, Teunissen C, Trojanowski JQ, Tumani H, Umek RM, Van Broeck B, Vanderstichele H, Vecsei L, Verbeek MM, Windisch M, Zhang J, Zetterberg H, Blennow K (2011) The Alzheimer's Association external quality control program for cerebrospinal fluid biomarkers. *Alzheimer's & dementia: the journal of the Alzheimer's Association* 7, 386-395..

[38] Oliver KG, Kettman JR, Fulton RJ. Multiplexed analysis of human cytokines by use of the FlowMetrix system. Clin Chem 1998;44: 2057–60.

[39] Olsson A, Vanderstichele H, Andreasen N, De Meyer G, Wallin A, Holmberg B, et al. Simultaneous measurement of beta-amyloid(1- 42), total tau, and phosphorylated tau (Thr181) in cerebrospinal fluid by the xMAP technology. Clin Chem 2005; 51:336–45.

[40] Mattsson N, Zetterberg H, Hansson O, Andreasen N, Parnetti L, Jonsson M, et al. CSF biomarkers and incipient Alzheimer disease in patients with mild cognitive impairment. JAMA 2009;302:385–93.

[41] Jongbloed W, Kester MI, van der Flier WM, Veerhuis R, Scheltens P, Blankenstein MA, Teunissen CE. Discriminatory and predictive capabilities of enzyme-linked immunosorbent assay and multiplex platforms in a longitudinal Alzheimer's disease study. Alzheimers Dement. 2012 Oct 27. (Epub ahead of print)

[42] Schipke CG, Prokop S, Heppner FL, Heuser I, Peters O. Comparison of immunosorbent assays for the quantification of biomarkers for Alzheimer's disease in human cerebrospinal fluid Dement Geriatr Cogn Disord. 2011;31(2):139-45.

[43] Teunissen CE, Verwey N a, Kester MI, van Uffelen K, Blankenstein M a (2010) Standardization of Assay Procedures for Analysis of the CSF Biomarkers Amyloid β((1-42)), Tau, and Phosphorylated Tau in Alzheimer's Disease: Report of an International Workshop. International journal of Alzheimer's disease 2010, Article ID 635053, 6 pages.

Chapter 9

Candidate Bio-Markers of Alzheimer's Disease

B.K. Binukumar and Harish C. Pant

Additional information is available at the end of the chapter

http://dx.doi.org/10.5772/55069

1. Introduction

Alzheimer's disease (AD) is a neurodegenerative disorder of the central nervous system characterized by a progressive loss of short-term memory accompanied by a gradual loss of cognitive functions (Ross et al., 2004). AD is among the most frequently encountered diseases in aging societies with an estimated 5million people in the United States and 17 million people worldwide suffering from the disease. It is expected that these numbers will quadruple by the year 2040, by which 1 out of 45 Americans will be affected, leading to a considerable public health burden (Fratiglioni et al., 1999). AD pathogenic mechanisms contributing to neuronal loss and brain dysfunction are still unclear. However, remarkable advances have taken place in understanding of both the genetics and molecular biological aspects of the intracellular processing of amyloid and tau and the changes leading to the pathologic formation of extracellular amyloid plaques and the intraneuronal aggregation of hyperphosphorylated tau into neurofibrillary tangles. This progress in our understanding of the molecular pathology has set the stage for clinically meaningful advances in the development of biomarkers.

Proper diagnosis is essential for instituting appropriate clinical management. While diagnostic accuracy for the disease has improved, the differential diagnosis of the disorder is still problematic. In the very early stages of the disease, frequently classified as mild cognitive impairment (MCI), delineating disease process from "normal ageing" may be difficult; in later stages of the disease, distinguishing AD from a number of neurodegenerative diseases associated with dementia may also be difficult. Furthermore, the disease progression is slow and there is variability of performance on clinical measures, making it difficult to monitor change effectively. Since disease modifying therapy is likely to be most effective early in the course of disease, early diagnosis is highly desirable before neurodegeneration becomes severe and widespread.

In clinical practice, the diagnosis of AD is still largely based on consensuscriteria combined with the exclusion of secondary causes of memory loss (Knopman et al., 2001; McKhann et al., 1984).Thus, there is an urgent and desperate need for a biomarker that can reliably prognose the disease. Biomarkers of AD occupy an essential place in recently formulated diagnostic criteria for AD, in which their role is to identify the pathophysiological processes underlying cognitive impairment or to help predict time to reach up to dementia. Criteria for a useful biomarker have been proposed by an international consensus group on molecular and biochemical markers of AD in 1998 (The Ronald and Nancy Reagan Research Institute of the Alzheimer's Association and the National Institute on Aging Working Group, 1998). According to these guidelines, a biomarker for AD should detect a manifestation of the fundamental neuropathology and be validated in neuropathologically-confirmed cases. Its sensitivity for detecting AD should exceed 80% and its specificity in differentiating between AD and other dementias should be higher than 80%. Ideally, a biomarker should also be reliable, reproducible, non-invasive, simple to perform, and inexpensive. One further role of particular interest to patients and clinicians dealing with AD is its ability to detect the disease at the earliest possible stage.

Based on growing body of evidence concerning the pathophysiology of AD, a number of putative biological markers of disease have been evaluated against clinical and neuropathological standards. Biomarkers are very useful for diagnosing and monitoring disease progression (Ward et al., 2007) and are important for patient selection, monitoring side-effects, aiding selection of appropriate patient treatment, and helping new drug discovery. For the clinical studies of AD therapeutics, there is an increasing need for diagnostic markers to ensure that therapies are targeted at the right patient population, to initiate early treatment when disease-modifying drugs will be available, and to monitor disease progression (Hye et al., 2006).

2. Biomarkers in CSF

One of the most promising sources of biomarkers in AD is the cerebrospinal fluid (CSF).The molecular changes in the brain extracellular and interstitial environments are reflected in CSF. The single-cell layer epithelium separating the two compartments allows a virtually unhindered flow of molecules from the brain towards the CSF. CSF biomarkers for AD should reflect the central pathogenic processes in the brain. Furthermore the CSF is accessible to trained clinicians using a relatively simple lumbar puncture (Fenton et al., 1994). Several studies have investigated CSF inflammatory markers, immunological mediators, neurotrophins, metalloproteinases or isoprostenes. Candidate CSF biomarkers include total tau (T-tau) as a marker for the neuronal degeneration (table 1), phosphorylated tau (P-tau) as a marker for tau hyperphosphorylation (table 2) and formation of tangles Aβ42 as a marker for Aβ metabolism and plaque formation (table 3, Blennow et al.,2003).

http://dx.doi.org/10.5772/55069

Category	Reference	Sensitivity range (100%) for AD versus controls	Methods	Study Title	Study population
Tau	Arai et al., 1995	80-90	ELISA	Tau in cerebrospinal fluid: a potential diagnostic marker in Alzheimer's disease	AD (n=70), non-AD (n=96) control (n=19)
Tau	Riemenschneider et al., 1996	90-100	ELISA	Cerebrospinal protein tau is elevated in early Alzheimer's disease.	AD(n=22), dementia(n=3) Healthy controls(HC)(n=19)
Tau	Shoiji et al., 1998	20-30	ELISA	Combination assay of CSF tau, A beta 1-40 and A beta 1-42(43) as a biochemical marker of Alzheimer's disease	sporadic AD(n=55), controls(n=34), non-AD dementia(n=23), other neurological diseases(n=45)
Tau	Kanai et al., 1998	30-40	ELISA	Longitudinal study of cerebrospinal fluid levels of tau, A beta1-40, and A beta1-42(43) in Alzheimer's disease: a study in Japan	AD(n=93), non-AD dementia(n=33) other neurological diseases (n=56), HC(n=54)
Tau	Tapiola et al., 1998	50-60	ELISA	CSF tau is related to apolipoprotein E genotype in early Alzheimer's disease.	Early AD(n=81), other dementia (n=43), non demented neurologic HC(n=33)
Tau	Kahle et al., 2000	50-60	ELISA	Combined assessment of tau and neuronal thread protein in Alzheimer's disease CSF	Probable AD(n=25), definite AD(n=5), non demented with PD (n=29), HC(n=16).
Tau	Sjögren et al., 2000	60-70	ELISA	Decreased CSF -amyloid42 in Alzheimer's disease and amyotrophic lateral sclerosis may reflect mismetabolism of -amyloid induced by separate mechanisms	AD (n = 19), FTD (n = 14), ALS (n = 11) PD(n = 15) HC(n = 17)
Tau	Shoji et al., 2002	50-60	ELISA	Cerebrospinal fluid tau in dementia disorders:a large scale multicenter study by a Japanese study group	AD(n=366), 168 non-AD dementia(n=168) HC(n=181).
Tau	Buerger et al., 2002	70-80	ELISA	Differential diagnosis of Alzheimer's disease with cerebrospinal fluid levels of tau protein phosphorylated at threonine 231	AD(n=82) FTD(n=26) VD(n=20) HC(n=21)
Tau	Riemenschneider et al., 2002	80-90	ELISA	Tau and Abeta42 protein in CSF of patients with frontotemporal degeneration	FTD(n=34), AD(n=74), HC(n=40).
Tau	Schönknecht et al., 2003	50-60	ELISA	Levels of total tau and tau protein phosphorylated at threonine 181 in patients with incipient and manifest Alzheimer's disease	manifest AD (n=43) Incipient AD(n=8) VD(n=16) HC(n=16)

Data from Blennow K, Hampel H (2003)

Table 1. CSF total tau (T-tau) as a diagnostic marker for AD

Catagory	Reference	Sensitivity (100%) for AD versus controls	Methods	Study Title	Study population
p- tau	Ishiguro etal., 1999	80-90	ELISA	Phosphorylated tau in human cerebrospinal fluid is a diagnostic marker for Alzheimer's disease.	AD (n=36) , Controls (n=30)
p- tau	Kohnken et al., 2000	80-90	ELISA	Detection of tau phosphorylated at threonine 231 in cerebrospinal fluid of Alzheimer's disease patients	AD(n=27), non-AD(n=31)
p- tau	Sjögren et al., 2001	40-50	ELISA	The cerebrospinal fluid levels of tau, growth-associated protein-43 and soluble amyloid precursor protein correlate in Alzheimer's disease, reflecting a common pathophysiological process	FTD(n = 14), AD(n = 47) VAD(n = 16), controls (n = 12)
p- tau	Itoh et al.,2001	90-100	ELISA	Large-scale, multicenter study of cerebrospinal fluid tau protein phosphorylated at serine 199 for the antemortem diagnosis of AD	AD(n = 236), non-AD (n = 239), controls (n = 95)
p- tau	Parnetti et al., 2001	80-90	ELISA	CSF phosphorylated tau is a possible marker for discriminating AD from dementiawith Lewy bodies. Phospho-Tau International Study Group	AD (n=80), DLB (n=43) Controls (n=40)
p-tau	Sjögren et al., 2002	50-60	ELISA	Decreased CSF -amyloid42 in Alzheimer's disease and amyotrophic lateral sclerosis may reflect mismetabolism of -amyloid induced by separate mechanisms.	AD (n = 19), FTD (n = 14), ALS (n = 11) PD(n = 15)
p- tau	Buerger et al., 2002	90-100	ELISA	CSF tau protein phosphorylated at threonine 231 correlates with cognitive decline in MCI subjects	MCI(n=77), probable AD (n=55) Control (n=30)
p-tau	Hu et al., 2002	90-100	ELISA	Levels of nonphosphorylated and phosphorylated tau in cerebrospinal fluid of Alzheimer's disease patients: an ultrasensitive bienzyme-substrate-recycle enzyme-linked immunosorbent assay.	AD (*n* = 30), VaD, (*n* = 18) non-AD (*n* = 13): depression (*n* = 3), malignant lymphoma (*n* = 2) control (*n* = 24)
p-tau	Schönknecht et al.,2003	60-70	ELISA	CSF phosphorylated tau is a possible marker for discriminating Alzheimer's disease from dementia with Lewy bodies. Phospho-Tau International Study Group	AD (n=80) DLB (n=43) Controls (n=40).

Data from Blennow K, Hampel H.(2003)

Table 2. CSF Phosphorylaterd tau (p-tau) as a diagnostic marker for AD

http://dx.doi.org/10.5772/55069

Catagory	Reference	Sensitivity (100%) for AD versus controls	Methods	Study Title	Study group
$A\beta_{1-42}$	Galasko et al ., 1998	70-80	ELISA	High cerebrospinal fluid tau and low amyloid beta42 levels in the clinical diagnosis of Alzheimer disease and relation to apolipoprotein E genotype	Probable AD(n=82), control (n=60) ND (n= 74)
$A\beta_{1-42}$	Andreasen et al., 1999	90-100	ELISA	Cerebrospinal fluid -amyloid(1-42) in Alzheimer's disease: differences between early- and late-onset Alzheimer disease and stability during the course of disease	AD (n=53) Control (n=21)
$A\beta_{1-42}$	Andreasen et al.,1999	90-100	ELISA	Sensitivity, specificity and stability of CSF t-tau in AD in a community-based patient sample.	AD (n= 407) Depression(n=28) control (n=65).
$A\beta_{1-42}$	Andreasen et al., 1999C	80-90	ELISA	Cerebrospinal fluid -amyloid(1-42) in Alzheimer's disease: differences between early- and late-onset Alzheimer disease and stability during the course of disease.	AD (n=53) Control (n= 21)
$A\beta_{1-42}$	Hulstaert et al., 1999	70-80	ELISA	Improved discrimination of AD patients using beta-amyloid(1-42) and tau levels in CSF.	AD (n=150) control (n= 100) ND (n=84),
$A\beta_{1-42}$	Otto et al., 2000	90-100	ELISA	Decreased beta-amyloid1-42 in cerebrospinal fluid of patients with Creutzfeldt-Jakob disease	CJD (n=27), AD(n=14), other dementia(n=19), NDC(n=20)
$A\beta_{1-42}$	Kapaki et al., 2001	70-80	ELISA	Highly increased CSF tau protein and decreased beta-amyloid (1-42) in sporadic CJD: a discrimination from Alzheimer's disease?	CJD (n=14), AD(n=38)controls (n=47).
$A\beta_{1-42}$	Sjögren et al., 2002	90-100	ELISA	Decreased CSF -amyloid42 in Alzheimer's disease and amyotrophic lateral sclerosis may reflect mismetabolism of -amyloid induced by separate mechanisms	AD (n = 19), FTD (n = 14), ALS (n = 11) PD (n = 15) controls (n = 17).

Data from Blennow K, Hampel H.(2003)

Table 3. CSF $A\beta_{1-42}$as a diagnostic marker for AD

2.1. Tau protein

One of the major neuropathological hallmarks of AD are neurofibrillary tangles composed of paired helical filaments (PHF). The principal protein subunit of PHF is abnormally phosphorylated tau (p-tau) (Iqbal et al., 1998). Physiologically, tau protein is located in neuronal axons, in components of the cytoskeleton and in the intracellular transport systems. Total-tau (t-tau) and truncated forms of monomeric and p-tau can be traced in the CSF. Using antibodies that detect all isoforms of tau proteins independent of phosphorylation, or specific phosphorylation Core biomarker candidates of Alzheimer's disease 251 sites, ELISA have been developed to measure t-tau and p-tau concentrations (Vandermeeren et al., 1993; Blennow et al., 2002, 1995; Hampel et al., 2003). CSF total tau protein in the differentiation between AD and normal aging. Total tau protein, thought to be a general marker of neuronal destruction, has been intensely studied in more than 2200 AD patients and 1000 age-matched elderly controls over the last 10 years (Sunderland et al., 2003, table 1). The most consistent finding is a statistically significant increase of CSF t-tau protein in AD. The mean level of CSF t-tau protein concentration is about 3 times higher in AD compared to elderly controls. A sensitivity and specificity level varies between studies primarily due to the different control groups used. Specificity levels between 65% and 86% and sensitivity levels between 40% and 86% have been found (Blennow et al., 2001, table 1). In several studies, a significant elevation was also found in patients with early dementia (Galasko et al., 1997; Kurz et al., 1998; Riemenschneider et al., 1997). In these studies of early dementia, the potential of CSF t-tau protein to discriminate between AD and normal aging appeared high, with average 75% sensitivity and 85% specificity. An age-associated increase of t-tau protein has been shown in nondemented subjects (Buerger et al., 2003; Sjogren et al., 2001b). Therefore, the effect of age should be considered when t-tau protein levels are employed diagnostically.

2.2. Phosphorylated tau (p-tau)

Tau protein exists in six isoforms of 352–441 amino acids in length that are subject to a variety of posttranslational modifications (Hanger et al., 2007) and, presumably, function. Of the 79 serine and threonine phosphorylation sites on the longest isoform of tau, 4R/2N, approximately 40 have been verified (Iqbal et al., 2010) of which 25 have been identified as sites of "abnormal phosphorylation" (Mazanetz et al., 2007). The phosphorylation state of tau is the net result of a balance of kinase and phosphatase activity. Much of the activity in tau-based drug discovery has been focused on selective finding inhibitors of "tau kinase", a combination of the activity of two serine/theronine kinases that can phosphorylate tau – glycogen synthase kinase 3 (GSK3; tau protein kinase I), cyclin-dependent kinase 5 (CDK5; tau protein kinase II) and a third kinase, extracellular signal-regulated kinase 2 (ERK2), from the possible 518 member kinase family, as a possible therapeutic approach to treating AD (Hanger et al.,2009 Mazanetz et al.,2007, Brunden et al., 2009). Other kinases that are possible targets to prevent tau hyperphosphorylation are casein kinase 1 (Hanger et al.,2007), AMP-activated protein kinase (AMPK) (Greco et al.,2009) and DYRK1A and AKAP-13 (Azorsa et al., 2010). From a biomarker perspective, t-tau, a generic measure of cortical axon damage associated with AD, multiple sclerosis (Hernandez et al., 2007, Bartosik-Psujek et al.,2006), stroke and Creuzfeldt-

Jacob disease, and p-tau are increased by three fold in the CSF of confirmed AD patients (Shaw et al.,2009). Of the 40 or so phosphorylation sites on tau, pThr181 (phosphothreonine-181), pSer199, pSer202/pThr205 (AT8, epitopes site), pSer214/pSer212 (AT100, epitopessite), pThr231/ pSer235 (TG3 site) and pSer396/pSer396 (PHF1 site)–have been associated with tau hyperphosphorylation and to screen NCEs for potential "tau kinase" inhibitory activity. While pSer199 and pThr231 (p-tau231) have been evaluated as CSF biomarkers (Buerger et al., 2002; Engelborghs et al., 2008., table 2), pThr181 (also designated as p-tau181 or P-Tau181P) is the most widely used CSF biomarker to assess tau hyperphosphorylation (Lewczuk et al., 2002; Hampel et al., 2004) having similar diagnostic accuracy to p-tau231 (Fagan et al., 2009, table 2). Like Ab42, the diagnostic value of both t-tau and p-tau181 has been questioned in terms of their specificity as AD biomarkers (Mattsson et al., 2009).

2.3. β-Amyloid-protein

Extracellular senile plaques consisting of beta-amyloid-protein (Aβ) are one of the histopathological hallmarks of AD (Hyman and Trojanowski., 1997). They are the source of a pathogenic protein with 42 amino acids (Aβ1–42) (Selkoe et al., 1993). Several groups have developed and studied different bioassays specifically designed for Ab1–42 protein (Arai et al., 1997c, Sunderland et al., 2003). The reduction in CSF Ab1–42 found in AD has been hypothesized to indirectly reflect the amyloid deposition in senile plaques (SP), resulting in lower CSF levels in AD. A marked reduction in CSF Ab1–42, however, is also found in CJD, even in cases without Ab-positive plaques (Kapaki et al., 2001; Otto et al., 2000., table 3).

To date, at least 900 patients with clinical AD and 500 healthy individuals have been enrolled in independent research studies (Andreasen et al., 2001; Andreasen et al., 1999; Galasko et al., 1998; Sunderland et al., 2003., table 3). The most consistent finding is a marked decrease in Aβ1–42 protein in AD (to approximately 50% of control levels). Using Ab1–42 protein alone yielded sensitivities varying from 78% to 100% (table 3) and specificities from 47% to 81% when distinguish AD from elderly controls. There is a pronounced overlap, however, between studiesfrom different groups. Based on recent data a cut-off-level of >500 pg=ml has been suggested to discriminate AD best from normal aging (Sjogren et al., 2001a). One study has documented a significant decrease in CSF Aβ1–42 protein in MCI subjects compared to controls, but this study had no follow-up measure (Andreasen et al., 1999a). A second study examined MCI patients who went on to develop AD. However, in this sample Aβ1–42 protein levels did not differ significantly from age-matched normal controls (Maruyama et al., 2001). Blennow et al (2003) found Ab1–42 protein to be an indicator of early identification of AD in MCI subjects taking potential confounding factors into account such as age, severity of cognitive decline, time of observation, apolipoprotein E epsilon (e) 4 (APOE e4) carrier status, and gender (Blennow et al., 2003).Studies correlating CSF Aβ1–42 protein concentrations with cognitive performance in AD have been contradictory. Cross-sectionally, the concentration of Aβ1–42 protein and cognitive measures were either inversely correlated (Kanai et al., 1998; Samuels et al., 1999) or no significant correlation was found (Andreasenet al., 1999b; Hulstaert et al., 1999; Okamura et al., 1999). In a rare longitudinal study, a decrease in CSF Aβ1–42 protein was documented overa three year follow-up period (Tapiola et al., 2000). A highly significant correlation between low CSF concentrations at baseline and follow up. In a separate study, no correlation was found between CSF levels and duration or severity of AD (Andreasen et al., 1999b).

2.4. Combination of CSF amyloid and tau phosphorylation

The current limitations of the predictive value of Aβ 42, t-tau and p-tau181 as AD biomarkers alone, these have been used together to develop a "CSF AD signature", again, with mixed results (Shaw et al., 2009;Mattsso et al., 2009;Kauwe et al., 2009;Mihaescu et al., 2010;Breno et al.,2008;De Meyer et al., 2010). While some studies indicate that the combination Aβ 42, t-tau and p-tau181 biomarker signature in CSF has high predictivity in identifying cases of prodromal AD in MCI patents (Shaw et al.,2009; Jack et al.,2010; Hansson et al., 2006), there is considerable intersite variability that can confound biomarker accuracy (Kauwe et al., 2009). Reduced CSF Aβ 42 and increased CSF p-tau181 concentrations – were used independently of a clinical diagnosis to stratify patient groups (De Meyer et al., 2010). This AD signature was found in 90%, 72%, and 36% of patients with AD, mild MCI, and cognitively normal groups respectively (De Meyer et al., 2010). The cognitively normal group with an AD signature were enriched in apolipoprotein E4 alleles. Validation of these findings in two further data sets showed that 64/68 (94% sensitivity) of autopsy-confirmed AD patients were classified with an AD signature while 57 MCI patients followed for 5 years had a sensitivity of 100% in progressing to AD based on their biomarker signature. The presence of a CSF AD signature in cognitively normal subjects was interpreted by the authors as an indication of AD pathology being present and detectable far earlier than previously envisioned in disease progression.

2.5. NF proteins

Neurofilaments (NFs) are neuron-specific intermediate filaments and serve as a major cytoskeletal component in neurons. In a mature mammalian neuron, NFs are co-assembled from three subunits, termed NF-H (high), NF-M (medium) and NF-L (low). As NFs are confined to the nervous system, they might be one of the best markers reflecting neuronal pathogenic changes seen in some neurological disorders, such as AD. In AD brain, the levels of phosphorylated NF-H/M (pNF-H/M) have been found to be markedly increased (Wang et al., 2001). Hu et al., (2002) found that, the levels of phosphorylated NF-H/M (pNF-H/M), non-phosphorylated NF-H/M (npNF-H/M) and NF-L were significantly higher (pNF-H/M,,12–24-fold; npNF-H/M,,3–4-fold) in neurologically healthy aged people than young individuals. In AD, the levels of npNF-H/M, and NF-L were similar to vascular dementia (VaD), and higher than in age-matched controls and the levels of pNF-H/M were significantly higher AD and ALS than in aged controls and VaD. Based on these findings, it is suggested that the increased level of total NF, p-NF proteins in CSF could be used as a marker for brain aging and neurodegenerative disorders in general, and the levels of pNF-H/M as a marker to discriminate AD from normal brain aging and as well as neurological conditions including VaD (Hu et al 2002).

Specific antibodies derived from aberrantly and hyperphosphorylated neuronal intermediate filament peptides from AD brain as bio markers for early AD detection

In addition to hyperphosphorylated- tau, recently we have demonstrated the direct evidence of aberrantly and hyperphosphorylated neuronal intermediated proteins (NF-M/H) as integral part of NFTs of AD brain using phosphoproteomics (Rudrabhatla et al., 2011., table 5). Although, NFs have been shown immunohistologically to be part of NFTs, there has been debate that the identity of NF proteins in NFTs is due to the cross-reactivity of phosphorylated NF antibodies with phospho-Tau. This study has provided a direct evidence on the identity of NFs in NFTs by immunochemical and mass spectrometric analysis. For these studies purified NFTs were used and liquid chromatography/tandem mass spectrometry of NFT tryptic digests were analysed (table 4-6). The phosphoproteomics of NFTs clearly identified NF-M phosphopeptides (table 5). Western blotting of purified tangles with SMI31 showed a 150-kDa band corresponding to phospho-NF-M, while RT97 antibodies detected phospho-NF-H. These observations suggest that expression of some of these genes is elevated in AD in addition to their phosphorylation. Apart from phosphor Tau, phosphopeptides corresponding to MAP1B to Ser1270, Ser1274, and Ser1779); and MAP2 (corresponding to Thr350, Ser1702, and Ser1706) were also identified (table 6). These studies independently demonstrate that NF and other microtubule proteins are part of NFTs in AD brains (Rudrabhatla et al., 2011). These promising findings call for further studies on the diagnostic potential of specific antibodies derived from aberrantly and hyperphosphorylated neuronal intermediate filament (NF-M/H) peptides from AD brain as bio markers for early AD detection

Phosphopeptide	Phosphorylation site
TPPAPKT*PPSSGEPPK	Thr181
TPPAPKTPPS*SGEPPK	Ser184
TPPAPKTPPSS*GEPPK	Ser185
VAVVRT*PPKS*PSSAK	Thr231, Ser235
SRT*PSLPT*PPTR	Thr212, Thr217
TPSLPT*PPTR	Thr217
TDHGAEIVYKS*PVVSGDTSPR	Ser396
TDHGAEIVYKSPVVS*GDTSPR	Ser400
TDHGAEIVYKS*PVVSGDT*SPR	Ser396, Thr403

Table 4. Phosphopeptides and phosphorylation sites identified in NFT Tau

Phosphopeptides	Phosphorylation sites
NF-M SPVPKS*PVEEAK	Ser685
NF-M KAES*PVKEEAVAEVVTITK	Ser736
NF-M VSGSPSS*GFRSQSWSR	Ser33
NF-H EPDDAKAKEPS*K	Ser942

Table 5. Phosphopeptides and phosphorylation sites identified in NF-M and NF-H

MAP	Sequence	Phosphorylation site
MAP1B	VLSPLRS*PPLIGSESAYESFLSADDK	Ser1274
MAP1B	VLSPLRS*PPLIGSESAYESFLSADDK	Ser1270
MAP1B	VLS*PLRSPPLIGSESAYESFLSADDK	Ser1270
MAP2	KIDLS*HVTS*KCGS*LK	Ser1702, Ser1706
MAP2	VAIIRT*PPKSPATPK	Thr350

Table 6. Phosphopeptides and phosphorylation sites identified in MAP1 and MAP2

2.6. Microtubule-associated proteins and vimentin

Microtubules are polymers of α- and β-tubulin dimers that mediate many functions in neurons, including organelle transport and cell shape establishment and maintenance as well as axonal elongation and growthcone steering in neurons. The polymerization, stabilization, and dynamic properties of microtubules are influenced by interactions with microtubule-associated proteins (MAPs). Members of this protein family are classified by size: high molecular mass proteins (MAP1A, MAP1B, MAP2a, and MAP2b) and intermediate molecular mass MAPs (MAP2c, MAP2d, and tau) (Gonzalez-Billault,C et al.,2004).

Increasing evidence highlights the critical outcome of MAP modification in cytoskeletal disorganization associated with the early stages of AD development. A decreased content of MAP1B and tau associated with cytoskeletal breakdown was found in the brains of AD patients compared with those of control individuals, suggesting a decreased capacity of microtubule assembly and stability (Nieto,A et.al 1989). These results are consistent with those of Iqbal et al. (1986) describing a decreased capacity in the in vitro microtubule assembly from brain extracts of AD patients. One study has shown an early decrease in MAP2 labeling within dendrites from AD brain (Adlard, P. A., and Vickers, J. C. 2002). Other studies have demonstrated that MAP1B and MAP2 co-localize with NFTs (Kosik et al., 1984; Takahashi, et al., 1991). Alonso et al. (1997) studied the associations of the Alzheimer-hyperphosphorylated tau (AD P-tau) with the high molecular weight MAPs (HMW-MAPs) MAP1 and MAP2. The author found that AD P aggregate with MAP1 and MAP2. The association of AD P-tau to the MAPs resulted in inhibition of MAP-promoted microtubule assembly. These studies suggested that the abnormally phosphorylated tau can sequester both normal tau and HMW-MAPs and disassemble microtubules.

Vimentin is a 57-kDa intermediate filament (IF) protein commonly found in mesodermally derived cells. In the healthy adult brain, vimentin is lacking in neurons and generally restricted to vascular endothelial cells and certain subpopulations of glial cells at specific brain locations. Eli et al (2009) found that Vimentin was localized to neuronal perikarya and dendrites in AD brain, with vimentin-immunopositive neurons prevalent in regions exhibiting intra- and extracellular beta-amyloid1-42 (Aβ42) deposition. Neuronal colocalization of vimentin and Aβ42 was common in the cerebral cortex, cerebellum and hippocampus (Eli et al., 2009). Our lab recently discovered that the protein tangles which are a hallmark of the disease involve at least three different proteins rather than just one (table 4-6). The discovery of these additional proteins, neurofilaments, MAP2 and Vimentin, should provide better understanding the biology and progression of the disease as well as provide additional biomarker at the early stage of the disease.

2.7. Other CSF biomarkers for AD

As the AD signature approach based on the amyloid and tau causality hypothesis of AD continues to evolve, other CSF biomarkers are also being assessed. These include CSF cytokines (Swardfager et al.,2010; Olson etal.,2010)– specifically TGFβ increases in AD CSF (Swardfager et al.,2010)– CSF proteomic profiles (Papassotiropoulos et al.,2006), clusterin (Thambisetty et al.,2010)and IgG antibodies from the adaptive immune system (Reddy et al.,2011) The latter is a field of intense research, despite the challenges in analyzing proteome profiles, and involves the study of differences in the CSF proteome in AD, MCI and control subject groups (Papassotiropoulos et al.,2006;Zhang et al.,2005; Castano et al 2006; Finehout et al.,2007; Marouf et al.,2009; Choi et al.,2010). One study (Maarouf et al.,2009) reported changes in a variety of CSF proteins including a-2-macroglobulin, α1-antichymotrypsin,a1-antitrypsin, complement and heat shock proteins, cathepsinD, enolase and creatine. The ADNI is also generating CSF proteomic profiles as part of its "Use of Targeted Multiplex Proteomic Strategies to Identify Plasma-Based Biomarkers in Alzheimer's Disease" (Miller et al., 2009).

3. Oxidized proteins: Potential candidate biomarkers in AD

Although the pathogenesis of AD is not yet fully known, it is clear that the disease is caused by a combination of risk factors. Among several hypotheses, oxidative stress is considered to play a significant role (Butterfield, 2007). Although CSF represents the most suitable biological fluid to study neurodegenerative diseases since it can reflect the biochemical changes occurring in brain, its analysis is not always easily feasible for a large scale screening, because the costs involved are enormous and procedures are invasive, uncomfortable and not without risk. For a full screening and early diagnosis, biomarkers easily detectable in biological samples, such as plasma, are needed. Up to now, the search for reliable biomarkers for AD in peripheral blood is very challenging because of difficulties with the standardization of the methods of analysis and the low reproducibility of the results. Although a set of plasma markers that differentiated AD from controls have been shown to be useful in predicting conversion from MCI to AD (Song., 2009), the study has not been yet verified by other researchers and the application of these candidate biomarkers have yet to achieve the diagnostic power, sensitivity, and reproducibility necessary for widespread use in a clinical setting. Oxidized proteins may represent potential candidate biomarkers for "oxidative stress diseases", such as AD.

The first report on protein oxidation in CSF samples was from Tohgi et al. (1999) who demonstrated that 3-nitrotyrosine moderately but significantly increased with advancing age, and showed a remarkable increase in patients with AD. As the free tyrosine concentration did not decrease, the increase in 3-nitrotyrosine with age or associated with AD did not appear to be directly related to an increase in free-nitrated tyrosines. Rather, the increased 3-nitrotyrosine was likely due to an increase in nitrated tyrosines in proteins or increased degradation of 3-nitrotyrosin containing proteins, which are highly vulnerable to degradation.The most reliable CSF markers in AD are Aβ42 and tau. Low CSF Aβ 42 is associated with amyloid pathology in the brain and high Tau is linked with neurofibrillary pathology (Frey etal. 2005). Most subjects with decreased CSF Aβ42 and high tau develop AD during the follow-up (Herukka et al., 2007). Therefore, these CSF markers may reflect brain pathology and identify preclinical AD. Interestingly, the levels of CSF Aβ42 showed a tendency to correlate positively with serum oxidative markers in the whole study population and with plasma nitrotyrosines in AD patients. Moreover, a negative correlation between CSF tau and serum nitrotyrosine levels was evidenced in controls (Korolainen et al., 2009). The correlation between CSF AD markers and blood oxidative markers may suggest that oxidative metabolism is changed in AD. This hypothesis is further supported by the finding of decreased CSF protein carbonylation in APOE ε4 carriers, which is considered an important risk factor for developing AD (Raber et al., 2004) and correlates with redox proteomics studies that identified metabolic proteins as oxidatively modified and dysfunctional (Choi et al., 2004).

Subsequently, Ahmed et al. (2005) measured in CSF the levels of protein glycation, oxidation and nitration. The authors found that the concentrations of 3-nitrotyrosine,Nε-carboxymethyl-lysine,3-deoxyglucosone-derived hydroimidazolone and N-formylkynurenine (as markers of protein glycation) were increased in subjects with AD. The Mini-Mental State Examination (MMSE) score correlated negatively with 3-nitrotyrosine residue concentration. These findings indicated that protein glycation, oxidation and nitration were increased in the CSF of subjects with AD. A combination of nitration and glycation adduct estimates of CSF may conceivably provide an indicator for the diagnosis of AD. Increased levels of protein aggregates in the form of fibrils together with increased lipid peroxidation have been shown, both in AD andMCI brain (Butterfield et al., 2010).

Advanced oxidation end products (AOEs,) during AD, colocalize with neurofibrillary tangles, senile plaques, microglia, and astrocytes and have been also measured in plasma. Advanced oxidation protein products (AOPPs), a relatively novel marker of oxidative damage, are considered as reliable markers to estimate the degree of oxidant-mediated protein damage. A significant increase in protein carbonyls in hippocampus (HP) and inferior parietal lobule (IPL) of AD subjects compared with age-matched controls was observed. Dityrosine and 3-NT total levels were reported to be elevated in the hippocampus, IPL, and neocortical regions of AD brain. Alterations in brain phospholipids pattern, a more specific assessment of lipid peroxidation, have been reported for AD brain (Lovell et al., 1995; Nitsch etal.,1992; Prasad etal., 1998). The levels of phosphatidylinositol (PI) and phosphatidylethanolamine (PE), rich in easily oxidizable PUFA, are decreased in AD brain. The levels of F(2)-isoprostanes [F(2)-IsoP], F(4)-neuroprostane[F(4)-NP], and isoprostane 8,12-iso-iPF2(α)-VI were also found to be increased in AD brain compared to controls (Montine et al.,2002; Mark et al,1999). An increase in free HNE has been demonstrated in amygdala, hippocampus, and parahippocampal gyrus of the AD brain compared with age matched controls (Markesbery.,1998). Several proteins mainly involved in energy metabolism pathways, pH regulation, and mitochondrial functionsamong others, were found carbonylated, HNE-bound or nitrated in AD brain (Sultana,

2006). Newman et al (2007) also reported that a number of proteins modified by glutathionylation in AD IPL.

Previous studies on CSF nitrite and nitrate levels in patients with AD have provided contradictory results, with some showing decreased nitrate levels (Kuiper.,1994), others showing unaltered nitrite/nitrate levels (Ikeda.,1995), and still others increased nitrate levels (Tohgi., 1998). However, another study from the same group showed that nitrite/nitrate levels in AD were stage-dependent, being elevated only in the early phase of AD and decreasing to control levels with disease progression (Tohgi., 1998). This finding was interpreted to reflect progressive reduction of neurons. In contrast, free 3-nitrotyrosine levels increased significantly in parallel with the severity of AD, suggesting that protein degradation increases with disease progression, resulting in increased release of free 3-nitrotyrosine from tyrosine residues that have been nitrated. 3-nitrotyrosine and the 3-nitrotyrosine/tyrosine ratios in the CSF, both of which are believed to reflect degradation of nitrated tyrosine-containing proteins, increased significantly with age and were remarkably higher in patients with AD than in controls.

A study by Choi et al. (2002) identified uniquely oxidized proteins in AD plasma. These authors applied two-dimensional gel electrophoresis (2DE) coupled with immunological staining of protein carbonyl and the oxidized proteins observed in the plasma of both AD subjects and non-AD controls were determined. However, the level of oxidation of these protein spots was markedly higher in the AD samples. They also found that the increased oxidation was not a generalized phenomenon. In the total protein stain profile, more than 300 spots were detected, but less than 20 spots were positive by immunostaining with anti-DNP antibody. Furthermore, of the seven proteins that were most intensively oxidized, their relative levels of oxidation differed. These studies found that fibrinogen gamma chain precursor and alpha 1 antitrypsinprecursor showed increased levels of carbonyl groups in AD comparedwith controls (Stief et al., 1989).

4. Identification of a new plasma biomarker of AD using metabolomics technology

Current metabolomics research involves the identification and quantification of hundreds to thousands of small-molecular-mass metabolites (<1,500 Daltons) in cells, tissues, or biological fluids. The aims of such studies are typically to understand new diagnosis biomarkers, to understand the mechanism of action of therapeutic compounds, and to uncover the pharmacodynamics and kinetic markers of drugs in patients and in preclinical in vivo and in vitro models (Wilcoxen et al., 2010). Lipidomics is one of the metabolomics approaches used to analyze lipid species in biological systems (Hu et al., 2009; Han et al., 2005; Han and Gross, 2003). Investigating lipid biochemistry using a lipidomics approach will not only provide insights into the specific roles of lipid molecular species in healthy individuals and patients but will also assist in identifying potential biomarkers for establishing preventive or therapeutic approaches for human health (Hu et al., 2009,Wenk.,2005; Rosenson.,2010). Lipidomics has recently captured attention, owing to the well-recognized roles of lipids in numerous human diseases such as diabetes, obesity, atherosclerosis, and AD (Wenk et al., 2005; Watson., 2006; Steinberg,. 2005; Sato et al., 2010). In support of the hypothesis that lipid dysfunction plays an important role in AD pathogenesis, previous studies with post-mortem brain tissue samples have demonstrated altered lipidomes at the different stage of AD pathogenesis. For example, multiple classes of sphingolipids are altered not only at the late stage of the disease but also at the earliest clinically recognizable stage of AD. All major classes of phospholipids are ubiquitously decreased at the late stage of AD. Among these, the levels of plasmalogen (a major component in nerve tissue membranes counting for up to 85% of ethanolamine glycerophospholipid, or ~30% of total phospholipids of these membranes) are gradually reduced as progress of AD severity (Han et al., 2011). Sato et al (2011) established a lipidomics method for comprehensive phospholipids evaluation that identified 31 phospholipids as AD biomarker candidates in human plasma using LC/MS (Satoet al., 2010). Moreover, additional studies have suggested that AD associates with other lipid metabolism pathways and lipid carrier proteins such as apoE (Bertram et al., 2008; Corder et al., 1993; Farrer et al., 1997; Strittmatter et al., 1993).

A very recent study by Sato et al (2011) were able to find a biomarker desmosterol that changes in AD compared with plasma from healthy elderly controls. They have shown that desmosterol plasma level and the desmosterol/cholesterol ratio in the same patients was significantly decreased. This study is the first report that plasma desmosterol levels are decreased in AD and MCI. And future studies are needed to confirm whether desmosterol could become an attractive plasma AD biomarker that could perhaps also be utilized for diagnosis and as well as for monitoring noninvasively the effect of future AD drugs on disease progression.

5. MicroRNAs as biomarkers for AD

MicroRNAs (miRNAs) are a class of small, endogenous, noncoding RNA molecules that serve as posttranscriptional regulators of gene expression (Lee etal.,1993;Giannakakis etal.,2007). miRNAs are acquiring important and determinant roles in the regulation of brain gene transcription in health and disease: the fact that approximately 80% of the human brain genome is transcribed into RNA, but only about 2% of the genome is transcribed into protein, underscores the potential of various levels of RNA signaling and epigenetic mechanisms to contribute to physiological gene control (Makeyevetal., 2008). In the last few years, miRNAs have been emerging as important regulators of various aspects of neuronal development and dysfunction (Gao.,2007; Lukiw.,2007). The role of miRNAs in neurodegenerative diseases has been investigated using miRNA microarray profiling in brain tissue samples derived from patients and controls. Using miRNA expression profiling in cortex samples from a well-characterized clinicopathological series of elderly controls, MCI subjects and AD patients, Wang et al (2008) identified miR-107 to be specifically decreased early in the course of AD. Computational analyses predicted BACE1 mRNA as a target of miR-107 and correlative mRNA expression studies confirmed its role in regulating BACE1 expression. An independent miRNA profiling study by Hebert et al (2008) confirmed the importance of BACE1 regulation by miRNAs. The presence of a modulation of miRNA in regions of brain targeted by AD neuropathology was further demonstrated (Lukiw et al., 2008; Lukiw., 2009), thus suggesting a specific involvement of miRNAs in pathogenetic signaling pathways associated with the AD process. Recent findings suggest that neuronal miRNA deregulation in response to an insult by Aβ may be an important factor contributing to the cascade of events leading to AD (Schonrock, et al., 2010). Of note, the upregulation of peripheral miRNAs in AD could contribute to the diminished plasma proteins reported to be predictive biomarkers for AD (Ray Set al., 2007). In addition, it has recently been reported that miRNAs can be detected in CSF: an altered regulation of miRNA expression in AD brains was paralleled by a modulation of miRNA levels in the CSF (Cogswell et al., 2008). These studies provide an initial hope that miRNAs could represent accessible biomarkers to support clinical diagnosis in the near future.

6. Timing and other influencing factors of biomarker use

Disease modifying drugs are likely to be most effective in the earlier stages of AD, before neurodegeneration is too severe and widespread, so trials for this type of drug will need to include AD cases in the earlier stages of the disease. Validated biomarkers that could enable accurate identification of AD pathology at an early stage would be of great use (Hampel et al., 2011). Alternatively, baseline biomarker measurements can be used for enrichment and stratification in proof-of concept studies, as well as for supporting go/no-go decision making of phase III trials. Biomarkers should be used in all stages of drug development including phase I, phase II and phase III. They can be used to enhance inclusion and exclusion criteria, for stratification. Biomarkers can also be used as outcome markers to detect treatment effects. Particularly, if biomarkers are intended to be used as surrogate endpoints in pivotal studies, they must have been qualified to be a substitute for a clinical standard of truth and as such reasonably predict a clinical meaningful outcome. Finally, biomarkers can be used to identify adverse effects. Nevertheless there are several pitfalls to be faced in the interpretation of biomarker data in AD drug development, such as the fact that biomarkers may be non-specific to AD, it may not be feasible to measure them in the appropriate system (i.e. the central nervous system) and the risk of over-interpreting biomarker data in phase II trials if statistical significance levels are not adjusted for multiple comparisons (Aisen, 2009). Failure to consider these issues could contribute to false conclusions and costly errors (Hampel et al., 2011; Hampel et al., 2004)

7. Conclusion and future directions

Several promising drug candidates with disease-modifying effect, such as Aβ immunotherapy, secretase modulators, and tau aggregation inhibitors, have now reached the stage of being tested in clinical trials. The promise of disease-modifying therapy has created a need for biomarkers to enable the clinical identification of the disease at an early stage. Early diagnosis will be of great importance since disease-modifying drugs are likely to be most effective in the earlier stages of the disease, before neurodegeneration is too severe and widespread. A large number of studies have demonstrated that tests based on

CSF t-tau protein, p-tau and CSF beta-amyloid1–42 have reasonable specificity and sensitivity when differentiating AD from normal aging. A smaller number of studies show similar accuracy when distinguishing AD from major depression. These tests may also be useful in detecting MCI patients who go on to develop AD.

Unfortunately, the value of these biomarkers to clinicians is limited, because they are not specific enough to accurately separate AD from other common forms of dementia, such as VaD and LBD. Sometimes the combination of both CSF t-tau protein and CSF Aβ1–42 markers does not markedly improve on their individual sensitivity. CSF p-tau, based on different phosphorylation epitopes of tau protein, has now been examined in a number of independent studies. Initial results are extremely promising, showing that different p-tau protein epitopes may substantially contribute to improved diagnostic accuracy of AD in comparison with healthy aged controls, elderly depressed patients and those with other types of dementia. Compared with CSF t-tau protein and CSF Ab1–42 markers, CSF p-tau is more specific and less influenced by age or degree of cognitive decline (Hampel et al., 2004). This has an important implication for the value of CSF p-tau to clinicians. If the marker becomes abnormal very early in the course of disease relatively independent from the degree of cognitive decline than the marker may be ideal as a diagnostic test. If, however, the marker is closely linked to current or future cognitive decline, then it may be better suited as a prognostic tool. Studies of all possible biomarkers to date in AD, suggest p-tau comes the closest to the ideal diagnostic marker. However, different epitopes of p-tau may have different strengths and weaknesses. CSF p-tau231 may be most useful in distinguishing AD from frontotemporal dementia (FTD). CSF p-tau181 may improve separation between AD and LBD. In addition, CSF p-tau231 may be the most useful prognostic marker candidates that predicts cognitive decline to AD in MCI subjects.Further studies are needed to decide whether detection of multiple phosphoepitopes may allow a distinct representation of AD related pathology at different stages of the disease (Augustinack et al., 2002).

NFTs contain aberrantly hyperphosphorylated Tau as paired helical filaments. Although NFs have been shown immunohistologically to be part of NFTs, there has been debate that the identity of NF proteins in NFTs is due to the cross-reactivity of phosphorylated NF antibodies with phospho-Tau. Our laboratory recently reported (Rudrabhatla et al., 2010, 2011) the direct evidence of NFs in NFTs. Moreover, neuronal death and degeneration may release fragments of these proteins into body fluids at sufficient levels to be easily detected by specific antibodies at early, preclinical stages of AD. A battery of antibodies to NF-specific phosphoepitopes and Tau in NFTs may offer a unique approach to the design of effective early biomarkers.

The rapidly developing fields of large-scale and massive-scale genomics, proteomics, and metabolomics are now joining functional neuroimaging, structural neuroimaging, and neuropsychometric contenders in the race to establish useful biomarkers of AD and other dementing illnesses. Redox proteomics studies have provided insights into the role of oxidative stress in AD pathology. Posttranslational modifications of brain proteins, induced by oxidative damage, lead to impairment and dysfunction of several cellular functions thus providing clues about important molecular basis of neurodegeneration associated to AD. In addition, these studies have identified specific therapeutic targets in this disorder. In recent years, growing studies have been focused to establish a direct link between tissue specific oxidation and systemic oxidative damage (Blennow et al., 2010; Korolainen et al 2010; Ahmed et al., 2005; Aksenov et al., 2001). Correlations between total levels of oxidation markers in the brain and in the periphery have been shown. Although some of the reported results in AD are controversial, most of them support the presence of peripheral oxidative damage and of a characteristic panel of systemic oxidation that correlates with the occurrence of the disease. Studies investigating oxidative stress outside of the CNS, particularly in blood, while prove the occurrence of oxidative reactions, are not fully elucidating the complex cascade of events. Thus, one hypothesis is that oxidative stress first develops in the periphery as a result of different causes, and then it will contribute to perturb neuronal homeostasis, either by increasing the production of ROS or by depleting antioxidant defense, which will eventually lead to oxidative damage of the brain and neurodegeneration. The development of new plasma biomarkers could facilitate early detection, risk assessment and therapeutic monitoring in AD. On the other hand, it is also possible to imagine that oxidative stress starts in the CNS where several different metabolic end-products are formed and released into the blood stream. In this context, an important issue is to perform further studies in order to investigate the timing of appearance of oxidative damage signatures at systemic level during the onset of AD early stages and the progression to late stages.

Recently, important steps have been accomplished but there is still a lot of work to be directed towards the discovery, testing and validation of a panel of novel and old assays that could serve all the requirements for ideal biomarkers. However, the emerging trend which results from the collection of multiple data from different source is the wide variability among different studies that led to contrasting results. Thus, there is an urgent need to standardize protocols for replicate experiments on large population, which may allow to better understanding the effect of systemic oxidative damage in the pathogenesis and progression of AD. Indeed, this is also evident by the lack of redox proteomics and microRNA studies applied to biological fluids. This approach has the power to search for specific microRNA and protein oxidative modification thus allowing the identification of altered miroRNA and protein in complex matrices such as body fluids, which may discriminate AD vs healthy condition.

There are several different reasons to support the development of more sensitive method to detect a biochemical marker in AD: to increase diagnostic accuracy; to identify MCI subjects who will progress to clinical AD; to monitor pharmacological and biological effects of drugs. There is an urgent need to add further peripheral markers of oxidative stress as useful diagnostic biomarker. There is clearly a growing interest among clinicians and basic scientists to tap on each other's expertise in the area of ageing neurobiology research. Such collaborations between geriatricians, neuroimaging specialists, neuropsychiatrists as well as molecular and cellular neurobiologists are being fostered. Further research is necessary to improve especially the early/differential biochemical diagnosis of AD. Some considerations need to be taken into account when designing future studies. These should include high numbers of relevant AD of different origin, a combination of biomarkers and other risk factors, long-term follow- up of patients and if possible neuropathological verification of the diagnosis. Standardization of methods seems critical to reducing inconsistency and increasing reliability. It is necessary to implement common protocols for sample preparation, experimental design and generation of proteomics data. Thus, global initiatives of standardization are of critical importance and large multicenter studies are needed to further define the added diagnostic value when multiple biomarker modalities are combined.

The essential goal in biomarker discovery studies is the identification of preclinical marker, which facilitates disease diagnosis at earlystages, is hoped that markers of prognosis will enable clinicians to monitor whether new candidate treatments of AD are working, effectively and inexpensively and assesses the response to treatments by the time that disease-modifying treatments become available in clinical practice.

Acknowledgement

This work is supported by NINDS/NIH intramural funds.

Author details

B.K. Binukumar and Harish C. Pant

Laboratory of Neurochemistry, NINDS, National Institutes of Health, Bethesda, Maryland, USA

References

[1] Adlard, P. A, & Vickers, J. C. (2002). Morphologically distinct plaque types differentially affect dendritic structure and organisation in the early and late stages ofAlzheimer's disease.ActaNeuropathol., 103, 377-383.

[2] Andreasen, N, Hesse, C, Davidsson, P, et al. Cerebrospinal fluid-amyloid(1-42) in Alzheimer's disease: differences between early- and late-onset Alzheimer disease and stability during the course of disease. Arch Neurol (1999). , 56, 673-80.

[3] Andreasen, N, Hesse, C, Davidsson, P, Minthon, L, & Wallin, . (1999b) Cerebrospinal fluid beta-amyloid (1-42) in Alzheimer disease: differences between early- and late-onset Alzheimer disease and stability during the course of disease. Arch Neurol 56: 673-680.

[4] Andreasen, N, Minthon, L, Clarberg, A, Davidsson, P, Gottfries, J, Vanmechelen, E, & Vanderstichele, . , specificity, and stability of CSF-tau in AD in a community-based patient sample. Neurology 53: 1488-1494

[5] Andreasen, N, Minthon, L, Clarberg, A, et al. Sensitivity, specificity and stability of CSF t-tau in AD in a community-based patient sample. Neurology (1999). , 53, 1488-94.

[6] Andreasen, N, Minthon, L, Davidsson, P, Vanmechelen, E, & Vanderstichele, . (2001) Evaluation of CSF-tau and CSF-A-beta-42 as diagnostic markers for Alzheimer disease in clinical practice. Arch Neurol 58: 373-379.

[7] Andreasen, N, Minthon, L, Vanmechelen, E, Vanderstichele, H, & Davidsson, . (1999a) Cerebrospinal fluid tau and A-beta42 as predictors of development of Alzheimer's disease in patients with mild cognitive impairment. NeurosciLett 273: 5-8.

[8] Arai, H, Higuchi, S, & Sasaki, H. and cerebrospinal fluid tau protein: implications for the clinical diagnosis of Alzheimer's disease. Gerontology , 43, 2-10.

[9] Arai, H, Terajima, M, Miura, M, et al. Tau in cerebrospinal fluid: a potential diagnostic marker in Alzheimer's disease. Ann Neurol (1995). , 38, 649-52.

[10] Azorsa, DO, Robeson, RH, Frost, D, Meechoovet, B, Brautigam, GR, & Dickey, . . 2008 . Genome-wide association analysis reveals putative Alzheimer's disease susceptibility loci in addition to APOE. Am. J. Hum. Genet.83 :623- 632.

[11] Blennow, K, & Hampel, H. (2003). Cerebrospinal fluid markers for incipient Alzheimer's disease.LancetNeurol 2003, 2(10): 605-613.

[12] Blennow, K, Vanmechelen, E, & Hampel, H. CSF total tau, A-beta42 and phosphorylated tau protein as biomarkers for Alzheimer's disease. MolNeurobiol(2002). , 24, 87-97.

[13] Blennow, K, Wallin, A, Ågren, H, Spenger, C, Siegfried, J, & Vanmechelen, E. Tau protein in cerebrospinal fluid: a biochemical diagnostic marker for axonal degeneration in Alzheimer's disease? Mol Chem Neuropathol (1995). , 26, 231-45.

[14] Blennow, K, Wallin, A, & Häger, O. Low frequency of post-lumbar puncture headache in demented patients. Acta Neurol Scand (1993). , 88, 221-23.

[15] Breno, S. O. Diniz, Jony A, Pinto Jr, Orestes Vicente Forlenz.Do CSF total tau,phosphorylated tau, and b-amyloid 42 help to predict progression of mild cognitive impairment to Alzheimer's disease? A systematic review and metaanalysis of the literature. World J Biol Psychiatry (2008). , 9, 172-82.

[16] Brunden, K. R, & Trojanowski, J. Q. Lee VMY. Advances in tau-focused drug discovery for Alzheimer's disease and related tauopathies. Nat Rev Drug Discov (2009). , 8, 783-93.

[17] Buerger, K, Teipel, S. J, Zinkowski, R, et al. CSF tau protein phosphorylated at threonine 231 correlates with cognitive decline in MCI subjects. Neurology (2002). , 59, 627-29.

[18] Buerger, K, Zinkowski, R, Teipel, S. J, Arai, H, Debernardis, J, Padberg, F, Faltraco, F, Goernitz, A, Tapiola, T, Rapoport, S. I, & Hampel, H. Differentiation of geriatric ma-

jor depression from Alzheimer's disease with CSF tau protein phosphorylated at threonine 231. Am J Psychiatry (2003). , 160, 376-379.

[19] Buerger, K, Zinkowski, R, Teipel, SJ, Tapiola, T, Arai, H, & Blennow, . .Differential-Castano EM, Roher AE, Esh CL, Kokjohn TA, Beach T. Comparative proteomics of cerebrospinal fluid in neuropathologically-confirmed Alzheimer's disease and non-demented elderly subjects. Neurol Res 2006;28:155-63.

[20] Choi, Y. S, Choe, L. H, & Lee, K. H. Recent cerebrospinal fluid biomarker studies of Alzheimer's disease.Exp Rev Proteome (2010). , 7, 919-29.

[21] Cogswell, JP, Ward, J, Taylor, IA, Waters, M, Shi, Y, Cannon, B, Kelnar, K, & Kemppainen, . .Identification of miRNA changes in Alzheimer's disease brain and CSF yields putative biomarkers and insights into disease pathways. J Alzheimers Dis 2008; 14: 27-41.

[22] Corder, E. H, Saunders, A. M, Strittmatter, W. J, Schmechel, D. E, Gaskell, P. C, Small, G. W, Roses, A. D, Haines, J. L, & Pericak-vance, M. A. (1993). Gene dose of apolipoprotein E type 4 allele and the risk of Alzheimer's disease in late onset families. Science ., 261, 921-923.

[23] Butterfield, D. A, & Bader, M. L. Lange, R. Sultana, Involvements of the lipid peroxidation product, HNE, in the pathogenesis and progression of Alzheimer's disease,Biochim. Biophys.Acta (2010). , 1801(2010), 924-929.

[24] Butterfield, D. A, Reed, T, Newman, S. F, & Sultana, R. Roles of amyloid beta-peptideassociated oxidative stress and brain protein modifications in the pathogenesis of Alzheimer's disease and mild cognitive impairment, Free Radic. Biol. Med. (2007). , 43(2007), 658-677.

[25] De Meyer, G, Shapiro, F, Vanderstichele, H, Vanmechelen, E, Engelborghs, S, De Deyn, P. P, et al. For the Alzheimer's disease neuroimaging initiative.Diagnosis-independent Alzheimer disease biomarker signature in cognitively normalelderly people. Arch Neurol (2010). , 67, 949-56.

[26] Engelborghs, S, & De Vreese, K. Van de Casteele T, Vanderstichele H, Van Everbroeck B, Cras P, Martin J-J, Vanmechelen E, De Deyn PP. Diagnostic performance of a CSF-biomarker panel in autopsy-confirmed dementia. Neurobiol Aging (2008). , 29, 1143-59.

[27] Song, F, Poljak, A, Smythe, G. A, & Sachdev, P. Plasma biomarkers for mild cognitive impairment and Alzheimer's disease, Brain Res. Rev. (2009). , 61(2009), 69-80.

[28] Fagan, A. M, Mintun, M. A, Shah, A. R, Alde, P, & Roe, C. M. Cerebrospinal fluid tau and ptau181 increase with cortical amyloid deposition in cognitively normal individuals: implications for future clinical trials of Alzheimer's disease.EMBOMol Med (2009). , 1, 371-80.

[29] Farrer, L. A, Cupples, L. A, Haines, J. L, Hyman, B, Kukull, W. A, Mayeux, R, Myers, R. H, & Pericak-vance, M. A. (1997). Effects of age, sex, and ethnicity on the associa-

tion betweenapolipoprotein E genotype and Alzheimer disease.A meta-analysis.APOE and Alzheimer Disease Meta AnalysisConsortium.J. Am. Med. Assoc., 278, 1349-1356.

[30] Fenton, G, Steffen, M, Sugarbaker, E, Miller, K, Swit, B, Green, P, & Charlton, R. (1994). The lumbar puncture- factors affecting success rate. Ann Neurol , 36(3), 544-545.

[31] Finehout, E. J, Franck, Z, Choe, L. H, Relkin, N, & Lee, K. H. Cerebrospinal fluid proteomic biomarkers for Alzheimer's disease. Ann Neurol (2007). , 61, 120-9.

[32] Fink, J. K, Jones, S. M, Esposito, C, & Wilkowski, J. (1996). Human microtubule-associated protein 1a (MAP1A) gene: genomic organization, cDNA sequence, anddevelopmental- andtissue-specific expression. Genomics , 35, 577-585.

[33] Fratiglioni, L, De Ronchi, D, & Agüero-torres, H. (1999). Worldwide prevalence and incidence of dementia.Drugs Aging. , 15(5), 365-75.

[34] Galasko, D, Chang, L, Motter, R, Clark, CM, Kaye, J, Knopman, D, Thomas, R, & Kholodenko, . . High cerebrospinal fluid tau and low amyloid-beta-42 levels in the clinical diagnosisof Alzheimer disease and relation to apolipoprotein E genotype. Arch Neurol 1998; 55: 937-945.

[35] Galasko, D, Clark, C, Chang, L, Miller, B, Green, R. C, Rotter, R, & Seubert, O. Assessment of CSF levels of tau protein in mildly demented patients with Alzheimer's disease. Neurology(1997). , 48, 632-635.

[36] Giannakakis, A, Coukos, G, Hatzigeorgiou, A, & Sandaltzopoulos, R. Zhang L: miRNA genetic alterations in human cancers. Expert OpinBiolTher (2007). , 7, 1375-1386.

[37] Gonzalez-billault, C, Jimenez-mateos, E. M, Caceres, A, Diaz-nido, J, & Avila, J. (2004). Microtubule-associated protein 1B function during normal development, regeneration, and pathological conditions in the nervous system. J Neurobiol. , 58(1), 48-59.

[38] Greco, S. J, Sarkar, S, Johnston, J. M, & Tezapsidis, N. Leptin regulates tau phosphorylation and amyloid through AMPK in neuronal cells. BiochemBiophys Res Commun (2009). , 380, 98-104.

[39] Tohgi, H, Abe, T, Yamazaki, K, Murata, T, Isobe, C, & Ishizaki, E. The cerebrospinal fluid oxidized NO metabolites, nitrite and nitrate, in Alzheimer's disease and vasculardementia of Binswanger type and multiple small infarct type, J. Neural Transm. (1998). , 105(1998), 1283-1291.

[40] Tohgi, H, Abe, T, Yamazaki, K, Murata, T, Ishizaki, E, & Isobe, C. Alterations of 3-nitrotyrosine concentration in the cerebrospinal fluid during aging and in patients with Alzheimer's disease, Neurosci. Lett. (1999). , 269(1999), 52-54.

[41] Frey, H. J, Mattila, K. M, Korolainen, M. A, & Pirttila, T. Problems associated with biological markers of Alzheimer's disease, Neurochem. Res. (2005). , 30(2005), 1501-1510.

[42] Hampel, H, Buerger, K, Zinkowski, R, Teipel, S. J, Goernitz, A, Andreasen, N, et al. Measurement of phosphorylated tau epitopes in the differential diagnosis of Alzheimer disease: a comparative cerebrospinal fluid study. Arch Gen Psychiatry (2004). , 61, 95-102.

[43] Hampel, H, Ornitz, G, & Urger, A, B. K ((2003). Advances in the development of biomarkers for Alzheimer's disease: from CSF total tau and Ab1-42 proteins to phosphorylated tau protein. Brain Res Bull , 61(3), 243-253.

[44] Hampel, H, Mitchell, A, Blennow, K, Frank, R. A, Brettschneider, S, Weller, L, & Möller, H. J. Core biological marker candidates of Alzheimer's disease- perspectives for diagnosis, predictionof outcome and reflection of biological activity.J Neural Transm. (2004). , 2004(111), 3-247.

[45] Han, X, & Gross, R. W. (2003). Global analyses of cellular lipidomes directly from crude extracts of biological samples by ESI mass spectrometry: a bridge to lipidomics.J. Lipid Res. , 44, 1071-1079.

[46] Han, X, & Gross, R. W. (2005). Shotgun lipidomics: electrospray ionization mass spectrometric analysis and quantitation of cellular lipidomes directly from crude extracts of biological samples. Mass Spectrom. Rev. , 24, 367-412.

[47] Han, X, Rozen, S, Boyle, S. H, Hellegers, C, Cheng, H, & Burke, J. R. Kaddurah-Daouk RMetabolomics in early Alzheimer's disease: identification of altered plasma sphingolipidome usingshotgun lipidomics. PLoS One. (2011). e21643.

[48] Hanger, D. P, Anderton, B. H, & Noble, W. Tau phosphorylation: the therapeutic challenge for neurodegenerative disease. Trends Mol Med (2009). , 15, 112-9.

[49] Hanger, D. P, Byers, H. L, Wray, S, Leung, K. Y, Saxton, M. J, Seereeram, A, et al. Novel phosphorylation sites in tau from Alzheimer brain support a role for casein kinase 1 in disease pathogenesis. J BiolChem (2007). , 282, 23645-54.

[50] Hansson, O, Zetterberg, H, Buchhave, P, Londos, E, Blennow, K, & Minthon, . .Association between CSF biomarkers and incipient Alzheimer's disease in patients with mild cognitive impairment: a follow-up study. Lancet Neurol 2006;5:228-34.

[51] HaraldHampelGordon Wilcock , Sandrine Andrieu , Paul Aisen f, KajBlennow , K. Broich Maria Carrillo , Nick C. Foxj, Giovanni B. Frisoni. Biomarkers for Alzheimer's disease therapeutic trials. Progress in Neurobiology 95 ((2011).

[52] Hébert, SS, Horré, K, Nicolaï, L, Papadopoulou, AS, Mandemakers, W, & Silahtaroglu, . , De Strooper B: Loss of microRNA cluster miR-29a/b-1 insporadic Alzheimer's disease correlates with increased BACE1/beta-secretaseexpressionProcNatlAcadSci USA 2008; 105: 6415-6420.

[53] Hernandez, F, & Avila, J. Tauopathies.Mol Life Sci (2007). Bartosik-Psujek H, Stelmasiak Z. The CSF levels of total-tau and phosphotau in patients with relapsing-remitting multiple sclerosis. J Neural Trans 2006;113:339-45., 64, 2219-33.

[54] Hu, C R, Van Der Heijden, M, Wang, J, Van Der Greef, T, & Hankemeier, G. Xu . (2009). Analytical strategies in lipidomics and applications in disease biomarker discovery.J. Chromatogr. B Analyt.Technol. Biomed. Life Sci. , 877, 2836-2846.

[55] Hu, Y. Y, He, S. S, Wang, X, et al. Levels of nonphosphorylated and phosphorylated tau in cerebrospinal fluid of Alzheimer's disease patients: an ultrasensitive bienzyme-substrate-recycle enzyme-linked immunosorbent assay. Am J Pathol (2002). , 160, 1269-78.

[56] Hulstaert, F, Blennow, K, Ivanoiu, A, Schoonderwaldt, HC, Riemenschneider, M, & De Deyn, . (1999) Improved discrimination of AD patients using beta-amyloid (1-42) and tau levels in CSF. Neurology 52: 1555-1562.

[57] Hye, A, Lynham, S, Thambisetty, M, Causevic, M, Campbell, J, Byers, H. L, Hooper, C, Rijsdijk, F, Tabrizi, S. J, Banner, S, et al. (2006). Proteome-based plasma biomarkers for Alzheimer's disease.Brain ., 129, 3042-3050.

[58] Hyman, B. T, & Trojanowski, J. Q. Consensus recommendations for the postmortem diagnosis of Alzheimer disease from the National Institute on Aging and the Reagan InstituteWorking Group on diagnostic criteria for the neuropathological assessment of Alzheimer disease. J NeuropatholExpNeurol.(1997). , 56, 1095-1097.

[59] Iqbal, K, Alonso, A. C, Gong, C. X, Khatoon, S, Pei, J. J, Wang, J. Z, & Grundke-iqbal, I. (1998). Mechanisms of neurofibrillary degeneration and the formation of neurofibrillary tangles. J Neural Transm [Suppl] , 53, 169-180.

[60] Iqbal, K, Liu, F, Gong, C-X, Alonso, A. D, & Grundke-iqbal, I. Mechanisms of tauinducedneurodegeneration. ActaNeuopathol (2010). , 118, 53-69.

[61] Iqbal, K, Grundke-iqbal, I, Zaidi, T, Merz, P. A, Wen, G. Y, & Shaikh, S. S. (1986). Defetive brain microtubule assembly in Alzheimer's diseases.. Lancet , 2, 421-426.

[62] Ishiguro, K, Ohno, H, Arai, H, et al. Phosphorylated tau in human cerebrospinal fluid is a diagnostic marker for Alzheimer's disease. Neurosci Lett (1999). , 270, 91-94.

[63] Itoh, N, Arai, H, Urakami, K, et al. Large-scale, multicenter study of cerebrospinal fluid tau protein phosphorylated at serine 199 for the antemortem diagnosis of Alzheimer's disease. Ann Neurol (2001). , 50, 150-56.

[64] Choi, J, Malakowsky, C. A, Talent, J. M, Conrad, C. C, & Gracy, R. W. Identification of oxidized plasma proteins in Alzheimer's disease, Biochem. Biophys. Res. Commun.(2002). , 293(2002), 1566-1570.

[65] Choi, J, Forster, M. J, Mcdonald, S. R, Weintraub, S. T, Carroll, C. A, & Gracy, R. W. Proteomic identification of specific oxidized proteins in ApoE-knockout mice: relevance to Alzheimer's disease, Free Radic. Biol. Med. (2004)., 36(2004), 1155-1162.

[66] Raber, J, Huang, Y, & Ashford, J. W. ApoE genotype accounts for the vast majority of AD risk and AD pathology, Neurobiol. Aging (2004)., 25(2004), 641-650.

[67] Jack Jr CRWiste HJ, Vemuri P, Weigand SD, Senjem ML, Zeng G, et al. Brain beta-amyloid measures and magnetic resonance imaging atrophy both predict time-to-progression from mild cognitive impairment to Alzheimer's disease. Brain (2010)., 133, 3336-48.

[68] Blennow, K, Hampel, H, Weiner, M, & Zetterberg, H. Cerebrospinal fluid and plasma biomarkers in Alzheimer disease, Nat. Rev. Neurol. (2010)., 6(2010), 131-144.

[69] Kahle, P. J, Jakowec, M, Teipel, S. J, et al. Combined assessment of tau and neuronal thread protein in Alzheimer's disease CSF. Neurology (2000)., 54, 1498-504.

[70] Kanai, M, Matsubara, E, Isoe, K, et al. Longitudinal study of cerebrospinal fluid levels of tau, A beta1-40, and A beta1-42(43) in Alzheimer's disease: a study in Japan. Ann Neurol (1998)., 44, 17-26.

[71] Kanai, M, Matsubara, E, Isoe, K, Urakami, K, Nakashima, K, Arai, H, Sasaki, H, Abe, K, & Iwatsubo, . , (1998) Longitudinal study of cerebrospinal fluid levels of tau, A-beta1-40,and A-beta1-42(43) in Alzheimer's disease: a study in Japan. Ann Neurol 44: 17-26.

[72] Kapaki, E K. K, Paraskevas, G. P, Michalopoulou, M, & Patsouris, E. (2001). Highly increased CSFtau protein and decreased beta-amyloid (1-42) in sporadic CJD: a discrimination from Alzheimer's disease? J NeurolNeurosurg Psychiatry , 71, 401-403.

[73] Kauwe JSKWang J, Mayo K, Morris JC, Anne M, Fagan AM, et al. Alzheimer's disease risk variants show association with cerebrospinal fluid amyloid beta. Neurogenetics (2009)., 10, 13-7.

[74] Knopman, D. S, Dekosky, S. T, Cummings, J. L, Chui, H, Corey-bloom, J, Relkin, N, Small, G. W, Miller, B, & Stevens, J. C. (2001). Practice parameter: diagnosis of dementia (an evidence-based review)- Report of the Quality Standards Subcommittee of the American Academy of Neurology. Neurology , 56(9), 1143-1153.

[75] Kochanek, P. M, Berger, R. P, Bayir, H, Wagner, A. K, Jenkins, L. W, & Clark, R. S. (2008). Biomarkers of primary and evolving damage in traumatic and ischemic brain injury: diagnosis, prognosis, probing mechanisms, and therapeutic decision making. Curr.Opin.Crit. Care ., 14, 135-141.

[76] Kohnken, R, Buerger, K, Zinkowski, R, et al. Detection of tau phosphorylated at threonine 231 in cerebrospinal fluid of Alzheimer's disease patients. Neurosci Lett (2000)., 287, 187-90.

[77] Kosik, K. S, Duffy, L. K, Dowling, M. M, Abraham, C, Mccluskey, A, & Selkoe, D. J. (1984). Microtubule-associated protein 2: monoclonal antibodies demonstrate the selective incorporation of certain epitopes into Alzheimer neurofibrillary tangles.ProcNatlAcad:, 7941-7945.

[78] Kurz, A, Riemenschneider, M, Buch, K, Willoch, F, Bartenstein, P, Muller, U, & Gud-er, W. (1998). Tau protein in cerebrospinal fluid is significantly increased at the earliest clinical stage of Alzheimer disease. Alzheimer Dis AssocDisord , 12, 372-377.

[79] Lee, R. C, & Feinbaum, R. L. Ambros V: The C. elegansheterochronic gene lin-4 encodes small RNAs with antisense complementarity to lin-14. Cell (1993)., 75, 843-854.

[80] Lewczuk, P, Esselmann, H, Bibl, M, Beck, G, Maler, J. M, Otto, M, et al. Tau protein phosphorylated at threonine 181 in CSF as a neurochemical biomarker in Alzheimer's disease. Original data and review of the literature.JMolNeurosci (2004). , 23, 115-22.

[81] Lukiw, W. J, & Zhao, Y. Cui JG: An NF-kB-sensitive micro RNA-146a-mediated inflammatory circuit in Alzheimer disease and in stressed human brain cells. J BiolChem (2008)., 283, 31315-31322.

[82] Lukiw WJ: Micro-RNA speciation in fetaladult and Alzheimer's disease hippocampus.Neuroreport (2007)., 18, 297-300.

[83] Ikeda, M, Sato, I, Yuasa, T, Miyatake, T, & Murota, S. Nitrite, nitrate and cGMP in the cerebrospinal fluid in degenerative neurologic diseases, J. Neural Transm. Gen. Sect. (1995)., 100(1995), 263-267.

[84] Korolainen, M. A, & Pirttila, T. Cerebrospinal fluid, serum and plasma protein oxidation in Alzheimer's disease, Acta Neurol. Scand. (2009)., 119(2009), 32-38.

[85] Korolainen, M. A, Nyman, T. A, Aittokallio, T, & Pirttila, T. An update on clinical proteomics in Alzheimer's research, J. Neurochem. (2010)., 112(2010), 1386-1414.

[86] Kuiper, M. A, Visser, J. J, Bergmans, P. L, Scheltens, P, & Wolters, E. C. Decreased cerebrospinal fluid nitrate levels in Parkinson's disease, Alzheimer's disease and multiple system atrophy patients, J. Neurol. Sci. (1994)., 121(1994), 46-49.

[87] Lovell, M. A, Ehmann, W. D, Butler, S. M, & Markesbery, W. R. Elevated thiobarbituric acid-reactive substances and antioxidant enzyme activity in the brain in Alzheimer's disease, Neurology (1995)., 45(1995), 1594-1601.

[88] Prasad, M. R, Lovell, M. A, Yatin, M, Dhillon, H, & Markesbery, W. R. Regional membrane phospholipid alterations in Alzheimer's disease, Neurochem. Res. (1998)., 23(1998), 81-88.

[89] Aksenov, M. Y, Aksenova, M. V, Butterfield, D. A, Geddes, J. W, & Markesbery, W. R. Protein oxidation in the brain in Alzheimer's disease, Neuroscience (2001). , 103(2001), 373-383.

[90] Maarouf, C. L, Andacht, T. M, Kokjohn, T. A, Castan, o E. M, Sue, L. I, Beach, T. G, et al. Proteomic analysis of Alzheimer's disease cerebrospinal fluid from neuropathologically diagnosed subjects.Curr Alzheimer Res (2009). , 6, 399-406.

[91] Makeyev, E. V. Maniatis T: Multilevel regulation of gene expression by microRNAs. Science (2008). Gao FB: Posttranscriptional control of neuronal development by microRNA networks. Nat Med 2007; 13: 1359-1362., 319, 1789-1790.

[92] Maruyama, M, Arai, H, Sugita, M, Tanji, H, Higuchi, M, Okamura, N, Matsui, T, Higuchi, S, Matsushita, S, Yoshida, H, & Sasaki, H. (2001). Cerebrospinal fluid amyloid beta(1-42) levelsin the mild cognitive impairment stage of Alzheimer's disease. ExpNeurol , 172, 433-436.

[93] Mattsson, N, Zetterberg, H, Hansson, O, Andreasen, N, Parnetti, L, Jonsson, M, et al. CSF biomarkers and incipient Alzheimer disease in patients with mild cognitive impairment. J Am Med Assoc (2009). , 302, 385-93.

[94] Mazanetz, M. P, & Fischer, P. M. Untangling tau hyperphosphorylation in drug design for neurodegenerative diseases. Nat Rev Drug Discov (2007). , 6, 464-79.

[95] Mckhann, G, Drachman, D, Folstein, M, Katzman, R, Price, D, & Stadlan, E. M. (1984). Clinical diagnosis of Alzheimer's disease: report of the NINCDS-ADRDA Work Group under the auspices of the Department of Health and Human Services Task Force on Alzheimer's disease. Neurology , 34, 939-944.

[96] Mihaescu, R, Detmar, S. B, Cornel, M. C, Van Der Flier, W. M, Heutink, P, Hol, E. M, et al. Translational research in genomics of Alzheimer's disease: a review of current practice and future perspectives. J Alzheimer Dis (2010). , 20, 967-80.

[97] Miller, G. Alzheimer's biomarker initiative hits its stride. Science (2009). , 326, 386-9.

[98] Ahmed, N, Ahmed, U, Thornalley, P. J, Hager, K, Fleischer, G, & Munch, G. Protein glycation, oxidation and nitration adduct residues and free adducts of cerebrospinal fluid in Alzheimer's disease and link to cognitive impairment, J. Neurochem.(2005). , 92(2005), 255-263.

[99] Nieto, A. Montejo de Garcini, E., and Avila, J. ((1989). Altered levels of microtubule-proteins in brains of Alzheimer's disease patients.ActaNeuropathol., 78, 47-51.

[100] Nishimura, T, Takeda, M, Nakamura, Y, et al. Basic and clinical studies on the measurement of tau protein in cerebrospinal fluid as a biological marker for Alzheimer's disease and related disorders: multicenter study in Japan. Methods Find Exp Clin Pharmacol (1998). , 20, 227-35.

[101] Okamura, N, Arai, H, Higuchi, M, Tashiro, M, Matsui, T, Itoh, M, Iwatsubo, T, Tomita, T, & Sasaki, H. (1999). Cerebrospinal fluid levels of amyloid beta-peptide 1-42, but not tau have positive correlation with brain glucose metabolism in humans. NeurosciLett , 273, 203-207.

[102] Olson, L, & Humpel, C. Growth factors and cytokines/chemokines as surrogate biomarkers in cerebrospinal fluid and blood for diagnosing Alzheimer's disease and mild cognitive impairment. ExpGerentol (2010). , 45, 41-6.

[103] Otto, M, Esselmann, H, Schulz-Shaeffer, W, Neumann, M, Schroter, A, Ratzka, P, Cepek, L, & Zerr, . (2000) Decreased beta-amyloid 1-42 in cerebrospinal fluid of patients with Creutzfeldt-Jakob disease. Neurology 54: 1099-1102

[104] Papassotiropoulos, A, Fountoulakis, M, Dunckley, T, & Stephan, D. A. Reiman EM Genetics, transcriptomics, and proteomics of Alzheimer's disease. J Clin Psychiatry (2006). , 67, 652-70.

[105] Parnetti, L, Lanari, A, Amici, S, Gallai, V, Vanmechelen, E, & Hulstaert, F. CSF phosphorylated tau is a possible marker for discriminating Alzheimer's disease from dementia with Lewy bodies. Phospho-Tau International Study Group. Neurol Sci (2001). , 22, 77-78.

[106] Sultana, R, Perluigi, M, & Butterfield, D. A. Protein oxidation and lipid peroxidation in brain of subjects with Alzheimer's disease: insights into mechanism of neurodegeneration from redox proteomics, Antioxid. Redox Signal. (2006). , 8(2006), 2021-2037.

[107] Mark, R. J, Fuson, K. S, & May, P. C. Characterization of 8-epiprostaglandin F2alpha as a marker of amyloid beta-peptide-induced oxidative damage, J. Neurochem. (1999). , 72(1999), 1146-1153.

[108] Nitsch, R. M, Blusztajn, J. K, Pittas, A. G, Slack, B. E, Growdon, J. H, & Wurtman, R. J. Evidence for a membrane defect in Alzheimer disease brain, Proc. Natl. Acad. Sci. U.S. A. (1992). , 89(1992), 1671-1675.

[109] Ray, S, Britschgi, M, Herbert, C, Takeda-uchimura, Y, Boxer, A, Blennow, K, Friedman, L. F, Galasko, D. R, Jutel, M, Karydas, A, Kaye, J. A, Leszek, J, Miller, B. L, Minthon, L, Quinn, J. F, Rabinovici, G. D, & Robinson, W. H. Classification and prediction of clinical Alzheimer's diagnosis based on plasma signaling proteins. Nat Med (2007). , 13, 1359-1362.

[110] Reddy, M. M, Wilson, R, Wilson, J, Connell, S, Gocke, A, Hynan, L, et al. Identification of candidate IgG biomarkers for Alzheimer's disease via combinatorial library screening. Cell (2011). , 144, 132-42.

[111] Riemenschneider, M, Buch, K, Schmolke, M, Kurz, A, & Guder, . (1997) Diagnosis of Alzheimer's disease with cerebrospinal fluid tau protein and aspartate aminotransferase. Lancet 350: 784.

[112] Riemenschneider, M, Buch, K, Schmolke, M, Kurz, A, & Guder, W. G. Cerebrospinal protein tau is elevated in early Alzheimer's disease. Neurosci Lett (1996). , 212, 209-11.

[113] Riemenschneider, M, Wagenpfeil, S, Diehl, J, et al. Tau and Abeta42 protein in CSF of patients with frontotemporal degeneration. Neurology (2002). , 58, 1622-28.

[114] Rosenson, R. S. (2010). New technologies personalize diagnostics and therapeutics. Curr.Atheroscler. Rep. , 12, 184-186.

[115] Ross, C. A, & Poirier, M. A. (2004). Protein aggregation and neurodegenerative disease.Nat. Med. 10 (Suppl.): , 10-17.

[116] Rudrabhatla, P, Grant, P, Jaffe, H, & Strong, M. J. Pant HCQuantitativephosphoproteomic analysis of neuronal intermediate filament proteins (NF-M/H) in Alzheimer's disease by iTRAQ.FASEB J. (2010). , 2010(11), 4396-407.

[117] Rudrabhatla, P, & Pant, H. C. Phosphorylation-specific peptidyl-prolyl isomerization of neuronal cytoskeletal proteins by Pin1: implications for therapeutics in neurodegeneration.JAlzheimers Dis. (2010). , 19(2), 389-403.

[118] Newman, S. F, Sultana, R, Perluigi, M, Coccia, R, Cai, J, Pierce, W. M, Klein, J. B, Turner, D. M, & Butterfield, D. A. An increase in S-glutathionylated proteins in the Alzheimer'sdisease inferior parietal lobule, a proteomics approach, J. Neurosci. Res. (2007). , 85(2007), 1506-1514.

[119] Herukka, S. K, Helisalmi, S, Hallikainen, M, Tervo, S, Soininen, H, & Pirttila, T. CSF Abeta42, Tau and phosphorylated Tau, APOE epsilon4 allele and MCI type in progressive MCI, Neurobiol. Aging (2007). , 28(2007), 507-514.

[120] Samuels, S. C S. J, Marin, D. B, Peskind, E. R, Younki, S. G, Greenberg, D. A, Schnur, E, Santoro, J, & Davis, K. L. (1999). CSF beta-amyloid, cognition, and APOE genotype in Alzheimer's disease.Neurology , 52, 547-551.

[121] Sanchez, C, Diaz-nido, J, & Avila, J. (2000). Phosphorylation of microtubule-associated protein 2 (MAP2) and its relevance for the regulation of the neuronal cytoskeleton function.ProgNeurobiol.;, 61(2), 133-68.

[122] Sato, Y, Nakamura, T, Aoshima, K, & Oda, Y. (2010). Quantitative and wide-ranging profi ling of phospholipids in human plasma by two-dimensional liquid hromatography/mass spectrometry. Anal. Chem. , 82, 9858-9864.

[123] Sato, Y, Suzuki, I, Nakamura, T, Bernier, F, Aoshima, K, & Oda, Y. Identification of a new plasma biomarker of Alzheimer's disease using metabolomics technology.J Lipid Res. (2012). Mar;, 53(3), 567-76.

[124] Schönknecht, P, Pantel, J, Hunt, A, et al. Levels of total tau and tau protein phosphorylated at threonine 181 in patients with incipient and manifest Alzheimer's disease. Neurosci Lett (2003). , 339, 172-74.

[125] Schonrock, N, Ke, Y. D, Humphreys, D, Staufenbiel, M, Ittner, L. M, & Preiss, T. Götz J: Neuronal microRNA deregulation in response to Alzheimer's disease amyloid-beta. PLoS One (2010). e11070.

[126] Sethi, P. Lukiw WJ: Micro-RNA abundance and stability in human brain: specific alterations in Alzheimer's disease temporal lobe neocortex. NeurosciLett (2009). , 459, 100-104.

[127] Shaw, L. M, Vanderstichele, H, Knapik-czajka, M, Clark, C. M, Aisen, P. S, Petersen, R. C, et al. Cerebrospinal fluid biomarker signature in Alzheimer's disease neuroimaging initiative studies. Ann Neurol (2009). , 65, 403-13.

[128] Shoji, M, Matsubara, E, Kanai, M, et al. Combination assay of CSF tau, A beta 1-40 and A beta 1-42(43) as a biochemical marker of Alzheimer's disease. J Neurol Sci (1998). , 158, 134-40.

[129] Shoji, M, Matsubara, E, Murakami, T, et al. Cerebrospinal fluid tau in dementia disorders: a large scale multicenter study by a Japanese study group. Neurobiol Aging (2002). , 23, 363-70.

[130] Sjögren, M, Davidsson, P, Gottfries, J, et al. The cerebrospinal fluid levels of tau, growth-associated protein-43 and soluble amyloid precursor protein correlate in Alzheimer's disease, reflecting a common pathophysiological process. Dement Geriatr Cogn Disord (2001). , 12, 257-64.

[131] Sjogren, M, Davidsson, P, Tullberg, M, Minthon, L, Wallin, A, Wikkelso, C, & Granerus, . (2001b) Both total and phosphorylated tau are increased in Alzheimer's disease. J NeurolNeurosurg Psychiatry 70: 624-630.

[132] Sjögren, M, Davidsson, P, Wallin, A, et al. Decreased CSF-amyloid42 in Alzheimer's disease and amyotrophic lateral sclerosis may reflect mismetabolism of-amyloid induced by separate mechanisms. Dementia Geriatr Cogn Disord (2002). , 13, 112-18.

[133] Sjogren, M, Minthon, L, Davidsson, P, Granerus, A. K, Clarberg, A, Vanderstichele, H, Vanmechelen, E, Wallin, A, & Blennow, K. (2000a). CSF levels of tau, beta-amyloid(1-42) and GAP-43 in frontotemporal dementia, other types of dementia and normal aging. J Neural Transm , 107, 563-579.

[134] Steinberg, D. (2005). Thematic review series: the pathogenesis of atherosclerosis.An interpretive history of the cholesterol controversy: part II: the early evidence linking hypercholesterolemia to coronary disease in humans. J. Lipid Res. , 46, 179-190.

[135] Strittmatter, W. J, Saunders, A. M, Schmechel, D, Pericak-vance, M, Enghild, J, Salvesen, G. S, & Roses, A. D. (1993). Apolipoprotein E: high-avidity binding to beta-amyloid and increased frequency of type 4 allele in late-onset familial Alzheimer disease. Proc. Natl.Acad. Sci. USA ., 90, 1977-1981.

[136] Sunderland, T, Linker, G, Mirza, N, Putnam, K. T, Friedman, D. L, Kimmel, L. H, Bergeson, J, Manetti, G. J, Zimmermann, M, Tang, B, Bartko, J. J, & Cohen, R. M. and increased Tau levels in cerebrospinal fluid of patients with Alzheimer disease. JAMA , 289(16), 2094-2103.

[137] Swardfager, W, Lanctot, K, Rothenburg, L, Wong, A, Cappell, J, & Hermann, N. A met-analysis of cytokines in Alzheimer's disease.Biol Psychiatry (2010). , 68, 930-41.

[138] Montine, T. J, Neely, M. D, Quinn, J. F, Beal, M. F, Markesbery, W. R, Roberts, L. J, & Morrow, J. D. Lipid peroxidation in aging brain and Alzheimer's disease, Free Radic.Biol. Med. (2002). , 33(2002), 620-626.

[139] Stief, T. W, Marx, R, & Heimburger, N. Oxidized fibrin(ogen) derivatives enhance the activity of tissue type plasminogen activator, Thromb. Res. (1989). , 56(1989), 221-228.

[140] Takahashi, H, Hirokawa, K, Ando, S, & Obata, K. (1991). Immunohistological study on brains of Alzheimer's disease using antibodies to fetal antigens, C-series gangliosides and microtubule-associated protein 5.ActaNeuropathol., 81, 626-631.

[141] Tapiola, T, Lehtovirta, M, Ramberg, J, et al. CSF tau is related to apolipoprotein E genotype in early Alzheimer's disease. Neurology (1998). , 50, 169-74.

[142] Tapiola, T, Pirttil, a T, Mehta, P. D, Alafuzoff, I, Lehtovirta, M, & Soininen, H. (2000). Relationship between apoE genotype and CSF beta-amyloid (1-42) and tau in patients with probable and definite Alzheimer's disease. Neurobiol Aging , 21, 735-740.

[143] Thambisetty, M, Simmons, A, Velayudhan, L, Hye, A, Campbell, J, Zhang, Y, et al. Association of plasma clusterin concentration with severity, pathology, and progression in Alzheimer disease. Arch Gen Psychiatry (2010). , 67, 739-48.

[144] The Ronald and Nancy Reagan Research Institute of the Alzheimer's Association and the National Institute on Aging Working Group ((1998). Consensus report of the Working Group on: Molecular and Biochemical Markers of Alzheimer's Disease-Neurobiol Aging , 19, 109-116.

[145] Vandermeeren, M, Mercken, M, Vanmechelen, E, & Six, J. van de Voorde A, Martin JJ, Cras P. Detection of tau proteins in normal and Alzheimer's disease cerebrospinal fluid with a sensitive sandwich enzyme-linked immunosorbent assay. J Neurochem (1993). , 61, 1828-1834.

[146] Markesbery, W. R, & Lovell, M. A. Four-hydroxynonenal, a product of lipid peroxidation, is increased in the brain in Alzheimer's disease, Neurobiol. Aging (1998). , 19(1998), 33-36.

[147] Wang, W. X, Rajeev, B. W, Stromberg, A. J, Ren, N, Tang, G, Huang, Q, & Rigoutsos, I. Nelson PT:The expression of microRNA miR-107 decreases early in Alzheimer's disease and may accelerate disease progression through regulation of beta-site amyloid precursor protein-cleaving enzyme 1. J Neurosci (2008). , 28, 1213-1223.

[148] Ward, M. Biomarkers for Alzheimer's disease. Expert Rev. Mol. Diagn.(2007). , 7, 635-646.

[149] Watson, A. D. Thematic review series: systems biology approaches to metabolic and cardiovascular disorders. Lipidomics: a global approach to lipid analysis in biological systems. J. Lipid Res.(2006). , 47, 2101-2111.

[150] Wenk, M. R. The emerging fi eld of lipidomics.Nat. Rev. Drug Discov(2005). , 4, 594-610.

[151] Wilcoxen, K. M, Uehara, T, Myint, T. T, Sato, Y, & Oda, Y. Practical metabolomics in drug discovery.Expert Opinion on Drug Discovery(2010). , 5, 249-263.

[152] Zhang, J, Goodlett, D. R, Quinn, J. F, Peskind, E, Kaye, J. A, Zhou, Y, et al. Quantitative proteomics of cerebrospinal fluid from patients with Alzheimer disease. J Alzheimers Dis (2005). , 7, 125-33.

Chapter 10

Using Magnetic Resonance Imaging in the Early Detection of Alzheimer's Disease

Emily J. Mason, Manus J. Donahue and
Brandon A. Ally

Additional information is available at the end of the chapter

http://dx.doi.org/10.5772/54445

1. Introduction

Alzheimer's disease (AD) is the most common form of dementia. While many strides have been made in elucidating the underlying causes of AD, studying the disorder *in vivo* has faced several hurdles: First, the structures affected by AD lie deep within the brain where biopsy is not practical. Second, animal models do not develop AD naturally, and genetically engineered models designed to mimic AD do not fully reproduce the human phenotypes [1-3]. Third, while studies using Positron Emission Tomography (PET) have been very useful for examining plaques and metabolic changes, they involve the injection of radioactive contrast agents. Many of these materials have short half-lives and must be created on-site, making PET very expensive and difficult to be performed at non-specialized centers. Finally, studies which examine cerebrospinal fluid (CSF) require participants to undergo an invasive and sometimes painful lumbar puncture, potentially on multiple occasions [4-7]

In contrast to other techniques, Magnetic Resonance (MR) offers a non-invasive method for analyzing structural and functional brain characteristics without the need for ionizing radiation. In other words, it can be performed in longitudinal studies without significant health concerns. Multiple scans can be performed quickly in the same testing session to assess tissue response to tasks or pharmacological administration. The scans are generally 2-5 minutes each and many analyses can be done post-hoc. Conveniently, most hospitals and clinics already possess the MR scanners at field strengths of 1.5 and 3.0 Tesla (T).

Many MR techniques have been used to understand the underlying pathology in patient populations already diagnosed with AD. Because MR studies require absolute stillness for several minutes, and some functional scans require the patient to focus on performing a difficult task, performing MR work in advanced AD cases is quite challenging and as such, most studies are limited to mild and very mild cases. While these studies are typically performed at a time when pathology is irreversible, the results of this work point to changes that may be apparent before cognitive decline has become clinically apparent. For this reason, studies that examine differences between people who will eventually develop AD and people who will not develop AD provide insight into both the cause and the physiology of the disease.

It is impossible to predict with certainty who will develop AD, but there are several factors that increase the risk. These at-risk populations include individuals in the prodromal stage of AD, termed amnestic mild cognitive impairment (aMCI), and people at a genetic risk for developing AD. A diagnosis of aMCI indicates that there is more memory decline than would be expected based on the person's age and education level, however memory impairment is not interfering with daily activities. It is estimated that 10-20% of people 65 and older have aMCI, and out of those 10-15% will progress to develop AD in 3-4 years. [8,9] Because approximately 30% of people diagnosed with aMCI will remain stable or improve over time, it is important to find biomarkers that will identify those most likely to progress to AD.

This chapter will focus on the use of MR in the early detection of AD. Major advances have been made in structural imaging of both gray and white matter using proton density, T1- and T2- weighted imaging, and Diffusion Tensor Imaging (DTI). Functional imaging in AD will also be reviewed, and Blood Oxygenation Level-Dependent (BOLD) functional Magnetic Resonance Imaging (fMRI) will be broken down into its primary contributors: Cerebral Blood Flow (CBF), Cerebral Blood Volume (CBV), and the Cerebral Metabolic Rate of Oxygen ($CMRO_2$). Finally, hemodynamic fMRI contrast can be complemented using measures of neurochemistry, including measuring the balance between excitatory (glutamatergic) and inhibitory (γ-aminobutyric acid; GABAergic) neurotransmission. This can be achieved with new single-voxel chemical imaging techniques such as Magnetic Resonance Spectroscopy (MRS), or more recently using multi-voxel MRS imaging (MRSi)

2. Basics of MRI

Before reviewing the work that has been done with MR, a brief overview of the theory behind MR should be covered. MR physics can essentially be understood using principles of classical physics, however for a more comprehensive understanding the reader is directed to an excellent review by Plewes and Kucharzck [4,10]. Briefly, MR takes advantage of the behavior of a system of protons in the presence of a magnetic field and how this behavior changes based on the micro- and macroscopic environment. Magnetic strength is generally reported in units of Tesla (T), and MRI scanners have very high field strengths. In human research, 1.5T, 3T, and 7T scanners are commonly used, though 1.5T and 3T scanners predominate the clinical setting. The magnet's strength and direction is represented by the vector B0 (see Figure 1), and lies along the Z-axis (generally from foot to head).

http://dx.doi.org/10.5772/54445

Due to the large amount of water that constitutes tissue (~80-99% depending on tissue type), most MR is specifically focused on the protons on water molecules. Protons have an intrinsic spin that in nature is oriented randomly. In the presence of a magnetic field however, these spins align themselves on average parallel or antiparallel to the axis of the field (Figure 1a). The number of protons aligned parallel to the field is very slightly larger than the number of protons aligned antiparallel, and it is this difference that produces the net magnetization vector in a voxel. When a radiofrequency (RF) pulse is applied at the proper frequency (Larmor frequency), the longitudinal (z) component of the magnetization vector is tipped away from the axis of the main magnetic field, but continues to spin around the longitudinal axis or "precess" (Figure 1b). When the pulse is removed, the longitudinal component of the magnetization vector will realign itself with the field with a unique time constant that varies with the local environment.

Manipulating the timing of the RF pulses controls the magnetization and creates the desired contrast. The most fundamental timing parameters of relevance are repetition time (TR), echo time (TE), and in some cases inversion time (TI). TR is the time between consecutive acquisitions, and TE is the time from the onset of the excitation pulse that is used for preparing the signal for detection to the signal refocusing and in most cases acquisition. In an inversion recovery pulse sequence, TI refers to the time between the inversion pulse and the excitation pulse. Importantly, simply by manipulating the timing of the above parameters a range of MR contrasts can be obtained with varying sensitivity to different tissue types. A simple pulse sequence indicating RF and gradient timing is illustrated in Figure 1c.

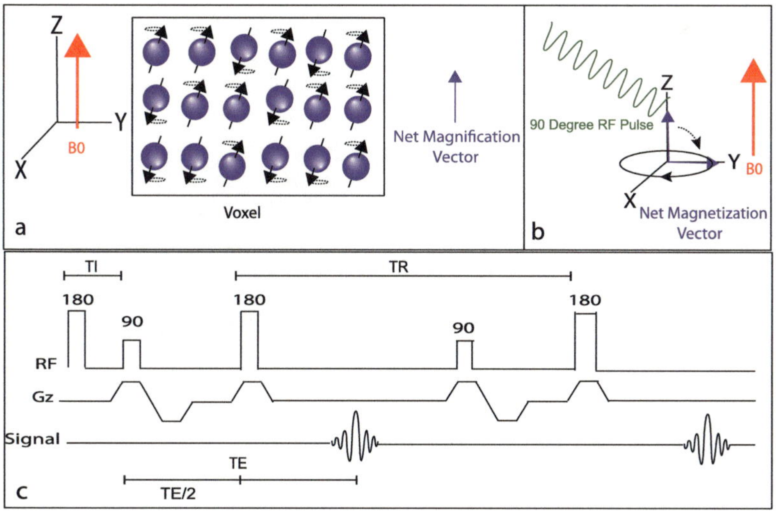

Figure 1. Physics underlying magnetic resonance. Hydrogen atoms align parallel and antiparallel to a strong magnetic field, producing a net magnification vector (a). When a radio frequency pulse is applied at the Larmor frequency, the net magnetization vector is tipped away from the main magnetic field (b). Example of a simple pulse sequence showing timing parameters of the application of radio frequency pulse (RF), the onset of gradients in the Z direction (Gz), and the timing of signal acquisition (Signal) (c).

In most cases, the detectible signal (S) that is measured in MRI is a combination of three primary factors: water proton density (C; ml tissue /100 ml water), magnetization in the longitudinal plane (M_Z) and magnetization in the transverse plane (M_{XY}):

$$S \propto C \bullet M_Z \bullet M_{XY} \tag{1}$$

The two major methods or "weighting" that are used for generating contrast are T1 and T2. T1 and T2 are independent measures and reflect different properties of the tissue of interest, with T1 governing the M_z term and T2 the M_{xy} term in Eq. 1 above. The time it takes for the magnetization to realign itself longitudinally is measured using T1 weighting (Figure 2a), and is achieved with a short TR and a short TE sequence. T1 is a constant that is unique for each tissue type and is equal to the point when 63% of longitudinal magnetization is recovered (Figure 2b). At the times selected for T1 imaging, there is a high amount of contrast between gray and white matter and therefore T1 weighted imaging is useful for viewing structural changes in the brain (Figure 2c).

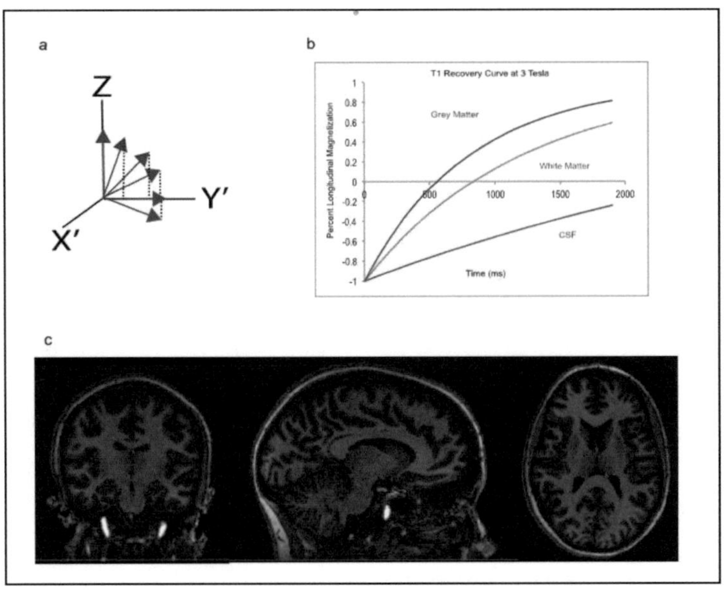

Figure 2. T1 weighted imaging. After removal of an RF pulse the magnetization vector recovers longitudinally (a). The recovery time is a constant for each tissue type based on the magnetic field strength that is applied (b). Example T1 weighted images (c).

The M_Z component of the magnetization vector is based on pulse timing as well as the T1 of tissue, and for magnetization following a pre-pulse with flip angle, α, is given by:

$$M_Z = \left(1 - \alpha e^{\frac{-TI}{T1}} + e^{\frac{-TR}{T1}}\right) \tag{2}$$

http://dx.doi.org/10.5772/54445

Note that in the absence of a prepulse (α=0), the TR determines the T1-weighting. When the RF pulse is applied, individual protons will also precess in synchrony in the transverse plane. When the pulse is removed, the protons will lose that synchrony or dephase, which results in a reduced M_{XY} (Figure 3a). This is referred to as T2 decay. Like T1, the T2 time constant is unique for each tissue (Figure 3b). Unlike T1, T2 weighting is achieved with a long TE and long TR.

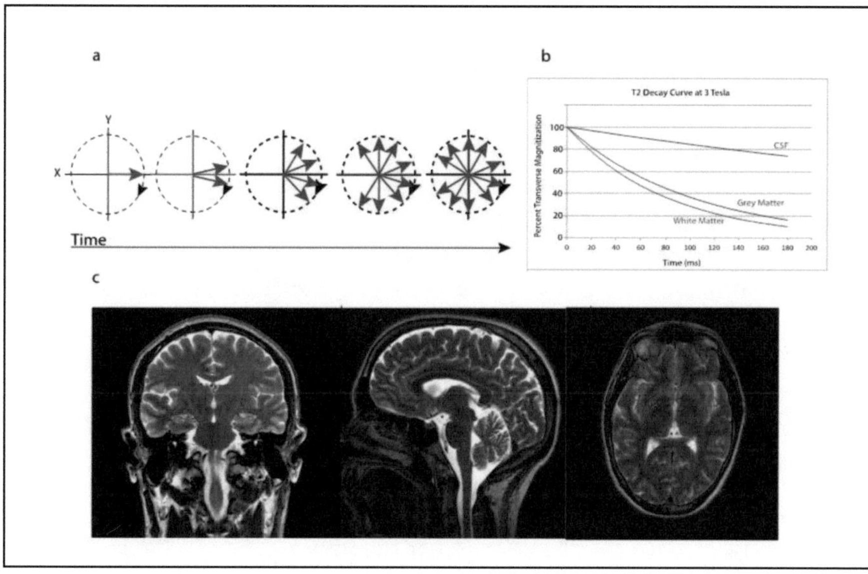

Figure 3. T2 weighted imaging. Protons lose synchrony after removal of an RF pulse (a). The amount of time it takes for protons to lose synchrony is a constant that is unique to each tissue type (b). Example of T2 weighted images (c).

The M_{XY} component of MRI is based on pulse timing as well as the T2 constant of the tissue area, and can be written:

$$M_{XY} = e^{-TE/T2} \tag{3}$$

The three equations can be combined to form one overall equation for the MR signal that takes into account both the T1 and the T2 properties of the tissue:

$$S \propto C \bullet \left(1 - \alpha e^{\frac{-TI}{T1}} + e^{\frac{-TR}{T1}}\right) \bullet e^{-TE/T2} \tag{4}$$

T1 and T2 components are each present whenever a proton is flipped out of alignment, but by manipulating the pulse sequences one can contribute to the signal more than the other. This is referred to as weighting. If neither the T1 nor the T2 signal contributes strongly to the signal, only the C component is left. These images are referred to as proton density images.

3. Structural imaging

By far, the most established use of MR is to examine the gross anatomy of the brain. With the right specifications, MR can provide a highly detailed three-dimensional image that allows for the examination of brain structures. Weighting is used to provide contrast for the tissue of interest.

3.1. Anatomical imaging

T1 weighted imaging is used to visualize structural changes in tissue. At a field strength of 3 Tesla, T1 weighted images can be acquired in about five minutes and have a resolution of approximately 1 mm^3.

The most significant differences reported in patients are atrophy of the structures in the medial temporal lobe (MTL) which typically follow the "Braak stages" of AD progression [11]. Briefly, pathology starts in the transentorhinal region (stages I and II), moves to the limbic region (stages III and IV) and ends in isocortical regions (stages V and VI). Studies that have been done in AD patients show that hippocampal and entorhinal cortex volume change, as well as temporal lobe morphology changes are the best measures to predict change over time [12]. A higher level of regional brain atrophy has also been associated with decreased levels of Aβ-42 and increased levels of phosphorylated tau in the CSF of AD patients [12].

In patients who have been diagnosed with aMCI, changes to the parahippocampal region are already apparent. It is up for debate whether the investigation of the entire brain or just volumes of interest (VOIs) are better at predicting conversion from aMCI to AD, but in a recent meta-analysis of work using data from the Alzheimer's Disease Neuroimaging Initiative (ADNI) only four methods were able to distinguish those who would convert more accurately than random chance. None of the four were more statistically reliable than the others, but three examined VOIs (Voxel-STAND, 57% sensitivity and 78% specificity; Voxel-COMPARE, 62% sensitivity and 67% specificity; Hippo-Volume, 62% sensitivity and 69% specificity) while only one examined the entire brain (Thickness-Direct, 32% sensitivity and 91% specificity) [11,13-15]. A protocol devised by Chincarini et al. to sample several VOIs has demonstrated a method of separating converters from non-converters with a sensitivity of 71% and a specificity of 65% [16,17]. Another method for predicting conversion is examining hippocampal shape, and Costafreda et. al. were able to develop a method with 77% sensitivity and 80% specificity. [18,19].

Patients that are at-risk for AD but have no cognitive deficit are much more difficult to identify. Most studies have been done in carriers of the ApoE ε4 allele, however it is important to remember that these studies have been cross sectional, and therefore may reflect a consequence of the gene that makes carriers more susceptible to AD, but not necessarily a stage of AD itself. There have been cortical thinning signatures identified in children, adolescent, and young adult carriers of the ε4 allele. These signatures reflect reductions in dorsolateral and medial prefrontal, lateral, temporal, and parietal cortices. [20-22]. Middle-aged carriers

http://dx.doi.org/10.5772/54445

of the ε4 allele were found to have a thinning of the cortex in the entorhinal region, subiculum, and other MTL structures, although the results were stronger in those with a family history of AD than those that carried the ε4 allele alone [23,24].

The detectible changes are not limited to atrophy. There have been several studies that have discovered an increase in gray matter in young adult carriers of the ε4 ellele. Increases were found in bilateral cerebellar, occipital, and thalamic regions as well as in the fusiform and right lingual gyri [22,25]. Recent work has also suggested that changes in the basal cholinergic forebrain may be detectible decades before cognitive impairment, although this study did not take into account genetic status [26].

One of the significant weaknesses of analyzing structural changes is that the regions of interest can vary in size even across healthy individuals. Longitudinal studies are the only way to control for this variability. Secondly, the atrophy of brain regions likely occurs secondary to functional changes. The assessment of atrophy alone gives little information as to the underlying factors that led to neuronal loss.

3.2. White matter imaging

Unlike T1 weighted imaging, T2 imaging relies on the dephasing of the magnetization vector in the transverse plane. T2 weighting, specifically FLuid Attenuated Inversion Recovery (FLAIR) imaging, is used to identify White Matter Hyperintensities (WMH), which are increased in AD [27]. In contrast, diffusion tensor imaging (DTI) is able to indirectly measure the integrity of myelin sheaths surrounding white matter tracts, and Susceptibility weighted imaging (SWI) is able to distinguish tissues at a high resolution based on several properties.
FLuid Attenuated Inversion Recovery (FLAIR) and Diffusion Tensor Imaging (DTI)

If simply T2 weighted imaging was used, the signal from Cerebrospinal Fluid (CSF) is strong and therefore very bright (T2 of CSF ~ 600 ms at 3T). This makes it difficult to see subtle abnormalities in the white matter regions that partial volume with CSF. FLAIR imaging nulls the signal from CSF so that the image is focused solely on the white matter. The first RF pulse inverts the magnetization by 180 degrees. Then, when the longitudinal magnetization for the CSF = 0, an excitation pulse and readout is applied. Because T1 of CSF (~4000 ms at 3T) is much longer than that of tissue (T1~700-1200 ms at 3T), residual tissue signal remains at the time of the CSF nulling.

DTI measures fractional anisotropy (FA), a quantitative measure of the coordinated movement of water molecules. FA assumes that the stronger a white matter tract is, the more likely the water molecules will be to move along the tract rather than sideways within the myelin sheath. If the myelin sheath is damaged it becomes easier for water molecules to diffuse through it, and the FA value will decrease.

The loss of white matter integrity, either through WMH or FA differences, may correlate with increasing cognitive impairment [28,29]. In AD populations reduced FA values have been found in frontal and temporal lobes, the posterior cingulum, the corpus callosum, the superior longitudinal fasciculus and the uncinate fasciculus [30]. Both WMH and FA have been found to distinguish normal aging from aMCI[31] and predict conversion from aMCI to AD[32]. Results have differed in whether they correlate with ApoE ε4 status, with some studies saying they do not [33,34], while several others say they do [35-37]. Note that the studies that claim white matter integrity correlates with ApoE ε4 status are more recent, and their ability to detect differences are likely more sensitive. White matter integrity has also been found to correlate with a family history of AD regardless of ApoE status [38,39].

White matter hyperintensities are associated with vascular abnormalities and therefore highly correlated with cardiovascular disease. For this reason, many clinicians will exclude a diagnosis of AD if there are many apparent WMH and instead diagnose the patient with vascular dementia [32]. Many non-amnestic MCI patients tend to have a higher degree of cardiovascular disease than those with aMCI or AD, however aMCI and AD patients have increased WMH scores. For this reason, increased WMH scores in cognitively impaired individuals is likely associated with neurological disease rather than vascular disease [32].

Susceptibility Weighted Imaging (SWI)

Susceptibility weighted imaging is a method that can discriminate tissue content with a high level of resolution based on the tissue's intrinsic magnetic properties. SWI uses T2* weighting along with magnitude and phase information to enhance contrast, and when combined with traditional MR weighting it can be used to detect small differences in susceptibility between blood and tissue. It is particularly useful for detecting cerebral microbleeds because it can exploit the magnetic properties of blood since the susceptibility effects from fully oxygenated (arterial) and partially de-oxygenated (venous) blood water, and tissue, varies greatly – especially at high field strength. It can also be used to measure the iron content of a tissue.

Microbleeds are inversely correlated with performance during cognitive testing in healthy older adults, although this finding has never reached significance in an AD population [13,14]. SWI would allow for improved visualization of microbleeds so that if there is a relationship between microbleeds and susceptibility to AD pathology, it can be recognized. Techniques are being developed that semi-automatically detect cerebral microbleeds with little human interference. These would significantly reduce the processing time and standardize the quantification of microbleeds across patients and imaging centers.

In addition to microbleeds, one marker of oxidative stress is an increase in a tissue's iron content. Iron levels are highly elevated in AD patients as well as those with aMCI, and it is thought that changes in iron content may be detectible decades before the onset of the disease [16]. There is a theory that Aβ deposition may occur as a cellular response to an increased level of iron, and this is one of the underlying causes of amyloid plaque formation[40]. SWI has been shown to be a promising method to non-invasively assess iron distribution, and determine if there is a link between iron accumulation and the onset of AD pathology [18].

SWI has only been used as a technique since 2004, which makes it very new technology. Although it has not yet been used in an at-risk population, SWI studies will likely be important tools in assessing AD risk.

3.3. Future of structural imaging

There is still a lot of work to be done in structural imaging. Most clinical studies to date have used 1.5 Tesla (T) scanners, however many medical centers now have 3T scanners and there are approximately 50 7T scanners worldwide. These high-field scanners allow for increased resolution, and provide better spatial resolution for observing structural changes in the same scan time. Although 7T scanners are not yet FDA approved for clinical use, they are already being utilized in neuroimaging research, including in patients with AD.

Many atrophy measurements are made either through a trained radiologist's visual assessment, or by manually tracing the area of interest. As such, the measurement of atrophy can be subjective, and is not always reproducible across testing site. In fact, one study found that the ability of radiologists to diagnose subjects based on atrophy alone had a specificity of 85% and a sensitivity of only 27% [20]. The introduction of FDA-approved methods that can automatically detect atrophy will create standardization of the field, and decrease variability across medical centers [41].

4. Functional imaging

While structural imaging is important to assess brain atrophy, the hope is that AD pathology will be identified before neuronal death so that atrophy can be prevented. One current theory is that one of the major components leading to amyloid and tau pathologies could be vascular changes [42]. Two of the risk factors for AD are mutated forms of APP, and the ApoE ε4 isoform and both of these factors are involved in cholesterol processing. The inability of a neuron to clear amyloid plaques may be prognostic and indicate impaired blood flow as a risk factor for AD. While it is not immediately apparent how blood flow is contributing to AD, some vascular changes are being evaluated through the use of hemodynamic-based functional imaging techniques.

4.1. BOLD fMRI

Functional magnetic resonance imaging, or fMRI is a way to gain insight into the functional processes occurring in the brain. Most fMRI modalities are based on the blood oxygenation level-dependent (BOLD) effect. This is an indirect method of tracking the activation or inactivation of brain regions relative to a baseline state, and is based on the idea that an active area will need more energy and consume more glucose and oxygen and therefore more blood will need to be directed to that area. More specifically, oxygenated and deoxygenated blood water have different intrinsic magnetic properties (oxygenated blood is diamagnetic and deoxygenated blood is paramagnetic) and therefore affect the T2 and T2* relaxation times of surrounding water in blood and tissue in different ways. Deoxygenated blood has a strong enough magnetic affect (paramagnetic) that it will distort the local field and decrease the signal intensity (i.e. shorten T2) of surrounding water for that region. Oxygenated blood will not have the same effect, and therefore regions containing more oxygenated blood will have higher signal intensity (longer T2). Importantly, during functional activation the cerebral blood flow increases by a large amount (20-100%) relative to the cerebral metabolic rate of oxygen consumption (CMRO2), resulting in a relative decrease in the concentration of deoxyhemoglobin in capillaries and veins. By comparing the signal intensities of regions at baseline (Figure 4a) and during a task (Figure 4b), the regions that have an increase in capillary and venous oxygenation can be visualized.

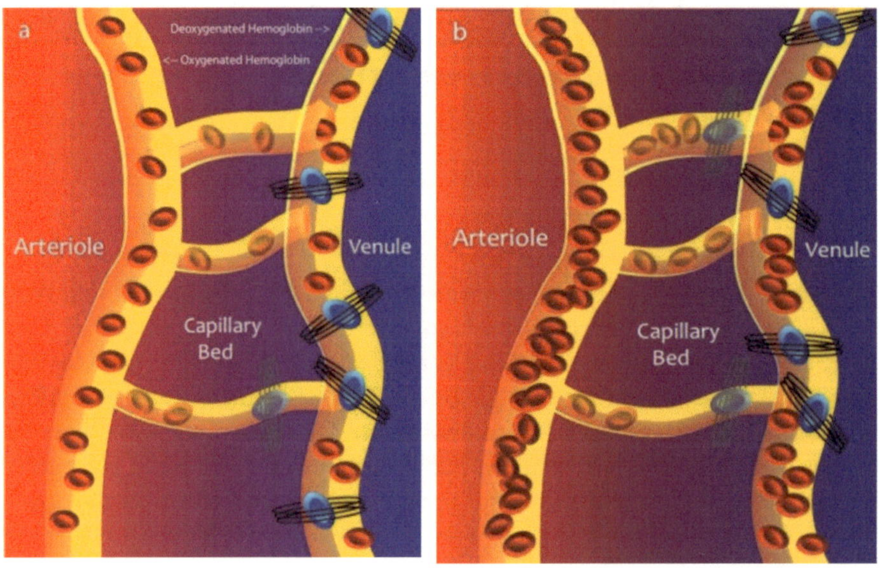

Figure 4. Blood flow at rest (a) and during activation (b)

BOLD imaging involves very fast sequences in order to visualize changes in functional activation on the timescale of the hemodynamic response. This rapid sequencing allows for a time resolution of approximately 2s. Total time required to perform a BOLD scan varies with the task being performed, but typically scans take 5-15 minutes.

There are two main types of fMRI: evoked (task-related) and spontaneous ("resting" state). Evoked fMRI is the more commonly performed test in which the same task is repeated many times with a baseline measurement taken between trials. Statistical tests (Z- and t-tests) are used to differentiate the regions activated during the task from those active at baseline. By contrast, spontaneous BOLD specifically measures synchrony of baseline signal fluctuations to determine how the brain is functionally connected.

http://dx.doi.org/10.5772/54445

Evoked BOLD fMRI

There are several established testing paradigms that have been designed to study memory. The most commonly used paradigms look specifically at either episodic or semantic memory. Episodic memories involve the recognition of autobiographical or cued information (e.g., faces, words, other visual stimuli) while semantic memory involves the recognition of a fact or information regardless of personal context (e.g., famous faces, geographical locations). Because episodic memory is highly affected by AD, many fMRI paradigms use an episodic memory task to elicit functional differences between patients and controls. While encoding a new memory, activation of the hippocampal and parahippocampal regions is decreased in mild AD patients compared to healthy controls [43]. In a block design face name paradigm, AD patients also show decreased hippocampal activation to novel stimuli compared to repeated comparisons [43].

A multitude of studies have been performed in asymptomatic carriers of ApoE ε4 with mixed results. In an extensive review of the literature by Trachtenberg et al, some claim that carriers have increased activation across brain structures while others claim the opposite[44]. Moreover, there have been reports of both increases and decreases of activation or that there is no significant effect at all of carrying the ApoE ε4 allele[44]. In each case, investigators have provided hypotheses to explain both increased and decreased activation in ApoE ε4 carriers: decreased activation can be easily explained by the fact that presymptomatic carriers are already accumulating AD pathology hallmarks before cognitive decline is experienced. These pathologies may be hindering the BOLD response in the specific areas that experience a decrease in activation, or they may be inhibiting areas that lie functionally upstream. In contrast, an increase in activation can be explained in two ways, which take into account AD pathology. For one, the accumulation of pathology may lead to the dedifferentiation of neural network such that many networks become involved in a specific process. This may in fact be a part of healthy aging [45] and could be found in young, presymptomatic carriers of ApoE ε4 because their brains are aging more rapidly. Alternatively, the brain may have a cognitive reserve that needs to "work harder" during a difficult task to perform at a normal level, and thus would have a higher amount of activation. Trachtenberg et al [44] argue that the populations tested in these studies are very young (20s and 30s) and have a great deal of time before they will begin to experience cognitive decline. He suggests instead that the possession of an ApoE ε4 allele leads to a fundamental difference in neurophysiology that could be contributing to this effect.

A growing body of evidence suggests that an episodic memory task may not be the best way to characterize memory loss because episodic memory declines as a part of healthy aging as well. Episodic memory tasks are also more difficult than semantic memory tasks, The work may therefore be experiencing a basement effect[45]. Semantic memory, in contrast, is affected very early in AD, but remains relatively untouched in the healthy aging process [45]. Most semantic memory tests involve the recognition of famous names and faces [45-47] or categorizing word lists [1,3]. These types of studies have shown an increase in activation and a decrease in deactivation the MTL regions of carriers of the ApoE ε4 allele.

Spontaneous BOLD fMRI

Resting state, or functional connectivity MRI (fcMRI) is a task-independent measurement of brain regions that fluctuate in their BOLD signal together, indicating that they are functionally connected. The Default Mode Network (DMN) is a collection of brain regions that seem to activate together while the brain is at rest, and are deactivated while the brain is engaged in a cognitive task. The DMN is composed of MTL and lateral frontal regions, particularly the posterior cingulate complex [4,6,7]. This network is altered in AD and is a potent biomarker for separating patients with AD from healthy controls [8], patients with aMCI from healthy controls [48], and genetically at-risk individuals from healthy controls [4].

Caveats to BOLD fMRI

Although BOLD fMRI is an important tool for research, there are some limitations to its clinical feasibility as a biomarker for future AD. To date, it has not successfully been used in predicting patient prognosis or trajectory. In terms of practicality, fMRI is expensive and requires extensive image processing, which will drive up the cost of any tests. It is also not completely reproducible across testing sites or days. Different equipment and software can create variables in data analysis across testing sites. Longitudinal studies can present difficulties because as they age, patients may develop comorbidities, or begin taking drugs that will interfere with the BOLD signal in a way unrelated to AD pathology. Even subtle changes can influence the BOLD signal such as recent alcohol [49] or caffeine [50] intake.

The biggest difficulty with BOLD fMRI is that it is generally not quantitative. Changes in blood oxygenation are based on three individual components: Cerebral Blood Flow (CBF), Cerebral Blood Volume (CBV), and the Cerebral Metabolic Rate of Oxygen ($CMRO_2$) [51]. Figure 5 represents the many ways that CBF, CBV, and $CMRO_2$ can contribute to the BOLD effect. It is impossible to determine which of these is contributing to a BOLD fluctuation with fMRI alone. For this reason, vascular imaging techniques are being developed that are able to quantitatively determine the physiological changes that are contributing to the BOLD signal. Techniques to quantify CBF and CBV have been validated and are gaining popularity. $CMRO_2$ methods are still in development and have not been used in an AD population and will therefore not be covered.

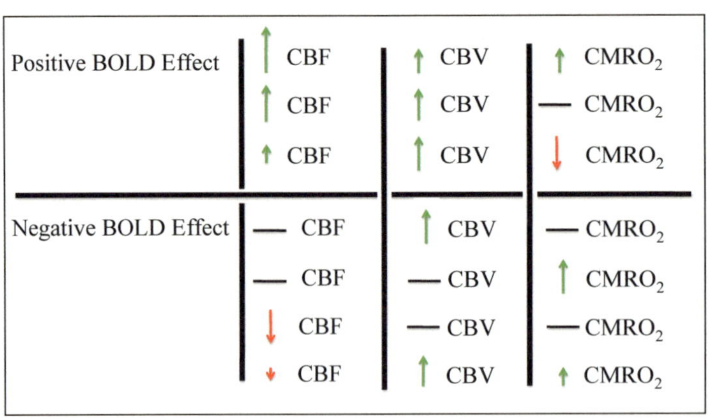

http://dx.doi.org/10.5772/54445

Figure 5. Positive and negative BOLD effects are influenced by CBF, CBV, and CMRO2 and it is not possible to distinguish which factor is contributing by only measuring BOLD.

4.2. Cerebral blood flow

Cerebral blood flow is a measurement of the rate of tissue perfusion, usually measured by the amount of blood that reaches a tissue per unit time (mL blood per 100 g tissue per minute) [52]. CBF has been quantified by Positron Emission Tomography (PET) [53,54] and Single Photon Emission Computed Tomography (SPECT) [10,55,56] but today it can also be quantified noninvasively using a technique called Arterial Spin Labeling (ASL). ASL uses a radiofrequency pulse to label blood water in an area outside of the region of interest, usually in the neck. After 1-2s, the labeled blood water flows into the imaging region and exchanges with tissue water and a tagged image can be obtained [51,57]. This image is compared with an image where the blood water is not labeled, and the difference between the two images provides a map proportional to CBF. As can be seen, ASL is analogous to tracer-based approaches such as 15O PET and Gadolinium-MRI, however the tracer is endogenous blood water as opposed to an exogenous contrast agents. Whole-brain ASL scans can be performed in less than 5 minutes with a spatial resolution of 3-5 mm.

In AD patients, deficits in CBF have been seen in the temporoparietal cortex, posterior cingulate cortex, and frontal cortex [57-59]. CBF as measured by ASL has been shown to be increased in aMCI patients but decreased pre-symptomatic carriers of ApoE ε4 [11,60]. The increase that is seen in aMCI has been attributed to compensatory mechanisms [60].

Often, changes in blood flow precede structural changes, but reduced CBF is not necessarily an indicator of vascular dysfunction. For instance, CBF alterations may be due to a lower metabolic demand, cardiac output, or blood pressure [10,61,62]. Longitudinal analysis of CBF in at-risk populations should be developed for its potential as a method for tracking disease progress or recognizing it before cognitive symptoms begin.

4.3. Cerebral blood volume

Cerebral blood volume measures the amount of blood per 100 mL brain tissue. It is an indirect measurement of the vascularization of brain regions, and is less dependent on the subject's respiration than CBF[11,15,63,64]. There are currently two major techniques that measure CBV: Dynamic Susceptibility Contrast MRI (DSC-MRI) and Vascular Space Occupancy MRI (VASO). DSC-MRI involves the injection of gadolinium as a contrast agent, and is the best validated measure. Unfortunately, the injection of gadolinium is dose-restricted because of its toxic effect on kidneys which limits its potential for longitudinal studies and older patient populations [17,65]. VASO is a completely non-invasive method of measuring CBV changes and has been gaining popularity in recent years. Unlike DSC-MRI, VASO uses endogenous blood water as a contrast agent. VASO can be performed by measuring the tissue signal with and without blood water nulled, and subtracting one image from the other. Although VASO is correlated with DSC-MRI there are some minor variations in the two measurements, suggesting that the underlying physiology may be different [19,63].

VASO has been applied to a mixed group of patients with aMCI and AD and found that there are CBV reductions in the frontal and parietal lobes. These reductions were most striking in white matter which suggests that any vascular component of AD is especially damaging to white matter compared to gray matter [21,22,61]. In the future, longitudinal studies should be performed in carriers of ApoE ε4 to determine if these white matter vascular deficiencies can be recognized at a young age.

5. Chemical imaging

Structural and functional imaging are important for assessing the damage caused by AD, but for designing therapeutics the ability to view changes at the macromolecular level would be highly beneficial. New techniques are being developed that can do just that. Magnetic Resonance Spectroscopy (MRS) can be done in a single voxel or across multiple voxels (MRS imaging, MRSi) to assess macromolecular concentration. Both are new techniques that are still being optimized, but will be extremely useful in understanding AD.

5.1. Magnetic resonance spectroscopy

MR imaging primarily measures signal from water protons, but in MR spectroscopy protons of various metabolites can be assessed at one time. Quantification is achieved by exciting a single voxel with a combination of RF pulses, and obtaining a free induction decay (FID) spectrum. When this spectrum is Fourier transformed, metabolites can be visualized due to their variability in chemical shift (Figure 6). Because the chemical shift of a single metabolite is constant, it will always peak at the same frequency (measured in parts per million, ppm). By calculating the area under the peak, the concentration of a metabolite relative to an internal standard can be obtained.

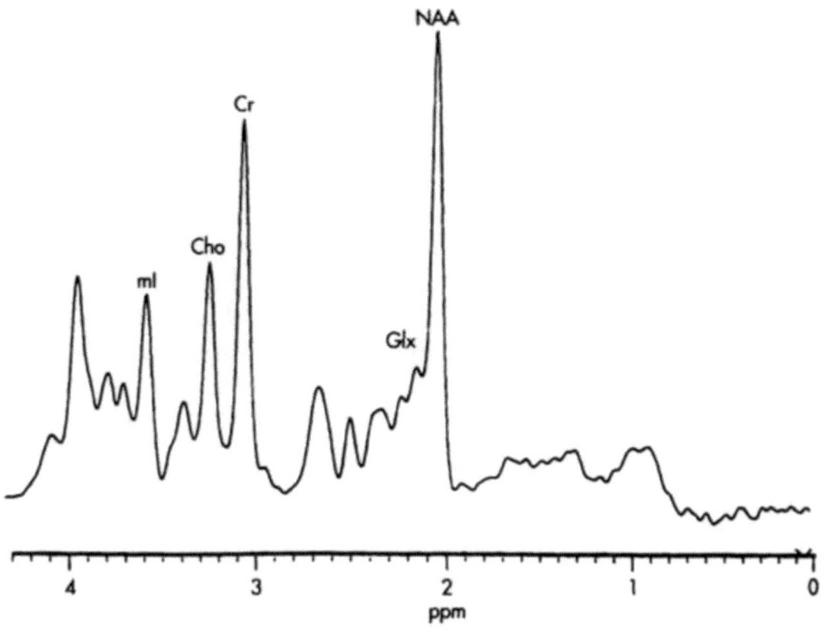

Figure 6. Example of chemical shift spectrum from a normal brain (from the University of Missouri-Kansas City Radiology Resident Resource Webpage

The most common macromolecules studied in neuroimaging are creatine (Cr) which is usually unaffected by disease and can act as an internal standard, *N*-acetyl-aspartate (NAA), a marker for neuronal health, myo-inositol (mI), a marker of gliosis [32,66], and choline (Cho). In AD, NAA is typically decreased in AD and mI is typically increased so NAA/Cr, mI/Cr and NAA/mI ratios are good markers of the disease with the ratio of NAA to mI being the strongest. The mI concentration has been found to be elevated in aMCI [33,34,67]. There is a trend that NAA is decreased in aMCI, however the effect is much more mild if it exists [35-37,68]. Glutamate (Glu) is the primary excitatory neurotransmitter, and is significantly reduced in AD [69] Gamma-amino butyric acid (GABA) is an inhibitory neurotransmitter, and its concentration may be decreased in AD [70]. It is possible to use MRS to estimate relative concentrations of both Glu and GABA *in vivo*, but due to their low concentrations compared to NAA and other metabolites, and the fact that signal from these metabolites is very close in frequency space to other metabolites of larger concentration, it is more difficult to identify them without suppressing or "editing" other signals. One of the common methods used to quantify GABA is a PRESS or MEGA-PRESS sequence which suppresses or edits signals from water, creatine, and other nearby metabolites so that the characteristic GABA peaks can be identified. For more information on the MEGA-PRESS sequence, see Waddell 2007 [71].

The importance of MRS research is clear, but there are some difficulties associated with it. To begin with, the scans take a long time to complete—more than ten minutes in some cases—and because the measurements are taken in a single voxel the subject must stay absolutely still throughout the scan. This is very difficult for young healthy subjects, and may be nearly impossible in older, demented subjects. Common sedation drugs such as propofol will change the levels of brain metabolites and should be avoided[72]. In premenopausal women GABA levels also vary depending on the stage of the menstrual cycle, and may introduce variability[73].

Typically, spectroscopy is done in the posterior cingulate or medial temporal cortices, but these are only affected by AD in late stages of the disease. It would be more helpful to study the smaller limbic areas that are affected sooner, but the voxel sizes typically used in spectroscopy are larger than many of these areas [66]. Falini et al developed a technique to perform spectroscopy across the entire brain and found that NAA levels are reduced in those with AD, however whole-brain spectroscopy is a non-specific marker [41,74]. These limitations will be overcome with higher field strength, advances in shimming algorithms, and improvements to computerized registration techniques [42,68].

5.2. Magnetic Resonance Spectroscopy imaging (MRSi)

MRSi is a technique that uses spectroscopy but applies it to voxels across the entire brain. The concentration of the chemical of interest corresponds to the brightness or color of the voxel in the image produced. It can achieve high spatial resolution (up to 0.25 cm^3), and when optimized can produce a wealth of information [44,75]. This technique has largely been developed for breast cancer imaging, and can identify chemical "hot spots" that are of use when categorizing a tumor. It has great potential as a technique for understanding AD.

6. Concluding remarks

There is still a long way to go before AD can be fully understood and treated. With magnetic resonance technologies, it is possible to observe changes before cognitive decline begins. A lot of work has been done with structural imaging of gray and white matter, and changes are detectible in ApoE ε4 carriers decades before the onset of symptoms. More longitudinal studies need to be performed to determine which of these changes will specifically lead to AD. Functional studies offer a window of the changes that occur before neuronal atrophy, but the specific vascular causes behind the BOLD effect need to be further studied. Finally, chemical imaging can provide a glimpse of the changes occurring at the molecular level, and by further developing and standardizing these measures there is much that can be learned.

Author details

Emily J. Mason[1*], Manus J. Donahue[2] and Brandon A. Ally[1]

*Address all correspondence to: emily.mason.1@vanderbilt.edu

http://dx.doi.org/10.5772/54445

1 Department of Neurology, Vanderbilt University, Nashville, TN, USA

2 Department of Radiology, Vanderbilt University, Nashville, TN, USA

References

[1] Lind J, Persson J, Ingvar M, Larsson A, Cruts M, Van Broeckhoven C, et al. Reduced functional brain activity response in cognitively intact apolipoprotein E epsilon4 carriers. Brain. 2006 May;129(Pt 5):1240–8.

[2] Wilcock DM. The usefulness and challenges of transgenic mouse models in the study of Alzheimer's disease. CNS Neurol Disord Drug Targets. 2010 Aug.;9(4):386–94.

[3] Persson J, Lind J, Larsson A, Ingvar M, Sleegers K, Van Broeckhoven C, et al. Altered deactivation in individuals with genetic risk for Alzheimer's disease. Neuropsychologia. 2008;46(6):1679–87.

[4] Fleisher AS, Sherzai A, Taylor C, Langbaum JBS, Chen K, Buxton RB. Resting-state BOLD networks versus task-associated functional MRI for distinguishing Alzheimer's disease risk groups. NeuroImage. 2009 Oct. 1;47(4):1678–90.

[5] Sinha G. Peering inside Alzheimer's brains. Nat. Biotechnol. 2011 May;:384–7.

[6] Filippini N, Macintosh BJ, Hough MG, Goodwin GM, Frisoni GB, Smith SM, et al. Distinct patterns of brain activity in young carriers of the APOE-epsilon4 allele. Proc Natl Acad Sci USA. 2009 Apr. 28;106(17):7209–14.

[7] Boly M, Phillips C, Tshibanda L, Vanhaudenhuyse A, Schabus M, Dang-Vu TT, et al. Intrinsic brain activity in altered states of consciousness: how conscious is the default mode of brain function? Ann N Y Acad Sci. 2008;1129:119–29.

[8] Greicius MD, Srivastava G, Reiss AL, Menon V. Default-mode network activity distinguishes Alzheimer's disease from healthy aging: evidence from functional MRI. Proc Natl Acad Sci USA. 2004 Mar. 30;101(13):4637–42.

[9] Alzheimer's Association. 2012 Alzheimer's disease facts and figures. Alzheimers Dement. 8th ed. 2012 Mar. 5;:131–68.

[10] Plewes DB, Kucharczyk W. Physics of MRI: a primer. J Magn Reson Imaging. 2012 May;35(5):1038–54.

[11] Braak H, Braak E. Neuropathological stageing of Alzheimer-related changes. Acta Neuropathol. 1991;82(4):239–59.

[12] Jack CR Jr., Bernstein MA, Borowski BJ, Gunter JL, Fox NC, Thompson PM, et al. Update on the Magnetic Resonance Imaging core of the Alzheimer's Disease Neuroimaging Initiative. Alzheimer's and Dementia. 2010 May;6(3):212–20.

[13] Poels MMF, Ikram MA, van der Lugt A, Hofman A, Niessen WJ, Krestin GP, et al. Cerebral microbleeds are associated with worse cognitive function: the Rotterdam Scan Study. Neurology. 2012 Jan. 31;78(5):326–33.

[14] Pettersen JA, Sathiyamoorthy G, Gao F-Q, Szilagyi G, Nadkarni NK, St George-Hyslop P, et al. Microbleed topography, leukoaraiosis, and cognition in probable Alzheimer disease from the Sunnybrook dementia study. Arch Neurol. 2008 Jun.;65(6): 790–5.

[15] Cuingnet R, Gerardin E, Tessieras J, Auzias G, Lehéricy S, Habert M-O, et al. Automatic classification of patients with Alzheimer's disease from structural MRI: a comparison of ten methods using the ADNI database. NeuroImage. 2011 May 15;56(2): 766–81.

[16] Smith MA, Zhu X, Tabaton M, Liu G, McKeel DW, Cohen ML, et al. Increased iron and free radical generation in preclinical Alzheimer disease and mild cognitive impairment. J Alzheimers Dis. 2010;19(1):363–72.

[17] Chincarini A, Bosco P, Calvini P, Gemme G, Esposito M, Olivieri C, et al. Local MRI analysis approach in the diagnosis of early and prodromal Alzheimer's disease. NeuroImage. 2011 Sep. 15;58(2):469–80.

[18] Hopp K, Popescu BFG, McCrea RPE, Harder SL, Robinson CA, Haacke ME, et al. Brain iron detected by SWI high pass filtered phase calibrated with synchrotron X-ray fluorescence. J Magn Reson Imaging. 2010 Jun.;31(6):1346–54.

[19] Costafreda SG, Dinov ID, Tu Z, Shi Y, Liu C-Y, Kloszewska I, et al. Automated hippocampal shape analysis predicts the onset of dementia in mild cognitive impairment. NeuroImage. 2011 May 1;56(1):212–9.

[20] Ringman JM, Pope W, Salamon N. Insensitivity of visual assessment of hippocampal atrophy in familial Alzheimer's disease. J Neurol. 2010 May 1;257(5):839–42.

[21] Shaw P, Lerch JP, Pruessner JC, Taylor KN, Rose AB, Greenstein D, et al. Cortical morphology in children and adolescents with different apolipoprotein E gene polymorphisms: an observational study. Lancet Neurol. 2007 Jun. 1;6(6):494–500.

[22] Alexander GE, Bergfield KL, Chen K, Reiman EM, Hanson KD, Lin L, et al. Gray matter network associated with risk for Alzheimer's disease in young to middle-aged adults. Neurobiology of aging. 2012 Dec.;33(12):2723–32.

[23] Donix M, Burggren AC, Suthana NA, Siddarth P, Ekstrom AD, Krupa AK, et al. Family history of Alzheimer's disease and hippocampal structure in healthy people. Am J Psychiatry. 2010 Nov. 1;167(11):1399–406.

[24] Donix M, Burggren AC, Suthana NA, Siddarth P, Ekstrom AD, Krupa AK, et al. Longitudinal changes in medial temporal cortical thickness in normal subjects with the APOE-4 polymorphism. NeuroImage. 2010 Oct. 15;53(1):37–43.

[25] Espeseth T, Westlye LT, Fjell AM, Walhovd KB, Rootwelt H, Reinvang I. Accelerated age-related cortical thinning in healthy carriers of apolipoprotein E epsilon 4. Neurobiology of aging. 2008 Mar. 1;29(3):329–40.

[26] Grothe M, Heinsen H, Teipel SJ. Atrophy of the cholinergic Basal forebrain over the adult age range and in early stages of Alzheimer's disease. Biol Psychiatry. 2012 May 1;71(9):805–13.

[27] Brickman AM, Honig LS, Scarmeas N, Tatarina O, Sanders L, Albert MS, et al. Measuring cerebral atrophy and white matter hyperintensity burden to predict the rate of cognitive decline in Alzheimer disease. Arch Neurol. 2008 Sep.;65(9):1202–8.

[28] Yoshita M, Fletcher E, Harvey D, Ortega M, Martinez O, Mungas DM, et al. Extent and distribution of white matter hyperintensities in normal aging, MCI, and AD. Neurology. 2006 Dec. 26;67(12):2192–8.

[29] Carmichael O, Schwarz C, Drucker D, Fletcher E, Harvey D, Beckett L, et al. Longitudinal changes in white matter disease and cognition in the first year of the Alzheimer disease neuroimaging initiative. Arch Neurol. 2010 Nov.;67(11):1370–8.

[30] Sexton CE, Kalu UG, Filippini N, Mackay CE, Ebmeier KP. A meta-analysis of diffusion tensor imaging in mild cognitive impairment and Alzheimer's disease. Neurobiology of aging. 2011 Dec.;32(12):2322.e5–18.

[31] Smith EE, Egorova S, Blacker D, Killiany RJ, Muzikansky A, Dickerson BC, et al. Magnetic resonance imaging white matter hyperintensities and brain volume in the prediction of mild cognitive impairment and dementia. Arch Neurol. 2008 Jan.;65(1): 94–100.

[32] Appel J, Potter E, Bhatia N, Shen Q, Zhao W, Greig MT, et al. Association of white matter hyperintensity measurements on brain MR imaging with cognitive status, medial temporal atrophy, and cardiovascular risk factors. American Journal of Neuroradiology. 2009 Nov.;30(10):1870–6.

[33] Hirono N, Yasuda M, Tanimukai S, Kitagaki H, Mori E. Effect of the apolipoprotein E epsilon4 allele on white matter hyperintensities in dementia. Stroke. 2000 Jun.;31(6): 1263–8.

[34] Sawada H, Udaka F, Izumi Y, Nishinaka K, Kawakami H, Nakamura S, et al. Cerebral white matter lesions are not associated with apoE genotype but with age and female sex in Alzheimer's disease. J. Neurol. Neurosurg. Psychiatr. 2000 May;68(5): 653–6.

[35] Persson J, Lind J, Larsson A, Ingvar M, Cruts M, Van Broeckhoven C, et al. Altered brain white matter integrity in healthy carriers of the APOE epsilon4 allele: a risk for AD? Neurology. 2006 Apr. 11;66(7):1029–33.

[36] Høgh P, Garde E, Mortensen EL, Jørgensen OS, Krabbe K, Waldemar G. The apolipoprotein E epsilon4-allele and antihypertensive treatment are associated with in-

creased risk of cerebral MRI white matter hyperintensities. Acta Neurol. Scand. 2007 Apr.;115(4):248–53.

[37] Ryan L, Walther K, Bendlin BB, Lue L-F, Walker DG, Glisky EL. Age-related differences in white matter integrity and cognitive function are related to APOE status. NeuroImage. 2011 Jan. 15;54(2):1565–77.

[38] Bendlin BB, Ries ML, Canu E, Sodhi A, Lazar M, Alexander AL, et al. White matter is altered with parental family history of Alzheimer's disease. Alzheimers Dement. 2010 Sep. 1;6(5):394–403.

[39] Smith CD, Chebrolu H, Andersen AH, Powell DA, Lovell MA, Xiong S, et al. White matter diffusion alterations in normal women at risk of Alzheimer's disease. Neurobiology of aging. 2010 Jul. 1;31(7):1122–31.

[40] Atwood CS, Obrenovich ME, Liu T, Chan H, Perry G, Smith MA, et al. Amyloid-beta: a chameleon walking in two worlds: a review of the trophic and toxic properties of amyloid-beta. Brain Res. Brain Res. Rev. 2003 Sep.;43(1):1–16.

[41] Brewer JB, Magda S, Airriess C, Smith ME. Fully-automated quantification of regional brain volumes for improved detection of focal atrophy in Alzheimer disease. American Journal of Neuroradiology. 2009 Mar. p. 578–80.

[42] la Torre de JC. Is Alzheimer's disease a neurodegenerative or a vascular disorder? Data, dogma, and dialectics. Lancet Neurol. 2004 Mar. 1;3(3):184–90.

[43] Sperling R. Functional MRI Studies of Associative Encoding in Normal Aging, Mild Cognitive Impairment, and Alzheimer's Disease. Ann N Y Acad Sci. 2007 Feb. 1;1097(1):146–55.

[44] Trachtenberg AJ, Filippini N, Mackay CE. The effects of APOE-ε4 on the BOLD response. NBA. Elsevier Inc; 2012 Feb. 1;33(2):323–34.

[45] Sugarman MA, Woodard JL, Nielson KA, Seidenberg M, Smith JC, Durgerian S, et al. Functional magnetic resonance imaging of semantic memory as a presymptomatic biomarker of Alzheimer's disease risk. Biochimica et Biophysica Acta (BBA) - Molecular Basis of Disease. 2012 Mar.;1822(3):442–56.

[46] Seidenberg M, Guidotti L, Nielson KA, Woodard JL, Durgerian S, Antuono P, et al. Semantic memory activation in individuals at risk for developing Alzheimer disease. Neurology. 2009 Aug. 25;73(8):612–20.

[47] Woodard JL, Seidenberg M, Nielson KA, Antuono P, Guidotti L, Durgerian S, et al. Semantic memory activation in amnestic mild cognitive impairment. Brain. 2009 Aug.;132(Pt 8):2068–78.

[48] Sorg C, Riedl V, Muhlau M, Calhoun VD, Eichele T, Laer L, et al. Selective changes of resting-state networks in individuals at risk for Alzheimer's disease. Proc Natl Acad Sci USA. 2007 Nov. 20;104(47):18760–5.

[49] Luchtmann M, Jachau K, Tempelmann C, Bernarding J. Alcohol induced region-dependent alterations of hemodynamic response: implications for the statistical interpretation of pharmacological fMRI studies. Exp Brain Res. 2010 Jul.;204(1):1–10.

[50] Koppelstaetter F, Poeppel TD, Siedentopf CM, Ischebeck A, Kolbitsch C, Mottaghy FM, et al. Caffeine and cognition in functional magnetic resonance imaging. J Alzheimers Dis. 2010;20 Suppl 1:S71–84.

[51] Donahue MJ, Blicher JU, Østergaard L, Feinberg DA, Macintosh BJ, Miller KL, et al. Cerebral blood flow, blood volume, and oxygen metabolism dynamics in human visual and motor cortex as measured by whole-brain multi-modal magnetic resonance imaging. J Cereb Blood Flow Metab. 2009 Nov.;29(11):1856–66.

[52] KETY SS, SCHMIDT CF. The nitrous oxide method for the quantitative determination of cerebral blood flow in man; theory, procedure and normal values. J. Clin. Invest. 1948 Jul.;27(4):476–83.

[53] Corder EH, Saunders AM, Strittmatter WJ, Schmechel DE, Gaskell PC, Small GW, et al. Gene dose of apolipoprotein E type 4 allele and the risk of Alzheimer's disease in late onset families. Science. 1993 Aug. 13;261(5123):921–3.

[54] Ishii K, Sasaki M, Yamaji S, Sakamoto S, Kitagaki H, Mori E. Demonstration of decreased posterior cingulate perfusion in mild Alzheimer's disease by means of H215O positron emission tomography. Eur J Nucl Med. 1997 Jun.;24(6):670–3.

[55] Bartenstein P, Minoshima S, Hirsch C, Buch K, Willoch F, Mösch D, et al. Quantitative assessment of cerebral blood flow in patients with Alzheimer's disease by SPECT. J. Nucl. Med. 1997 Jul.;38(7):1095–101.

[56] Kogure D, Matsuda H, Ohnishi T, Asada T, Uno M, Kunihiro T, et al. Longitudinal evaluation of early Alzheimer's disease using brain perfusion SPECT. J. Nucl. Med. 2000 Jul.;41(7):1155–62.

[57] Schmitz BL, Aschoff AJ, Hoffmann MHK, Grön G. Advantages and pitfalls in 3T MR brain imaging: a pictorial review. AJNR Am J Neuroradiol. 2005 Oct.;26(9):2229–37.

[58] Alsop DC, Detre JA, Grossman M. Assessment of cerebral blood flow in Alzheimer's disease by spin-labeled magnetic resonance imaging. Ann Neurol. 2000 Jan.;47(1):93–100.

[59] Johnson NA, Jahng G-H, Weiner MW, Miller BL, Chui HC, Jagust WJ, et al. Pattern of cerebral hypoperfusion in Alzheimer disease and mild cognitive impairment measured with arterial spin-labeling MR imaging: initial experience. Radiology. 2005 Mar.;234(3):851–9.

[60] Kim SM, Kim MJ, Rhee HY, Ryu C-W, Kim EJ, Petersen ET, et al. Regional cerebral perfusion in patients with Alzheimer's disease and mild cognitive impairment: effect of APOE Epsilon4 allele. Neuroradiology. 2012 Jul. 25.

[61] Uh J, Lewis-Amezcua K, Martin-Cook K, Cheng Y, Weiner M, Diaz-Arrastia R, et al. Cerebral blood volume in Alzheimer's disease and correlation with tissue structural integrity. Neurobiology of aging. 2010 Dec.;31(12):2038–46.

[62] Vernooij MD M, Smits MD M. Structural Neuroimaging in Aging and Alzheimer's Disease. Neuroimaging Clinics of NA. Elsevier Inc; 2012 Feb. 1;22(1):33–55.

[63] Lu H, Law M, Johnson G, Ge Y, Van Zijl PCM, Helpern JA. Novel approach to the measurement of absolute cerebral blood volume using vascular-space-occupancy magnetic resonance imaging. Magn Reson Med. 2005 Dec. 1;54(6):1403–11.

[64] Grubb RL, Raichle ME, Eichling JO, Ter-Pogossian MM. The effects of changes in PaCO2 on cerebral blood volume, blood flow, and vascular mean transit time. Stroke. 1974 Sep.;5(5):630–9.

[65] Donahue MJ, Strother MK, Hendrikse J. Novel MRI approaches for assessing cerebral hemodynamics in ischemic cerebrovascular disease. Stroke. 2012 Mar.;43(3):903–15.

[66] Kantarci K. 1H magnetic resonance spectroscopy in dementia. Br J Radiol. 2007 Dec.; 80 Spec No 2:S146–52.

[67] Kantarci K, Smith GE, Ivnik RJ, Petersen RC, Boeve BF, Knopman DS, et al. 1H magnetic resonance spectroscopy, cognitive function, and apolipoprotein E genotype in normal aging, mild cognitive impairment and Alzheimer's disease. J Int Neuropsychol Soc. 2002 Nov.;8(7):934–42.

[68] Schott JM, Frost C, Macmanus DG, Ibrahim F, Waldman AD, Fox NC. Short echo time proton magnetic resonance spectroscopy in Alzheimer's disease: a longitudinal multiple time point study. Brain. 2010 Nov. 1;133(11):3315–22.

[69] Selkoe DJ. Alzheimer's disease is a synaptic failure. Science. 2002 Oct. 25;298(5594): 789–91.

[70] Limon A, Reyes-Ruiz JM, Miledi R. Loss of functional GABAA receptors in the Alzheimer diseased brain. Proc Natl Acad Sci USA. 2012 Jun. 19;109(25):10071–6.

[71] Waddell KW, Avison MJ, Joers JM, Gore JC. A practical guide to robust detection of GABA in human brain by J-difference spectroscopy at 3 T using a standard volume coil. Magn Reson Imaging. 2007 Sep.;25(7):1032–8.

[72] Zhang H, Wang W, Gao W, Ge Y, Zhang J, Wu S, et al. Effect of propofol on the levels of neurotransmitters in normal human brain: A magnetic resonance spectroscopy study. Neurosci Lett. 2009 Dec.;467(3):247–51.

[73] Harada M, Kubo H, Nose A, Nishitani H, Matsuda T. Measurement of variation in the human cerebral GABA level by in vivo MEGA-editing proton MR spectroscopy using a clinical 3 T instrument and its dependence on brain region and the female menstrual cycle. Hum. Brain Mapp. 2011 May;32(5):828–33.

[74] Falini A, Bozzali M, Magnani G, Pero G, Gambini A, Benedetti B, et al. A whole brain MR spectroscopy study from patients with Alzheimer's disease and mild cognitive impairment. NeuroImage. 2005 Jul. 15;26(4):1159–63.

[75] Hu J, Feng W, Hua J, Jiang Q, Xuan Y, Li T, et al. A high spatial resolution in vivo 1H magnetic resonance spectroscopic imaging technique for the human breast at 3 T. Med Phys. 2009 Nov.;36(11):4870–7.

Section 3

Therapy

Potential Therapeutic Strategies to Prevent the Progression of Alzheimer to Disease States

Ester Aso and Isidre Ferrer

Additional information is available at the end of the chapter

http://dx.doi.org/10.5772/54783

1. Introduction

Alzheimer is an age-dependent neurodegenerative process distinct from normal aging and characterized morphologically by the presence of senile plaques and neurofibrillary tangles, which progress from the brain stem and inner parts of the temporal lobes to most the telencephalon.

Senile plaques are mainly composed of different species of fibrillar β-amyloid (Aβ), a product of the cleavage of the β-amyloid precursor protein (APP), and they are surrounded by dystrophic neurites, reactive astrocytes and microglia. Aβ fibrillar deposits also occur in diffuse plaques, subpial deposits and in the wall of the cerebral and meningeal blood vessels in the form of amyloid angiopathy. A substantial part of β-amyloid is not fibrillar but soluble and forms oligomers of differing complexity which are toxic to nerve cells.

Neurofibrillary tangles are mainly composed of various isoforms of tau protein, which is hyper-phosphorylated and nitrated. It has an altered conformation and is truncated at different sites through the action of a combination of several proteolytic enzymes giving rise to species of low molecular weight which are toxic to nerve cells. Abnormal tau deposition also occurs in the dystrophic neurites of senile plaques and within the small neuronal processes, resulting in the formation of neuropil threads.

The mechanisms of disease progression are not completely understood but Aβ initiates the pathological process in the small percentage of familial cases due to mutations in genes encoding APP, presenilin 1 and presenilin 2, the latter involved in the cleavage of APP, and potentiates tau phosphorylation in sporadic cases that represent the majority of affected individuals (β-amyloid cascade hypothesis). Moreover, Aβ act as a seed of new β-amyloid production and deposition under appropriate settings, and abnormal tau promotes the production and deposition of hyper-phosphorylated tau. Therefore, Aβ and hyper-phosphorylated tau promote the progression of the process and this may occur in an exponential way once these abnormal proteins are accumulated in the brain.

In addition to these pathological hallmarks, multiple alterations play roles in the degenerative process. Several genetic factors, such as apolipoprotein ε4 (APOE4), and external factors, such as vascular and circulatory alterations and repeated cerebral traumatisms, among others, facilitate disease progression in sporadic forms. Furthermore, metabolic components mainly, but not merely, associated with aging have a cardinal influence, including mitochondrial defects and energy production deficiencies, production of free radicals (oxidative and nitrosative reactive species: ROS and NOS) and oxidative and nitrosative damage, increased reticulum stress damage, altered composition of membranes, inflammatory responses and impaired function of degradation pathways such as autophagy and ubiquitin-proteasome system.

It has been proven that the degenerative process, at least the presence of neurofibrillary tangles, starts in middle age in selected nuclei of the brain stem and entorhinal cortex, and then progresses to other parts of the brain. Instrumental stages of Braak cover stages I and II with involvement of the entorhinal and transentorhinal cortices; stages II and IV also affect the hippocampus and limbic system together with the basal nucleus of Meynert; and stages V and VI involve the whole brain although neurofibrillary tangles are not found in selected regions such as the cerebellar cortex and the dentate gyrus. The distribution of senile plaques is a bit different as they first appear in the orbitofrontal cortex and temporal cortex and then progress to the whole convexity.

A concomitant decline in neuronal organization occurs most often in parallel with senile plaques and neurofibrillary tangles manifested as synaptic dysfunction and synaptic loss, and neuronal death and progressive isolation of remaining neurons.

An important observation is that about 80% of individuals aged 65 years have Alzheimer-related changes, at least at stages I-III, whereas only 5% have cognitive impairment and dementia. About 25% of individuals aged 85 years suffer from cognitive impairment and dementia of Alzheimer type. Stages I-IV are often silent with no clinical symptoms. Cognitive impairment and dementia usually occur at stages V and VI when the neurodegenerative process is very advanced. Importantly, the progression from stage I to stage IV may last decades, whereas the progression to stages V and VI is much more rapid. Therefore, Alzheimer is a well-tolerated degenerative process during a relatively long period of time, but it may have devastating effects once thresholds are crossed. Moreover, clinical symptoms may be complicated by concomitant vascular pathology.

Several attempts have been made to predict the evolution to disease states. Neuroimaging, including high resolution and functional magnetic resonance imaging, positron emission tomography and the use of relative selective markers of β-amyloid and tau deposition in the brain, together with reduced levels of Aβ and increased index of phospho-tau/total tau in the cerebrospinal fluid, are common complementary probes (biomarkers) in addition to the data provided by the neuropsychological examination. Unfortunately, these tests, at present, detect relatively advanced stages of the process in pathological terms.

It is very illustrating to visualize under the microscope how a brain at middle stages of the degenerative process has been working without apparent neurological deficits during life. The adaptive capacities of the brain in coping with current functions in spite of the decrepitude of composition and organization resulting from the chronic progression of the degenerative process are impressive.

Taking into consideration this scenario, it is compulsory to increase understanding of the first stages of the degenerative process and to act on selective targets before the appearance of clinical symptoms.

The present review is not a mere list of putative treatments of Alzheimer's disease (AD) but rather an approach to learning about observations made on experimental models and early stages of disease aimed at curbing or retarding disease progression on the basis of definite rationales. It is also our aim to encourage the consideration of Alzheimer as a degenerative process not necessarily leading to dementia [1]. This concept has important clinical implications as it supports early preventive measures in the population at risk (i.e. persons over 50 years) even in the absence of clinical symptoms.

2. Experimental therapeutic strategies to prevent Alzheimer progression to Alzheimer Disease (AD) states

Several reviews have focused on various aspects related to habits and dietary elements which may act as protective factors against AD, including physical and mental exercise, low caloric intake, various diets with low fat content, and vitamin complements [2, 3]. It is worth noting that neuropathological studies in old-aged individuals usually present combined pathologies, and combination of Alzheimer changes and vascular lesions are very common [4]. It is well documented that vascular pathology potentiates primary neurodegenerative pathology and that vascular factors may be causative of cognitive impairment and dementia [5]. Therefore, therapies geared to reduce vascular risk factors are also protective factors against AD clinical manifestations.

2.1. Targeting Aβ

Most of the current drug development for the prevention or treatment of AD is based on the β-amyloid cascade hypothesis and aims at reducing the levels of Aβ in the brain. Overproduction, aggregation and deposition of the Aβ peptide begin before the onset of symptoms and they are considered an essential early event in AD pathogenesis. Thus, targeting these early Aβ alterations is assumed to reduce the progression to disease states. The different strategies developed to achieve this objective include decreasing Aβ production through modulating secretase activity, interfering with Aβ aggregation, and promoting Aβ clearance.

2.1.1. *Secretase-targeting therapies*

APP is processed in the brain exclusively by three membrane-bound proteases, α-, β- and γ-secretase. Therefore, specifically modifying such enzyme activity should result in a reduction of Aβ production [6].

- *α-secretase activators*: α-secretase initiates the non-amyloidogenic pathway by cleaving APP within the Aβ sequence, thereby preventing the production of Aβ and producing a non-toxic form of APP derivative which is neuroprotective and growth- promoting [7]. Therefore, compounds that stimulate α-secretase activity could become an attractive strategy to reduce Aβ production. In fact, some indirect methods of promoting α-secretase activity, such as the stimulation of the protein kinase C (PKC) or Mitogen-activated protein kinases (MAPK) pathways, the use of α-7-nicotinic acetylcholine (ACh) receptor and 5-hydroxi-tryptamine (5-HT) receptor 4 agonists, and γ-aminobutyric acid A receptor modulators, result in α-secretase-mediated cleavage of APP and reduced Aβ levels *in vivo* [8]. However, the development of a direct activator of α-secretase as a drug treatment for AD seems premature because of the lack of knowledge about the consequences of chronic up-regulation of α-secretase-mediated cleavage on other substrates [6].
- *β-secretase inhibitors*: the β-secretase enzyme initiates the amyloidogenic pathway, cleaving APP at the amino terminus of the Aβ peptide. Further cleavage of the resulting carboxy-terminal fragment by γ-secretase results in the release of Aβ. β-secretase activity is specifically mediated by the β-site APP cleaving enzyme 1 (BACE1), which is also involved in the processing of numerous substrates in addition to APP. The research of drugs inhibiting BACE1 activity was encouraged by studies revealing that the expression of mutated BACE1 reduces amyloidogenesis and cognitive impairment in APP transgenic mice [9, 10]. The first generation of BACE1 inhibitors was peptide-based mimetics of the APP β-cleavage site. Unfortunately, these compounds exhibited some difficulties because of the large substrate binding site of BACE1 and because of the difficulty in crossing the blood–brain barrier (BBB) and penetrating the plasma and endosomal membranes to gain access to the intracellular compartments where endogenous BACE1 plays its function. Recently, non-peptide small-molecule BACE1 inhibitors have been reported to improve bioavailability and to lower cerebral Aβ levels in animal models of AD [11, 12]. However, the involvement of BACE1 in other important physiological processes raises concerns about minimizing the potential adverse effects derived from generalized BACE1 inhibition.
- *γ-secretase inhibitors (GSIs)*: γ-secretase is a complex composed of presenilin 1 and presenilin 2 (PS1 and PS2) forming the catalytic core and three accessory proteins, anterior pharynx-defective 1 (APH-1), nicastrin and presenilin enhancer protein 2 (PEN2). The γ-secretase complex displays a high degree of subunit heterogeneity and little is known about the physiological roles of the diverse complexes and how they process different trans-membrane substrates in addition to APP. This heterogeneity suggests that selective targeting of one particular subunit might be a more effective treatment strategy than non-selective γ-secretase inhibition [13]. Thus, removal of APH-1B and APH-1C isoforms in a mouse model of AD decreased Aβ plaque formation and improved behavioral deficits [14]. A number of orally bioavailable and brain-penetrating GSIs have been shown to decrease Aβ production

and deposition in APP mouse models and in humans [15-17]. However, target-based toxicity of GSIs has been a major obstacle to the clinical development of these compounds. In fact, two large Phase III clinical trials of *Semagacestat*, the only GSI extensively studied in AD, were prematurely interrupted because of the observation of detrimental cognitive and functional effects of the drug [18]. Several dozen γ-secretase substrates have been identified, including Notch1 trans-membrane receptor, which plays an important role in a variety of developmental and physiological processes by controlling cell fate decisions. To overcome these toxicity issues, pharmaceutical companies have been trying to develop a second generation of 'Notch-sparing' GSIs, which revealed beneficial effects in *in vitro* and in animal models of AD [19-21]. They are currently under clinical studies. Such 'Notch-sparing' GSIs have higher pharmacological selectivity than the first GSIs probably due to the distinct binding to the substrate docking site on γ-secretase of Notch and APP. Identification of several γ-secretase inhibitors has been reviewed elsewhere [22].

2.1.2. Aβ degrading enzymes

Almost 20 enzymes are currently known to contribute to Aβ degradation in the brain, although the most studied are two zinc metalloproteases, neprilysin (NEP) and insulin-degrading enzyme (IDE). NEP is one of the major Aβ-degrading enzymes in the brain [23] and NEP levels are decreased in the brain of AD and animal models [24, 25]. Lentiviral delivery of the NEP gene to the brain of AD transgenic mice reduced Aβ pathology [26]. A number of subsequent studies with NEP and other related peptidases such as endothelin-converting enzymes 1 and 2 (ECE-1 and ECE-2) further supported this observation [27]. Similarly, over-expression of IDE in neurons significantly reduces brain Aβ levels, prevents Aβ plaque formation and its associated cytopathology, and rescues the premature lethality present in these particular APP transgenic mice [28]. A growing body of evidence has been accumulated supporting the potential therapeutic properties of IDE in AD [29].

Other specific Aβ-cleaving proteases such as angiotensin-converting enzyme (ACE), matrix metalloproteinase-9 (MMP-9) and the serine protease plasmin, which have distinct sub-cellular localizations and differential responses to aging, oxidative stress and pharmacological agents, are also potential candidates to become novel therapeutic strategies for AD prevention and treatment [27].

Targeting the delivery of these compounds to the brain remains a major challenge. The most promising current approaches include peripheral administration of agents that enhance the activity of Aβ-degrading enzymes and direct intra-cerebral release of enzymes by convection-enhanced delivery. Genetic procedures geared at increasing cerebral expression of Aβ-degrading enzymes may offer additional advantages [30].

2.1.3. Decreasing Aβ aggregation

Compounds that suppress the aggregation or reduce the stability of Aβ oligomers may bind monomers in order to attenuate formation of both the oligomeric and senile plaque fibrillar Aβ constituents. One of the amyloid-binding drugs more extensively studied in animal models and AD patients is tramiprosate (3-amino-1-propanesulfonic acid; Alzhemed). Tramiprosate was effective in reducing Aβ polymerisation *in vitro*, inhibiting the formation of neurotoxic aggregates, and decreasing Aβ plaque formation in animal models [31]. However, recent phase III clinical trials did not produce any significant improvement in cognition in AD patients chronically treated with tramiprosate in spite of the significant reduction in hippocampus volume loss [32]. Similarly, some other compounds known to inhibit Aβ aggregation and fibril formation showed positive effects in animal and *in vitro* models of AD but failed to produce conclusive results in human clinical trials. This is the case with scyllo-inositol and PBT2. Scyllo-inositol inhibited cognitive deficits in TgCRND8 mice and significantly ameliorated disease pathology, even in animals at advanced stages of AD-like pathology, without interfering with endogenous phosphatidylinositol lipid production [33, 34]. Yet a phase II clinical trial failed in supporting or refuting a benefit of scyllo-inositol in mild to moderate AD patients [35]. PBT2 is a copper/zinc ionophore which targets metal-induced aggregation of Aβ. When given orally to two models of Aβ-bearing transgenic mice, PTB2 was able to markedly decrease soluble brain Aβ levels within hours and to improve cognitive performance within days [36]. These results correlated with a rapid cognitive improvement in AD patients in a recent phase IIa clinical trial [37], an observation that argues for large-scale testing of PBT2 for AD.

Another promising recent experimental approach is the use of dendrimers as agents interfering with Aβ fibrilization. Dendrimers are globular branched polymers, typically symmetric around the core with a spherical three-dimensional morphology. Their chemical structure allows dendrimers to couple to active amyloid species through hundreds of possible sites. Dendrimers have been shown to be able to modulate Aβ peptide aggregation by interfering in different ways with the polymerization process, including fibril breaking, inhibition of fibril formation and acceleration of fibril formation [38, 39]. However, some dendrimers assayed in amyloidogenic systems are toxic to cells. The development of non-toxic glycodendrimers, which reduce toxicity by clumping fibrils together [40], opens the possibility of using dendrimers with low intrinsic toxicity in AD. Additional difficulties in dendrimer administration involve the crossing of the BBB so as to reach their targets in the brain.

2.1.4. Facilitating Aβ clearance: Immunotherapy against Aβ

Active and passive immunotherapy against Aβ peptide has been explored as a therapeutic approach to stimulate the clearance of Aβ in the brain at the preclinical and clinical stages of the disease in animal models. Pioneering studies proved that vaccination of young APP transgenic mice using a synthetic aggregated form of $A\beta_{42}$ (AN-1792) effectively prevented Aβ plaque formation, neuritic dystrophy and astrogliosis in adult brains [41]. Subsequent studies further demonstrated improvement of memory loss in those APP transgenic mice vaccinated against Aβ [42, 43]. Different models, methods and ways of administration showed the beneficial effects of active and passive immunization in animal models of AD. Nevertheless, the phase II trial in humans was discontinued because of the occurrence of aseptic meningoencephalitis in a number of cases [44-46]. The cause of the meningoencephalitis was a concomitant T-cell-mediated autoimmune response [45, 46]. Moreover, several studies in APP transgenic mice have reported an increased risk of microhemorrhages at sites of cerebrovascular Aβ deposits [47]. Yet important conclusions were drawn from the studies in humans: immunization reduced the number of Aβ plaques and the number of dystrophic neurites, including tau phosphorylation around plaques, but not Aβ burden in blood vessels; however, immunization increased intracerebral levels of soluble Aβ [48-50].

New vaccines containing immunodominant B-cell epitopes of Aβ [51] and recognizing other Aβ residues [52, 53], and the use of passive immunization with deglycosylated antibodies [54] have demonstrated positive effects in the clearance of Aβ without causing inflammatory response or hemorrhages in animal models of AD [55]. These findings have prompted new clinical trials which are currently evaluating the toxicity and effectiveness of at least ten vaccines in mild-to-moderate AD patients worldwide [56]. While vaccines hold great hope as AD therapies, it is important to stress that immunization at pre-symptomatic stages is essential in order to avoid the irreversible brain damage occurring even at the early symptomatic stages [57].

2.2. Targeting tau

The interest in tau-related therapies is still emerging and very few clinical studies are underway, in part because of the difficulties encountered with anti-Aβ strategies that captured most efforts in the two last decades, but also because of the challenging identification of tractable therapeutic targets related to tau. Current research in the prevention of tau pathology developed in animal models of AD has resulted in some promising results [58]. Main rationales in tau pathology are based on: 1: inhibition of tau aggregation, 2: reduction of tau phosphorylation by inhibition of tau kinases or activation of phosphatases (including PP2a activity), 3: reduction of tau levels by increasing tau degradation or by using active immunization, and 4: stabilization of microtubule [59].

2.2.1. Inhibition of tau aggregation

Some compounds that are known to inhibit tau-tau interactions have been tested as agents aimed at slowing Alzheimer progression to disease states. Among them, phenothiaziazine methylene blue inhibits tau-tau interactions, is neuroprotective and is able to facilitate soluble tau clearance in a mouse model of human tauopathy [60, 61]. Moreover, phenothiaziazine methylene blue has shown beneficial effects in a phase II clinical trial conducted for one year [62]. Another promising inhibitor of tau aggregation is the immunosuppressant FK506, which exerts its beneficial effects in transgenic mice by directly binding tau to the FK506 binding protein 52 and by modulating microglial activation [63, 64].

However, some concerns araise from the use of tau aggregation inhibitors in that at least some tau aggregation inhibitors enhance the formation of potentially toxic tau oligomers [65].

2.2.2. Reduction of tau hyperphosphorylation

Kinases which participate in the phosphorylation of tau and phosphatases which dephosphorylate tau are clear putative therapeutic targets for AD [66]. The most widely studied tau kinases in AD pathogenesis are Glycogen synthase kinase 3 beta (GSK-3β) and Cyclin-dependent kinase (CDK5) [67, 68]. Several GSK-3β inhibitors, including lithium, aloisines, flavopiridol, hymenialdisine, paullones, and staurosporine, are under active investigation and development [69]. Lithium revealed some promising results when administered in transgenic mice expressing the P301L human 4R0N tau at pre-symptomatic stages; it improved behavior and reduced the levels of phosphorylation, aggregation and insoluble tau in transgenic mice [70]. However, several concerns have arisen in relation of the use of GSK-3β in the treatment of AD; these are based on the fact that lithium lacks specificity over GSK-3β activity and it has a narrow safety margin [71]. Moreover, GSK-3β acts on multiple metabolic pathways that are also impaired with unknown consequences after chronic treatment.

CDK5 inhibitors prevent Aβ-induced tau hyper-phosphorylation and cell death *in vitro* [72, 73]. A recent *in vivo* study further demonstrates that inhibition of CDK5 activates GSK-3β, which plays a more dominant role in overall tau phosphorylation than does CDK5 [74]. Thus, considering that CDK5 inhibitors might be unable to reverse abnormal hyper-phosphorylation of tau and treat neurofibrillary degeneration because of the interplay between CDK5 and GSK-3β, as well as the essential role played by CDK5 in multiple cell signaling pathways [75], the interest of such compounds as a tau-targeting therapy for AD is limited.

Another approach to reverse tau hyper-phosphorylation is up-regulation of tau phosphatases [66]. The major tau phosphatase, PP2A, is down-regulated in AD brain. In consequence, correcting PP2A levels is the primary target to be considered. Among the compounds known to reverse PP2A inhibition, memantine is the most outstanding because of the demonstrated clinical benefit in AD. In an animal model, memantine was able to reverse okadaic acid–induced PP2A inhibition and to prevent tau hyper-phosphorylation, restoring MAP2 expression [76]. Similarly, melatonin has also been shown to restore PP2A activity and reverse tau hyper-phosphorylation, both *in vitro* and in experimental animals [77]. One important concern in considering PP2A as a potential therapeutic target is that all protein phosphatases have much broader substrate specificities than protein kinases. Thus, more undesirable effects might be expected than when using kinase inhibitors [66]. A further intriguing point is that PP2A function and activity depend on multiple subunits and cofactors which are dysregulated in AD [78]. It is not clear how all these elements can be resolved to result in maintained balanced activity.

2.2.3. *Reduction of tau levels*

A potential alternative to modulate tau phosphorylation is reducing overall tau levels [58]. Experiments carried out in genetically-modified mice expressing reduced tau levels revealed diminished cognitive impairment and Aβ-induced neuronal damage [79-81]. An alternative method to reduce tau levels could is by targeting molecules that regulate the expression or clearance of tau. Tau can be degraded via the ubiquitin-proteasome system and the lysosomal pathways. Reduction of the levels of the tau ubiquitin-ligase CHIP increases the accumulation of tau aggregates in JNPL3 mice, suggesting that increasing the expression of CHIP could result in reduced tau levels [82]. Acetylation of tau inhibits its degradation [83], alters its microtubule binding, and enhances aggregation [84]. Thus, the combination of tau acetylation inhibition and ubiquitination-proteasome enhancement might produce a synergy that lowers the levels of pathogenic tau species.

Tau degradation can also be enhanced by immunization. Active immunization targeting phosphorylated tau reduces filamentous tau inclusions and neuronal dysfunction in JNPL3 transgenic mice [85, 86]. Moreover, recent studies have raised the possibility of modulating tau pathology by passive immunization revealing reduced behavioral impairment and tau pathology in two transgenic models of taupathies [87].

2.2.4. Microtubule stabilizers

Since microtubule disruption occurs in several models of AD and is associated with tau dysfunction, microtubule stabilizers have been assayed in preclinical and clinical trials for AD [88]. The anti-mitotic drug paclitaxel prevents Aβ-induced toxicity in cell culture [89], as well as axonal transport deficits and behavioral impairments in tau transgenic mice [90]. Unfortunately, paclitaxel is a P-glycoprotein substrate and it has very low capacity to cross the BBB, making it unsuitable for the treatment of human tauopathies. Epothilone D, which has better BBB permeability, improves microtubule density and cognition in tau transgenic mice [91]. Finally, the peptide NAP stabilizes microtubules and reduces tau hyper-phosphorylation [92]. NAP can be administered intra-nasally and has shown promising results in a phase II clinical trial [93].

2.3. Oxidative stress

Several pieces of evidence demonstrate that oxidative stress precedes other hallmarks of the neurodegenerative process in human brains and animal models of AD, including Aβ deposition, NFT formation, and metabolic dysfunction and cognitive decline. It plays a functional role in the pathogenesis of the disease [94-100]. These findings sustain the possibility of using anti-oxidants in the prevention and treatment of Alzheimer [101, 102]. Several studies in AD transgenic mouse models support the potential beneficial effect of antioxidant compounds as preventive drugs.

2.3.1. Naturally-occurring anti-oxidants

Several nutritional antioxidants such as resveratrol, curcumin, epigallocatechin gallate, L-acetyl-carnitine, RRR-α-tocopherol (vitamin E) and ascorbic acid (vitamin C) have been tested to counteract oxidative stress-induced brain damage in AD.

- *Resveratrol* is a polyphenolic compound found in grapes, berries and peanuts with well known anti-oxidant, anti-cancer, anti-inflammatory and estrogenic activities. *In vitro* and animal experiments reveal that resveratrol protects against Aβ toxicity by promoting the non-amyloidogenic cleavage of APP, thus enhancing the clearance of Aβ peptides by promoting their degradation through the ubiquitin-proteasome system, as well as reducing neuronal damage by decreasing the expression of inducible nitric oxide synthase (iNOS) and cyclooxigenase 2 (COX-2), and the pro-apoptotic factors Bax and c-Jun N-terminal kinase (JNK). Moreover, the capacity of resveratrol to induce the over-expression of sirtuins, proteins having a role in cell survival, probably contributes to its neuroprotective effect [103, 104].

- *Curcumin* is a polyphenolic compound present in the rhizome of *Curcuma longa*, commonly used as a spice to color and flavor food, which has anti-inflammatory, anti-carcinogenic and anti-infectious properties. The first evidence of a protective role of curcumin in AD was derived from epidemiological studies based on populations subjected to a curcumin-enriched diet. Additionally, *in vitro* studies have shown that curcumin protects neurons from Aβ toxicity whereas the use of AD transgenic mouse models show that curcumin suppresses inflammation and oxidative damage as well as accelerating the Aβ rate of clearance and inhibiting Aβ aggregation. Curcumin is considered a bi-functional anti-oxidant because it is a direct scavenger of oxidants as well as a long-lasting protector promoting the expression of cytoprotective proteins through the induction of Nrf2-dependent genes [105, 106]. Regrettably, no significant improvement in cognitive function between placebo and curcumin-treated groups has been observed in the only two clinical trials carried out until now [107].

- *Epigallocatechin gallate (EGCG)* is a polyphenolic flavonoid encountered in green tea. Human epidemiological and animal data suggest that tea may decrease the incidence of dementia and AD. EGCG has been demonstrated to exert its neuroprotective activity by reducing Aβ production and inflammation, and increasing mitochondrial stabilization, iron chelation and ROS scavenging [108]. However, to date no clinical trials have been performed to verify whether EGCG neuroprotective/neurorestorative actions can be successfully translated into human beings.

- *Acetyl-L-Carnitine (ALC)* is a natural compound found in red meat whose biological role is to facilitate the transport of fatty acids to the mitochondria. Thus, the main mechanism of action of ALC is the improvement of mitochondrial respiration, which allows the neurons to produce the necessary ATP to maintain normal membrane potential. Yet ALC is neuro-protective through a variety of additional effects, including an increase in protein kinase C activity and modulation of synaptic plasticity by counteracting the loss of NMDA receptors in the neuronal membrane and by increasing the production of neurotrophins [105]. Moreover, ALC reduces Aβ toxicity in primary cortical neuronal cultures by increasing both heme-oxygenase 1 (HO-1) and heat-shock protein 70 (Hsp70) expression, probably through transcription factor Nrf2. In two clinical studies, ALC administered for one year significantly reduced cognitive decline in early-onset AD patients [109, 110] thus sustaining the potential use of ALC in AD prevention and treatment at early stages.

- *RRR-a-tocopherol (Vitamin E)* is probably the most important lipid-soluble natural antioxi-dant in mammalian cells. Most vegetable oils, nuts and some fruits are important dietary sources of vitamin E. The interest in evaluating its potential beneficial properties in AD is also sustained by its known ability to cross the BBB and to accumulate in the central nervous system. Deficiency in the α-tocopherol transfer protein mediating vitamin E activity induces an increase in brain lipid peroxidation, earlier and more severe cognitive dysfunction, and increased Aβ deposits in the brain of Tg2576 mice; this phenotype was ameliorated with vitamin E supplementation [111]. However, although epidemiological studies have demonstrated that increasing the intake of fruit and vegetables rich in vitamins prevents or retards the onset of AD, clinical trials for vitamin E treatment have revealed paradoxical results: whereas vitamin E supplementation partially prevents the memory loss associated with the progression of the disease in some cases, the same treatment was detrimental in others [112].

- *Ascorbic acid (Vitamin C)* is an essential nutrient since it acts as a cofactor in elemental enzymatic reactions, but in contrast to most of organisms, humans are not able to synthesize ascorbic acid. The main dietary source of vitamin C is fresh fruit and vegetables. The main interest in vitamin C for the treatment of neurodegenerative processes is related to its potent anti-oxidant properties. Some studies have revealed that vitamin C supplementation reduces oxidative stress, and mitigates Aβ oligomer formation and behavioral decline, but it did not decrease plaque deposition in AD mouse models [113, 114]. Despite epidemiological studies reporting reduced prevalence and incidence of AD in consumers of vitamin supplements [115], meta-analyses revealed the risks of chronic consumption of high doses of vitamin C thus discouraging its routine use in AD. [116]

- *Egb76* is a standardized *Ginkgo biloba* extract already approved in some countries as symptomatic treatment for dementia although the evidence for its effectiveness remains inconclusive [117]. However, Egb761 has anti-oxidant properties, inhibits Aβ oligomerization *in vitro*, reduces impaired memory and learning capacities and enhances hippocampal neurogenesis in AD transgenic mice [118]. For these reasons, *Ginkgo biloba* extract is currently under evaluation as a preventive drug in AD.

In spite of the experimental evidence of beneficial effects of natural anti-oxidants in cultured cells and transgenic models, clinical studies have demonstrated only minimal effect in humans probably due to the bioavailability and pharmacokinetics of these substances [102, 105]. What's more, a slight acceleration in cognitive decline has been observed in patients treated for 16 weeks with a cocktail of natural antioxidants [119].

2.3.2. *Mitochondrial antioxidants*

In contrast to other antioxidants, those designed to target the free radical damage to mitochondria provide greater therapeutic potential.

- *Lipoic acid (LA)* is a naturally-occurring precursor of an essential cofactor of many mitochondrial enzymes, including pyruvate dehydrogenase and alpha-ketoglutarate dehydrogenase, which is found in almost all foods. LA has been shown to present a variety of properties that can interfere with pathogenic processes of AD. LA increases ACh production, stimulates glucose uptake, protects against Aβ toxicity, chelates redox-active transition metals, scavenges reactive oxygen species (ROS) and induces anti-oxidant protective enzymes probably through the activation of the transcription factor Nrf2. Via the same mechanisms, down-regulation of redox-sensitive inflammatory processes is also achieved [120]. Data from cell culture and animal models suggest that LA can be combined with other dietary anti-oxidants to synergistically decrease oxidative stress, inflammation, Aβ levels, and thus provide a combined benefit in the treatment of AD. However, clinical benefits after LA administration were quite small in patients with mild or moderate dementia [121].

- *N-acetyl-cysteine (NAC)* is a precursor of glutathione (GSH), the most abundant endogenous anti-oxidant. NAC acts itself as an anti-oxidant by directly interacting with free radicals, as well as by increasing GSH levels. NAC protects against Aβ-induced cognitive deficits by decreasing the associated oxidative stress and related neuroinflammation, but also by activating anti-apoptotic signaling pathways in neuronal cultures [122]. Late-stage AD patients supplemented with NAC over a period of six months showed significantly improved performance in some cognitive tasks, although levels of oxidative stress in peripheral blood did not differ significantly from untreated patients [123].

- *Coenzyme Q_{10}(CoQ_{10})* is a small electron-carrier of the respiratory chain with anti-oxidant properties due to its role in carrying high-energy electrons from complex I to complex II during oxidative phosphorylation. CoQ_{10} and its analogues, idebenone and mitoquinone (or MitoQ), have been widely used for the treatment of mitochondrial disorders, as well as for the treatment of Friedreich's ataxia, and they are also being tested in other neurodegenerative disorders such as amyotrophic lateral sclerosis, and Huntington's, Parkinson's and Alzheimer's diseases [124]. CoQ_{10} reduces oxidative stress damage and Aβ plaque burden, and ameliorates behavioral performance in mouse models of AD [125, 126]. However, CoQ_{10} presents two major weaknesses. First, the function of the enzyme is entirely dependent on the electron transport chain (ETC) which is usually damaged in AD mitochondria. Second, CoQ_{10} does not efficiently cross the BBB when administered systemically, being unable to directly protect neurons from damage. Consequently, CoQ_{10} derivatives such as MitoQ, which is a more soluble compound able to penetrate the BBB and that does not depend on ETC, are seen to offer more promising results [127].

2.4. Inflammation

There is a general consensus that neuroinflammation is a prominent feature in AD with activated microglia being one of the main manifestations. Neuroinflammation is a complex process that has both beneficial effects, in terms of maintaining brain homeostasis after various kinds of insults, and detrimental effects when sustained chronically [128]. This latter situation is what occurs in AD, in which neuroinflammation is driven by different mechanisms including Aβ production and plaque formation, tau pathology, oxidative stress, and autocrine and paracrine release of cytokines and other inflammatory molecules which contribute to a feed-forward spiral favoring the self-propagation of neuroinflammation.

Early epidemiological studies suggesting that long-term use of antiinflammatories might reduce the risk for developing AD [129] prompted several studies designed to evaluate the preventive properties of non-steroid anti-inflammatory drugs (NSAIDs). The main NSAID mechanism of action is to inhibit the activity of cyclooxigenase-1 and -2 (COX-1 and COX-2) which are the enzymes responsible of the production of prostaglandins and other inflammatory agents [130]. The administration of the NSAID ibuprofen at early stages of the pathological process resulted in the reduction of the Aβ burden, dystrophic neurites and activated microglia in at least three different AD transgenic models [131-134]. Another study indicated that ibuprofen was effective even in older mice once lesions are well established [135]. Other NSAIDs such as indomethacin and nimuselide exhibit milder effects compared to ibuprofen in the Tg2576 mice [136, 137]. In contrast, the selective COX-2 inhibitor celecoxib failed to reduce the inflammatory burden and, even worse, increased the $A\beta_{42}$ levels when administered to young Tg2576 mice [138].

In spite of the promising results in animal models and the data from retrospective human epidemiological studies identifying long-term use of NSAIDs as being protective against AD, prospective clinical trials have not confirmed the efficiency of this group of drugs in the amelioration of symptoms and in the progression of AD [139].

Other anti-inflammatory agents such as trifusal have been shown to be beneficial in certain AD transgenic mice models [140].

2.5. Energetic failure: Metabolic deficiency and mitochondrial impairment

Several findings indicate that brain glucose hypometabolism, deficient bioenergetics and mitochondrial dysfunction precede clinical symptoms in AD [1, 141-143]. The energetic failure observed even in the prodromal phase of the Alzheimer process is thought to be produced by the combination of mitochondria dysfunction, alteration of energy metabolism at pore-mitochondrial level, and increase in energetic demands of altered nerve cells. Thus, strategies to improve brain energy supply and to preserve mitochondrial functions becomes relevant in the prevention of progression to disease states [1, 144-146].

2.5.1. Metabolic deficiency

The primary fuel for the brain under normal conditions is glucose, whereas the energetic contribution made by fatty acids is minor. Therefore, facilitation of energy metabolism and energy availability has been assayed in animal models and AD by facilitating glucose metabolism and shifting towards the use of alternative fuels.

- *Targeting reduced glucose metabolism*: Reduction in the utilization of glucose in AD [147] can be due to several causes including deficient insulin signaling, impairment in glucose transport mechanisms and dysfunction in glycolysis. Preclinical studies in animal models of AD have revealed some beneficial effects of anti-diabetic treatments. Thus, the use of the insulin sensitizer rosiglitazone, an activator of peroxisome-proliferator-activated receptor gamma (PPARγ) receptor, resulted in the rescue of behavioral deficits and insulin responsiveness in Tg2576 mice [148, 149]. Similarly, exendin-4, an antidiabetic agent that stimulates the insulin signaling pathway through activation of glucagon-like peptide -1 (GLP1) receptors, shows beneficial effects in AD, and reduces brain soluble Aβ levels, amyloid plaque burden, and cognitive impairment in treated APP/PS1 transgenic mice [150, 151]. Therefore, it seems that the positive effects of targeting insulin signaling in AD are related to the role played by insulin receptor in memory formation, inflammation and Aβ neuroprotective effects rather than to the facilitation of glucose transport into the brain [149, 150]. This hypothesis seems also to be supported by a recent study revealing that insulin did not ameliorate the disruption of energetic homeostasis induced by Aβ oligomers in cultured neurons [152]. In the end, clinical trials designed to test whether PPARγ agonists could be beneficial in AD patients provided negative results [153].

- *Shift to alternative energy source*: Under metabolically challenging conditions neurons can utilize acetyl-CoA generated from ketone body metabolism, produced distally in the liver or locally in the brain by glial cells. In this way, ketone bodies can bypass defects in glucose metabolism and enter the tricarboxylic acid cycle in the mitochondria of neurons as a source of ATP. The use of ketogenic diets reduces Aβ40 and Aβ42 levels in young AD transgenic mice [154] and enhances mitochondrial bioenergetic capacity, reducing Aβ generation and increasing mechanisms of Aβ clearance in a mouse model of AD [155]. The ketogenic compound AC-1202 administered in patients with AD has shown a significant improvement in some cognitive parameters more notable in individuals APOE4(-) [156]. Another possible alternative source of ATP is creatine. Preliminary studies have shown that creatine has protective effects against Aβ *in vitro* [157] and against injury *in vivo* by maintaining ATP levels and mitochondrial function [158], suggesting a potential therapeutic effect of creatine supplementation in AD.

2.5.2. Mitochondrial dysfunction

In addition to the already discussed antioxidant compounds, other potential drugs targeting mitochondrial dysfunction in AD are available. Several findings point towards a role for Aβ toxicity in the mitochondrial dysfunction found in AD.

The progressive Aβ accumulation in mitochondria is associated with diminished enzymatic activity of respiratory chain complexes (III and IV) and reduction in the rate of oxygen consumption, contributing to cellular dysfunction in AD [159]. Aβ in mitochondria binds to Aβ-binding alcohol dehydrogenase (ABAD) to block ABAD activity, increasing the production of ROS, reducing the mitochondrial membrane potential and the activity of the respiratory chain complex IV, and ultimately leading to a decrease in ATP levels [160]. In fact, double transgenic mice over-expressing mutated APP and ABAD exhibit exaggerated oxidative stress and memory impairment [160]. Therefore, compounds designed to block Aβ-ABAD interactions are considered putative therapeutic agents in AD. In line with this hypothesis, a recent study has shown that AG18051, a novel small ABAD-specific compound inhibitor, partially blocked the Aβ-ABAD interaction, prevented the Aβ42-induced down-regulation of ABAD activity and protected cultured neurons against Aβ42 toxicity by reducing Aβ42-induced impairment of mitochondrial function and oxidative stress [161]. Furthermore, the introduction of an ABAD-decoy peptide into transgenic APP mice reduces Aβ-ABAD interaction and protects against Aβ-mediated mitochondrial toxicity [162].

Another line of research suggests that drugs that activate ATP-sensitive potassium (K_{ATP}) channels present in the mitochondrial inner membrane exhibit therapeutic potential in the treatment of AD, as K_{ATP} channels are activated when cellular ATP levels fall below a critical value thereby reducing excitability so as to maintain ion homeostasis and preserve ATP levels [163]. Long-term administration of diazoxide improves neuronal bioenergetics, suppresses Aβ and tau pathologies, and ameliorates memory deficits in the 3xTgAD mouse model of AD [164].

Finally, another potential drug in the treatment of AD that acts on mitochondrial pathways is latrepirdine, also known as Dimebon™ [165]. Latrepirdine reduces Aβ-induced mitochondrial impairment and increases the threshold of inductors to mitochondrial pore transition, making mitochondria more resistant to lipid peroxidation and increasing neuronal survival *in vitro* [166-168]. The interest in developing latrepirdine as a drug against AD is also supported by its multiple potential mechanism of action apart from mitochondrial effects, including anti-excitotoxic agent, inhibitor of AChE, channel-regulatior and neurotrophic stimulator [165]. A preliminary clinical trial revealed that latrepirdine was safe and well tolerated, and significantly improved the clinical course of the disease in patients with mild-to-moderate AD [169]. Current phase III clinical trials are already being conducted [165].

2.6. Neurotransmitter dysfunction

The alteration of several transmitter systems is assumed to trigger both cognitive and neuropsychiatric symptoms in AD. A number of *post-mortem* studies indicate that neurotransmitter systems are not uniformly affected in AD. Thus, while cholinergic, serotonergic and glutamatergic deficits are present at relatively early stages of AD, dopaminergic and GABAergic systems appear to be affected later [170].

2.6.1. Cholinergic system

A large body of evidence has shown that basal forebrain cholinergic neurons are vulnerable to AD leading to a progressive cholinergic denervation of the cerebral neocortex [171, 172]. Taking into account the involvement of this system in the cognitive processing of memory and attention, the current attempts in cholinergic therapy in AD are justified [172, 173]. The various cholinergic strategies include the use of ACh precursors, inhibitors of cholinesterases, muscarinic and nicotinic agonists, and ACh releasers, in addition to the rescue of cholinergic function by nerve growth factor (NGF) which is reviewed in section 2.8.

- *ACh precursor.* Animal studies report that choline and lecithin increased the production of brain ACh which argues for their use in the treatment of cholinergic deficits in AD. However, evidence from randomized trials did not sustain this hypothesis [174].

- *Cholinesterase inhibitors (ChEIs).* Physostigmine, tacrine and derivatives donepezil, galantamine and rivastigmine have been tested in AD patients during the last three decades. Their therapeutic properties have been profusely reviewed [172, 175-177] and for this reason a detailed revision of ChEIs is beyond the scope of this chapter. Nevertheless, it is worth briefly indicating additional mechanisms of action of these compounds beyond inhibition of cholinesterases, including increase of nicotinc ACh receptor expression, facilitation of APP processing and attenuation of Aβ-induced toxicity [173, 178]. In spite of the fact that their efficacy has been proved in several clinical trials, only approximately 50% of patients respond positively. This limited effect of ChEIs on cognitive decline, together with the occurrence of undesirable side-effects such as diarrhea, nausea, insomnia, fatigue and loss of appetite, reduces the therapeutic capacities of ChEIs.

- *Muscarinic receptor 1 agonist.* The cholinergic deficiency in AD appears to be mainly pre-synaptic. Thus, the pharmacological stimulation of the post-synaptic M1 muscarinic receptors, which are preserved until late stages of AD, may balance the degeneration of pre-synaptic cholinergic terminals unable to properly synthesize and release ACh [173]. In fact, the selective M1 agonist AF267B reduces memory impairment, Aβ42 levels, and tau hyper-phosphorylation in AD triple transgenic mice [179], corroborating some early studies *in vitro* [180, 181]. This selective agonist is currently under clinical evaluation for safety and tolerability and a number of other M1 agonists are being investigated [173].

- *Nicotinic agonists.* Preclinical studies in animal models and some pilot studies in AD have shown that the activation of pre-synaptic nicotinic ACh receptors may reduce cognitive impairment by increasing ACh release and may have beneficial effects on Aβ metabolism [182, 183]. Thus, chronic nicotine treatment results in a significant reduction in plaque burden and in cortical Aβ concentrations in Tg2575/PS1-A246E mice [184]. However, nicotine exacerbates tau pathology in 3xTg-AD mice [185]. These apparently contradictory results may be due to the presence of several subtypes of nicotinic receptors, the activation of which may have disparate effects in AD. Therefore, more specific nicotine agonists are needed to act exclusively on determinate subtypes of nicotinic receptor [186]. In this line, α7 nAChR gene delivery into mouse hippocampal neurons leads to functional receptor expression and improves spatial memory-related performance and hyperphosphorylation of tau [187]. Regarding α4β2 nicotinic receptor, the selective agonist cytisine inhibits Aβ cytotoxicity in cortical neurons [188].

- *ACh releasers.* Facilitation of ACh release can be achieved with depolarizing agents of the cholinergic neurons acting via potassium-channel blockade as happens with linopirdine and analogues [189] or by the blockade of the pre-synaptic inhibitory M2 muscarinic receptor via specific antagonists [190, 191]. However, clinical trials using linopirdine did not demonstrate effectiveness in improving cognitive function [192]. On the other hand, certain selective M2 antagonists, such as SCH-57790 and SC-72788, restore memory impairments in animal models that mimic to some extent the cholinergic failure in AD [193]. It must be kept in mind that the potential benefit of M2 antagonists is limited because of the progressive pre-synaptic cholinergic degeneration in AD and because of the possible side-effects derived from the blockade of peripheral M2 receptors including cardiac M2 receptors.

2.6.2. Glutamatergic system

Low concentrations of Aβ oligomers are able to activate certain glutamate receptors including NMDA receptors. The activation of NMDA receptors may increase glutamate activity, raise intracellular Ca2+ concentration and promote excitotoxicity and neuronal damage [194, 195]. Another process contributing to the excessive glutamate activity in AD is the impairment of glial cells to remove glutamate form the synaptic cleft possibly due to the action of free radicals on the glutamate transporter 1 (GLT-1) [196]. Glutamatergic activation, in turn, may disrupt synaptic plasticity promoting long term depression (LTD) and inhibiting long term potentiation (LTP) of 2-amino-3-(5-methyl-3-oxo-1,2-oxazol-4-yl)propanoic acid (AMPA) receptor-mediated synaptic transmission [197]. The associated persistent reduction in the number of

http://dx.doi.org/10.5772/54783

functional synaptic AMPA receptors reduces fast excitatory transmission and eventually triggers spine retraction and synaptic loss [198]. Moreover, glutamate receptors are not only involved in the process of Aβ-mediated synaptic dysfunction but also play important roles in Aβ production [199, 200].

Based on these observations, several studies have been designed in an attempt to correct glutamatergic dysfunction in AD, including the modulation of both AMPA and NMDA receptors [201]. First attempts were carried out with AMPAKines [202], which are drugs that prolong the action of glutamate on AMPA receptors by increasing their sensitivity. Interestingly, AMPAKines proved effective in restoring cognitive deficits in aging rats [203, 204]. These compounds were tested in AD patients [205]. The modulation of the NMDA receptor was assessed via the glycine co-agonist site in rats with disrupted glutamatergic temporal systems resulting in improved learning and memory [206]. Preliminary clinical studies suggested some promising effects in AD [207] but full-scale trials have not yet been initiated.

The most relevant glutamatergic strategy against AD is the non-competitive NMDA antagonist memantine [201, 208], which has succeeded in clinical trials in moderate and severe AD as reviewed in detail elsewhere [209, 210]. Several studies performed in animal models of AD corroborate the beneficial properties of memantine as a symptomatological and neuroprotective treatment in AD [211-215]. Nevertheless, memantine has no benefits in cases with mild AD [216] suggesting that this drug is not a good choice for preventing the progression to disease states.

2.6.3. Serotonergic system

Loss of serotonergic nerve terminals in AD was described several years ago [217, 218]. Although the suggested serotonergic dysfunction was initially related almost exclusively with the neuropsychiatric symptoms of AD, including anxiety, irritability, fear and depression, recent studies have demonstrated that serotonin signaling also plays an important role in cognition and in the development of Aβ and tau pathologies [219].

Antidepressant compounds, acting through serotonin signaling, result in cognitive improvements and reduce the levels of Aβ and tau pathology in animal models of AD [220, 221]. Similar compounds reduce amyloid burden in humans [221]. Additional serotonergic compounds that are currently being investigated in AD are 5-hydroxytryptamine (5-HT or serotonin) receptors: 5-HT_1 and 5-HT_6 antagonists, and 5-HT_4 agonists. The 5-HT_{1A} antagonist lecozotan (SRA-333) enhances cognition in primates and is now being tested in AD [222-224]. The pro-cognitive effects of 5-HT_{1A} antagonists are probably due to the facilitation of glutamategic and cholinergic transmission after reduction of the inhibitory effects of serotonin. Similarly, 5-HT_6 antagonists improve cognitive performance in animal models and human beings by modulating multiple neurotransmitter systems [225]. These properties mark 5-HT_6 antagonists as potential symptomatic drugs in AD. In addition, 5-HT_4 receptor agonists are neuroprotective, modulating the production of Aβ, and have the property of ameliorating cognitive deficits [226, 227].

2.7. Synaptic dysfunction

Synaptic dysfunction and failure are processes that occur early in the Alzheimer process and progress during the course of the disease from an initially reversible functionally-responsive stage of down-regulated synaptic function to stages irreversibly associated with degeneration.

These alterations are manifested early as impaired metabotropic glutamate receptor/phospholipase C signaling pathway [230] and up-regulation of adenosine receptors in the frontal cortex in AD [231].

The initial reversible stages are important targets for protective treatments to slow progression and preserve cognitive and functional abilities [232, 233]. *In vivo* and *in vitro* studies have demonstrated that high levels of Aβ impair structural and functional plasticity of synapses by affecting the balance between excitation and inhibition and contributing to the destabilization of neuronal networks, eventually causing synaptic loss [234]. Two main designs have been proposed to antagonize synaptic plasticity-disrupting actions of Aβ oligomers in preclinical AD: maintenance of the structure and fluidity of the lipid membranes forming the synaptic buttons, and stimulation of synaptic plasticity by neurotrophic factors.

Minor changes in the fluidity of phospholipidic membranes might have an important impact on the function of synapses by influencing neurotransmitter receptor activity. In fact, AD brains exhibit altered lipid composition of lipid rafts, key membrane microdomains that facilitate the transfer of substrates and protein-protein and lipid-protein interactions, as a result of the abnormally low levels of n-3 long-chain polyunsaturated fatty acids, mainly docosahexaenoic acid (DHA), increasing viscosity and energy consumption and contributing to synaptic dysfunction [142, 235]. Abnormal lipid raft composition may also modify the activity of key enzymes that modulate the cleavage of APP to form toxic Aβ. Thus, the preservation of adequate membrane composition has become an alternative way to prevent the deleterious effect of Aβ at the synapses. DHA is a major lipid constituent of synaptic end-sites and its delivery is a prerequisite for the conversion of nerve growth cones to mature synapses [236]. Numerous epidemiological studies have highlighted the beneficial influence of DHA on the preservation of synaptic function and memory capacity in aged individuals or after Aβ exposure, whereas DHA deficiency is presented as a risk factor for AD [237]. Moreover, a number of studies have reported the beneficial effects of dietary DHA supplementation on cognition and synaptic integrity in various AD models [238]. According to thes evidence, DHA, which can be synthesized or obtained directly from fish oil, appear to be one of the most valuable diet ingredients whose neuroprotective properties contribute to preventing AD.

Cytidine 5'-diphosphocholine, CDP-choline, or citicoline is an essential intermediate in the biosynthetic pathway of structural phospholipids in cell membranes, particularly phosphatidylcholine. Chronic administration has been beneficial in patients with mild cognitive impairment [239].

Another emerging potential line to preserve synaptic function is the targeting of scaffolding proteins that modulate neurotransmitter receptor activity at the synapses. Scaffolding proteins stabilize post-synaptic receptors at the spines in close proximity to their intracellular signaling proteins, phosphatases and kinases, thereby facilitating signal-transduction cascades. Evidence from *in vitro* cell and animal models of AD indicates that reductions in the post-synaptic density membrane-associated guanylate kinase (PSD-MAGUK) proteins are linked to synaptic dysfunction that might trigger plastic changes at early stages of the Alzheimer process [240]. However, specific molecules that affect interactions between scaffolding proteins and neurotransmitter receptors are still in development and further research is necessary to evaluate their potential benefit in AD.

2.8. Neurotrophic factors

Neurotrophins represent a family of proteins that play a pivotal role in the mechanisms underlying neuronal survival, differentiation, modulation of dendritic branching and dendritic spine morphology as well as synaptic plasticity and apoptosis [241]. All the members of the neurotrophin family, including NGF, brain-derived neurotrophic factor (BDNF) and neurotrophins 3 to 7, transduce their biological effects by interacting with two types of cell surface receptors, the tyrosine kinase receptor (Trk) and the p75 pan-neurotrophin receptor ($p75^{NTR}$) [241]. Other growth factor families also related to synaptic plasticity include the cytokine family of growth factors, the transforming growth factor-β (TGFβ) family, the fibroblast growth factor family and the insulin-like growth factor family. Evidence accumulated during recent years suggests that targeting neurotrophic factor signaling can retard nerve cell degeneration and to some extent preserve synaptic function. The most studied neurotrophic factors in AD are NGF, BDNF and TGFβ1.

- *NGF*: Mature basal forebrain cholinergic neurons are highly dependent on the availability of NGF for the maintenance of their biochemical and morphological phenotype, and for survival after lesions or variegated insults [242, 243]. For this reason, exploitation of NGF activity on cholinergic neurons may provide an attractive therapeutic option for preventing cholinergic cell degeneration in AD. Levels of proNGF, the precursor form of NGF, are highly elevated in AD brains and animal models, a feature that may be associated with a reduced conversion to NGF and augmented degradation of mature NGF. These combined effects have been interpreted as causative of cholinergic atrophy in AD [244]. A role for Aβ peptide in the induction of such NGF altered metabolism has been described [245]. Minocycline, a second-generation tetracycline antibiotic known to potentiate NGF activity, is able to normalize proNGF levels and to reverse the increased activity of the NGF-degrading enzyme matrix metalloproteinase 9, as well as to increase the expression of iNOS and microglial activation, leading to improved cognitive behavior in a transgenic mouse model of AD [245]. Yet a disturbing finding is the demonstration of AD proNGF when compared to proNGF of control individuals [246-248]. Whether this abnormal form of AD-related proNGF has any impact on the pathogenesis of AD needs further investigation. Another putative therapy is the use NGF, but NGF does not readily cross the BBB and requires intra-cerebroventricular infusion to reach targeted brain areas. Pilot clinical trials were discontinued because of the side-effects of NGF infusions [249]. Therefore, the development of NGF therapy is constrained by the need to achieve adequate concentrations in the relevant brain areas with susceptible target neurons while preventing unwanted adverse effects in non-target regions or cells. Alternative strategies that are currently under development include gene therapy and nasal delivery of recombinant forms of NGF, the use of small molecules with NGF agonist activity, NGF synthesis inducers, NGF processing modulators, and proNGF antagonists [250].

- *BDNF*: This neurotrophin is normally produced in the cerebral cortex with high levels in the entorhinal cortex and hippocampus in adulthood [241]. BDNF levels are reduced in the cerebral cortex and hippocampus in AD [251-254]. Several studies have shown beneficial effects of BDNF in animal models of AD [255]. For instance, sustained BDNF gene delivery using viral vectors after disease onset resulted in elevated BDNF levels in the entorhinal cortex and hippocampus which were associated with improvement in learning and memory, and with restoration of most genes altered as a result of mutant APP expression in that specific transgenic mice model [256]. Similar results were obtained in a different mouse model of AD, and in aged rats and primates by using distinct BDNF delivery systems [256, 257]. It is worth pointing out that BDNF did not change β-amyloid plaque density in any case suggesting that the therapeutic effects of BDNF occur independently of direct action on APP processing. However, the multiple variegated effects of BDNF on neuronal function also raise the hypothetical possibility that unintended adverse effects of BDNF may limit its clinical efficacy in AD [256]. An additional point must be considered; BDNF signaling pathway is also altered in AD as TrkB expression is reduced and truncated TrkB is highly expressed in astrocytes at least in advanced stages of the disease [251]. Therefore, regarding BDNF function in AD, there is not only an alteration in the expression of BDNF but also an impaired downstream pathway that may corrupt the signal of the trophic factor acting on inappropriate receptors. Preliminary clinical trials are currently in progress to evaluate the safety and efficacy of BDNF.
- *TGFβ1*: Astrocytes and microglia are the major sources of TGF-β1 in the injured brain [258, 259]. Impaired TGF-β1 signaling has been demonstrated in AD brain, particularly at the early phase of the disease; this is associated with Aβ pathology and neurofibrillary tangle formation in animal models [260]. Reduced TGF-β1 seems to induce microglial activation [259] and ectopic cell-cycle re-activation in neurons [261]. Several drugs may induce TGF-β1 release by glial cells, including estrogens [262], mGlu2/3 agonists [263], lithium [264], the antidepressant venlafaxine [265] and glatiramer, which is a synthetic amino acid co-polymer currently approved for the treatment of multiple sclerosis [266]. All of them have neuroprotective effects in different *in vitro* and *in vivo* models of AD pathology [260]. Additionally, small molecules with specific TGF-β1-like activity are being developed as neuroprotectors [267].

A final point must be considered. A generalized sprouting is produced around β-amyloid deposits in senile plaques in both humans and in animal models [268-270]. The reasons for such sprouting are not well defined but amyloid species may play a trigger role. In any case, trophic factors might increase aberrant sprouting at the senile plaques through receptors expressed at these localizations.

2.9. Autophagy

Autophagy is a catabolic process occurring in all cell types in which the machinery of the lysosome degrades cellular components such as long-lived or damaged proteins and organelles. Thus, a failure of autophagy in neurons results in the accumulation of aggregate-prone proteins that might exacerbate neurodegenerative process [271, 272]. Autophagy is also implicated in the accumulation of altered mitochondria and polymorphous inclusions in the dystrophic neurites around amyloid plaques [273-278].

Indeed, autophagic dysfunction is implicated in the progression of Alzheimer from the earliest stage, when a defective lysosomal clearance of autophagic substrates and impaired autophagy initiation occurs and leads to massive buildup of incompletely digested substrates within dystrophic axons and dendrites [279]. The pharmacological induction of 'preserved' autophagy might enhance the clearance of intracytoplasmic aggregate-prone proteins and therefore ameliorate pathology [272]. Attempts to restore more normal lysosomal proteolysis and autophagy efficiency in mouse models of AD pathology have revealed promising therapeutic effects on neuronal function and cognitive performance, demonstrating the relevance of the failure of autophagy in the pathogenesis of AD, and the potential of autophagy modulation as a therapeutic strategy. Autophagy induction with the mTOR-inhibiting drug rapamycin in young mice resulted in a reduction in Aβ plaques, NFT and cognitive deficits in the adulthood in two different models of AD [280-283]. Interestingly, rapamycin did not alter any of those parameters when administered in old animals once the pathology was established, highlighting the importance of early treatmenting in the disease progression [282]. However, the kinase mTOR plays an important role in multiple signaling pathways apart from negatively regulating autophagy [284]. Therefore, rapamycin treatment is also a putative inducer of undesirable side-effects. Other drugs including lithium, sodium valproate and carbamazepine acting have ben proved to induce autophagy through the inhibition of of inositol monophosphatase in an mTOR-independent pathway [285]. These compunds reveal positive effects by reducing the accumulation and toxic effects of aggregation-prone proteins in cell models as well as by protecting against neurodegeneration in *in vivo* models of Huntington's disease [286]. Further research is needed to learn whether they can also be useful tools in the treatment of AD.

2.10. Multi-target treatments

Considering the multifactorial etiology of AD, and the numerous and complex pathological mechanisms involved in the progression of the disease, it is quite reasonable that treatments targeting a single causal or modifying factor may have limited benefits. Therefore, growing interest is focused on therapeutic agents with pleiotropic activity, which will be able to target, in parallel, several processes affected in AD [287, 288]. Several compounds already mentioned in the previous sections fulfill these properties, such as DHA which presents anti-inflammatory, anti-oxidant, neuroprotective and anti-tau phosphorylation properties apart from the modulation of synaptic membrane composition [289], and curcumin, which in addition to anti-oxidant properties also exhibits anti-inflammatory and Aβ- and tau-binding properties [106]. Similarly, rosiglitazone and dimebon are known to produce beneficial effects through insulin receptor signaling modulation and mitochondrial protection [153, 165]. Other multi-target potential treatments currently under development for AD are based on the use of the following compounds:

- *Caffeine*: This is one of the most consumed psychoactive drugs which mainly acts blocking adenosine receptors 1 and 2 [290, 291]. In addition, caffeine reduces amyloid burden in animal models of AD [292, 293]. Epidemiological studies in humans have also shown protection against cognitive decline [294-296].
- *Estrogen*: This steroid hormone is known to play an important role in neuronal survival, mitochondrial function, neuroinflammation and cognition, with important neuroprotective effects [297-299]. Some of the neuroprotective actions mediated by estrogens are related to the insulin-like growth factor-1 (IGF-1) signaling pathway [300]. Several studies in animal models of AD have revealed therapeutic properties of estrogen against the progression of the disease. For instance, the treatment of ovariectomized 3xTg-AD mice with estrogen resulted in prevention of the increased Aβ accumulation and worsening memory performance induced by the depletion of sex steroid hormones [301]. Clinical and epidemiological studies in AD support the beneficial effets of estrogens [302]. However, a critical factor for success in estrogen therapy for AD is the age at the initiation of the treatment; the efficacy of estrogens is greatest in younger women and in women who initiated the estrogen therapy at the time of menopause [303].
- *Cannabinoids*: The natural compounds derived from *Cannabis sativa* or synthetic compounds acting on endogenous cannabinoid system have emerged as potential agents against several neurodegenerative processes [305]. Cannabinoids offer a multi-faceted approach for the treatment of AD as the stimulation of the widely brain-expressed cannabinoid receptors provides neuroprotection against Aβ [305, 306] and reduces neuroinflammation [306-308] and tau phosphorylation [306, 309] in AD-like transgenic mice. In addition, cannabinoids support brain repair mechanisms by augmenting neurotrophin expression and enhancing neurogenesis [310]. Moreover, cannabinoids are able to reduce Aβ-dependent oxidative stress [311] and Aβ-mediated lysosomal destabilization related to apoptosis [312]. In addition, some cannabinoids are able to inhibit acetylcholinesterase activity [313]. It is worth stressing that molecular achievements of cannabinoids are accompanied by cognitive improvement and reduction of several degenerative markers in two different animal models of AD [306, 308]. Examination of the potential beneficial effects of chronic administration of low doses of cannabinoids with little psychotropic effect at early stages of the degenerative process in humans seems very promising.
- *Erythropoietin (EPO) and derivatives*: EPO is effective in neuroprotection against ischemia and traumatic brain injury [314]. In addition, animal studies reveal that EPO both reduces tau phosphorylation through modulation of PI3K/Akt-GSK-3beta pathway [315] and protects against Aβ-induced cell death through anti-oxidant mechanisms [316]. An additional characteristic of EPO that confers potential utility in AD is the specific effect on cognition: EPO enhances hippocampal LTP and memory by modulating plasticity, synaptic connectivity and activity of memory-related neuronal networks [317]. In spite of these benefits, chronic administration of EPO is problematic because of the concomitant excessive erythropoiesis. In this sense, some new derivatives of EPO that do not bind to the classical EPO

receptor (carbamylated EPO) or that have such a brief half-life in the circulation that they do not stimulate erythropoiesis (asialo EPO and neuro EPO) have demonstrated neuroprotective activities without the potential adverse effects on circulation associated with EPO [318]. Therefore, these new compounds are considered as potential treatments in AD.

- *Statins*: Evidence has accumulated that a high cholesterol level may increase the risk of developing AD and that the use of statins to treat hyper-cholesterolemia is useful in treating and preventing AD [319]. Statins reduce the production of cholesterol and isoprenoid intermediates. These isoprenoids modulate the turnover of small GTPase molecules that are essential in numerous cell-signaling pathways, including vesicular trafficking and inflammation [320]. Thus, statins reduce the production of Aβ by disrupting secretase enzyme function and by curbing neuroinflammation in experimental models of AD [321, 322].
- *Ladostigil* is a dual acetylcholine-butyrylcholineesterase and brain selective monoamine oxidase (MAO)-A and -B inhibitor *in vivo*. Interest in this compound in AD treatment research is sustained by the potential increase in brain cholinergic activity properties but also by the capacity of ladostigil to prevent gliosis and oxidative-nitrosative stress damage. Moreover, ladostigil has been demonstrated to possess potent anti-apoptotic and neuroprotective properties *in vitro* and in various neurodegenerative animal models including AD transgenic mice [323]. These neuroprotective activities involve regulation of APP processing, activation of protein kinase C and mitogen-activated protein kinase signaling pathways, inhibition of neuronal death markers, prevention of the fall in mitochondrial membrane potential, up-regulation of neurotrophic factors, and anti-oxidative activity.
- *Huperzine A* is an extract of the Chinese plant *Huperzia serrata*. Huperzine A is a selective potent inhibitor of AChE [324]. In addition, some studies have shown that huperzine A may shift APP metabolism towards the non-amyloidogenic α-secretase pathway [325]. In addition, huperzine A reduces glutamate-induced cytotoxicity by antagonizing cerebral NMDA receptors [326]. Finally, huperzine A reverses or attenuates cognitive deficits in some animal models of AD [325]. Large-scale, randomized, placebo-controlled trials are necessary to establish the role of huperzine A in the treatment of AD [327].
- *Phytochemicals* as curcumin, catechins and resveratrol beyond their antioxidant activity are also involved in antiamyloidogenic, anti-inflammatory mechanisms and inhibitors of NFkappaB [328-330].
- *Celastrol* is another compound whicha appears to have multiple functions as anti-inflammatory, anti-oxidant and reductor of amyloouid via BACE 1 [331, 332].

3. Concluding remarks

Main targets of therapeutic intervention at early stages of Alzheimer are summarized in Figure 1. Based on the presently available data several conclusions can be drawn. Combination therapies with drugs targeting different pathological factors or the use of multi-target compounds appear to be the most effective strategy in the treatment of the neurodegenerative process in Alzheimer. Most potential experimental therapies exhibit the highest efficiency when applied during the pre-symptomatic phase of the disease. Therefore, it is essential to develop diagnostic tools to detect Alzheimer at early stages. Moreover, considering that Alzheimer, as a degenerative process not necessarily leading to dementia, affects a large percentage of individuals in the sixth decade of life, it would be wise to introduce habits and low-cost, safe treatments to prevent the progression of Alzheimer early in life, as occurs in artheriosclerosis, to transform AD into a chronic, incomplete and non-devastating disease thereby allowing for normal life in the elderly.

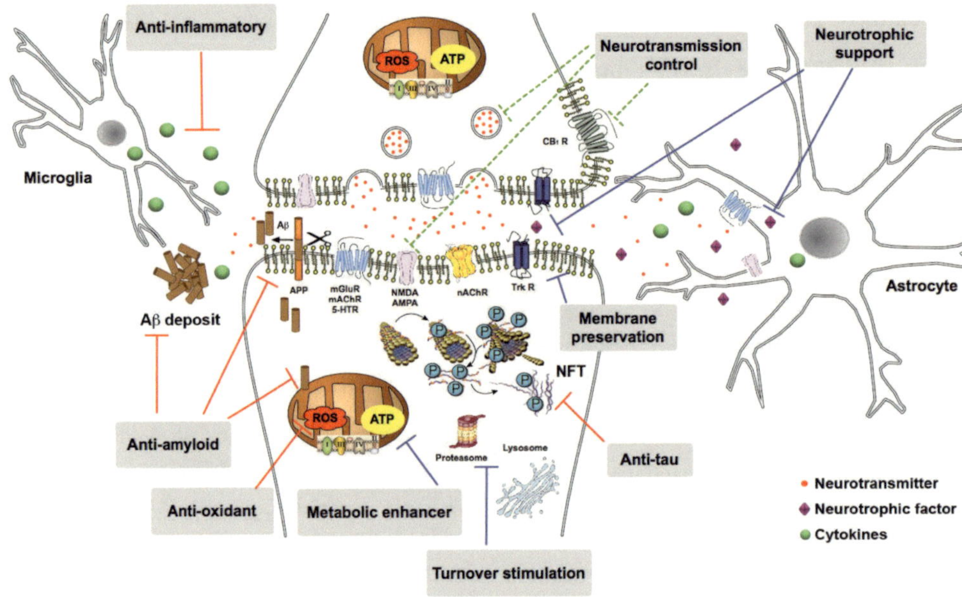

Figure 1. Schematic representation of the main cellular targets that are currently under development to prevent or retard the progression of Alzheimer to disease states. Most of the experimental approaches are designed to block or mitigate (red lines) pathological events occurring at the earliest stages, including abnormal Aβ and tau aggregation, chronic inflammatory responses, and oxidative stress damage. Other strategies (blue lines) aim at stimulating the metabolism to reduce Alzheimer's energetic failure as well as to promote intrinsic mechanisms that protect or repair cellular damage, including synaptic plasticity, preservation of the lipid membrane composition, and the promotion of damaged protein and organelle turnover. Therapeutic approaches based on the modulation of neurotransmission (green dashed lines) are designed to bypass deficient cholinergic neurotransmission whereas other compounds aim to block glutamatergic excitotoxicity. Considering the complex scenario of the Alzheimer neurodegenerative process, multi-target therapies applied at early stages of the disease appear to be the most effective strategy.

In addition to these general conclusions, several points deserve a particular comment. Recognition of the genotypic background, clinical and neuropathological subtypes and different pace of clinical manifestations is important to refine personalized treatments [333-335]. This includes modifications of the treatment as Alzheimer is not a mere accumulation of defects but rather a combination of deficiencies and plastic changes that imply shifts in molecular pathways with disease progression. Drugs and treatments beneficious at first stages of the degenerative process may be harmful at advanced stages. Special effort must be put into practice to learn about the combination of drugs at which determinate time for every particular individual.

Acknowledgements

Parts of the work used in this review were supported by the project BESAD-P (Instituto Carlos III), Mutua Madrileña and Agrupación Mútua. We wish to thank T. Yohannan for editorial assistance.

Author details

Ester Aso and Isidre Ferrer*

*Address all correspondence to: 8082ifa@gmail.com

Institut de Neuropatologia, Hospital Universitari de Bellvitge, Universitat de Barcelona, CIBERNED, Spain

References

[1] Ferrer I. Defining Alzheimer as a common age-related neurodegenerative process not inevitably leading to dementia. Prog Neurobiol. 2012; 97: 38-51.

[2] Petot GJ, Friedland RP. Lipids, diet and Alzheimer disease: an extended summary. J Neurol Sci. 2004; 226: 31-3.

[3] Luchsinger JAQ, Tang Noble JM, Scarmeas N. Diet and Alzheimer's disease. Curr Neurol Neurosci Rep. 2007; 7: 366-72.

[4] Kovacs GG, Alafuzoff I, Al-Sarraj S, Arzberger T, Bogdanovic N, Capellari S, Ferrer I, Gelpi E, Kövari V, Kretzschmar H, Nagy Z, Parchi P, Seilhean D, Soininen H, Troakes C, Budka H. Mixed brain pathologies in dementia: the brainNet Europe consortium experience. Dementia. 2008; 26: 343-50.

[5] Ferrer I. Cognitive impairment of vasxcular origin: Neuropathology of cognitive impairment of vascular origin. J Neurol Sci. 2010; 299-339-49.

[6] De Strooper B, Vassar R, Golde T. The secretases: enzymes with therapeutic potential in Alzheimer disease. Nat Rev Neurol. 2010; 6: 99-107

[7] Ring S, Weyer SW, Kilian SB, Waldron E, Pietrzik CU, Filippov MA, Herms J,Buchholz C, Eckman CB, Korte M, Wolfer DP, Müller UC. The secreted beta-amyloid precursor

protein ectodomain APPs alpha is sufficient to rescue the anatomical, behavioral, and electrophysiological abnormalities of APP-deficient mice. J Neurosci. 2007; 27: 7817-26.

[8] Bandyopadhyay S, Goldstein LE, Lahiri DK, Rogers JT. Role of the APP non-amyloidogenic signaling pathway and targeting alpha-secretase as an alternative drug target for treatment of Alzheimer's disease. Curr Med Chem. 2007; 14: 2848-64.

[9] Laird FM, Cai H, Savonenko AV, Farah MH, He K, Melnikova T, Wen H, Chiang HC, Xu G, Koliatsos VE, Borchelt DR, Price DL, Lee HK, Wong PC. BACE1, a major determinant of selective vulnerability of the brain to amyloid-beta amyloidogenesis, is essential for cognitive, emotional, and synaptic functions. J Neurosci. 2005; 25:11693-709.

[10] McConlogue L, Buttini M, Anderson JP, Brigham EF, Chen KS, Freedman SB, Games D, Johnson-Wood K, Lee M, Zeller M, Liu W, Motter R, Sinha S. Partial reduction of BACE1 has dramatic effects on Alzheimer plaque and synaptic pathology in APP Transgenic Mice. J Biol Chem. 2007; 282: 26326-34.

[11] Hills ID, Vacca JP. Progress toward a practical BACE-1 inhibitor. Curr Opin Drug Discov Devel. 2007; 10: 383-91.

[12] Rajendran L, Schneider A, Schlechtingen G, Weidlich S, Ries J, Braxmeier T, Schwille P, Schulz JB, Schroeder C, Simons M, Jennings G, Knölker HJ, Simons K. Efficient inhibition of the Alzheimer's disease beta-secretase by membrane targeting. Science. 2008; 320: 520-3.

[13] Serneels L, Van Biervliet J, Craessaerts K, Dejaegere T, Horré K, Van Houtvin T, Esselmann H, Paul S, Schäfer MK, Berezovska O, Hyman BT, Sprangers B, Sciot R, Moons L, Jucker M, Yang Z, May PC, Karran E, Wiltfang J, D'Hooge R, De Strooper B. gamma-Secretase heterogeneity in the Aph1 subunit: relevance for Alzheimer's disease. Science. 2009; 324: 639-42.

[14] Serneels L, Dejaegere T, Craessaerts K, Horré K, Jorissen E, Tousseyn T, Hébert S, Coolen M, Martens G, Zwijsen A, Annaert W, Hartmann D, De Strooper B. Differential contribution of the three Aph1 genes to gamma-secretase activity in vivo. Proc Natl Acad Sci U S A. 2005; 102:1719-24.

[15] Dovey HF, John V, Anderson JP, Chen LZ, de Saint Andrieu P, Fang LY, Freedman SB, Folmer B, Goldbach E, Holsztynska EJ, Hu KL, Johnson-Wood KL, Kennedy SL, Kholodenko D, Knops JE, Latimer LH, Lee M, Liao Z, Lieberburg IM, Motter RN, Mutter LC, Nietz J, Quinn KP, Sacchi KL, Seubert PA, Shopp GM, Thorsett ED, Tung JS, Wu J, Yang S, Yin CT, Schenk DB, May PC, Altstiel LD, Bender MH, Boggs LN, Britton TC, Clemens JC, Czilli DL, Dieckman-McGinty DK, Droste JJ, Fuson KS, Gitter BD, Hyslop PA, Johnstone EM, Li WY, Little SP, Mabry TE, Miller FD, Audia JE. Functional gamma-secretase inhibitors reduce beta-amyloid peptide levels in brain. J Neurochem. 2001; 76: 173-81.

[16] Abramowski D, Wiederhold KH, Furrer U, Jaton AL, Neuenschwander A, Runser MJ, Danner S, Reichwald J, Ammaturo D, Staab D, Stoeckli M, Rueeger H, Neumann U,

Staufenbiel M. Dynamics of Abeta turnover and deposition in different beta-amyloid precursor protein transgenic mouse models following gamma-secretase inhibition. J Pharmacol Exp Ther. 2008; 327: 411-24.

[17] Bateman RJ, Siemers ER, Mawuenyega KG, Wen G, Browning KR, Sigurdson WC, Yarasheski KE, Friedrich SW, Demattos RB, May PC, Paul SM, Holtzman DM. A gamma-secretase inhibitor decreases amyloid-beta production in the central nervous system. Ann Neurol. 2009; 66: 48-54.

[18] Schor NF. What the halted phase III γ-secretase inhibitor trial may (or may not) be telling us. Ann Neurol. 2011; 69: 237-9.

[19] Netzer WJ, Dou F, Cai D, Veach D, Jean S, Li Y, Bornmann WG, Clarkson B, Xu H, Greengard P. Gleevec inhibits beta-amyloid production but not Notch cleavage. Proc Natl Acad Sci USA. 2003; 100:12444-9.

[20] Mayer SC, Kreft AF, Harrison B, Abou-Gharbia M, Antane M, Aschmies S, Atchison K, Chlenov M, Cole DC, Comery T, Diamantidis G, Ellingboe J, Fan K, Galante R, Gonzales C, Ho DM, Hoke ME, Hu Y, Huryn D, Jain U, Jin M, Kremer K, Kubrak D, Lin M, Lu P, Magolda R, Martone R, Moore W, Oganesian A, Pangalos MN, Porte A, Reinhart P, Resnick L, Riddell DR, Sonnenberg-Reines J, Stock JR, Sun SC, Wagner E, Wang T, Woller K, Xu Z, Zaleska MM, Zeldis J, Zhang M, Zhou H, Jacobsen JS. Discovery of begacestat, a Notch-1-sparing gamma-secretase inhibitor for the treatment of Alzheimer's disease. J Med Chem. 2008; 51: 7348-51.

[21] Borgegard T, Juréus A, Olsson F, Rosqvist S, Sabirsh A, Rotticci D, Paulsen K,Klintenberg R, Yan H, Waldman M, Stromberg K, Nord J, Johansson J, Regner A,Parpal S, Malinowsky D, Radesater AC, Li T, Singh R, Eriksson H, Lundkvist J. First and second generation γ-secretase modulators (GSMs) modulate amyloid-β (Aβ) peptide production through different mechanisms. J Biol Chem. 2012; 287:11810-9.

[22] D'Onofrio G, Panza F, Frisardi V, Solfrizzi V, Imbimbo BP, Paroni G, Cascavilla L, Seripa D, Pilotto A. Advances in the identification of γ-secretase inhibitors for the treatment of Alzheimer's disease. Expert Opin Drug Discov. 2012; 7: 19-37.

[23] Shirotani K, Tsubuki S, Iwata N, Takaki Y, Harigaya W, Maruyama K, Kiryu-Seo S, Iwata H, Tomita T, Iwatsubo T, Saiudo TC. Neprilysin degrades both amyloid beta peptides 1-40 and 142 most rapidly and efficiently among thiorphan- and phosphoramidon-sensitive endopeptidases. J Biol Chem. 2001; 276: 21895-901.

[24] Iwata N, Takaki Y, Fukami S, Tsubuki S, Saido TC. Region-specific reduction of A beta-degrading endopeptidase, neprilysin, in mouse hippocampus upon aging. J Neurosci Res. 2002; 70: 493-500.

[25] Wang DS, Iwata N, Hama E, Saido TC, Dickson DW. Oxidized neprilysin in aging and Alzheimer's disease brains. Biochem Biophys Res Commun. 2003; 310: 236-41.

[26] Marr RA, Rockenstein E, Mukherjee A, Kindy MS, Hersh LB, Gage FH, Verma IM, Masliah E. Neprilysin gene transfer reduces human amyloid pathology in transgenic mice. J Neurosci. 2003; 23: 1992-6.

[27] Nalivaeva NN, Beckett C, Belyaev ND, Turner AJ. Are amyloid-degrading enzymes viable therapeutic targets in Alzheimer's disease? J Neurochem. 2012; 120 Suppl 1:167-85.

[28] Leissring MA, Farris W, Chang AY, Walsh DM, Wu X, Sun X, Frosch MP, Selkoe DJ. Enhanced proteolysis of beta-amyloid in APP transgenic mice prevents plaque formation, secondary pathology, and premature death. Neuron. 2003; 40: 1087-93.

[29] Qiu WQ, Folstein MF. Insulin, insulin-degrading enzyme and amyloid-beta peptide in Alzheimer's disease: review and hypothesis. Neurobiol Aging. 2006; 27: 190-8.

[30] Miners JS, Barua N, Kehoe PG, Gill S, Love S. Aβ-degrading enzymes: potential for treatment of Alzheimer disease. J Neuropathol Exp Neurol. 2011; 70: 944-59.

[31] Aisen PS, Gauthier S, Vellas B, Briand R, Saumier D, Laurin J, Garceau D. Alzhemed: a potential treatment for Alzheimer's disease. Curr Alzheimer Res. 2007; 4: 473-8.

[32] Aisen PS, Gauthier S, Ferris SH, Saumier D, Haine D, Garceau D, Duong A, Suhy J, Oh J, Lau WC, Sampalis J. Tramiprosate in mild-to-moderate Alzheimer's disease _ a randomized, double-blind, placebo-controlled, multi-centre study (The Alphase study). Arch Med Sci. 2011; 7: 102-11.

[33] Fenili D, Brown M, Rappaport R, McLaurin J. Properties of scyllo-inositol as a therapeutic treatment of AD-like pathology. J Mol Med (Berl). 2007; 85: 603-11.

[34] Hawkes CA, Deng LH, Shaw JE, Nitz M, McLaurin J. Small molecule beta-amyloid inhibitors that stabilize protofibrillar structures in vitro improve cognition and pathology in a mouse model of Alzheimer's disease. Eur J Neurosci. 2010; 31: 203-13.

[35] Salloway S, Sperling R, Keren R, Porsteinsson AP, van Dyck CH, Tariot PN, Gilman S, Arnold D, Abushakra S, Hernandez C, Crans G, Liang E, Quinn G, Bairu M, Pastrak A, Cedarbaum JM; ELND005-AD201 Investigators. A phase 2 randomized trial of ELND005, scyllo-inositol, in mild to moderate Alzheimer disease. Neurology. 2011; 77: 1253-62.

[36] Adlard PA, Cherny RA, Finkelstein DI, Gautier E, Robb E, Cortes M, Volitakis I, Liu X, Smith JP, Perez K, Laughton K, Li QX, Charman SA, Nicolazzo JA, Wilkins S, Deleva K, Lynch T, Kok G, Ritchie CW, Tanzi RE, Cappai R, Masters CL, Barnham KJ, Bush AI. Rapid restoration of cognition in Alzheimer's transgenic mice with 8-hydroxy quinoline analogs is associated with decreased interstitial Abeta. Neuron. 2008 59: 43-55.

[37] Faux NG, Ritchie CW, Gunn A, Rembach A, Tsatsanis A, Bedo J, Harrison J, Lannfelt L, Blennow K, Zetterberg H, Ingelsson M, Masters CL, Tanzi RE, Cummings JL, Herd

CM, Bush AI. PBT2 rapidly improves cognition in Alzheimer's Disease: additional phase II analyses. J Alzheimers Dis. 2010; 20: 509-16.

[38] Klajnert B, Cladera J, Bryszewska M. Molecular interactions of dendrimers with amyloid peptides: pH dependence. Biomacromolecules. 2006; 7: 2186-91.

[39] Klajnert B, Cortijo-Arellano M, Cladera J, Bryszewska M. Influence of dendrimer's structure on its activity against amyloid fibril formation. Biochem Biophys Res Commun. 2006; 345: 21-8.

[40] Klementieva O, Benseny-Cases N, Gella A, Appelhans D, Voit B, Cladera J. Dense shell glycodendrimers as potential nontoxic anti-amyloidogenic agents in Alzheimer's disease. Amyloid-dendrimer aggregates morphology and cell toxicity. Biomacromolecules. 2011; 12: 3903-9.

[41] Schenk D, Barbour R, Dunn W, Gordon G, Grajeda H, Guido T, Hu K, Huang J, Johnson-Wood K, Khan K, Kholodenko D, Lee M, Liao Z, Lieberburg I, Motter R, Mutter L, Soriano F, Shopp G, Vasquez N, Vandevert C, Walker S, Wogulis M, Yednock T, Games D, Seubert P. Immunization with amyloid-beta attenuates Alzheimer-disease-like pathology in the PDAPP mouse. Nature. 1999; 400:173-7.

[42] Janus C, Pearson J, McLaurin J, Mathews PM, Jiang Y, Schmidt SD, Chishti MA, Horne P, Heslin D, French J, Mount HT, Nixon RA, Mercken M, Bergeron C, Fraser PE, St George-Hyslop P, Westaway D. A beta peptide immunization reduces behavioural impairment and plaques in a model of Alzheimer's disease. Nature. 2000; 408: 979-82.

[43] Morgan D, Diamond DM, Gottschall PE, Ugen KE, Dickey C, Hardy J, Duff K, Jantzen P, DiCarlo G, Wilcock D, Connor K, Hatcher J, Hope C, Gordon M, Arendash GW. A beta peptide vaccination prevents memory loss in an animal model of Alzheimer's disease. Nature. 2000; 408: 982-5.

[44] Orgogozo JM, Gilman S, Dartigues JF, Laurent B, Puel M, Kirby LC, Jouanny P, Dubois B, Eisner L, Flitman S, Michel BF, Boada M, Frank A, Hock C. Subacute meningoencephalitis in a subset of patients with AD after Abeta42 immunization. Neurology. 2003; 61: 46-54.

[45] Nicoll JA, Wilkinson D, Holmes C, Steart P, Markham H, Weller RO. Neuropathology of human Alzheimer disease after immunization with amyloid-beta peptide: a case report. Nat Med. 2003; 9: 448-52.

[46] Ferrer I, Boada Rovira M, Sánchez Guerra ML, Rey MJ, Costa-Jussá F. Neuropathology and pathogenesis of encephalitis following amyloid-beta immunization in Alzheimer's disease. Brain Pathol. 2004; 14: 11-20.

[47] Meyer-Luehmann M, Mora JR, Mielke M, Spires-Jones TL, de Calignon A, von Andrian UH, Hyman BT. T cell mediated cerebral hemorrhages and microhemorrhages during passive Abeta immunization in APPPS1 transgenic mice. Mol Neurodegener. 2011; 6: 22.

[48] Patton RL, Kalback WM, Esh CL, Kokjohn TA, Van Vickle GD, Luehrs DC, Kuo YM, Lopez J, Brune D, Ferrer I, Masliah E, Newel AJ, Beach TG, Castaño EM, Roher AE. Amyloid-beta peptide remnants in AN-1792-immunized Alzheimer's disease patients: a biochemical analysis. Am J Pathol. 2006; 169: 1048-63.

[49] Nicoll JA, Barton E, Boche D, Neal JW, Ferrer I, Thompson P, Vlachouli C, Wilkinson D, Bayer A, Games D, Seubert P, Schenk D, Holmes C. Abeta species removal after abeta42 immunization. J Neuropathol Exp Neurol. 2006 ; 65: 1040-8.

[50] Serrano-Pozo A, William CM, Ferrer I, Uro-Coste E, Delisle MB, Maurage CA, Hock C, Nitsch RM, Masliah E, Growdon JH, Frosch MP, Hyman BT. Beneficial effect of human anti-amyloid-beta active immunization on neurite morphology and tau pathology. Brain. 2010; 133: 1312-27.

[51] Agadjanyan MG, Ghochikyan A, Petrushina I, Vasilevko V, Movsesyan N, Mkrtichyan M, Saing T, Cribbs DH. Prototype Alzheimer's disease vaccine using the immunodominant B cell epitope from beta-amyloid and promiscuous T cell epitope pan HLA DR-binding peptide. J Immunol. 2005; 174:1580-6.

[52] McLaurin J, Cecal R, Kierstead ME, Tian X, Phinney AL, Manea M, French JE, Lambermon MH, Darabie AA, Brown ME, Janus C, Chishti MA, Horne P, Westaway D, Fraser PE, Mount HT, Przybylski M, St George-Hyslop P. Therapeutically effective antibodies against amyloid-beta peptide target amyloid-beta residues 4-10 and inhibit cytotoxicity and fibrillogenesis. Nat Med. 2002; 8: 1263-9.

[53] Lemere CA, Maier M, Jiang L, Peng Y, Seabrook TJ. Amyloid-beta immunotherapy for the prevention and treatment of Alzheimer disease: lessons from mice, monkeys, and humans. Rejuvenation Res. 2006; 9: 77-84.

[54] Wilcock DM, Alamed J, Gottschall PE, Grimm J, Rosenthal A, Pons J, Ronan V, Symmonds K, Gordon MN, Morgan D. Deglycosylated anti-amyloid-beta antibodies eliminate cognitive deficits and reduce parenchymal amyloid with minimal vascular consequences in aged amyloid precursor protein transgenic mice. J Neurosci. 2006; 26: 5340-6.

[55] Solomon B, Frenkel D. Immunotherapy for Alzheimer's disease. Neuropharmacology. 2010; 59: 303-9.

[56] Delrieu J, Ousset PJ, Caillaud C, Vellas B. 'Clinical trials in Alzheimer's disease': immunotherapy approaches. J Neurochem. 2012; 120 Suppl 1:186-93.

[57] Golde TE, Schneider LS, Koo EH. Anti-aβ therapeutics in Alzheimer's disease: the need for a paradigm shift. Neuron. 2011; 69: 203-13.

[58] Morris M, Maeda S, Vossel K, Mucke L. The many faces of tau. Neuron. 2011; 70: 410-26.

[59] Huang Y, Mucke L. Alzheimer mechanisms and therapeuthic strategies. Cell 2012; 148: 1204-22.

[60] Wischik CM, Edwards PC, Lai RY, Roth M, Harrington CR. Selective inhibition of Alzheimer disease-like tau aggregation by phenothiazines. Proc Natl Acad Sci USA. 1996; 93:11213-8.

[61] O'Leary JC 3rd, Li Q, Marinec P, Blair LJ, Congdon EE, Johnson AG, Jinwal UK, Koren J 3rd, Jones JR, Kraft C, Peters M, Abisambra JF, Duff KE, Weeber EJ, Gestwicki JE, Dickey CA. Phenothiazine-mediated rescue of cognition in tau transgenic mice requires neuroprotection and reduced soluble tau burden. Mol Neurodegener. 2010; 5: 45.

[62] Gura T. Hope in Alzheimer's fight emerges from unexpected places. Nat Med. 2008; 14: 894.

[63] Yoshiyama Y, Higuchi M, Zhang B, Huang SM, Iwata N, Saido TC, Maeda J, Suhara T, Trojanowski JQ, Lee VM. Synapse loss and microglial activation precede tangles in a P301S tauopathy mouse model. Neuron. 2007; 53: 337-51.

[64] Chambraud B, Sardin E, Giustiniani J, Dounane O, Schumacher M, Goedert M, Baulieu EE. A role for FKBP52 in Tau protein function. Proc Natl Acad Sci U S A. 2010; 107: 2658-63.

[65] Taniguchi S, Suzuki N, Masuda M, Hisanaga S, Iwatsubo T, Goedert M, Hasegawa M. Inhibition of heparin-induced tau filament formation by phenothiazines, polyphenols, and porphyrins. J Biol Chem. 2005; 280: 7614-23.

[66] Gong CX, Iqbal K. Hyperphosphorylation of microtubule-associated protein tau: a promising therapeutic target for Alzheimer disease. Curr Med Chem. 2008; 15: 2321-8.

[67] Mi K, Johnson GV. The role of tau phosphorylation in the pathogenesis of Alzheimer's disease. Curr Alzheimer Res. 2006; 3: 449-63.

[68] Hernández F, de Barreda EG, Fuster-Matanzo A, Goñi-Oliver P, Lucas JJ, Avila J. The role of GSK3 in Alzheimer disease. Brain Res Bull. 2009; 80: 248-50.

[69] Mazanetz MP, Fischer PM. Untangling tau hyperphosphorylation in drug design for neurodegenerative diseases. Nat Rev Drug Discov. 2007; 6: 464-79.

[70] Noble W, Planel E, Zehr C, Olm V, Meyerson J, Suleman F, Gaynor K, Wang L, LaFrancois J, Feinstein B, Burns M, Krishnamurthy P, Wen Y, Bhat R, Lewis J, Dickson D, Duff K. Inhibition of glycogen synthase kinase-3 by lithium correlates with reduced tauopathy and degeneration in vivo. Proc Natl Acad Sci U S A. 2005; 102: 6990-5.

[71] Grandjean EM, Aubry JM. Lithium: updated human knowledge using an evidence-based approach. Part II: Clinical pharmacology and therapeutic monitoring. CNS Drugs. 2009; 23: 331-49.

[72] Alvarez A, Toro R, Cáceres A, Maccioni RB. Inhibition of tau phosphorylating protein kinase cdk5 prevents beta-amyloid-induced neuronal death. FEBS Lett. 1999; 459: 421-6

[73] Zheng YL, Kesavapany S, Gravell M, Hamilton RS, Schubert M, Amin N, Albers W, Grant P, Pant HC. A Cdk5 inhibitory peptide reduces tau hyperphosphorylation and apoptosis in neurons. EMBO J. 2005; 24: 209-20.

[74] Wen Y, Planel E, Herman M, Figueroa HY, Wang L, Liu L, Lau LF, Yu WH, Duff KE. Interplay between cyclin-dependent kinase 5 and glycogen synthase kinase 3 beta mediated by neuregulin signaling leads to differential effects on tau phosphorylation and amyloid precursor protein processing. J Neurosci. 2008; 28: 2624-32.

[75] Cheung ZH, Ip NY. Cdk5: a multifaceted kinase in neurodegenerative diseases. Trends Cell Biol. 2012; 22: 169-75.

[76] Li L, Sengupta A, Haque N, Grundke-Iqbal I, Iqbal K. Memantine inhibits and reverses the Alzheimer type abnormal hyperphosphorylation of tau and associated neurodegeneration. FEBS Lett. 2004; 566: 261-9.

[77] Cheng Y, Feng Z, Zhang QZ, Zhang JT. Beneficial effects of melatonin in experimental models of Alzheimer disease. Acta Pharmacol Sin. 2006; 27: 129-39.

[78] Torrent L, Ferrer I. PP2A and Alzheimer disease. Curr Alzheimer Res. 2012; 9: 248-56.

[79] Ittner LM, Ke YD, Delerue F, Bi M, Gladbach A, van Eersel J, Wölfing H, Chieng BC, Christie MJ, Napier IA, Eckert A, Staufenbiel M, Hardeman E, Götz J. Dendritic function of tau mediates amyloid-beta toxicity in Alzheimer's disease mouse models. Cell. 2010 ; 142: 387-97.

[80] Roberson ED, Scearce-Levie K, Palop JJ, Yan F, Cheng IH, Wu T, Gerstein H, Yu GQ, Mucke L. Reducing endogenous tau ameliorates amyloid beta-induced deficits in an Alzheimer's disease mouse model. Science. 2007; 316: 750-4.

[81] Roberson ED, Halabisky B, Yoo JW, Yao J, Chin J, Yan F, Wu T, Hamto P, Devidze N, Yu GQ, Palop JJ, Noebels JL, Mucke L. Amyloid-β/Fyn-induced synaptic, network, and cognitive impairments depend on tau levels in multiple mouse models of Alzheimer's disease. J Neurosci. 2011; 31: 700-11.

[82] Sahara N, Murayama M, Mizoroki T, Urushitani M, Imai Y, Takahashi R, Murata S, Tanaka K, Takashima A. In vivo evidence of CHIP up-regulation attenuating tau aggregation. J Neurochem. 2005; 94:1254-63.

[83] Min SW, Cho SH, Zhou Y, Schroeder S, Haroutunian V, Seeley WW, Huang EJ, Shen Y, Masliah E, Mukherjee C, Meyers D, Cole PA, Ott M, Gan L. Acetylation of tau inhibits its degradation and contributes to tauopathy. Neuron. 2010; 67: 953-66.

[84] Cohen TJ, Guo JL, Hurtado DE, Kwong LK, Mills IP, Trojanowski JQ, Lee VM. The acetylation of tau inhibits its function and promotes pathological tau aggregation. Nat Commun. 2011; 2: 252.

[85] Asuni AA, Boutajangout A, Quartermain D, Sigurdsson EM. Immunotherapy targeting pathological tau conformers in atangle mouse model reduces brain pathology with associated functional improvements. J Neurosci. 2007; 27: 9115-29.

[86] Boimel M, Grigoriades N, Lourbopoulos A, Haber E, Abramsky O, Rosennmann H. Efficacy and safety of immunization with phosphorylated tau against neurofibrillary tangles in mice. Exp Neurol 2010; 224: 472-85.

[87] Chai X, Wu S, Murray TK, Kinley R, Cella CV, Sims H, Buckner N, Hanmer J, Davies P, O'Neill MJ, Hutton ML, Citron M. Passive immunization with anti-Tau antibodies in two transgenic models: reduction of Tau pathology and delay of disease progression. J Biol Chem. 2011; 286: 34457-67.

[88] Brunden KR, Yao Y, Potuzak JS, Ferrer NI, Ballatore C, James MJ, Hogan AM, Trojanowski JQ, Smith AB 3rd, Lee VM. The characterization of microtubule-stabilizing drugs as possible therapeutic agents for Alzheimer's disease and related tauopathies. Pharmacol Res. 2011; 63: 341-51.

[89] Zempel H, Thies E, Mandelkow E, Mandelkow EM. Abeta oligomers cause localized Ca(2+) elevation, missorting of endogenous Tau into dendrites, Tau phosphorylation, and destruction of microtubules and spines. J Neurosci. 2010; 30: 11938-50.

[90] Zhang B, Maiti A, Shively S, Lakhani F, McDonald-Jones G, Bruce J, Lee EB, Xie SX, Joyce S, Li C, Toleikis PM, Lee VM, Trojanowski JQ. Microtubule-binding drugs offset tau sequestration by stabilizing microtubules and reversing fast axonal transport deficits in a tauopathy model. Proc Natl Acad Sci USA. 2005; 102:: 227-31.

[91] Brunden KR, Zhang B, Carroll J, Yao Y, Potuzak JS, Hogan AM, Iba M, James MJ, Xie SX, Ballatore C, Smith AB 3rd, Lee VM, Trojanowski JQ. Epothilone D improves microtubule density, axonal integrity, and cognition in a transgenic mouse model of tauopathy. J Neurosci. 2010; 30:13861-6.

[92] Vulih-Shultzman I, Pinhasov A, Mandel S, Grigoriadis N, Touloumi O, Pittel Z, Gozes I. Activity-dependent neuroprotective protein snippet NAP reduces tau hyperphosphorylation and enhances learning in a novel transgenic mouse model. J Pharmacol Exp Ther. 2007; 323: 438-49.

[93] Gozes I, Stewart A, Morimoto B, Fox A, Sutherland K, Schmeche D. Addressing Alzheimer's disease tangles: from NAP to AL-108. Curr Alzheimer Res. 2009; 6: 455-60.

[94] Nunomura A, Perry G, Aliev G, Hirai K, Takeda A, Balraj EK, Jones PK, Ghanbari H, Wataya T, Shimohama S, Chiba S, Atwood CS, Petersen RB, Smith MA. Oxidative damage is the earliest event in Alzheimer disease. J Neuropathol Exp Neurol. 2001; 60:759-67.

[95] Nunomura A, Perry G, Pappolla MA, Friedland RP, Hirai K, Chiba S, Smith MA. Neuronal oxidative stress precedes amyloid-beta deposition in Down syndrome. J Neuropathol Exp Neurol. 2000; 59: 1011-7

[96] Perry G, Smith MA. Is oxidative damage central to the pathogenesis of Alzheimer disease? Acta Neurol Belg. 1998; 98:175-9.

[97] Praticò D, Uryu K, Leight S, Trojanoswki JQ, Lee VM. Increased lipid peroxidation precedes amyloid plaque formation in an animal model of Alzheimer amyloidosis. J Neurosci. 2001; 21: 4183-7.

[98] Praticò D, Clark CM, Liun F, Rokach J, Lee VY, Trojanowski JQ. Increase of brain oxidative stress in mild cognitive impairment: a possible predictor of Alzheimer disease. Arch Neurol. 2002 59(6):972-6. Erratum in: Arch Neurol 2002; 59:1475.

[99] Martínez A, Portero-Otin M, Pamplona R, Ferrer I. Protein targets of oxidative damage in human neurodegenerative diseases with abnormal protein aggregates. Brain Pathol. 2010; 20: 281-97.

[100] Terni B, Boada J, Portero-Otin M, Pamplona R, Ferrer I. Mitochondrial ATP-synthase in the entorhinal cortex is a target of oxidative stress at stages I/II of Alzheimer's disease pathology. Brain Pathol. 2010; 20: 222-33.

[101] Praticò D. Evidence of oxidative stress in Alzheimer's disease brain and antioxidant therapy: lights and shadows. Ann N Y Acad Sci. 2008; 1147: 70-8.

[102] Bonda DJ, Wang X, Perry G, Nunomura A, Tabaton M, Zhu X, Smith MA. Oxidative stress in Alzheimer disease: a possibility for prevention. Neuropharmacology. 2010; 59: 290-4

[103] Richard T, Pawlus AD, Iglésias ML, Pedrot E, Waffo-Teguo P, Mérillon JM, Monti JP. Neuroprotective properties of resveratrol and derivatives. Ann N Y Acad Sci. 2011; 1215: 103-8.

[104] Li F, Gong Q, Dong H, Shi J. Resveratrol, a neuroprotective supplement for Alzheimer's disease. Curr Pharm Des. 2012; 18: 27-33.

[105] Mancuso C, Bates TE, Butterfield DA, Calafato S, Cornelius C, De Lorenzo A, Dinkova Kostova AT, Calabrese V. Natural antioxidants in Alzheimer's disease. Expert Opin Investig Drugs. 2007; 16:1921-31.

[106] Belkacemi A, Doggui S, Dao L, Ramassamy C. Challenges associated with curcumin therapy in Alzheimer disease. Expert Rev Mol Med. 2011; 13:e34.

[107] Hamaguchi T, Ono K, Yamada M. REVIEW: Curcumin and Alzheimer's disease. CNS Neurosci Ther. 2010; 16: 285-97.

[108] Mandel SA, Amit T, Weinreb O, Reznichenko L, Youdim MB. Simultaneous manipulation of multiple brain targets by green tea catechins: a potential neuroprotective strategy for Alzheimer and Parkinson diseases. CNS Neurosci Ther. 2008; 14: 352-65.

[109] Spagnoli A, Lucca U, Menasce G, Bandera L, Cizza G, Forloni G, Tettamanti M, Frattura L, Tiraboschi P, Comelli M, et al. Long-term acetyl-L-carnitine treatment in Alzheimer's disease. Neurology. 1991; 41: 1726-32.

[110] Montgomery SA, Thal LJ, Amrein R. Meta-analysis of double blind randomized controlled clinical trials of acetyl-L-carnitine versus placebo in the treatment of mild cognitive impairment and mild Alzheimer's disease. Int Clin Psychopharmacol. 2003; 18: 61-71.

[111] Nishida Y, Yokota T, Takahashi T, Uchihara T, Jishage K, Mizusawa H. Deletion of vitamin E enhances phenotype of Alzheimer disease model mouse. Biochem Biophys Res Commun. 2006; 350: 530-6.

[112] Viña J, LLoret A, Giraldo E, Badia MC, Alonso MD. Antioxidant pathways in Alzheimer's disease: possibilities of intervention. Curr Pharm Des 2011; 17: 3861-4.

[113] Harrison FE, Hosseini AH, McDonald MP, May JM. Vitamin C reduces spatial learning deficits in middle-aged and very old APP/PSEN1 transgenic and wild-type mice. Pharmacol Biochem Behav. 2009; 93: 443-50.

[114] Murakami K, Murata N, Ozawa Y, Kinoshita N, Irie K, Shirasawa T, Shimizu T. Vitamin C restores behavioral deficits and amyloid- oligomerization without affecting plaque formation in a mouse model of Alzheimer's disease. J Alzheimers Dis. 2011; 26: 7-18.

[115] Zandi PP, Anthony JC, Khachaturian AS, Stone SV, Gustafson D, Tschanz JT, Norton MC, Welsh-Bohmer KA, Breitner JC; Cache County Study Group. Reduced risk of Alzheimer disease in users of antioxidant vitamin supplements: the Cache County Study. Arch Neurol. 2004; 61: 82-8

[116] Boothby LA, Doering PL. Vitamin C and vitamin E for Alzheimer's disease. Ann Pharmacother. 2005; 39: 2073-80.

[117] Birks J, Grimley Evans J. Ginkgo biloba for cognitive impairment and dementia. Cochrane Database Syst Rev. 2009; (1):CD003120.

[118] Tchantchou F, Xu Y, Wu Y, Christen Y, Luo Y. EGb 761 enhances adult hippocampal neurogenesis and phosphorylation of CREB in transgenic mouse model of Alzheimer's disease. FASEB J. 2007; 21: 2400-8.

[119] Galasko DR, Peskind E, Clark CM, Quinn JF, Ringman JM, Jicha GA, Cotman C, Cottrell B, Montine TJ, Thomas RG, Aisen P; for the Alzheimer's Disease Cooperative Study. Antioxidants for Alzheimer disease: a randomized clinical trial with cerebrospinal fluid biomarker measures. Arch Neurol. 2012 Mar 19.

[120] Holmquist L, Stuchbury G, Berbaum K, Muscat S, Young S, Hager K, Engel J, Münch G. Lipoic acid as a novel treatment for Alzheimer's disease and related dementias. Pharmacol Ther. 2007; 113:154-64.

[121] Maczurek A, Hager K, Kenklies M, Sharman M, Martins R, Engel J, Carlson DA, Münch G. Lipoic acid as an anti-inflammatory and neuroprotective treatment for Alzheimer's disease. Adv Drug Deliv Rev. 2008; 60: 1463-70.

[122] Pocernich CB, Butterfield DA. Elevation of glutathione as a therapeutic strategy in Alzheimer disease. Biochim Biophys Acta. 2012; 1822: 625-30.

[123] Adair JC, Knoefel JE, Morgan N. Controlled trial of N-acetylcysteine for patients with probable Alzheimer's disease. Neurology. 2001; 578: 1515-7.

[124] Orsucci D, Mancuso M, Ienco EC, LoGerfo A, Siciliano G. Targeting mitochondrial dysfunction and neurodegeneration by means of coenzyme Q10 and its analogues. Curr Med Chem. 2011; 18: 4053-64

[125] Beal MF. Mitochondrial dysfunction and oxidative damage in Alzheimer's and Parkinson's diseases and coenzyme Q10 as a potential treatment. J Bioenerg Biomembr. 2004; 36: 381-6.

[126] Dumont M, Kipiani K, Yu F, Wille E, Katz M, Calingasan NY, Gouras GK, Lin MT, Beal MF. Coenzyme Q10 decreases amyloid pathology and improves behavior in a transgenic mouse model of Alzheimer's disease. J Alzheimers Dis. 2011; 27: 211-23.

[127] McManus MJ, Murphy MP, Franklin JL. The mitochondria-targeted antioxidant MitoQ prevents loss of spatial memory retention and early neuropathology in a transgenic mouse model of Alzheimer's disease. J Neurosci. 2011; 31:15703-15.

[128] Hensley K. Neuroinflammation in Alzheimer's disease: mechanisms, pathologic consequences, and potential for therapeutic manipulation. J Alzheimers Dis. 2010; 21:1-14.

[129] McGeer PL, McGeer E, Rogers J, Sibley J. Anti-inflammatory drugs and Alzheimer disease. Lancet. 1990; 335:1037.

[130] Kaufmann WE, Andreasson KI, Isakson PC, Worley PF. Cyclooxygenases and the central nervous system. Prostaglandins. 1997; 54: 601-24.

[131] Lim GP, Yang F, Chu T, Chen P, Beech W, Teter B, Tran T, Ubeda O, Ashe KH, Frautschy SA, Cole GM. Ibuprofen suppresses plaque pathology and inflammation in a mouse model for Alzheimer's disease. J Neurosci. 2000; 20: 5709-14.

[132] Jantzen PT, Connor KE, DiCarlo G, Wenk GL, Wallace JL, Rojiani AM, Coppola D, Morgan D, Gordon MN. Microglial activation and beta -amyloid deposit reduction caused by a nitric oxide-releasing nonsteroidal anti-inflammatory drug in amyloid precursor protein plus presenilin-1 transgenic mice. J Neurosci. 2002; 22: 2246-54.

[133] Yan Q, Zhang J, Liu H, Babu-Khan S, Vassar R, Biere AL, Citron M, Landreth G. Anti-inflammatory drug therapy alters beta-amyloid processing and deposition in an animal model of Alzheimer's disease. J Neurosci. 2003; 23: 7504-9.

[134] Heneka MT, Sastre M, Dumitrescu-Ozimek L, Hanke A, Dewachter I, Kuiperi C, O'Banion K, Klockgether T, Van Leuven F, Landreth GE. Acute treatment with the PPARgamma agonist pioglitazone and ibuprofen reduces glial inflammation and Abeta1-42 levels in APPV717I transgenic mice. Brain. 2005; 128: 1442-53.

[135] Lim GP, Yang F, Chu T, Gahtan E, Ubeda O, Beech W, Overmier JB, Hsiao-Ashec K, Frautschy SA, Cole GM. Ibuprofen effects on Alzheimer pathology and open field activity in APPsw transgenic mice. Neurobiol Aging. 2001; 22: 983-91.

[136] Quinn J, Montine T, Morrow J, Woodward WR, Kulhanek D, Eckenstein F. Inflammation and cerebral amyloidosis are disconnected in an animal model of Alzheimer's disease. J Neuroimmunol. 2003; 137: 32-41.

[137] Sung S, Yang H, Uryu K, Lee EB, Zhao L, Shineman D, Trojanowski JQ, Lee VM, Praticò D. Modulation of nuclear factor-kappa B activity by indomethacin influences A beta levels but not A beta precursor protein metabolism in a model of Alzheimer's disease. Am J Pathol. 2004; 165: 2197-206.

[138] Kukar T, Murphy MP, Eriksen JL, Sagi SA, Weggen S, Smith TE, Ladd T, Khan MA, Kache R, Beard J, Dodson M, Merit S, Ozols VV, Anastasiadis PZ, Das P, Fauq A, Koo EH, Golde TE. Diverse compounds mimic Alzheimer disease-causing mutations by augmenting Abeta42 production. Nat Med. 2005; 11: 545-50.

[139] Jaturapatporn D, Isaac MG, McCleery J, Tabet N. Aspirin, steroidal and non-steroidal anti-inflammatory drugs for the treatment of Alzheimer's disease. Cochrane Database Syst Rev. 2012; CD006378.

[140] Coma M, Serenó L, Da Rocha-Souto B, Scotton TC, España J, Sánchez MB, Rodríguez M, Agulló J, Guardia-Laguarta C, Garcia-Alloza M, Borrelli LA, Clarimón J,Lleó A, Bacskai BJ, Saura CA, Hyman BT, Gómez-Isla T. Triflusal reduces dense-core plaque load, associated axonal alterations and inflammatory changes, and rescues cognition in a transgenic mouse model of Alzheimer's disease. Neurobiol Dis. 2010; 38: 482-91.

[141] Mosconi L, Pupi A, De Leon MJ. Brain glucose hypometabolism and oxidative stress in preclinical Alzheimer's disease. Ann NY Acad Sci 2008; 147: 180-95.

[142] Ferrer I. Altered mitochondria, energy metabolism, voltage-dependent anion channel, and lipid rafts converge to exhaust neurons in Alzheimer's disease. J Bioenerg Biomembr. 2009; 41: 425-31.

[143] Ferreira IL, Resende R, Ferreiro E, Rego AC, Pereira CF.Multiple defects in energy metabolism in Alzheimer's disease. Curr Drug Targets. 2010; 11: 1193-206.

[144] Ankarcrona M, Mangialasche F, Winblad B. Rethinking Alzheimer's disease therapy: are mitochondria the key? J Alzheimers Dis. 2010; 20 Suppl 2: S579-90

[145] Cunnane S, Nugent S, Roy M, Courchesne-Loyer A, Croteau E, Tremblay S, Castellano A, Pifferi F, Bocti C, Paquet N, Begdouri H, Bentourkia M, Turcotte E, Allard M, Barberger-Gateau P, Fulop T, Rapoport SI. Brain fuel metabolism, aging, and Alzheimer's disease. Nutrition. 2011; 27: 3-20.

[146] Kapogiannis D, Mattson MP. Disrupted energy metabolism and neuronal circuit dysfunction in cognitive impairment and Alzheimer's disease. Lancet Neurol. 2011; 10: 187-98.

[147] Jagust WJ, Seab JP, Huesman RH, Valk PE, Mathis CA, Reed BR, Coxson PG, Budinger TF. Diminished glucose transport in Alzheimer's disease: dynamic PET studies. J Cereb Blood Flow Metab. 1991; 11: 323-30.

[148] Pedersen WA, Flynn ER. Insulin resistance contributes to aberrant stress responses in the Tg2576 mouse model of Alzheimer's disease. Neurobiol Dis 2004; 17: 500-6.

[149] Landreth G, Jiang Q, Mandrekar S, Heneka M. PPARgamma agonists as therapeutics for the treatment of Alzheimer's disease. Neurotherapeutics. 2008; 5: 481-9.

[150] Bak AM, Egefjord L, Gejl M, Steffensen C, Stecher CW, Smidt K, Brock B, Rungby J. Targeting amyloid-beta by glucagon-like peptide -1 GLP-1) in Alzheimer's disease and diabetes. Expert Opin Ther Targets. 2011; 15: 1153-62.

[151] Bomfim TR, Forny-Germano L, Sathler LB, Brito-Moreira J, Houzel JC, Decker H, Silverman MA, Kazi H, Melo HM, McClean PL, Holscher C, Arnold SE, Talbot K, Klein WL, Munoz DP, Ferreira ST, De Felice FG. An anti-diabetes agent protects the mouse brain from defective insulin signaling caused by Alzheimer's disease-associated Aβ oligomers. J Clin Invest. 2012; 122: 1339-53.

[152] Miichi Y, Sakurai T, Akisaki T, Yokono K. Effects of insulin and amyloid β(1-42) oligomers on glucose incorporation and mitochondrial function in cultured rat hippocampal neurons. Geriatr Gerontol Int. 2011; 11: 517-24.

[153] Miller BW, Willett KC, Desilets AR. Rosiglitazone and pioglitazone for the treatment of Alzheimer's disease. Ann Pharmacother. 2011; 45: 1416-24.

[154] Van der Auwera I, Wera S, Van Leuven F, Henderson ST. A ketogenic diet reduces amyloid beta 40 and 42 in a mouse model of Alzheimer's disease. Nutr Metab. 2005; 2: 28.

[155] Yao J, Chen S, Mao Z, Cadenas E, Brinton RD. 2-Deoxy-D-glucose treatment induces ketogenesis, sustains mitochondrial function, and reduces pathology in female mouse model of Alzheimer's disease. PLoS One. 2011; 6:e21788.

[156] Henderson ST, Vogel JL, Barr LJ, Garvin F, Jones JJ, Costantini LC. Study of the ketogenic agent AC-1202 in mild to moderate Alzheimer's disease: a randomized, double-blind, placebo-controlled, multicenter trial. Nutr Metab. 2009; 6:31.

[157] Brewer GJ, Wallimann TW. Protective effect of the energy precursor creatine against toxicity of glutamate and beta-amyloid in rat hippocampal neurons. J Neurochem. 2000; 74: 1968-78.

[158] Sullivan PG, Geiger JD, Mattson MP, Scheff SW. Dietary supplement creatine protects against traumatic brain injury. Ann Neurol. 2000; 48: 723-9.

[159] Caspersen C, Wang N, Yao J, Sosunov A, Chen X, Lustbader JW, Xu HW, Stern D, McKhann G, Yan SD. Mitochondrial Abeta: a potential focal point for neuronal metabolic dysfunction in Alzheimer's disease. FASEB J. 2005; 19: 2040-1.

[160] Lustbader JW, Cirilli M, Lin C, Xu HW, Takuma K, Wang N, Caspersen C, Chen X, Pollak S, Chaney M, Trinchese F, Liu S, Gunn-Moore F, Lue LF, Walker DG, Kuppusamy P, Zewier ZL, Arancio O, Stern D, Yan SS, Wu H. ABAD directly links Abeta to mitochondrial toxicity in Alzheimer's disease. Science. 2004; 304: 448-52.

[161] Lim YA, Grimm A, Giese M, Mensah-Nyagan AG, Villafranca JE, Ittner LM, Eckert A, Götz J. Inhibition of the mitochondrial enzyme ABAD restores the amyloid-β-mediated deregulation of estradiol. PLoS One. 2011; 6: e28887

[162] Yao J, Du H, Yan S, Fang F, Wang C, Lue LF, Guo L, Chen D, Stern DM, Gunn Moore FJ, Xi Chen J, Arancio O, Yan SS. Inhibition of amyloid-beta (Abeta)peptide-binding alcohol dehydrogenase-Abeta interaction reduces Abeta accumulation and improves mitochondrial function in a mouse model of Alzheimer's disease. J Neurosci. 2011; 31: 2313-20.

[163] Yamada K, Inagaki N. Neuroprotection by KATP channels. J Mol Cell Cardiol.2005 ; 38: 945-9.

[164] Liu D, Pitta M, Lee JH, Ray B, Lahiri DK, Furukawa K, Mughal M, Jiang H, Villarreal J, Cutler RG, Greig NH, Mattson MP. The KATP channel activator diazoxide ameliorates amyloid-β and tau pathologies and improves memory in the 3xTgAD mouse model of Alzheimer's disease. J Alzheimers Dis. 2010; 22: 443-57.

[165] Sabbagh MN, Shill HA. Latrepirdine, a potential novel treatment for Alzheimer's disease and Huntington's chorea. Curr Opin Investig Drugs. 2010; 11: 80-91.

[166] Bachurin S, Lermontova N, Shevtzova E, Serkova T, Kireeva E. Comparative study of Tacrine and Dimebon action on mitochondrial permeability transition and β-amyloid-induced neurotoxicity. J Neurochem. 1999; 73(Suppl S): S185.

[167] Lermontova NN, Redkozubov AE, Shevtsova EF, Serkova TP, Kireeva EG, Bachurin SO.Dimebon and tacrine inhibit neurotoxic action of β-amyloid in culture and block L-type Ca2+ channels. Bull Exp Biol Med. 2001; 132:1079–83.

[168] Shevtsova EP, Grigoriev VV, Kireeva EG, Koroleva IV, Bachurin SO. Dimebon as mitoprotective and antiaging drug. Biochim Biophys Acta. 2006 (Suppl S) Abs P2.3.4.

[169] Doody RS, Gavrilova SI, Sano M, Thomas RG, Aisen PS, Bachurin SO, Seely L, Hung D; dimebon investigators. Effect of dimebon on cognition, activities of daily living, behaviour, and global function in patients with mild-to-moderate Alzheimer's disease: a randomised, double-blind, placebo-controlled study. Lancet. 2008; 372: 207-15.

[170] Francis PT, Ramírez MJ, Lai MK. Neurochemical basis for symptomatic treatment of Alzheimer's disease. Neuropharmacology. 2010; 59: 221-9.

[171] Geula C, Nagykery N, Nicholas A, Wu CK. Cholinergic neuronal and axonal abnormalities are present early in aging and in Alzheimer disease. J Neuropathol Exp Neurol. 2008; 67: 309-18.

[172] Mufson EJ, Counts SE, Perez SE, Ginsberg SD. Cholinergic system during the progression of Alzheimer's disease: therapeutic implications. Expert Rev Neurother. 2008; 8: 1703-18.

[173] Fisher A. Cholinergic treatments with emphasis on m1 muscarinic agonists as potential disease-modifying agents for Alzheimer's disease. Neurotherapeutics. 2008; 5: 433-42.

[174] Higgins JP, Flicker L. Lecithin for dementia and cognitive impairment. Cochrane Database Syst Rev. 2003; CD001015.

[175] Birks J. Cholinesterase inhibitors for Alzheimer's disease. Cochrane Database Syst Rev. 2006; (1):CD005593.

[176] Wilcock GK, Dawbarn D. Current pharmacological approaches to treating Alzheimer's disease. In: Neurobiology of Alzheimer's Disease. Third edition. Edited by David Dawbarn and Shelley J. Allen. Oxford University Press. 2007. Pp 359-390.

[177] Herrmann N, Chau SA, Kircanski I, Lanctôt KL. Current and emerging drug treatment options for Alzheimer's disease: a systematic review. Drugs. 2011; 71: 2031-65.

[178] Fischer W, Wictorin K, Björklund A, Williams LR, Varon S, Gage FH. Amelioration of cholinergic neuron atrophy and spatial memory impairment in aged rats by nerve growth factor. Nature. 1987; 329: 65-8.

[179] Caccamo A, Oddo S, Billings LM, Green KN, Martinez-Coria H, Fisher A, LaFerla FM. M1 receptors play a central role in modulating AD-like pathology in transgenic mice. Neuron. 2006; 49: 671-82.

[180] Nitsch RM, Slack BE, Wurtman RJ, Growdon JH. Release of Alzheimer amyloid precursor derivatives stimulated by activation of muscarinic acetylcholine receptors. Science. 1992; 258: 304-7.

[181] Wolf BA, Wertkin AM, Jolly YC, Yasuda RP, Wolfe BB, Konrad RJ, Manning D, Ravi S, Williamson JR, Lee VM. Muscarinic regulation of Alzheimer's disease amyloid precursor protein secretion and amyloid beta-protein production in human neuronal NT2N cells. J Biol Chem. 1995; 270: 4916-22.

[182] Woodruff-Pak DS, Gould TJ. Neuronal nicotinic acetylcholine receptors: involvement in Alzheimer's disease and schizophrenia. Behav Cogn Neurosci Rev. 2002; 1: 5-20.

[183] Parri RH, Dineley TK. Nicotinic acetylcholine receptor interaction with beta-amyloid: molecular, cellular, and physiological consequences. Curr Alzheimer Res. 2010; 7: 27-39.

[184] Nordberg A, Hellström-Lindahl E, Lee M, Johnson M, Mousavi M, Hall R, Perry E, Bednar I, Court J. Chronic nicotine treatment reduces beta-amyloidosis in the brain of a mouse model of Alzheimer's disease (APPsw). J Neurochem. 2002; 81:655-8.

[185] Oddo S, Caccamo A, Green KN, Liang K, Tran L, Chen Y, Leslie FM, LaFerla FM. Chronic nicotine administration exacerbates tau pathology in a transgenic model of Alzheimer's disease. Proc Natl Acad Sci U S A. 2005; 102: 3046-51.

[186] Haydar SN, Dunlop J. Neuronal nicotinic acetylcholine receptors - targets for the development of drugs to treat cognitive impairment associated with schizophrenia and Alzheimer's disease. Curr Top Med Chem. 2010; 10:144-52.

[187] Ren K, Thinschmidt J, Liu J, Ai L, Papke RL, King MA, Hughes JA, Meyer EM. alpha7 Nicotinic receptor gene delivery into mouse hippocampal neurons leads to functional receptor expression, improved spatial memory-related performance, and tau hyper-phosphorylation. Neuroscience. 2007; 145: 314-22

[188] Kihara T, Shimohama S, Urushitani M, Sawada H, Kimura J, Kume T, Maeda T, Akaike A. Stimulation of alpha4beta2 nicotinic acetylcholine receptors inhibits beta-amyloid toxicity. Brain Res. 1998; 792: 331-4.

[189] Tam SW, Zaczek R. Linopirdine. A depolarization-activated releaser of transmitters for treatment of dementia. Adv Exp Med Biol. 1995; 363:47-56.

[190] Lachowicz JE, Duffy RA, Ruperto V, Kozlowski J, Zhou G, Clader J, Billard W, Binch H 3rd, Crosby G, Cohen-Williams M, Strader CD, Coffin V. Facilitation of acetylcholine release and improvement in cognition by a selective M2 muscarinic antagonist, SCH 72788. Life Sci. 2001; 68: 2585-92.

[191] Clader JW, Wang Y. Muscarinic receptor agonists and antagonists in the treatment of Alzheimer's disease. Curr Pharm Des. 2005; 11: 3353-61.

[192] Rockwood K, Beattie BL, Eastwood MR, Feldman H, Mohr E, Pryse-Phillips W, Gauthier S. A randomized, controlled trial of linopirdine in the treatment of Alzheimer's disease. Can J Neurol Sci. 1997; 24:140-5.

[193] Boyle CD, Lachowicz JE. Orally active and selective benzylidene ketal M2 muscarinic receptor antagonists for the treatment of Alzheimer's disease. Drug Dev Res 2002; 56: 310 –20.

[194] Palop JJ, Mucke L. Amyloid-beta-induced neuronal dysfunction in Alzheimer's disease: from synapses toward neural networks. Nat Neurosci. 2010; 13: 812-8.

[195] Hu NW, Ondrejcak T, Rowan MJ. Glutamate receptors in preclinical rserarch on Alzheimer's disease: update on recent advances. Pharmacol Biochem Behav 2012; 100: 855-62.

[196] Keller JN, Mark RJ, Bruce AJ, Blanc E, Rothstein JD, Uchida K, Waeg G, Mattson MP. 4-Hydroxynonenal, an aldehydic product of membrane lipid peroxidation, impairs glutamate transport and mitochondrial function in synaptosomes. Neuroscience. 1997; 80: 685-96.

[197] Li S, Hong S, Shepardson NE, Walsh DM, Shankar GM, Selkoe D. Soluble oligomers of amyloid Beta protein facilitate hippocampal long-term depression by disrupting neuronal glutamate uptake. Neuron. 2009; 62: 788-801.

[198] Cissé M, Halabisky B, Harris J, Devidze N, Dubal DB, Sun B, Orr A, Lotz G, Kim DH, Hamto P, Ho K, Yu GQ, Mucke L. Reversing EphB2 depletion rescues cognitive functions in Alzheimer model. Nature. 2011; 469: 47-52.

[199] Hoey SE, Williams RJ, Perkinton MS. Synaptic NMDA receptor activation stimulates alpha-secretase amyloid precursor protein processing and inhibits amyloid-beta production. J Neurosci. 2009; 29: 4442-60.

[200] Bordji K, Becerril-Ortega J, Nicole O, Buisson A. Activation of extrasynaptic, but not synaptic, NMDA receptors modifies amyloid precursor protein expression pattern and increases amyloid-ß production. J Neurosci. 2010; 30:15927-42.

[201] Francis PT. Glutamatergic approaches to the treatment of cognitive and behavioural symptoms of Alzheimer's disease. Neurodegener Dis. 2008; 5: 241-3.

[202] Lynch G, Gall CM. Glutamate-based therapeutic approaches: ampakines. Curr Opin Pharmacol. 2006; 6: 82-8.

[203] Granger R, Deadwyler S, Davis M, Moskovitz B, Kessler M, Rogers G, Lynch G. Facilitation of glutamate receptors reverses an age-associated memory impairment in rats. Synapse. 1996; 22: 332-7.

[204] Bartolini L, Casamenti F, Pepeu G. Aniracetam restores object recognition impaired by age, scopolamine, and nucleus basalis lesions. Pharmacol Biochem Behav. 1996; 53: 277-83.

[205] Johnson SA, Simmon VF. Randomized, double-blind, placebo-controlled international clinical trial of the Ampakine CX516 in elderly participants with mild cognitive impairment: a progress report. J Mol Neurosci. 2002; 19: 197-200.

[206] Myhrer T, Paulsen RE. Infusion of D-cycloserine into temporal-hippocampal areas and restoration of mnemonic function in rats with disrupted glutamatergic temporal systems. Eur J Pharmacol. 1997; 328: 1-7.

[207] Schwartz BL, Hashtroudi S, Herting RL, Schwartz P, Deutsch SI. d-Cycloserine enhances implicit memory in Alzheimer patients. Neurology. 1996; 46: 420-4.

[208] Parsons CG, Stöffler A, Danysz W. Memantine: a NMDA receptor antagonist that improves memory by restoration of homeostasis in the glutamatergic system—too little activation is bad, too much is even worse. Neuropharmacology. 2007; 53: 699-723.

[209] Reisberg B, Doody R, Stöffler A, Schmitt F, Ferris S, Möbius HJ; Memantine Study Group. Memantine in moderate-to-severe Alzheimer's disease. N Engl J Med. 2003; 348:1333-41.

[210] McKeage K. Memantine: a review of its use in moderate to severe Alzheimer's disease. CNS Drugs. 2009; 23: 881-97.

[211] Danysz W, Parsons CG. The NMDA receptor antagonist memantine as asymptomatological and neuroprotective treatment for Alzheimer's disease: preclinical evidence. Int J Geriatr Psychiatry. 2003; 18(Suppl 1): S23-32.

[212] Dong H, Yuede CM, Coughlan C, Lewis B, Csernansky JG. Effects of memantine on neuronal structure and conditioned fear in the Tg2576 mouse model of Alzheimer's disease. Neuropsychopharmacology. 2008; 33: 3226-36.

[213] Scholtzova H, Wadghiri YZ, Douadi M, Sigurdsson EM, Li YS, Quartermain D, Banerjee P, Wisniewski T. Memantine leads to behavioral improvement and amyloid reduction in Alzheimer's-disease-model transgenic mice shown as by micromagnetic resonance imaging. J Neurosci Res. 2008; 86: 2784-91.

[214] Martinez-Coria H, Green KN, Billings LM, Kitazawa M, Albrecht M, Rammes G, Parsons CG, Gupta S, Banerjee P, LaFerla FM. Memantine improves cognition and reduces Alzheimer's-like neuropathology in transgenic mice. Am J Pathol. 2010; 176: 870-80.

[215] Filali M, Lalonde R, Rivest S. Subchronic memantine administration on spatial learning, exploratory activity, and nest-building in an APP/PS1 mouse model of Alzheimer's disease. Neuropharmacology. 2011; 60: 930-6.

[216] Schneider LS, Dagerman KS, Higgins JP, McShane R. Lack of evidence for the efficacy of memantine in mild Alzheimer disease. Arch Neurol. 2011; 68: 991-8.

[217] Bowen DM, Allen SJ, Benton JS, Goodhardt MJ, Haan EA, Palmer AM, Sims NR, Smith CC, Spillane JA, Esiri MM, Neary D, Snowdon JS, Wilcock GK, Davison AN. Biochemical assessment of serotonergic and cholinergic dysfunction and cerebral atrophy in Alzheimer's disease. J Neurochem. 1983; 41: 266-72.

[218] Arai H, Ichimiya Y, Kosaka K, Moroji T, Iizuka R. Neurotransmitter changes in early- and late-onset Alzheimer-type dementia. Prog Neuropsychopharmacol Biol Psychiatry. 1992; 16: 883-90.

[219] Geldenhuys WJ, Van der Schyf CJ. Role of serotonin in Alzheimer's disease: a new therapeutic target? CNS Drugs. 2011; 25: 765-81.

[220] Nelson RL, Guo Z, Halagappa VM, Pearson M, Gray AJ, Matsuoka Y, Brown M, Martin B, Iyun T, Maudsley S, Clark RF, Mattson MP. Prophylactic treatment with paroxetine ameliorates behavioral deficits and retards the development of amyloid and tau pathologies in 3xTgAD mice. Exp Neurol. 2007; 205:166-76.

[221] Cirrito JR, Disabato BM, Restivo JL, Verges DK, Goebel WD, Sathyan A, Hayreh D, D'Angelo G, Benzinger T, Yoon H, Kim J, Morris JC, Mintun MA, Sheline YI. Serotonin signaling is associated with lower amyloid-β levels and plaques in transgenic mice and humans. Proc Natl Acad Sci U S A. 2011; 108: 14968-73.

[222] Schechter LE, Dawson LA, Harder JA. The potential utility of 5-HT1A receptor antagonists in the treatment of cognitive dysfunction associated with Alzheimer s disease. Curr Pharm Des. 2002; 8:139-45.

[223] Schechter LE, Smith DL, Rosenzweig-Lipson S, Sukoff SJ, Dawson LA, Marquis K, Jones D, Piesla M, Andree T, Nawoschik S, Harder JA, Womack MD, Buccafusco J, Terry AV, Hoebel B, Rada P, Kelly M, Abou-Gharbia M, Barrett JE, Childers W. Lecozotan (SRA-333): a selective serotonin 1A receptor antagonist that enhances the stimulated release of glutamate and acetylcholine in the hippocampus and possesses cognitive-enhancing properties. J Pharmacol Exp Ther. 2005; 314:1274-89.

[224] Patat A, Parks V, Raje S, Plotka A, Chassard D, Le Coz F. Safety, tolerability, pharmacokinetics and pharmacodynamics of ascending single and multiple doses of lecozotan in healthy young and elderly subjects. Br J Clin Pharmacol. 2009; 67: 299-308.

[225] Upton N, Chuang TT, Hunter AJ, Virley DJ. 5-HT6 receptor antagonists as novel cognitive enhancing agents for Alzheimer's disease. Neurotherapeutics 2008; 5: 458-69.

[226] Cho S, Hu Y. Activation of 5-HT4 receptors inhibits secretion of beta-amyloid peptides and increases neuronal survival. Exp Neurol. 2007; 203: 274-8.

[227] Russo O, Cachard-Chastel M, Rivière C, Giner M, Soulier JL, Berthouze M, Richard T, Monti JP, Sicsic S, Lezoualc'h F, Berque-Bestel I. Design, synthesis, and biological evaluation of new 5-HT4 receptor agonists: application as amyloid cascade modulators and potential therapeutic utility in Alzheimer's disease. J Med Chem. 2009; 52: 2214-25.

[228] Knafo S, Alonso-Nanclares L, Gonzalez-Soriano J, Merino-Serrais P, Fernaud-Espinosa I, Ferrer I, DeFelipe J. Widespread changes in dendritic spines in a model of Alzheimer's disease. Cereb Cortex. 2009; 19: 586-92.

[229] Smith DL, Pozueta J, Gong B, Arancio O, Shelanski M. Reversal of long-term dendritic spine alterations in Alzheimer disease models. PNAS 2009; 106: 16877-82.

[230] Albasanz JL, Dalfó E, Ferrer I, Martín M. Impaired metabotropic glutamate receptor/ phospholipase C signaling pathway in the cerebral cortex in Alzheimer's disease and dementia with Lewy bodies correlates with stage of Alzheimer's-disease-related changes. Neurobiol Dis. 2005; 20: 685-93.

[231] Albasanz JL, Perez S, Barrachina M, Ferrer I, Martín M. Up-regulation of adenosine receptors in the frontal cortex in Alzheimer's disease. Brain Pathol. 2008; 18: 211-9.

[232] Coleman P, Federoff H, Kurlan R. A focus on the synapse for neuroprotection in Alzheimer disease and other dementias. Neurology. 2004; 63:1155-62.

[233] Arendt T. Alzheimer's disease as a disorder of mechanisms underlying structural brain self-organization. Neuroscience. 2001; 102: 723-65.

[234] Palop JJ, Mucke L. Synaptic depression and aberrant excitatory network activity in Alzheimer's disease: two faces of the same coin? Neuromolecular Med. 2010; 12: 48-55.

[235] Martin V, Fabelo N, Santpere G, Puig B, Marín R, Ferrer I, Diaz M. Lipid alterations in lipid rafts from Alzheimer's disease human brain córtex. J Alzheimers Dis 2010; 19: 489-502.

[236] Darios F, Davletov B. Omega-3 and omega-6 fatty acids stimulate cell membrane expansion by acting on syntaxin 3. Nature. 2006; 440: 813-7.

[237] Florent-Béchard S, Desbène C, Garcia P, Allouche A, Youssef I, Escanyé MC, Koziel V, Hanse M, Malaplate-Armand C, Stenger C, Kriem B, Yen-Potin FT, Olivier JL, Pillot T, Oster T. The essential role of lipids in Alzheimer's disease. Biochimie. 2009; 91: 804-9.

[238] Oster T, Pillot T. Docosahexaenoic acid and synaptic protection in Alzheimer's disease mice. Biochim Biophys Acta. 2010; 1801: 791-8.

[239] Secades JJ, Lorenzo JL. Citicoline: pharmacological and clinical review, 2006 update. Methods Find Exp Clin Pharmacol. 2006; Suppl B:1-56.

[240] Proctor DT, Coulson EJ, Dodd PR. Post-synaptic scaffolding protein interactions with glutamate receptors in synaptic dysfunction and Alzheimer's disease. Prog Neurobiol. 2011; 93: 509-21.

[241] Kaplan DR, Miller FD. Neurotrophin signal transduction in the nervous system. Curr Opin Neurobiol. 2000; 10: 381-91.

[242] Montero CN, Hefti F. Rescue of lesioned septal cholinergic neurons by nerve growth factor: specificity and requirement for chronic treatment. J Neurosci. 1988; 8: 2986-99.

[243] Allard S, Leon WC, Pakavathkumar P, Bruno MA, Ribeiro-da-Silva A, Cuello AC. Impact of the NGF maturation and degradation pathway on the cortical cholinergic system phenotype. J Neurosci. 2012; 32: 2002-12.

[244] Cuello AC, Bruno MA, Allard S, Leon W, Iulita MF. Cholinergic involvement in Alzheimer's disease. A link with NGF maturation and degradation. J Mol Neurosci. 2010; 40: 230-5.

[245] Bruno MA, Leon WC, Fragoso G, Mushynski WE, Almazan G, Cuello AC. Amyloid beta-induced nerve growth factor dysmetabolism in Alzheimer disease. J Neuropathol Exp Neurol. 2009; 68: 857-69.

[246] Pedraza CE, Podlesniy P, Vidal N, Arévalo JC, Lee R, Hempstead B, Ferrer I, Iglesias M, Espinet C. Pro-NGF isolated from the human brain affected by Alzheimer's disease induces neuronal apoptosis mediated by p75NTR. Am J Pathol. 2005; 166: 533-43.

[247] Podlesniy P, Kichev A, Pedraza C, Saurat J, Encinas M, Perez B, Ferrer I, Espinet C. Pro-NGF from Alzheimer's disease and normal human brain displays distinctive abilities to induce processing and nuclear translocation of intracellular domain of p75NTR and apoptosis. Am J Pathol. 2006; 169:119-31.

[248] Kichev A, Ilieva EV, Piñol-Ripoll G, Podlesniy P, Ferrer I, Portero-Otín M, Pamplona R, Espinet C. Cell death and learning impairment in mice caused by in vitro modified

pro-NGF can be related to its increased oxidative modifications in Alzheimer disease. Am J Pathol. 2009; 175: 2574-85.

[249] Eriksdotter Jönhagen M, Nordberg A, Amberla K, Bäckman L, Ebendal T, Meyerson B, Olson L, Seiger, Shigeta M, Theodorsson E, Viitanen M, Winblad B, Wahlund LO. Intracerebroventricular infusion of nerve growth factor in three patients with Alzheimer's disease. Dement Geriatr Cogn Disord. 1998; 9: 246-57.

[250] Cattaneo A, Capsoni S, Paoletti F. Towards noninvasive nerve growth factor therapies for Alzheimer's disease. J Alzheimers Dis. 2008; 15:255-83.

[251] Ferrer I, Marín C, Rey MJ, Ribalta T, Goutan E, Blanco R, Tolosa E, Martí E. BDNF and full-length and truncated TrkB expression in Alzheimer disease. Implications in therapeutic strategies. J Neuropathol Exp Neurol. 1999; 58: 729-39.

[252] Connor B, Young D, Yan Q, Faull RL, Synek B, Dragunow M. Brain-derived neurotrophic factor is reduced in Alzheimer's disease. Brain Res Mol Brain Res. 1997; 49: 71-81.

[253] Holsinger RM, Schnarr J, Henry P, Castelo VT, Fahnestock M. Quantitation of BDNF mRNA in human parietal cortex by competitive reverse transcription-polymerase chain reaction: decreased levels in Alzheimer's disease. Brain Res Mol Brain Res. 2000; 76: 347-54.

[254] Hock C, Heese K, Hulette C, Rosenberg C, Otten U. Region-specific neurotrophin imbalances in Alzheimer disease: decreased levels of brain-derived neurotrophic factor and increased levels of nerve growth factor in hippocampus and cortical areas. Arch. Neurol 2000; 57: 846–51.

[255] Nagahara AH, Tuszynski MH. Potential therapeutic uses of BDNF in neurological and psychiatric disorders. Nat Rev Drug Discov. 2011; 10: 209-19.

[256] Nagahara AH, Merrill DA, Coppola G, Tsukada S, Schroeder BE, Shaked GM, Wang L, Blesch A, Kim A, Conner JM, Rockenstein E, Chao MV, Koo EH, Geschwind D, Masliah E, Chiba AA, Tuszynski MH. Neuroprotective effects of brain-derived neurotrophic factor in rodent and primate models of Alzheimer's disease. Nat Med. 2009; 15: 331-7.

[257] Blurton-Jones M, Kitazawa M, Martinez-Coria H, Castello NA, Müller FJ, Loring JF, Yamasaki TR, Poon WW, Green KN, LaFerla FM. Neural stem cells improve cognition via BDNF in a transgenic model of Alzheimer disease. Proc Natl Acad Sci U S A. 2009; 106: 13594-9.

[258] Finch CE, Laping NJ, Morgan TE, Nichols NR, Pasinetti GM. TGF-β1 is an organizer of response to neurodegeneration. J Cell Biochem. 1993; 53: 314–22.

[259] Brionne TC, Tesseur I, Masliah E, Wyss Coray T. Loss of TGF-β1 leads to increased neuronal cell death and microgliosis in mouse brain. Neuron. 2003; 40:1133–45.

[260] Caraci F, Spampinato S, Sortino MA, Bosco P, Battaglia G, Bruno V, Drago F, Nicoletti F, Copani A. Dysfunction of TGF-β1 signaling in Alzheimer's disease: perspectives for neuroprotection. Cell Tissue Res. 2012 347;: 291-301.

[261] Caraci F, Battaglia G, Busceti C, Biagioni F, Mastroiacovo F, Bosco P, Drago F, Nicoletti F, Sortino MA, Copani A. TGF-beta 1 protects against Abeta-neurotoxicity via the phosphatidylinositol-3-kinase pathway. Neurobiol Dis. 2008; 30: 234-42.

[262] Sortino MA, Chisari M, Merlo S, Vancheri C, Caruso M, Nicoletti F, Canonico PL, Copani A. Glia mediates the neuroprotective action of estradiol on beta-amyloid-induced neuronal death. Endocrinology. 2004; 145: 5080–6.

[263] Bruno V, Battaglia G, Casabona G, Copani A, Caciagli F, Nicoletti F. Neuroprotection by glial metabotropic glutamate receptors is mediated by transforming growth factor-beta. J Neurosci. 1998; 18: 9594–600.

[264] Caraci F, Battaglia G, Bruno V, Bosco P, Carbonaro V, Giuffrida ML, Drago F, Sortino MA, Nicoletti F, Copani A. TGF-beta1 pathway as a new target for neuroprotection in Alzheimer's disease. CNS Neurosci Ther. 2009; 17: 237–249.

[265] Vollmar P, Haghikia A, Dermietzel R, Faustmann PM. Venlafaxine exhibits an anti-inflammatory effect in an inflammatory co-culture model. Int J Neuropsychopharmacol. 2008; 11:111-7.

[266] Arnon R, Aharoni R. Mechanism of action of glatiramer acetate in multiple sclerosis and its potential for the development of new applications. Proc Natl Acad Sci USA. 2004; 101 (Suppl 2): 14593–8.

[267] Zhang H, Zou K, Tesseur I, Wyss-Coray T. Small molecule tgf-beta mimetics as potential neuroprotective factors. Curr Alzheimer Res. 2005; 2: 183-6.

[268] Scheibel AB, Tomiyasu U. Dendritic sprouting in Alzheimer's presenile dementia. Exp Neurol. 1978; 60:1-8.

[269] Ferrer I, Aymami A, Rovira A, Grau Veciana JM. Growth of abnormal neurites in atypical Alzheimer's disease. A study with the Golgi method. Acta Neuropathol. 1983; 59:167-70.

[270] Arendt T. Synaptic degeneration in Alzheimer's disease. Acta Neuropathol. 2009; 118: 167-79.

[271] Barnett A, Brewer GJ. Autophagy in aging and Alzheimer's disease: pathologic or protective? J Alzheimers Dis. 2011; 25: 385-94.

[272] Harris H, Rubinsztein DC. Control of autophagy as a therapy for neurodegenerative disease. Nat Rev Neurol. 2011; 8: 108-17.

[273] Nixon RA, Wegiel J, Kumar A, Yu WH, Peterhoff C, Cataldo A, Cuervo AM. Extensive involvement of autophagy in Alzheimer disease: an immuno-electron microscopy study. J Neuropathol Exp Neurol. 2005; 64: 113-22.

[274] Barrachina M, Maes T, Buesa C, Ferrer I. Lysosome-associated membrane protein 1 (LAMP-1) in Alzheimer's disease. Neuropathol Appl Neurobiol. 2006; 32: 505-16.

[275] Li L, Zhang X, Le W. Autophagy dysfunction in Alzheimer's disease. Neurodegener Dis. 2010; 7: 265-71.

[276] Moreira PI, Santos RX, Zhu X, Lee HG, Smith MA, Casadesus G, Perry G. Autophagy in Alzheimer's disease. Expert Rev Neurother. 2010; 10: 1209-18.

[277] Lee S, Sato Y, Nixon RA. Primary lysosomal dysfunction causes cargo-specific deficits of axonal transport leading toAlzheimer-like neuritic dystrophy. Autophagy. 2011; 7: 1562-3.

[278] Sanchez-Varo R, Trujillo-Estrada L, Sanchez-Mejias E, Torres M, Baglietto-Vargas D, Moreno-Gonzalez I, De Castro V, Jimenez S, Ruano D, Vizuete M, Davila JC, Garcia-Verdugo JM, Jimenez AJ, Vitorica J, Gutierrez A. Abnormal accumulation of autophagic vesicles correlates with axonal and synaptic pathology in young Alzheimer's mice hippocampus. Acta Neuropathol. 2012; 123: 53-70.

[279] Nixon RA, Yang DS. Autophagy failure in Alzheimer's disease--locating the primary defect. Neurobiol Dis. 2011; 43: 38-45.

[280] Caccamo A, Majumder S, Richardson A, Strong R, Oddo S. Molecular interplay between mammalian target of rapamycin (mTOR), amyloid-beta, and Tau: effects on cognitive impairments. J Biol Chem. 2010; 285: 13107-20.

[281] Spilman P, Podlutskaya N, Hart MJ, Debnath J, Gorostiza O, Bredesen D, Richardson A, Strong R, Galvan V. Inhibition of mTOR by rapamycin abolishes cognitive deficits and reduces amyloid-beta levels in a mouse model of Alzheimer's disease. PLoS One. 2010; 5: e9979.

[282] Majumder S, Richardson A, Strong R, Oddo S. Inducing autophagy by rapamycin before, but not after, the formation of plaques and tangles ameliorates cognitive deficits. PLoS One. 2011; 6: e25416.

[283] Yang DS, Stavrides P, Mohan PS, Kaushik S, Kumar A, Ohno M, Schmidt SD, Wesson D, Bandyopadhyay U, Jiang Y, Pawlik M, Peterhoff CM, Yang AJ, Wilson DA, St George-Hyslop P, Westaway D, Mathews PM, Levy E, Cuervo AM, Nixon RA.Reversal of autophagy dysfunction in the TgCRND mouse model of Alzheimer's disease ameliorates amyloid pathologies and memory deficits. Brain. 2011; 134: 258-77.

[284] Laplante M, Sabatini DM. mTOR signaling in growth control and disease. Cell. 2012; 149: 274-93.

[285] Sarkar S, Floto RA, Berger Z, Imarisio S, Cordenier A, Pasco M, Cook LJ, Rubinsztein DC. Lithium induces autophagy by inhibiting inositol monophosphatase. J Cell Biol. 2005; 170:1101-11.

[286] Williams A, Sarkar S, Cuddon P, Ttofi EK, Saiki S, Siddiqi FH, Jahreiss L, Fleming A, Pask D, Goldsmith P, O'Kane CJ, Floto RA, Rubinsztein DC. Novel targets for Hun-

tington's disease in an mTOR-independent autophagy pathway. Nat Chem Biol. 2008; 4: 295-305.

[287] Frautschy SA, Cole GM. Why pleiotropic interventions are needed for Alzheimer's disease. Mol Neurobiol. 2010; 41: 392-409.

[288] Bajda M, Guzior N, Ignasik M, Malawska B. Multi-target-directed ligands in Alzheimer's disease treatment. Curr Med Chem. 2011; 18: 4949-75.

[289] Hashimoto M, Hossain S. Neuroprotective and ameliorative actions of polyunsaturated fatty acids against neuronal diseases: beneficial effect of docosahexaenoic acid on cognitive decline in Alzheimer's disease. J Pharmacol Sci. 2011; 116: 150-62.

[290] Fredholm BB, Battig K, Holmen J, Nehlig A, Zvartau EE. Actions of caffeine in the brain with special reference to factors that contribute to its widespread use. Pharmacol Rev. 1999; 51: 83-133.

[291] Marques S, Batalha VL, Vaqueiro Lops L, Fleming Outeiro T. Modulating Alzheimer's disease through caffeine: a putative link to epigenetics. J Alzheimers Dis 2011; 24: 161-71.

[292] Arendash GW, Scleif W, Rezai-Zadech K, Jackson EK, Zacharia LC, Cracchiolo JR, Shippy D, Tan J. Caffeine protects Alzheimer's mice against cognitive impairmenmt and reduces brain beta-amyloid production. Neuroscience (2006) 142: 941-52.

[293] Dall'Igna OP, Fett P, Gomes MW, Souza DO, Cunha RA, Lara DR. Caffeine and adenosine A (2a) receptor antagonists prevent beta-amyloid (25-30)-induced cognitive deficits in mice. Exp Neurol. 2007; 203: 241-5.

[294] Ritchie K, Carriere I, de Mendonca A, Portet F, Dartigues JF, Rouaud O, Barberger-Gateau P, Ancelin ML. The neuroprotective effects of caffeine: a prospective population study. Neurology. 2007; 69: 536-45.

[295] Santos C, Lunet N, Azevedo A, de Mendonca A, Richtie K, Barros H. Caffeine intake and dementia: systematic review and meta-analysis. J Alzheimers Dis. 2010; suppl 1: S187-204.

[296] Eskelinen MH, Kivipelto M. Caffeine as a protective factor in dementia and Alzheimer's disease. J Alzheimers Dis 2010; 20 suppl 1: S167-74.

[297] Singh M, Dykens JA, Simpkins JW. Novel mechanisms for estrogen-induced neuroprotection. Exp Biol Med. 2006; 231: 514-21.

[298] Pike CJ, Carroll JC, Rosario ER, Barron AM. Protective actions of sex steroid hormones in Alzheimer's disease. Front Neuroendocrinol. 2009; 30: 239-58.

[299] Correia SC, Santos RX, Cardoso S, Carvalho C, Santos MS, Oliveira CR, Moreira PI. Effects of estrogen in the brain: is it a neuroprotective agent in Alzheimer's disease? Curr Aging Sci. 2010; 3:113-26.

[300] Alonso A, Gonzalez C. Neuroprotective role of estrogens: relationship with insulin/ IGF-1 signaling. Front Biosci. 2012; 4: 607-19.

[301] Carroll JC, Rosario ER, Chang L, Stanczyk FZ, Oddo S, LaFerla FM, Pike CJ. Progesterone and estrogen regulate Alzheimer-like neuropathology in female 3xTg-AD mice. J Neurosci. 2007; 27:13357-65.

[302] Fillit H, Weinreb H, Cholst I, Luine V, McEwen B, Amador R, Zabriskie J. Observations in a preliminary open trial of estradiol therapy for senile dementia-Alzheimer's type. Psychoneuroendocrinology. 1986; 11: 337–45.

[303] Craig MC, Murphy DG. Estrogen therapy and Alzheimer's dementia. Ann N Y Acad Sci. 2010; 1205: 245-53.

[304] Campbell VA, Gowran A. Alzheimer's disease: taking the edge off with cannabinoids? Br J Pharmacol 2007; 152: 655-62.

[305] Van Der Stelt M, Mazzola C, Espositp G, Mathias I, Petrosino S, De Filippis D et al. Endocannabinoids and b-amyloid-induced neurotoxicity in vivo: effect of pharmacological elevation of endocannabinoid levels. Cell Mol Life Sci. 2006; 63: 1410–24.

[306] Aso E, Palomer E, Juvés S, Maldonado R, Muñoz FJ, Ferrer I. CB1 agonist ACEA protects neurons and reduces the cognitive impairment of AβPP/PS1 mice. J Alzheimers Dis. 2012; 30: 439-59.

[307] Ramírez BG, Blázquez C, Gómez del Pulgar T, Guzmán M, de Ceballos ML. Prevention of Alzheimer's disease pathology by cannabinoids: neuroprotection mediated by blockade of microglial activation. J Neurosci. 2005; 25:1904-13.

[308] Martín-Moreno AM, Brera B, Spuch C, Carro E, García-García L, Delgado M, Pozo MA, Innamorato NG, Cuadrado A, Ceballos ML. Prolonged oral cannabinoid administration prevents neuroinflammation, lowers β-amyloid levels and improves cognitive performance in Tg APP 2576 mice. J Neuroinflammation. 2012; 9:8.

[309] Esposito G, De Filippis D, Carnuccio R, Izzo AA, Iuvone T. The marijuana component cannabidiol inhibits beta-amyloid-induced tau protein hyperphosphorylation through Wnt/beta-catenin pathway rescue in PC12 cells. J Mol Med 2006; 84: 253.8.

[310] Galve-Roperh I, Aguada T, Palazuelos J, Guzman M. The endocannabinoid system and neurogenesis in health and disease. Neuroscientist 2007; 13: 109–14.

[311] Harvey BS, Ohlsson KS, Mååg JL, Musgrave IF, Smid SD. Contrasting protective effects of cannabinoids against oxidative stress and amyloid-β evoked neurotoxicity in vitro. Neurotoxicology. 2012; 33: 138-46.

[312] Noonan J, Tanveer R, Klompas A, Gowran A, McKiernan J, Campbell VA. Endocannabinoids prevent β-amyloid-mediated lysosomal destabilization in cultured neurons. J Biol Chem. 2010; 285: 38543-54.

[313] Eubanks LM, Rogers CJ, Beuscher AE 4th, Koob GF, Olson AJ, Dickerson TJ, Janda KD. A molecular link between the active component of marijuana and Alzheimer's disease pathology. Mol Pharm. 2006; 3: 773-7.

[314] Sirén AL, Fasshauer T, Bartels C, Ehrenreich H. Therapeutic potential of erythropoietin and its structural or functional variants in the nervous system. Neurotherapeutics. 2009; 6: 108-27.

[315] Sun ZK, Yang HQ, Pan J, Zhen H, Wang ZQ, Chen SD, Ding JQ. Protective effects of erythropoietin on tau phosphorylation induced by beta-amyloid. J Neurosci Res. 2008; 86: 3018-27.

[316] Li G, Ma R, Huang C, Tang Q, Fu Q, Liu H, Hu B, Xiang J. Protective effect of erythropoietin on beta-amyloid-induced PC12 cell death through antioxidant mechanisms. Neurosci Lett. 2008; 442:143-7.

[317] Adamcio B, Sargin D, Stradomska A, Medrihan L, Gertler C, Theis F, Zhang M, Müller M, Hassouna I, Hannke K, Sperling S, Radyushkin K, El-Kordi A, Schulze L, Ronnenberg A, Wolf F, Brose N, Rhee JS, Zhang W, Ehrenreich H. Erythropoietin enhances hippocampal long-term potentiation and memory. BMC Biol. 2008; 6:37.

[318] Ponce LL, Navarro JC, Ahmed O, Robertson CS. Erythropoietin neuroprotection with traumatic brain injury. Pathophysiology. 2012 Mar 13.

[319] Shepardson NE, Shankar GM, Selkoe DJ. Cholesterol level and statin use in Alzheimer disease: I. Review of epidemiological and preclinical studies. Arch Neurol. 2011; 68: 1239-44.

[320] Pac-Soo C, Lloyd DG, Vizcaychipi MP, Ma D. Statins: the role in the treatment and prevention of Alzheimer's neurodegeneration. J Alzheimers Dis. 2011; 27: 1-10.

[321] Chauhan NB, Siegel GJ, Feinstein DL. Effects of lovastatin and pravastatin on amyloid processing and inflammatory response in TgCRND8 brain. Neurochem Res. 2004; 29: 1897-911.

[322] Li L, Cao D, Kim H, Lester R, Fukuchi K. Simvastatin enhances learning and memory independent of amyloid load in mice. Ann Neurol. 2006; 60: 729-39.

[323] Weinreb O, Amit T, Bar-Am O, Youdim MB. Ladostigil: a novel multimodal neuroprotective drug with cholinesterase and brain-selective monoamine oxidase inhibitory activities for Alzheimer's disease treatment. Curr Drug Targets. 2012; 13: 483-94.

[324] Wang R, Yan H, Tang XC. Progress in studies of huperzine A, a natural cholinesterase inhibitor from Chinese herbal medicine. Acta Pharmacol Sin. 2006; 27:1-26.

[325] Peng Y, Lee DY, Jiang L, Ma Z, Schachter SC, Lemere CA. Huperzine A regulates amyloid precursor protein processing via protein kinase C and mitogen-activated protein kinase pathways in neuroblastoma SK-N-SH cells over-expressing wild type human amyloid precursor protein 695. Neuroscience. 2007; 150: 386-95.

[326] Ved HS, Koenig ML, Dave JR, Doctor BP. Huperzine A, a potential therapeutic agent for dementia, reduces neuronal cell death caused by glutamate. Neuroreport. 1997; 8: 963-8.

[327] Li J, Wu HM, Zhou RL, Liu GJ, Dong BR. Huperzine A for Alzheimer's disease. Cochrane Database Syst Rev. 2008; 16:CD005592.

[328] Huang TC, Lu KT, Wo YY, Wu YJ, Yang YL. Resveratrol protects rats from Aβ-induced neurotoxicity by the reduction of iNOS expression and lipid peroxidation. PLoS One. 2011; 6: e29102.

[329] Li F, Gong Q, Dong H, Shi J. Resveratrol, a neuroprotective supplement for Alzheimer's disease. Curr Pharm Des. 2012; 18: 27-33.

[330] Davinelli S, Sapere N, Zella D, Bracale R, Intrieri M, Scapagnini G. Pleiotropic protective effects of phytochemicals in Alzheimer's disease. Oxid Med Cell Longev. 2012; 2012:386527.

[331] Allison AC, Cacabelos R, Lombardi VR, Alvarez XA, Vigo C. Celastrol, a potent antioxidant and anti-inflammatory drug, as a possible treatment for Alzheimer'sdisease.

[332] Neuropsychopharmacol Biol Psychiatry. 2001; 25: 1341-1357.

[333] Paris D, Ganey NJ, Laporte V, Patel NS, Beaulieu-Abdelahad D, Bachmeier C, March A, Ait-Ghezala G, Mullan MJ. Reduction of beta-amyloid pathology by celastrol in a transgenic mouse model of Alzheimer'sdisease. J Neuroinflammation. 2010;7: 17.

[334] Murray ME, Graff-Radford NR, Ross OA, Petersen RC, Duara R, Dickson DW. Neuropathologically defined subtypes of Alzheimer's disease with distinct clinical characteristics: a retrospective study. Lancet Neurol. 2011; 10: 785-796.

[335] Reiman EM, Langbaum JB, Fleisher AS, Caselli RJ, Chen K, Ayutyanont N, Quiroz YT, Kosik KS, Lopera F, Tariot PN.Alzheimer's Prevention Initiative: a plan to accelerate the evaluation of presymptomatic treatments. J Alzheimers Dis. 2011; 26 Suppl 3:321-329.

[336] Henderson ST, Poirier J. Pharmacogenetic analysis of the effects of polymorphisms in APOE, IDE and IL1B on a ketone body based therapeutic on cognition in mild to moderate Alzheimer's disease; a randomized, double-blind, placebo-controlled study. BMC Med Genet. 2011; 12:137.

Chapter 12

Animal Assisted Therapy and Activities in Alzheimer's Disease

Sibel Cevizci, Halil Murat Sen, Fahri Güneş and Elif Karaahmet

Additional information is available at the end of the chapter

http://dx.doi.org/10.5772/54504

1. Introduction

Animal-Assisted Therapy (AAT) or *Pet Therapy* is a supportive goal-oriented intervention which is mainly result from human and animal interaction. [1]- [6] In this treatment process, a health professional/patients' doctor have to determine which animal model should be accompanied with a specific clinical goal. This interventions can be followed by physical therapists, neurologist, psychiatrist, veterinary public health specialists, psychologist, occupational therapists, provided that they have taken a certification in AAT. In addition, all therapy processes should be followed by patients' doctor according to the suggestions of AAT specialist.

Although there are so many approach about the effect mechanism of AAT, it is known that the human and animal interaction is the basis for all of them. The positive-constructive bond result from between human and animal interaction is the key point to initiate the effect mechanism of AAT. This curative effect starts to work four basic mechanism including psychological stimulation, emotional, playing, and physical according to the Ballarini. [4] However all of these mechanisms are different therapy ways, they can become interpenetrate with each others. The important point is that, it is supposed that the psychosomatic effects which give rise to curative features of AAT occurs when these mechanisms start to work. All of the mechanism together revealed that psychosomatic effects of human-animal bond and interaction in people taking an AAT and AAA. [5], [6]

Lafrance et al., reported that patients' social and verbal behaviors have been improved in a presence of a therapy dog. [7] Nathans et al., revealed that Animal Assisted Therapy can be used for improving anhedonia in patients with schizophrenia. In addition, they have found that AAT can be beneficial for rehabilitation of life quality and psycho-social behaviors. [8]

Different researchers have reported that AAT should be considered planning of the treatment of individual with dementia. [1], [9]- [12]

The interaction between an animal and human result in an increase neurochemicals initiating a decrease in blood pressure and relaxation. This relationship may be beneficial for ameliorating agitate behavior and psychological symptoms of dementia. In another study, it has been reported that aquarium assisted therapy may be beneficial for increasing eating behavior of aged people living in a nursing home. [10] Richeson revealed that AAT can be increase social interactions by initiating decrease the agitate behaviors of patients with dementia. [12] Kongable et al., observed that a therapy dog increased patients' some social behaviors such as smile, laugh, look, touch, verbalization. [13]

In aged people, AAT are used for ameliorating agitate behaviors, psychological, occupational, social and physical disorders especially in Alzheimer and Dementia. [14]- [20] People with Alzheimer may have an easier time decoding the simple repetitive, non-verbal actions of a dog. Animals can act as transitional objects, allowing people to first establish a bond with them and then extend this bond to people. Most of the study results revealed that AAT especially dog therapy had an "calming effect" on the patients with dementia and Alzheimer disease. [15]- [17], [20] This effect can be helpful as a communication link during therapy sessions and also decrease agitation behaviors. It is well known that incidence of aggression, agitation, social withdrawal, depression, and psychotic disorders are growing problems in Alzheimer disease for special care units, staff and family members of patients. Furthermore, environmental factors in nursing home or other health care units have been become increasingly forcible barrier for therapy of Alzheimer disease. In this conditions, AAT and other animal activities may be helpful to cope with these difficulties by presenting a different aspect.

AAT should be more commonly used in the world through increasing awareness of public health services about beneficials of companion animal and activities. Especially, AAT can be used for improving health disorders of aged people with physical-mental and social disabilities such as Alzheimer, dementia, aphasia, anxiety, depression, stres, schizophrenia, and feeling of loneliness, quality of life. An aquarium assisted therapy may be a good starting point to learn about benefits and facilities of AAT in developing countries like Turkey which have more lower the socio-economic groups than the developed countries.

Main principle of AAT is based on using psychosomatic effects, which appear as results of biological-physical-chemical changes during human and animal interactions. [4] Feeding animals or being together with animals cause these effects to appear, and play an important role in recovery of mental, social and physical health. [21] The strength of bonding between humans and animals has been revealed in a survey study, which is conducted on 14 veterinarians and 117 patients in Ontario. In the study, patients, whose pets are died, have received a survey to define causes and effects of their worries by a phone call or e-mail. Of 30% of participants has been observed to have severe worries. [22] This strong bonding between humans and animals can also affect physical and mental health, and sometimes death or loss of an animal can be so effective that it can change a subject's life. [23] Dog, horse and dolphin are the most commonly preferred animal species in animal assisted therapy.

There are also studies indicating that keeping an animal has positive effects on the community health. [24] Heady et. al. reported that AAT caused decreasing national health costs. [25] Governments have been recently realized the significance of interaction between humans and animals as well as the contributions into human health, life quality and economy. Many countries have passed laws, which are a new understanding to allow keeping animals in apartments for rent, so as to support pet owners. Positive measures are taken in many European countries to keep pets in houses by laws. [26] AAT is to benefit from animal companionship during a targeted therapy in order to facilitate achievement of optimum results in patients, and to support the therapy. It provides very positive effects like providing adaptations of subjects to stressful situations and hospital environments; decreasing anxiety, stress, pain and blood pressure; increasing mobility and muscle activity. It has been shown that guiding animals increase physical activity, help in prevention of some moods like loneliness and depression, improve daily life activities and provide a social support by increasing the life quality. [27]- [29]

2. Benefits of animal companionship for therapy from past to present

Close relationships between humans and animals are way back to the prehistoric ages. By using DNA techniques, it has been demonstrated that dogs might have been domesticated 100,000 years ago. [30] Animals have been used to improve emotional and functional conditions of humans since ancient Greeks. Ancient Greeks have used dog drawings in their therapeutic temples, and they have provided melancholic people to ride on horses so as to get rid of their diseased souls. These applications have been used later also by Romans. [31] A dog showing the way to a blind man is drawn on armor in Pompeii historical ruins. [32]

The first studies, which have shown animal assistance in therapy, were performed to recover behaviors of mentally ill people in 1792 in York Retreat in United Kingdom by using farm animals. [3] Florence Nightingale defined the significance of assisting animals for therapy as: "Especially during treatment of a patient with a chronic illness, a small pet is a perfect friend for the patient". [32]

Dogs were used in rehabilitation after the World War I, in the first half of the 20th century. To improve moods of American army officers, who experienced depression related to the war, dogs were given to them to keep in company. [33] In the same period, thousands of dogs were trained under a program to support blinded soldiers in Germany. In 1931, "Guiding Dogs Society" was established for blind people. Currently, dogs are being trained in order to support people with hearing problems; to alert people with seizures before the symptoms are started; and to support people with severe physical problems.

Similar applications have been widely spread all over the world, so they have helped thousands of people with disabilities to live freely. Lane et. al. have reported that this ability of dogs was very amazing, and this social support that they have provided for people they have accompanied was very significant. [34]

Since 1980s, animal assisted therapies, which have been performed by planning and an experienced team, have been shown to improve social functions and to be beneficial especially in elderly people, so studies about this issue have been supported. [35]- [37] Therefore, when it was 1990s, study results of many articles are published from different populations. [28], [29], [38]- [40] Sable explained in the manuscript how, especially dogs and cats, could contribute into well being of family members, with whom they lived all their lives, emotionally and socially. [39]

As mentioned before, the first scientific studies indicating effects of human and animal interactions have been conducted in the second half of 20th century. UK originated Society for Companion Animal Studies (SCAS) is established in 1979, whereas the international organization, named International Association of Human-Animal Interaction Organization (IAHAIO) is established in 1990. IAHAIO is an affiliation of the World Health Organization, and it functions as a conductor organ among non-governmental organizations and other affiliations. The most marked point in the studies belonging to 2000s is that animal assisted therapy has been used against specific diseases, and evaluation of human-animal interaction results. [1], [23], [41]- [44]

Current patient healthcare methods, which are developing and containing evidence based interventions, are faced with some problems. Along with conventional treatments, complementary and adjuvant treatments are also included in these methods. Animal assisted therapy (AAT) is discussed as a supportive treatment approach with positive effects on life quality and health. [45]

3. Action mechanism in animal assisted therapies

Gagnon et. al. defined animal assisted therapy as a clinical intervention method, which has aimed to establish natural and improving bonding between humans and animals, and is applied for both preventive and therapeutic requirements. [46] Animal assisted therapy (AAT) can be applied through different action mechanisms in respect with the disease type and individual characteristics. Five factors directing the mechanism are psychological impulse, emotional, physical and playing mechanisms. [4] Although these mechanisms are defined separately, they cannot be considered independent from each other for functioning and developing of psychosomatic effects. The most important point in the treatment is human-animal interaction. This interaction constitutes a strong emotional background. It has been reported result benefits would depend on the strength of the emotional interactions.

In another words, confident, positive and sedative bonding between a human and an animal can trigger beneficial mechanisms by affecting secretions of adrenaline (epinephrine) and other corticosteroid hormones or stress hormones (like cortisol etc.); decreasing arterial blood pressure, cardiac and respiratory rates. Emotional, psychological impulse, playing and physical mechanisms used in AAT applications cause psychosomatic effects.

Understanding of "play" principle is quite important in animal assisted therapy. Ballarini reported that activities like "entertainment" and especially "laughing" are parts of the bonding

http://dx.doi.org/10.5772/54504

between humans and animals. When an ill person plays with a cat or laughs at a dog's behavior, an increase in the healing potential of that illness is initiated. As playing increases mobility, it is a good physical activity source. [4] Haubenhofer and Kirchengast measured cortisol levels in saliva of dogs, which were involved in animal assisted interventions and therapies to investigate their physiological reactions. Cortisol levels, which were monitored during therapy sessions in the earlier time periods of day, were reported to be higher than those measured after the therapy and in the control periods. The study results showed that therapeutic work was physiologically activating for the dogs. [47] At this point, it may be considered that these physiologically changes occurred in dogs can result in positive reactions in humans during animal assisted therapies and activities. But, further research is needed to indicate whether these positive effects related to the animal assisted therapies or not.

We have already mentioned that action mechanism of AAT is based on positive-healing bonding, which has occurred by human-animal interaction, and psychological, emotional, playing and physical mechanisms, which have caused physical and biochemical reactions by activation of this bonding. [4], [46] Key structures activating these mechanisms in patients should be structured according to mainly four theories. These are touching, biophilia hypothesis, learning and cognitive theories. [48] In animal assisted therapy applications, all types of applications, which are performed according to these four theories, can provide various benefits.

Touching theory provides a special and continuous bonding between patient and animal at the first contact. The aim of this bonding is generally due to searching for closeness and tendency to preserve this closeness instinctively. It is normal that such a bonding occurs between an Alzheimer patient and a therapy dog. Because, may be, this is the first time that the patient has met another living organism without any prejudice, without verbal communication and agitated behaviors, and which has accepted him/her as he/she is. In this situation, patient firstly feels comfortable, and a trained dog will allow the patient to direct to itself first by expanding its limits, and allow the patient to touch it. Generally this initial contact in therapies is started with patient directing to the dog and touching it. During therapy period in this comfortable-caring treatment environment, many supportive benefits for clinical treatment compliance (being the leading one), relatives of patients, and healthcare personnel have been achieved.

Another important concept in therapies is *biophilia hypothesis*. As it has been mentioned in this review before, this concept defends that there is an instinctive, strong bonding between humans and all other living organisms, and both sides are in need of his strong bonding in order to survive. According to biophilia concept (short definition may be enthusiasm for life) human beings get in contact with the environment and all living creatures around genetically due to the human nature. This symbiotic relationship was started in the past, and continued in the present by contacting and keeping dogs, cats (the leading animals), other farm animals. As feeling of ownership has affected humans negatively in time, animals have been the mainly damaged side of this relationship. Especially animals, which we are calling currently domesticated, have moved away from their natural environments, and instead of living with humans, or accompanying humans, they have got under protection of humans. All other living creatures that human being as not felt close to himself, or could not domesticate or has not get under protection have remained as "Undomesticated-Wild". The reasons why we mention these philosophical approaches is the context of animal assisted therapies especially ethically, are applications, which are performed with animal companionship, and we would very much emphasize to use "living with the company of animals" term rather than "pet ownership" or "keeping an animal". Thus, "living with the company of animals" will be developed. May be this approach will help to develop the awareness of "living with somebody/living creature that is ill" rather than "having an ill relative". Then, experiencing the pure form of animal-human interaction at the beginning, and providing patient and his/her relatives to share this humane environment may reveal many positive effects, which we have not known or defined yet.

Learning theory, which is a model in psychology, defends that human beings give various responses to his/her surroundings by the learning principle. In AAT, the learning principle of the patient is triggered in a more human way; so a patient with Alzheimer´s disease can show some behaviors that he or she has started to forget, without the degree of forgetting, in the same way again, or can show some behaviors for longer times without forgetting. For example, while feeding fish in the aquarium, their eating desire may be increased or they remember eating behavior and eat some food; while feeding a dog, they may start to use hand skills, so that these will help them to improve slightly their daily life activities etc. *This interaction with animals may be perceived as a more human approach than verbal reminding of healthcare personnel and/or patient's relatives or verbal commands of caregivers what to do. While healthcare personnel and/or patient caregivers can be under intensive stress and may unintentionally pronounce these commands at higher and sharp voice tones, and they may even say/behave in agitated ways for patients.* Therefore, animal assisted therapies and activities can be a good supportive way in long term therapy and care for individuals with chronic diseases like Alzheimer´s disease. *Cognitive theory*, which is another model in psychology, tries to explain human behaviors by investigating how human beings gain, process, and store the knowledge. Main headings in cognitive approach, which investigates perception of knowledge, processing of knowledge, and switching into behaviors, are perception language, attention, memory, problem solving, decision making-judging and intelligence.

As animals do not have any expectations and demands from humans at their first contacts, patients feel self-confidence, and they may feel that everything is under their controls. [48] Therefore, animals do not react like us when they meet a healthy or ill person. We, humans, tend to perceive, remember, shape up, judge with the previously learned concepts, and even show verbal-physical behaviors, when we first meet a healthy or ill person or any living being. This situation is quickly sensed and perceived by the opposite side. When a dog meets a blind, limb or amnestic person in the street, it will behave as if it has met a healthy individual. However, when we meet people with health problems in the street, we define them as "he has got no arm!", "he is blind!", "Is he a lunatic?", "ill person", and we imply our thoughts sometimes with words or sometimes with our behaviors. Due to these reasons, animal assisted therapies naturally eradicate negative conditions like these, and they provide a more humane surrounding for therapies of subjects with chronic diseases; they support them; they increase adaptation potentials of patients and their relatives to difficult therapy periods, and they improve their life qualities. After all, we should remembered that the aforementioned paragraphs are theoretical concepts which try to comprise biology, sociology, psychology and philosophy to explain some of the effects AAT on humans in general, not only for patients with Alzheimer's disease.

4. Fields of Animal Assisted Therapies (AAT)

According to medical studies and field screenings, it is evident that AAT has relaxing and supportive effects on humans. Recoveries obtained in some diseases through these positive interactions are listed in Table 1. [49], [34]- [39], [50] , [51]

Decreased anxiety and depression
Increased self-esteem
Increased impulse for communication
Decreased blood pressure
Increase in required motivation for recovery
Decrease in analgesic requirement in some patients, who have had previous operations
Improvement in communication with other patients or hospital personnel

Table 1. Main improvements observed in AAT applied subjects

This supportive therapy with various services is being provided to more than 35000 patients in more than 100 healthcare service units in San Francisco. Subjects mainly benefited from these services are as follows: *Children treated in pediatric clinic; AIDS patients; patients, who require acute care and physical rehabilitation services; children with conduct disorder and physical problems; subjects staying at hospitals (patients, their relatives and hospital personnel), patients with mental diseases.* Public health organizations currently provide various services with dogs suitable for therapies. Samples for some application fields of AAT are given in Table 2 regarding human health improvement and development. [4], [52]

As Ballarini has mentioned, AAT is no longer a mysterious application, but currently it has become a treatment option, which is applied for supportive aims, and has resulted in positive outcomes in many diseases. In recent years, AAT has gained more attention all over the world, and it is being preferred as a complimentary and supportive method to improve life quality and health in some therapies, during which various problems have arisen. [45], [53], [54] Therefore, many studies have been performed to establish its scientific background, and different AAT models are being developed. Dolphin assisted therapy is one of these, and it is employed as an adjunctive method in various diseases (Table 3). [55], [56] During therapies, it has been observed that dolphins have tried to communicate with ill subjects by increasing their sound levels. [57]

For psychological training	
In children with poor or underdeveloped socialization attitudes,	
In conduct disorders,	
In children with low academic success and low self-esteem	
To decrease hostile behaviors	
In jails	
In mental institutions with convicts	
In reformatory schools	
Psychiatric conditions	
Mild or moderate autism	
In treatment and prevention of depression symptoms in old people	
Anxiety	
Neuro-psychological tension	
Medical interventions	
In recovery periods of diseases	
Arterial hypertension	
Cardiopathies	
Chronic muscle-nervous system diseases	
Different motor disorder therapies and rehabilitation	

Table 2. Application fields of AAT

Autism
Down syndrome
Rett syndrome
Depression (non-endogenous type)
Neurotic disorder
Brain trauma (without cramp syndrome)
Brain paralysis (without cramp syndrome)
Cerebral palsy in children
Childhood neurosis like fobby, enuresis and asthenia
Environmental conduct disorders
Support for post-coma treatment
Severe psychological and complex trauma
Cephalgia
Chronic fatigue syndrome
Delayed speech development
Delayed psychological development
Chronic diseases

Table 3. Some medical and mental health problems for application of dolphin therapy

5. AAT use in some chronic diseases

Since Alzheimer´s disease is generally observed in elderly people, it may be concomitant with some other chronic diseases. Among these diseases, cardiovascular diseases are the leading ones. Conducted studies have indicated that systolic blood pressure and plasma triglyceride levels are lower in pet owner subjects when compared with the non-owners. [38] In Odendaal's study, neurochemicals (β-endorphin, oxytocin, prolactin, phenylacetic acid, dopamine, cortisol) related to drop down of blood pressure were evaluated between 18 subjects and 18 dogs before and after the positive interactions. Statistically significant data ($p<0.05$) have indicated that neurochemicals related to blood pressure are increased in both groups and attention behavior function is increased after AAT except cortisol (cortisol was low significantly in humans, but this decrease was not found to be significantly in dogs. [58] It has been reported in studies of another chronic disease, namely cancer, that AAT had positive effects both on patients and their relatives. [46], [59], [60] The positive effects are reported as decreased stress and anxiety; compliance with treatment and improvement in adaptation; relaxation; better nutrition; physical activity; socialization; participitating in new activities; verbalization of fright and concerns; decreased nervousness; increased feeling of happiness; thus improvement in life quality. [46], [60]

Similar results have been obtained in studies performed on disabled subjects. [61]- [64] Especially achieved improvements were increased non-verbal interactions, physical activities, and daily life activities leading to increased life quality. Although these studies have been performed commonly in children with widespread developmental disorders, it should also be considered that Alzheimer patients may have various disabilities, which would lower their life quality, so their daily life activities may be limited according to the stage and severity of disease. When evaluated in this aspect, animal assisted therapies will provide significant benefits.

In a study performed on AIDS patients, it has been reported that cat assisted therapy has supported patients' communications with their families and friends, and has provided prevention from the feeling of loneliness.

6. Psychological and psychiatric diseases

Animal assisted therapies are especially employed in hospitalized children and Alzheimer patients to decrease stress. Animal companionship is employed in anxiety, refusal of therapy, refusal of eating and decreasing other agitated behaviors, treatments of various psychological and psychiatric disorders o provide treatment compliance and to increase the life quality. Patients, who are hospitalized in rehabilitation centers are scheduled for weekly or monthly therapy programs with trained animals, so physical, emotional, social and cognitive benefit of AAT are used. It has been reported that blood pressure and cardiac rate are decreased, cortisol (stress hormone) is markedly decreased, and pain sensation is decreased.

Animal assisted therapy has been shown to be effective in patients with speech disorders like aphasia, schizophrenia and dementia (Table 4). [3], [7], [8], [12], [51]

Reference	Patients, study group	Pet therapy model	Results
Macauley BL, 2006[3]	Three men with aphasia from left-hemisphere strokes and during AAT therapy with a 8 year old neutered male Newfoundland dog participated into the study.	Dog therapy	Dog may act as an excellent catalyst to motivate the client to talk and provide an atmosphere of unconditional acceptance for the speech disorders and brain injuries.
LaFrance C et al, 2007[7]	A 61-year old male with non-fluent aphasia and a left cerebral vascular accident. A therapy dog was 5 year old tetriever.	Dog therapy	In condition with the dog and dog handler, it was found that both social verbal and non-verbal behaviors markedly increased in patient.
Nathans-Barel I et al, 2005[8]	Patients with hedonic tone of 10 chronic schizophrenia participated in 10 weekly sessions of AAT was compared to control group treated without animal.	Dog therapy	In AAT group, significant improvements of hedonic tone compared to control. It was observed that an increasing in use of leisure time and motivation.
Richeson N, 2003[12]	15 nursing home residents with dementia participated in a daily AAT for three weeks.	Dog therapy	Significant decrease in agitated behaviors and statistically significant increase in social interaction.
Kovács Z, 2004[51]	Seven schizophrenic patients living in a social institute participated into the study for 9 month treatment period. Each weekly therapeutic session was 50 min.	Dog therapy	AAT was found to be helpful in daily life activities and rehabilitation of schizophrenic patients. Significant improvement in domestic and health activities.

Table 4. Dog therapy models in aphasia, schizophrenia and dementia.

Nathan reported from his study that animal assisted therapy improved anhedonia in chronic schizophrenia patients. Anhedonia is one of the negative symptoms of dementia, and it is the main phenomenon related to poor social functionality and development of treatment resistance. In an active study performed with dogs, significant improvement has been observed in anhedonia in AAT group when compared with the controls. As a result of the study, it has been reported that animal assisted therapy might contribute in life quality and psychosocial rehabilitation of chronic schizophrenia patients.[8]

http://dx.doi.org/10.5772/54504

Antonioli and Reveley observed in their randomized, controlled study that depression symptoms were observed to be improved in the 2nd week of treatment in patients with mild-moderate depression. Antonioli responded the comment indicating that patient number was limited and study population was a specific group as this dolphin study has indicated that, according to "Biophilia" hypothesis, interaction between animals and humans could be beneficial in their natural environments. [65], [66] "Biophilia" term is first defined by psychologist Erich, and is based on "affection level, which is required for mental health and emotional well-being". [67] Kellert and Wilson improved biophilia concept, and stated that human health and well-being were related to interactions with the natural environments. [68]

7. How can a dog assisted therapy be beneficial for therapy in Alzheimer patients?

It may cause decreased agitation, improvement in the mood, and increased communication with the surrounding: Alzheimer patients may experience different clinical symptoms at different disease stages. Generally as the disease is progressed, they isolate themselves from their surroundings, family members, friends, healthcare personnel; they become quieter and less mobile. In this stage, an accompanying therapy dog may even become the only communication bridge to continue the interaction with their surroundings. Sometimes patients may end up the silence on a dog's touch or behaviors; they may smile, talk a few words, and even they may be involved more with their surroundings.

Indoor and outdoor safety problems are most commonly encountered problems in some patients. With the accompanying well-trained dog, the patient can feel more secure. Since the dog can estimate behaviors of the patient, it may warn the patient and his /her relatives and/or healthcare personnel before and/or during the behaviors. A guiding dog may prevent the patient, who would like to leave his/her surrounding (home or nursery home) without informing anybody, from many dangers he/she would be confronted with. When the patient come to the top of the ladder, the dog may inform the patient about his/her position, how he/she should act or what he/she should do next by barking or behaving differently non-verbally without agitating the patient. It may protect the patient while crossing the street. The dog guiding a patient, who will forget the way home or the address of his/her home, can lead the patient home safely and in good health.

Aquarium assisted therapy studies have revealed that eating habits of Alzheimer patients are improved by feeding fish. Moreover aquarium assisted activities improve hand skills as well as they increase socialization of patients. Various mood disorders like nervousness, agitation, unhappiness, very quietness, and loneliness may be observed in subjects with dementia, who live in nursery homes. Aquariums at nursery homes may attract attention of subjects in these crowded environments, they may provide relaxation and happiness for them as well as they may help people live in more humane environments by decreasing work load and stress also for relatives of patients and healthcare personnel. Aquariums may help all individuals to share the same environment with the underwater creatures.

AAT is especially effective in elderly subjects with cognitive disorders like Alzheimer disease. Patients with dementia usually experience various degrees of agitation mainly in the evening. This situation, known as "sundowning", is not only stressful for patients, but can also be challenging for the healthcare personnel. Even touching an animal may decrease anxiety during challenging evening hours, and increase calmness/well-being feelings.

It has been observed that responses have been achieved in patients with advanced dementia by animal assisted therapies. Some patients with dementia may develop better and easier communications with animals when compared with humans. A pet can listen to a patient with dementia without judging. In guiding dog visits in AAT program, dogs may allow patients to come near to them and play with them. It has been reported that dog assisted therapies may help these exercises to be happier and more motivating experiences in patients, who are recommended to take a walk. These patients are also reported to have improved life quality, and socialization desires when compared with patients, who have not kept or lived with animals.

A therapy dog provides the Alzheimer patient a unique communication and love bonding, which can be re-shaped according to the target whichever animal assisted therapy is required, and various physical, mental and social health benefits can be achieved. Fish, cat, dog, horse or tortoise may present human benefits, which we cannot presume for Alzheimer patients, and by supporting patients' treatment compliances, they provide that patient relatives and healthcare personnel serve under more positive conditions. To provide the most benefit from AAT or AAA, in especially dog therapies, "resident" or "visiting" models can be used together for patients with dementia and Alzheimer´s disease. [14], [15], [18] It is not clearly explored which therapy model more useful than the other one. [9] In another review written by Williams and Jenkins reported that animal visitings to nursing-care units can provide various benefits including relaxation, improving of apathy and decreasing in agitation, aggression behavior and blood pressure for both patients and their caregivers, relatives. [18] According to the Churchill et al., a therapy dog can reduce some agitation behaviors of Alzheimer patients with especially sundown syndrome, and also help increasing social behaviors and calm down. [16]

Studies shown that environmental factors or changes in Alzheimer's disease special care units can be effect on patients' behavioral health outcomes including aggression, resident agitation, social withdrawal, depression, psychotic problems. [69], [70] That is why, treatment procedures should be planned and managed considering a balanced combination of pharmacologic, behavioral and environmental options in order to improve health, behavior and quality of life of patients with Alzheimer's disease. [70] It is important that physicians who are playing a key role in recognizing problems and arranging suitable treatment for their patients should consider alternative treatment options based on social and recreational interventions including meditation, validation therapy, reality orientation, reminiscence therapy, sensory interventions (therapeutic touch and massage therapy, aromatherapy, music therapy, dance therapy, light therapy, multisensory stimulation therapy), social contact (animal-assisted therapy, simulated presence therapy), exercise, art therapy and Montessori-based activities. [71], [72] In addition, most of the AAT studies have been focused on dog, cat and other small animal activities. It is not well-known that animal assisted therapies with farm animals may have positive effects on self-efficacy and coping ability among psychiatric patients. [73]

http://dx.doi.org/10.5772/54504

As displayed on Table 5, AAT especially dog therapies can be used successively as a preventive and interventional method in patients with Alzheimers' disease and dementia. Also, recent studies have shown that AAT may be beneficial to improve for various psychiatric diseases including Alzheimer, dementia, depression, anxiety, addiction, schizophrenia, autism spectrum disorder. [74]- [79]

Authors	Patients or study group	Pet therapy model	Results	Study design
Moretti F, et al. 2011	Over 84 age patients with dementia, depression and psychosis Pet group (n=10) Control group (n=11)	Dog therapy	Comparing to the control group, improvements as below was observed in the pet group: Decreasing of depression symptoms at 50% level and increasing 4.5 times in mini mental scores.	Methodological Study (6 weeks)
McCabe BW, et al. 2002	Patients with Alzheimer in a special care unit	Resident dog therapy in a special care unit	Significantly decreasing of problem behaviors at the end of the 4 weeks.	Methodological study (4 weeks)
Edwards NE and Beck AM, et al. 2002	62 patients with Alzheimer living a special care unit	Aquarium therapy used for improving nutrition intake behaviors	Since 2th weeks, nutritional intake behavior increased significantly and this increase kept on during 6 weeks. Over 16 week period, it was observed that patients had needed less nutritional supplements than baseline. Finally, authors indicated that dog therapy can provide health care cost savings (personal communication).	Methodological study (Follow-up) (6 weeks)
Fritz CL, et al. 1996	244 caregivers working with Alzheimer patients in Northern California. 124 caregivers contact with pets. 120 caregivers didn't contact with pets included into the control group.	Man and women contacted with pets regular (dog or cat)	It was observed that man who were attached to dogs scored better psychological health than men who had no pets. While, women less than 40 years old attached to cats were scored better some psychological health than women same aged and had no pets, women aged 40 to 59 years attached to dogs scored worse of life satisfaction and depression than women in the same age and had no pets.	Case-control study

Authors	Patients or study group	Pet therapy model	Results	Study design
Fritz CL, et al. 1995	64 Alzheimer patients living in a private nursing home.	Pet-therapy group: 34 patients contact with pets Control group: 34 patients didn't contact with pets.	It was observed that, verbal aggression and anxiety was reported less in patients exposed to companion animals than patients didn't exposed to pets.	Methodological study
Tribet J, et al. 2008	2 female and one male patients in a nursing home diagnosed with severe dementia.	A dog therapy used 15 times over 9 months. A therapy performed in the same place for 30 min, once a week.	Psychological benefits obtained from the study as follows: *Calming effect* was observed on the patients, which is this effect provided that communication link would be needed during therapy sessions. With the dogs' unconditional acceptance *increased patients' self-esteem* need to pateints felt theirselfs was in more secure environment. Addition, it was observed that their *social behaviours increased* by touching dog and its non-verbal communication.	Prospective-qualitative study
Kanamori M, et al. 2001	7 patients with senile dementia and 20 patients enrolled into the control group in an adult day care center.	AAT was used for 6 weeks. Before and after AAT was evaluated mini mental state, activities of daily living, behavioral pathology and salivary CgA.	The average mini mental state exam score was more higher than baseline, activities of daily living was more higher than baseline, behavioral pathology was more lower than baseline and finally salivary CgA was found to be decreasing tendency. Several methods can be used in order to show useful effects of AAT in patients with dementia as determined in this study by Kanamori M, et al.	Methodological study

Table 5. Animal Assisted Therapy Studies in patients with Alzheimer´s disease and other dementia

According to the literature, number of studies recommending animal assisted therapies in clinical and social medicine practices in elderly people with dementia, Alzheimer´s disease, ability losses, mental health problems and conduct disorders, cognitive problems, physical and functional health problems have been increased rapidly. [1-3], [63] Targeted acquisitions in AAT applications can be classified under five headings as social, psychological, training, physical and motivational. Moreover, what we expect from all applications in a patient with Alzheimer's disease are mainly physiological improvements, better focusing on environment, enabling physical contact, interaction with surroundings, improvements in nutritional behaviors, socialization, acceptance, motivation, increased physical activity, stress, decreased mood disorders like depression, and agitation, enjoying, and decreased feeling of loneliness.

8. Risks of AAT and Their managements

In USA, 60% of the population has at least one pet at home. Patients and animals participating in AAT require special care for prevention of zoonotic diseases, hypersensitivity reactions and injuries during visits. Therefore, the maximum benefit obtained from this therapy method depends on the multidisciplinary team work of a veterinarian specialist, a veterinarian public health specialist, a medical doctor, and an experienced therapist. [49], [80] Animal assisted therapy performed at treatment centers should always be performed following by a structured program, under the recommended guides, and targeted at the objectives of the program. [49] Hamsworth and Pizer reported after they investigated studies, which evaluated interactions with animals, and risk factors for zoonosis in immunocomprimised children, and guidelines that information obtained from specialists were not adequately evidence-based. Keeping an animal is beneficial for prevention and development of emotional and physical health. However, guidelines are also required to conduct treatments. [81]

Minimization of risks in such applications depends upon a careful planning with multidisciplinary approaches, written protocols, personnel training, documentation, and investigations. Veterinarian public health practices, which will be performed in this field, are important sources to keep risks endangering human and animal health at minimum levels. Especially veterinarians should choose the appropriate animal for therapy of each patient group according to temperament and behaviors of animals, perform the care for each animal, work for prevention of zoonotic diseases, and suggest an appropriate interaction model for the therapy. [32] Infection controlling policies and regulations should be obeyed in treatment and prevention of zoonotic diseases, so that animal assisted therapies will be more widespread. If measures for risk prevention are taken, then AAT applications can be performed safely. [82], [83]

In studies, where risk analyses have been performed, people interacting with pets have been observed to have benefits for their health. It has been reported from regions, where risks were not significantly high, controlled environmental conditions are provided especially in Europe and North America, potential benefits are reported in treatments with animals kept at home or at hospitals. Guidelines have been developed to limit infection risk during applications and to perform safe treatments. [84]- [86]

In addition to guidelines used during treatments, supportive units have also been established. Animal Assisted Crisis Response (AACR) unit is one of these. This unit provides services in how to struggle with the impending crises for assigned healthcare personnel, consultants and other trainers during animal assisted therapies. [87] Efficiency of these studies depends upon conductance of communication between the related units with a mutual language and a multidisciplinary approach. The most commonly encountered crises issues may be animal behavior, infection risk, and patient-trainer dispute.

Before starting animal assisted therapy and during its' all procedures, it is always remembered that AAT should be performed according to the guidelines in order to prevent risks including adverse reactions of patients, animals, physicians, caregivers, nurses, health personnels, and also relatives of patients, infectious diseases, bitings, etc. it is well clearly explained that AAT should be arranged, managed and performed by a specialist team including patients' physician, veterinary surgeon, psychologist, occupational therapist, expert caregivers, specialist nurses. Therefore, especially veterinary students should be trained about animal assisted therapies, activities and first of all human-animal bond during their undergraduate and postgraduate education. [88]- [91] At this point, according to the Timmins, a veterinary family practice conception can be helpful to understand and contribute human-animal bond from the theoretical framework into the practice for providing needs of patients. [92]

During applications, issues like increased work intensity of the personnel, zoonotic diseases, comfort and care of animals are considered. [93] These may be prevented by well-planned programming. [94] Disease risk can be easily prevented by regular animal health controls, and follow up of individuals. In developing countries like Turkey, animal assisted therapy is not practiced as a specialty filed, yet. Only limited services can be provided according to positive outcomes of human-animal interactions. But recently, an international project (Animals in Therapy Education) have been implemented for 2 years among different institutions from Turkey, Italy and France with financial supporting by European Union LLP Grundtvig Program for aged people. This project intends to design a collection of best practices related to implementation of pet therapy on aged people. As a result of this project will also ease the transfer of pet therapy practices through the comparison and the evaluation of different solutions adopted in the countries involved among partners from Italy, France and Turkey. [95]

9. Conclusion

In this present review, some information about what animal assisted therapies are, application fields, mechanism of action, sample applications for Alzheimer patients, and risk control in AAT, and some recommendations are suggested. It has been observed that this supportive therapeutic approach has been aimed at "complete well-being of individuals physically, socially and mentally as well as improvements of these well-being conditions", which is always emphasized in public health aspect. However, there are still some questions without clear answers, such as AAT is also effective in group therapies as it has been in individualized therapy; how temperament and other features of assisting animal should be. Whatever types the program is, temperaments of all animals should be tested; they should be examined by a veterinarian; and listening-learning training should be performed with patients.

When AAT is practiced according to guidelines, appropriate ethical principles, then it will be an effective supportive treatment option for improvement of human health, life quality, and especially preservation of health state of individuals. However, as it has been undertaken in this present review, it is believed that studies related to animal assisted therapies are required also in our country to evaluate its efficacies in different patient groups correctly.

Author details

Sibel Cevizci[1*], Halil Murat Sen[2], Fahri Güneş[3] and Elif Karaahmet[4]

*Address all correspondence to: cevizci.sibel@gmail.com

1 Canakkale Onsekiz Mart University, School of Medicine, Department of Public Health, Canakkale, Turkey

2 Canakkale Onsekiz Mart University, School of Medicine, Department of Neurology, Canakkale, Turkey

3 Canakkale Onsekiz Mart University, School of Medicine, Department of Internal Medicine, Canakkale, Turkey

4 Canakkale Onsekiz Mart University, School of Medicine, Department of Psychiatry, Canakkale, Turkey

References

[1] Laun, L. Benefits of pet therapy in dementia. Home Healthc Nurse (2003). , 21, 49-52.

[2] Sockalingam, S, Li, M, Krishnadev, U, et al. Use of animal-assisted therapy in the rehabilitation of an assault victim with a concurrent mood disorder. Issues Ment Health Nurs (2008). , 29, 73-84.

[3] Macauley, B. L. Animal-assisted therapy for persons with aphasia: A pilot study. J Rehabil Res Dev (2006). , 43, 357-366.

[4] Ballarini, G. Pet therapy Animals in Human Therapy. Conference Report. Acta Bio Medica (2003). , 74, 97-100.

[5] Cevizci, S, Erginöz, E, & Baltas, Z. A new assisted therapy concept for improving of mental health- Animal assisted therapy. Nobel Med (2009). , 5(1), 4-9.

[6] Cevizci, S, Erginöz, E, & Baltas, Z. Animal assisted therapy for improving human health. TAF Prev Med Bull (2009). , 8(3), 263-272.

[7] LaFrance CGarcia LJ, Labreche J. The effect of a therapy dog on the communication skills of an adult with aphasia. J Commun Disord (2007). , 40(3), 215-224.

[8] Nathans-barel, I, Feldman, P, Berger, B, et al. Animal-assisted therapy ameliorates anhedonia in schizophrenia patients. A controlled pilot study. Psychother Psychosom (2005). , 74(1), 31-35.

[9] Filan, S. L, & Llewellyn-jones, R. H. Animal-assisted therapy for dementia: a review of the literature. Int Psychogeriatr (2006). , 18(4), 597-611.

[10] Edwards, N. E, & Beck, A. M. Animal-assisted therapy and nutrition in Alzheimer's disease. West J Nurs Res (2002). , 24(6), 697-712.

[11] Libin, A, & Cohen-mansfield, J. Therapeutic robocat for nursing home residents with dementia: preliminary inquiry. Am J Alzheimers Dis Other Demen (2004). , 19(2), 111-116.

[12] Richeson, N. Effects of animal-assisted therapy on agitated behaviors and social interactions of older adults with dementia. Am J Alzheimers Dis Other Demen (2003). , 18(6), 353-358.

[13] Kongable, L. G, Buckwalter, K. C, & Stolley, J. M. The effects of pet therapy on the social behavior of institutionalized Alzheimer's clients. Arch Psychiatr Nurs. (1989). , 3(4), 191-8.

[14] Perkins, J, Bartlett, H, Travers, C, & Rand, J. Dog-assisted therapy for older people with dementia: a review. Australas J Ageing. (2008). , 27(4), 177-82.

[15] Tribet, J, Boucharlat, M, & Myslinski, M. Animal-assisted therapy for people suffering from severe dementia. Encephale. (2008). , 34(2), 183-6.

[16] Churchill, M, Safaoui, J, Mccabe, B. W, & Baun, M. M. Using a therapy dog to alleviate the agitation and desocialization of people with Alzheimer's disease. J Psychosoc Nurs Ment Health Serv. (1999). , 37(4), 16-22.

[17] Mccabe, B. W, Baun, M. M, Speich, D, & Agrawal, S. Resident dog in the Alzheimer's special care unit. West J Nurs Res. (2002). , 24(6), 684-96.

[18] Williams, E, & Jenkins, R. Dog visitation therapy in dementia care: a literature review. Nurs Older People. (2008). , 20(8), 31-5.

[19] Kanamori, M, Suzuki, M, Yamamoto, K, Kanda, M, Matsui, Y, Kojima, E, Fukawa, H, Sugita, T, & Oshiro, H. A day care program and evaluation of animal-assisted therapy (AAT) for the elderly with senile dementia. Am J Alzheimers Dis Other Demen. (2001). , 16(4), 234-9.

[20] Cevizci, S. AAT in Turkiye. ATE: Animals in Therapy Education, European Community, LLP Grundtvig Program. Second Project Meeting, Istanbul, Turkiye, March (2011). , 3-4.

[21] Friedmann, E, & Son, H. The human-companion animal bond: how human benefit. Vet Clin North Am Small Anim Pract (2009). , 39(2), 293-326.

[22] Adams, C. L, Bonnett, B. N, & Meek, A. H. Predictors of owner response to companion animal death in 177 clients from 14 practices in Ontario. J Am Vet Med Assoc (2000). , 217(9), 1303-1309.

[23] Clements, P. T, Benasutti, K. M, & Carmone, A. Support for bereaved owners of pets. Perspect Psychiatr Care (2003). , 39(2), 49-54.

[24] Serpell, J. Beneficial effects of pet ownership on some aspects of human health and behaviour. Journal of the Royal Society of Medicine (1991). , 84, 717-720.

[25] Headey, B, Grabka, N. A, F, Zheung, M, & Pets, R. and human health in Australia, China and Germany: evidence from three continents. 10th International IAHAIO Conference on Human-Animal Interactions. Glasgow, UK, (2004).

[26] Bryant, I, & Mcbride, A. Pets, Policies and Tenants: Report on PATHWAY Housing provider 'Pet Policy' Survey. London, Dogs Trust. (2004).

[27] Dembicki, D, & Anderson, J. Pet ownership may be a factor in improved health of the elderly. J Nutr Elder (1996). , 15(3), 15-31.

[28] Raina, P, Waltner-toews, D, Bonnett, B, et al. Influence of companion animals on the physical and psychological health of older people: an analysis of a one-year longitudinal study. J Am Geriatr Soc (1999). , 47(3), 323-329.

[29] Friedmann, E, & Thomas, S. A. Pet ownership, social support, and one-year survival after acute myocardial infarction in the Cardiac Arrhythmia Suppression Trial (CAST). Am J Cardiol (1995). , 76(17), 1213-1217.

[30] Vila, C, Savolainen, P, Maldonado, J. E, et al. Multiple and ancient origins of the domestic dog. Science (1997). , 276, 1687-1689.

[31] Rennie, A. The therapeutic relationship between animals and humans. SCAS Journal (1997). IX;, 1-4.

[32] Ormerod, E. J. Edney ATB, Foster SJ, Whyham MC. Therapeutic applications of the human-companion animal bond. Veterinary Record (2005). , 157, 689-691.

[33] Bustad, L. The role of pets in therapeutic programmes, historic perspectives. In The Waltham Book of Human-Animal Interaction: Benefits and Responsibility of Pet Ownership. Ed I. Robinson. Oxford, Pergamon Press. (1995). , 55-57.

[34] Lane, D. R, Mcnicholas, J, & Collis, G. M. Dogs for the disabled: benefits to recipients and welfare of the dog. Applied Animal Behaviour Science (1998). , 59, 49-60.

[35] Ryder, E. L. Pets and the elderly. A social work perspective. Vet Clin North Am Small Anim Pract (1985). , 15(2), 333-343.

[36] Beck, A. M. The therapeutic use of animals. Vet Clin North Am Small Anim Pract (1985). , 15(2), 365-75.

[37] Messent, P. R. Pets as social facilitators. Vet Clin North Am Small Anim Pract (1985). , 15(2), 387-393.

[38] Anderson, W. P, Reid, C. M, & Jennings, G. L. Pet ownership and risk factors for cardiovascular disease. Med J Aust (1992). , 157(5), 298-301.

[39] Sable, P. Pets, attachment, and well-being across the life cycle. Soc Work (1995). , 40(3), 334-341.

[40] Graf, S. The elderly and their pets. Supportive and problematic aspects and implications for care. A descriptive study. Pflege (1999). , 12(2), 101-111.

[41] Johnson, R. A, & Meadows, R. L. Older Latinos, pets, and health. West J Nurs Res (2002). , 24(6), 609-620.

[42] Shore, E. R, Douglas, D. K, & Riley, M. L. What's in it for the companion animal? Pet attachment and college students' behaviors toward pets. J Appl Anim Welf Sci (2005). , 8(1), 1-11.

[43] Neidhart, L, & Boyd, R. Companion animal adoption study. J Appl Anim Welf Sci (2002). , 5(3), 175-192.

[44] Wright, J. D, Kritz-silverstein, D, Morton, D. J, et al. Pet Ownership and Blood Pressure in Old Age. Epidemiology (2007). , 18(5), 613-618.

[45] Cole, K. M, & Gawlinski, A. Animal-assisted therapy: the human-animal bond. AACN Clin Issues (2000). , 11(1), 139-149.

[46] Gagnon, J, Bouchard, F, Landry, M, et al. Implementing a hospital-based animal therapy program for children with cancer: a descriptive study. Can Oncol Nurs J (2004). , 14(4), 217-222.

[47] Haubenhofer, D. K, & Kirchengast, S. Physiological arousal for companion dogs working with their owners in animal-assisted activities and animal-assisted therapy. J Appl Anim Welf Sci (2006). , 9(2), 165-172.

[48] Fine, A. H. Handbook on Animal-Assisted Therapy: Theoratical Foundations and Guidlines for Practice. Chapter 2. Kruger AK, Serpell JA. Animal-Assisted Interventions in Mental Health: Definitions and Theoretical Foundations. S: 0-12369-484-1Press, (2006). by Elsevier. http://www.scribd.com/doc/76130150/1/CHAPTER-1#page=40Access time: 03.06.2012], 21-38.

[49] Jofré, M L. Animal-assisted therapy in health care facilities. Rev Chilena Infectol (2005). , 22(3), 257-263.

[50] http://wwwsfspca.org/info_rack/aat.pdf

[51] Kovács, Z, Kis, R, Rózsa, S, & Rózsa, L. Animal-assisted therapy for middle-aged schizophrenic patients living in a social institution. A pilot study. Clin Rehabil (2004). , 18(5), 483-486.

[52] Niksa, E. The use of animal-assisted therapy in psychiatric nursing: the story of Timmy and Buddy. J Psychosoc Nurs Ment Health Serv (2007). , 45(6), 56-58.

[53] Connor, K, & Miller, J. Help from our animal friends. Nurs Manage (2000). , 31(7), 42-6.

[54] Connor, K, & Miller, J. Animal-assisted therapy: an in-depth look. Dimens Crit Care Nurs (2000). , 19(3), 20-26.

[55] Brensing, K, Linke, K, & Todt, D. Can dolphins heal by ultrasound? J Theor Biol (2003). , 225(1), 99-105.

[56] http://www.dolphinchildtherapy.com/index.asp?langid=70000&location=1#indikationen

[57] Akiyama, J, & Ohta, M. Increased number of whistles of bottlenose dolphins, Tursiops truncatus, arising from interaction with people. J Vet Med Sci (2007). , 69(2), 165-170.

[58] Odendaal, J. S. Animal-assisted therapy-Magic or medicine? J Psychosom Res. (2000). , 49(4), 275-80.

[59] Johnson, R. A, Meadows, R. L, Haubner, J. S, & Sevedge, K. Animal-assisted activity among patients with cancer: effects on mood, fatigue, self-perceived health, and sense of coherence. Oncol Nurs Forum (2008). , 35(2), 225-32.

[60] Sobo, E. J, Eng, B, & Kassity-krich, N. Canine visitation (pet) therapy: pilot data on decreases in child pain perception. J Holist Nurs. (2006). , 24(1), 51-7.

[61] Esteves, S. W, & Stokes, T. Social Effects of a Dog's Presence on Children with Disabilities. Anthrozoos (2008). , 21(1), 5-15.

[62] Yorke, J, Adams, C, & Coady, N. Therapeutic Value of Equine-Human Bonding in Recovery from Trauma. Anthrozoös (2008). , 21(1), 17-30.

[63] Lotan, M. Alternative therapeutic intervention for individuals with Rett syndrome. Scientific World Journal (2007). , 7, 698-714.

[64] Burrows, K. E, Adams, C. L, & Spiers, J. Sentinels of safety: service dogs ensure safety and enhance freedom and well-being for families with autistic children. Qual Health Res. (2008). , 18(12), 1642-1649.

[65] Basil, B, & Mathews, M. Human and animal health: strengthening the link: methodological concerns about animal facilitated therapy with dolphins. BMJ (2005).

[66] Antonioli, C, & Reveley, M. A. Randomised controlled trial of animal facilitated therapy with dolphins in the treatment of depression. BMJ (2005).

[67] Kellert, S. R. Kinship to mastery. Biophilia in human evolution and development. Washington DC:Island Press (1997). , 1997, 3-115.

[68] Kellert, S. R, & Wilson, E. O. Thebiophilia hypothesis. Washington DC: Island Press, (1993).

[69] Sloane, P. D, Mitchell, C. M, Preisser, J. S, Phillips, C, Commander, C, & Burker, E. Environmental correlates of resident agitation in Alzheimer's disease special care units. J Am Geriatr Soc. (1998). , 46(7), 862-9.

[70] Zeisel, J, Silverstein, N. M, Hyde, J, Levkoff, S, Lawton, M. P, & Holmes, W. Environmental correlates to behavioral health outcomes in Alzheimer's special care units. Gerontologist. (2003). , 43(5), 697-711.

[71] Teri, L, & Logsdon, R. Assessment and management of behavioral disturbances in Alzheimer's disease. Compr Ther. (1990). , 16(5), 36-42.

[72] Manepalli, J, Desai, A, & Sharma, P. Psychosocial-Environmental Treatments for Alzheimer's Disease. Primary Psychiatry. (2009). , 16(6), 39-47.

[73] Berget, B, Ekeberg, O, & Braastad, B. O. Animal-assisted therapy with farm animals for persons with psychiatric disorders: effects on self-efficacy, coping ability and quality of life, a randomized controlled trial. Clin Pract Epidemiol Ment Health. (2008).

[74] Rossetti, J, & King, C. Use of animal-assisted therapy with psychiatric patients. J Psychosoc Nurs Ment Health Serv. (2010). , 48(11), 44-8.

[75] Knisely, J. S, Barker, S. B, & Barker, R. T. Research on benefits of canine-assisted therapy for adults in nonmilitary settings. US Army Med Dep J. (2012). , 2012, 30-7.

[76] Bánszky, N, Kardos, E, Rózsa, L, & Gerevich, J. The psychiatric aspects of animal assisted therapy]. Psychiatr Hung. (2012). , 27(3), 180-90.

[77] Javelot, H, Antoine-bernard, E, Garat, J, Javelot, T, Weiner, L, & Mervelay, V. Snoezelen and animal-assisted therapy in dementia patients]. Soins Gerontol. (2012).

[78] Marcus, D. A. Complementary medicine in cancer care: adding a therapy dog to the team. Curr Pain Headache Rep. (2012). , 16(4), 289-91.

[79] Aoki, J, Iwahashi, K, Ishigooka, J, Fukamauchi, F, Numajiri, M, Ohtani, N, & Ohta, M. Evaluation of cerebral activity in the prefrontal cortex in mood [affective] disorders during animal-assisted therapy (AAT) by near-infrared spectroscopy (NIRS): A pilot study. Int J Psychiatry Clin Pract. (2012). , 16(3), 205-13.

[80] Hoff, G. L, Brawley, J, & Johnson, K. Companion animal issues and the physician. South Med J (1999). , 92(7), 651-659.

[81] Hemsworth, S, & Pizer, B. Pet ownership in immunocompromised children-a review of the literature and survey of existing guidelines. Eur J Oncol Nurs (2006). , 10(2), 117-27.

[82] Guay, D. R. Pet-assisted therapy in the nursing home setting: potential for zoonosis. Am J Infect Control (2001). , 29(3), 178-186.

[83] Brickel, C. M. The therapeutic roles of cat mascots with a hospital-based geriatric population: a staff survey. Gerontologist (1979). , 19, 368-372.

[84] Writing Panel of Working GroupLefebvre SL et al. Guidelines for animal-assisted interventions in health care facilities. Am J Infect Control (2008). , 36(2), 78-85.

[85] DiSalvo HHaiduven D, Johnson N, et al. Who let the dogs out? Infection control did: utility of dogs in health care settings and infection control aspects. Am J Infect Control (2006). , 34(5), 301-307.

[86] Brodie, S. J, Biley, F. C, & Shewring, M. An exploration of the potential risks associated with using pet therapy in healthcare settings. J Clin Nurs (2002). , 11(4), 444-456.

[87] Greenbaum, S. D. Introduction to working with Animal Assisted Crisis Response animal handler teams. Int J Emerg Ment Health. (2006). , 8(1), 49-63.

[88] Schaffer, C. B. Enhancing human-animal relationships through veterinary medical instruction in animal-assisted therapy and animal-assisted activities. J Vet Med Educ. (2008). , 35(4), 503-10.

[89] Sherman, B. L, & Serpell, J. A. Training veterinary students in animal behavior to preserve the human-animal bond. J Vet Med Educ. (2008). , 35(4), 496-502.

[90] Wensley, S. P. Animal welfare and the human-animal bond: considerations for veterinary faculty, students, and practitioners. J Vet Med Educ. (2008). , 35(4), 532-9.

[91] Ormerod, E. J. Bond-centered veterinary practice: lessons for veterinary faculty and students. J Vet Med Educ. (2008). , 35(4), 545-52.

[92] Timmins, R. P. The contribution of animals to human well-being: a veterinary family practice perspective. J Vet Med Educ. (2008). , 35(4), 540-4.

[93] Khan, M. A, & Farrag, N. Animal assisted activity and infection control implications in a healthcare setting. Journal of Hospital Infection (2000). , 46, 4-11.

[94] Jorgenson, J. Therapeutic uses of companion animals in health care. Journal of Nursing Scholarship (1997). , 29, 249-254.

[95] ATE: Animals in Therapy Educationhttp://www.forsas.it/ate/Sito%20Eng/Ate_en.pdfAccess time: 12.07.(2012).

Section 4

Epidemiology, Clinical Presentation and Prevention

Chapter 13

Epidemiology of Alzheimer's Disease

Weili Xu, Camilla Ferrari and Hui-Xin Wang

Additional information is available at the end of the chapter

http://dx.doi.org/10.5772/54398

1. Introduction

1.1. Global aging

The aging of populations has become a worldwide phenomenon [1]. In 1990, 26 nations had more than two million elderly citizens aged 65 years and older, and the projections indicate that an additional 34 countries will join the list by 2030. In 2000, the number of old people (65+ years) in the world was estimated to be 420 million and it was projected to be nearly one billion by 2030, with the proportion of old people increasing from 7 to 12%. The largest increase in absolute numbers of old people will occur in developing countries; it will almost triple from 249 million in 2000 to an estimated 690 million in 2030. The developing regions' sharing the worldwide aging population will increase from 59 to 71% [2]. Developed countries, which have already shown a dramatic increase in people over 65 years of age will experience a progressive aging of the elderly population. Underlying global population aging is a process known as the "demographic transition" in which mortality and then fertility decline [3]. Decreasing fertility and lengthening life expectancy have together reshaped the age structure of the population in most regions of the planet by shifting relative weight from younger to older groups.

Both developed and developing countries will face the challenge of coping with a high frequency of chronic conditions, such as dementia, which is a characteristic of aging societies. These conditions impair the ability of older persons to function optimally in the community and reduce well-being among affected individuals and their families. Further, these conditions are associated with significant health care costs that must be sustained by the society at large. Thus, the global trend in the phenomenon of population aging has a dramatic impact on public health, healthcare financing and delivery systems throughout the world [4]. Due to the aging of the population, dementia has become a major challenge to elderly care and public health.

1.2. Dementia and Alzheimer's disease

Dementia is defined as a clinical syndrome, and characterized by the development of multiple cognitive deficits that are severe enough to interfere with daily functioning, including social and professional functioning. The cognitive deficits include memory impairment and at least one of the other cognitive domains, such as aphasia, apraxia, agnosia or disturbances in executive functioning [5, 6]. Alzheimer's disease is the most common cause of dementia in the elderly, accounting for 60-70% of all demented cases [7]. Alzheimer's disease is strictly a neuropathological diagnosis determined by the presence of neurofibrillary tangles and senile plaques in the brain of patients with dementia. The disease frequently starts with memory impairment, but is invariably followed by a progressive global cognitive impairment [8]. Vascular dementia is the second most common cause of dementia in the elderly after Alzheimer's disease. Vascular dementia is defined as loss of cognitive function resulting from ischemic, hypoperfusive, or haemorrhagic brain lesions due to cerebrovascular disease or cardiovascular pathology. Diagnosis of vascular dementia requires cognitive impairment; vascular brain lesions, often predominantly subcortical, as demonstrated by brain imaging; a temporal link between stroke and dementia; and exclusion of other causes of dementia [9]. The combination of Alzheimer's disease and vascular dementia pathological changes in the brains of older people are extremely common, making mixed dementia probably the most common type of dementia [10].

Alzheimer's disease was first identified more than 100 years ago, but research into its symptoms, causes, risk factors and treatment has gained momentum only in the last 30 years. Although research has revealed a great deal about Alzheimer's, the precise physiologic changes that trigger the development of Alzheimer's disease largely remain unknown. The only exceptions are certain rare, inherited forms of the disease caused by known genetic mutations. Alzheimer's disease affects people in different ways, but the most common symptom pattern begins with gradually worsening ability to remember new information. This occurs because disruption of brain cell function usually begins in brain regions involved in forming new memories. As damage spreads, individuals experience other difficulties. The following are warning signs of Alzheimer's disease: memory loss that disrupts daily life; challenges in planning or solving problems; difficulty completing familiar tasks at home, at work or at leisure; confusion with time or place; trouble understanding visual images and spatial relationships; new problems with words in speaking or writing; misplacing things and losing the ability to retrace steps; decreased or poor judgment; withdrawal from work or social activities; and changes in mood and personality. As the disease progresses, the individual's cognitive and functional abilities decline. In advanced Alzheimer's disease, people need help with basic activities of daily living, such as bathing, dressing, eating and using the bathroom. Those in the final stages of the disease lose their ability to communicate, fail to recognize loved ones and become bed-bound and reliant on around-the-clock care. When an individual has difficulty moving because of Alzheimer's disease, they are more vulnerable to infections, including pneumonia (infection of the lungs).

2. Occurrence of Alzheimer's disease

The occurrence of a disease can be measured as proportion of people affected by the disease in a defined population at a specific time point (prevalence), or as number of new cases that occur during a specific time period in a population at risk for developing that disease (incidence). The prevalence reflects the public health burden of the disease, whereas the incidence indicates the risk of developing that disease. The prevalence is determined by both incidence and duration of the disease, and in certain circumstances, the prevalence may be estimated as incidence × average disease duration.

2.1. Prevalence

Based on the available epidemiological data, a group of experts estimated that 24.3 million people have dementia today, with 4.6 million new cases of dementia every year (one new case every 7 seconds). The number of people affected will double every 20 years to 81.1 million by 2040 [11]. Similar estimates have been reported previously [12]. Most people with dementia live in developing countries. China and its western Pacific neighbours have the highest number of people with dementia (6 million), followed by the European Union (5.0 million), USA (2.9 million), and India (1.5 million). The rates of increase in the number of dementia cases are not uniform across the world; numbers in developed countries are forecasted to increase by 100% between 2001 and 2040, but to increase by more than 300% in India, China, and other south Asian and western Pacific countries [11]. About 70% of these cases were attributed to Alzheimer's disease [11, 13]. The pooled data of population-based studies in Europe suggests that the age-standardized prevalence in people 65+ years old was 6.4 % for dementia and 4.4 % for Alzheimer's disease [14]. In the US, a study of a national representative sample of people aged >70 years yielded a prevalence for Alzheimer's disease of 9.7 % [15].

Worldwide, the global prevalence of dementia was estimated to be 3.9 % in people aged 60+ years, with the regional prevalence being 1.6 % in Africa, 4.0 % in China and Western Pacific regions, 4.6 % in Latin America, 5.4 % in Western Europe, and 6.4 % in North America [11]. A meta-analysis including 18 studies from China during 1990-2010 showed prevalence of Alzheimer's disease of 1.9% [16]. More than 25 million people in the world are currently affected by dementia, most suffering from Alzheimer's disease, with around 5 million new cases occurring every year [11]. The number of people with dementia is anticipated to double every 20 years. Despite different inclusion criteria, several meta-analyses and nationwide surveys have yielded roughly similar age-specific prevalence of AD across regions (Figure 1) [17]. The age-specific prevalence of Alzheimer's disease almost doubles every 5 years after aged 65. Among developed nations, approximately 1 in 10 older people aged ≥ 65 is affected by some degree of dementia, whereas more than one third of very old people aged ≥85 years may have dementia-related symptoms and signs [18, 19]. There is a similar pattern of dementia subtypes across the world, with Alzheimer's disease and vascular dementia, the two most common forms of dementia, accounting for 50 % to 70 % and 15 % to 25 %, respectively, of all dementia cases.

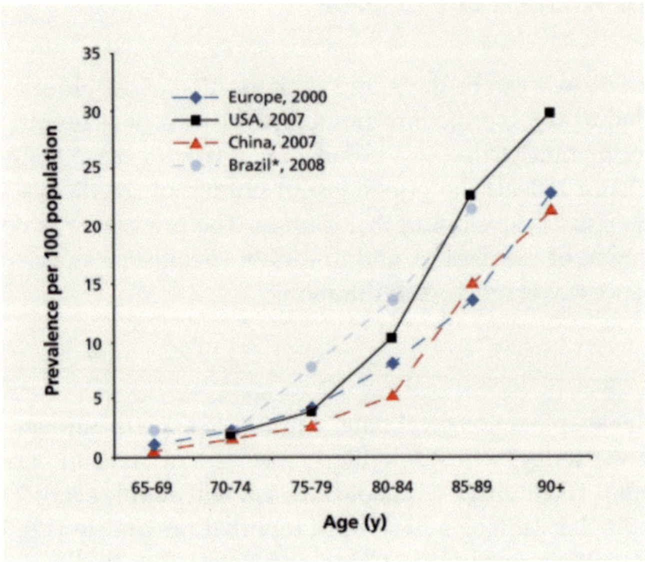

Figure 1. Age-specific prevalence of Alzheimer's disease (per 100 population) across continents and countries. *prevalence of all types of dementia [17].

Epidemiological research of dementia and AD in low- and middle-income countries has drawn much attention in recent years. A systematic review estimated that the overall prevalence of Alzheimer's disease in developing countries was 3.4 % (95 % CI,1.6 % - 5.0 %) [20]. The prevalence of dementia (DSM-IV criteria) in people aged 65+ years in seven developing nations varied widely from less than 0.5 % to more than 6 %, which is substantially lower than in developed countries [21]. Indeed, the prevalence rates of dementia in India and rural Latin America were approximately a quarter of the rates in European countries. However, the prevalence of AD in persons 65+ years in urban areas of China was 3.5 %, and even higher (4.8 %) after post-hoc correction for negative screening errors [22], which is generally comparable with those from Western nations. Similar prevalence rates of dementia were also reported from the urban populations of Latin American nations such as Havana in Cuba (6.4 %) and São Paulo in Brazil (5.1 %) [20, 23, 24].

2.2. Incidence

The global annual incidence of dementia is around 7.5 per 1,000 persons [11]. The incidence rate of dementia increases exponentially with age, from approximately one per 1,000 person-year in people aged 60-64 years to more than 70 per 1,000 person-year in 90+ year-olds. The incidence rates of dementia across regions are quite similar in the younger-old (<75 years), but greater variations are seen among the older ages [25]. Slightly lower rates have been detected in the USA in comparison with Europe and Asia, and this is possibly due to differences in the study designs and the case ascertainment procedures. The pooled incidence rate of Alzheimer's disease among people 65+ years of age in Europe was 19.4 per 1000 person-year [26]. The pooled data from two large-scale community-based studies of people aged ≥65 years in the US Seattle and Baltimore areas yielded an incidence rate for Alzheimer's disease of 15.0 (male, 13.0; female, 16.9) per 1000 person-year [27, 28]. The incidence rate of Alzheimer's disease increases almost exponentially with increasing age until 85 years of age (Figure 2) [17]. A consistently exponential increase, with advancing age in Alzheimer incidence suggests that Alzheimer's disease is an inevitable consequence of aging, whereas a convergence to or a decline at certain age may suggest that very old people may have reduced vulnerability, owing perhaps to genetic or environmental factors. The Cache County Study further found that the incidence of AD increased with age, peaked, and then started to decline at extreme old ages for both men and women [29]. However, some meta-analyses and large-scale studies in Europe provided no evidence for the potential decline in the incidence of dementia and Alzheimer's disease among the oldest-old age groups [26, 30, 31]. The apparent decline suggested in some studies may be an artifact of poor response rate and survival effect in these very old age groups. Several studies from Europe observed a higher incidence rate of Alzheimer's disease among women than men, especially among the oldest-old age groups, whereas studies in North America found no significant gender difference [17].

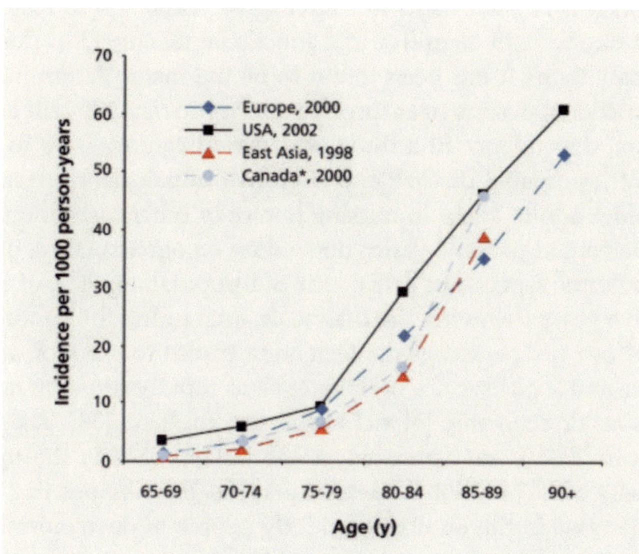

Figure 2. Age-specific incidence of Alzheimer's disease (per 1 000 person years) across continents and countries. *incidence of all types of dementia [17].

There appears to be some geographic variations in the incidence of Alzheimer's disease. The pooled data of eight European studies suggested a geographical dissociation across Europe, with higher incidence rates being found among the oldest-old people of north-western countries than among southern countries [26]. The incidence rates of Alzheimer's disease were reported to be slightly lower in North America than in Europe. Differences in methodology (e.g., differences in study design and procedure of case ascertainment), rather than real different regional distributions of the disease, may be partly responsible for the geographic variations. The study using identical methods in UK found no evidence of variation in dementia incidence among five areas in England and Wales [30]. Studies have confirmed that AD incidence in developing countries is generally lower than in North America and Europe. For example, the incidence rate of AD among people aged 65+ years was 7.7 per 1 000 person-year in Brazil and 3.2 per 1 000 person-year in India [20, 32].

3. Prognosis and impact

Dementia is one of the leading causes of death in older people. However, death certificates grossly underreport its cause, even when multiple underlying causes of death are taken into account. The community-based follow-up studies could provide reliable data on mortality. In the Swedish Kungsholmen Project of people aged 75 years or over, the mortality rate of dementia was 2.4 per 100 person-year; 70% of incident dementia cases died within five years following the diagnosis. In three years, more than 50% of the dementia cases reached the severe stage. In the Kungsholmen Project, the proportion of severe dementia among prevalent cases increased from 19% at baseline to 48% after three years, and to 78% after seven years. This progression is due to both cognitive and functional decline [33]. Dementia is strongly associated with disability as it has been found to be the major determinant of developing dependence and functional decline over three years. Approximately half of the persons who developed functional dependence in a three year period can attribute to dementia [34]. In industrialised countries, mental disease and cognitive impairment are the most prevalent disorders among older adults living in nursing homes or other institutions. However, institutionalisation of demented patients varies depending on age structure, urban or rural residence, and other cultural aspects. In a 75+ year old population, 70% of incident dementia cases died in the five years following the diagnosis, accounting for a mortality rate specific for dementia of 2.4 per 100 person-years. Dementia triples the risk of death [35]. The demands of healthcare and social service of the huge and rapidly growing numbers of dementia patients have a major economic impact at the societal level [36]. The worldwide direct costs for dementia in 2003 were estimated at 156 billion USD in the main scenario of a worldwide prevalence of 27.7 million demented persons. It is obvious that due to these costs and the expected increase in the number of elderly people in developing countries, the dementing conditions will present a great challenge [37,38].

4. Risk and protective factors

Alzheimer's disease is multifactorial disorder that is determined by genetic and environmental factors as well as their interactions. Population-based prospective study is the major epidemiological approach to identifying influential factors for chronic multifactorial diseases such as dementia, in which the life-course approach should be taken into consideration. Age is the most powerful determinant of Alzheimer's disease, and gene mutations contribute to a small proportion of all cases. The strong association of Alzheimer's disease with increasing age may partially reflect the cumulative effect of different risk and protective factors over the lifespan, including the effect of complex interactions of genetic susceptibility, psychosocial factors, biological factors, and environmental exposures experienced over the lifespan. Evidence from epidemiological, neuroimaging, and neuropathological research, supports the role of genetic, vascular, and psychosocial factors in the development of Alzheimer's disease, whereas evidence for the etiologic role of dietary or nutritional factors, occupational exposures, and inflammation is less clear [39].

4.1. Genetic factors

Mutations in amyloid precursor protein, presenilin-1, and presenilin-2 genes can cause early-onset familial Alzheimer's disease that account for no more than 5% of all cases. The majority of AD cases are sporadic, with considerable heterogeneity in their risk profiles and neuropathological features.

4.1.1. Apolipoprotein E ε4 (APOE ε4)

The *APOE* ε4 allele is the only established susceptibility gene for both early- and late-onset Alzheimer's disease, and is a susceptibility gene, being neither necessary nor sufficient for the development of Alzheimer's disease. *APOE* ε4 is one of three common forms (ε2, ε3 and ε4) of the *APOE* gene, which provides the blue print for a protein that carries cholesterol in the bloodstream. Everyone inherits one form of the *APOE* gene from each parent. Those who inherit one *APOE* ε4 gene have increased risk of developing Alzheimer's disease and of developing it at an earlier age than those who inherit the ε2 or ε3 forms of the *APOE* gene [40]. Those who inherit two *APOE*-ε4 genes have an even higher risk. Unlike inheriting a known genetic mutation for Alzheimer's disease, inheriting one or two copies of this form of the *APOE* gene does not guarantee that an individual will develop Alzheimer's disease. The risk effect of the *APOE* ε4 allele decreases with increasing age, and after age 75, 15–20% of Alzheimer's cases are attributable to *APOE* genotype [41]. Several other genes have been examined as possible candidates, but the reports are sporadic, and the results are inconsistent [42].

However, not all (4-carriers develop dementia. Studies have demonstrated that high education, active leisure activities, or maintaining vascular health seems to reduce the risk of dementia related to APOE ε4 [40, 41]. The ε4-carriers with these characteristics appear to have similar dementia-free survival time to non ε4-carriers. Further, the obese related FTO gene may interact with *APOE* ε4 to increase the risk of Alzheimer's disease [44].

4.1.2. Family history

Individuals who have a parent, brother or sister with Alzheimer's are more likely to develop the disease than those who do not have a first-degree relative with Alzheimer's [45-47]. Those who have more than one first-degree relative with Alzheimer's disease are at even higher risk of developing the disease [48]. When diseases run in families, heredity (genetics), shared environmental and /or lifestyle factors or both may play a role.

4.2. Biological risk factors

Increasing age is a well-established risk factor for Alzheimer's disease. The incidence of Alzheimer's disease almost doubles with every 5 years of age [49, 50]. Female sex is often associated with an increased risk of AD, especially at the oldest-old age [25]. Men seem to be at greater risk for vascular dementia than women [51].

4.3. Vascular disorders and risk factors

A number of vascular risk factors and disorders have been linked to Alzheimer's disease, but some factors may have a differential association with the risk of Alzheimer's disease depending on the age when the exposure is assessed.

4.3.1. Blood pressure

Several studies have consistently reported an association between midlife high blood pressure and increased risk of dementia and Alzheimer's disease [52, 53]. Hypertension has been linked to neurodegenerative markers in the brain, suggesting that long-term high blood pressure may play a causal role in the neurodegenerative process itself or by causing brain atrophy. In very old people, the deleterious effect of high blood pressure is less evident, whereas low blood pressure seems to be predictive of dementia and Alzheimer's disease. As dementia has a long latent period, low blood pressure may be a sign of impending illness [54], which was confirmed by the longitudinal data from the Kungsholmen Project, suggesting the involvement of late life low blood pressure and cerebral hypo-perfusion in the development of dementia and Alzheimer's disease [55]. All these findings suggest that the relation of blood pressure to dementia may be age-dependent [25].

Recent follow-up studies have suggested that the protective effect of antihypertensive therapy on dementia and AD may depend on the duration of treatment and the age when people take the medications; the more evident efficacy was seen among young-old people (i.e., <75 years) and those with long-term treatment [56, 57]. Evidence from clinical trials of antihypertensive therapy and dementia is summarized in the section on intervention trials towards primary prevention. Antihypertensive treatment may protect against dementia and AD by postponing atherosclerotic process, reducing the number of cerebrovascular lesions, and improving cerebral perfusion [52]. It has also been suggested that some antihypertensive agents (e.g., calcium-channel antagonists) may have neuroprotective effects. The recent neuropathological study found substantially less Alzheimer neuropathological changes (i.e., neuritic plaque and neurofibrillary tangle densities) in the medicated hypertension group than non-hypertensive group, which may reflect a salutary effect of antihypertensive therapy against Alzheimer's disease-associated neuropathology [57].

4.3.2. Cardiovascular disease

A healthy heart helps ensure that enough blood is pumped through blood vessels to the brain. The follow-up data of the Cardiovascular Health Study showed that cardiovascular disease was associated with an increased risk of Alzheimer's disease, especially in people with peripheral arterial disease [58], suggesting that extensive peripheral atherosclerosis is a risk factor for Alzheimer's disease. Other cardiovascular diseases, such as heart failure and atrial fibrillation, have been independently related to increased risk of dementia. In the Kungsholmen Project, heart failure was associated with a more than 80% increased risk of dementia and Alzheimer's disease [59].

4.3.3. Cerebrovascular disease

Cerebrovascular changes such as haemorrhagic infarcts, small and large ischemic cortical infarcts, vasculo-pathie, and white matter changes all increase the risk of dementia [13]. Systematic reviews of population-based studies reveal an approximately two- to four-fold increased risk of incident dementia associated with clinical stroke (post-stroke dementia). Multiple cerebral infarcts, recurrent and strategic strokes are main risk factors for post-stroke dementia. Silent stroke and white matter lesions detected on neuroimaging are associated with increased risk of dementia and cognitive decline. Spontaneous cerebral emboli were related to both AD and VaD. Some studies reported an association of stroke with Alzheimer's disease and cognitive decline [60]. Cerebral vascular lesions may interact with neurodegenerative lesions to produce a dementia syndrome in individuals not having sufficient neurodegenerative damages to express dementia [25]. Neuropathological studies suggested that cerebrovascular lesions, atherosclerosis, and neurodegenerative changes in the brain often coexist, and may be coincident processes converging to cause additive damage to the aging brain and to promote clinical expression of the dementia syndrome [61].

4.3.4. Diabetes mellitus

A potential link between diabetes and cognitive impairment was first reported more than 80 years ago. The association of diabetes with these cognitive changes is now well established [62]. There is substantial evidence suggesting that type 2 diabetes is associated with cognitive impairment involving both memory and executive function [63-65]. Several large longitudinal population-based studies have also shown that the rate of cognitive decline is accelerated in elderly people with type 2 diabetes [66]. An increased risk of not only vascular dementia but also neurodegenerative type dementia among persons with diabetes has been reported in several longitudinal studies [67-70], and the risk effect was confirmed by a systematic review [71]. Midlife diabetes or a longer duration of diabetes may play a crucial role in dementia and Alzheimer's disease [68, 72]. Overall, diabetes leads to a 20-70% greater decline in cognitive performance, and a 60% higher risk of dementia [73]. In addition, borderline or prediabetes or impaired glucose tolerance, is also linked to an increased risk of dementia and Alzheimer's disease in very old people [74].

4.3.5. Overweight and obesity

Similar to hypertension, recent studies suggested a lifespan-dependent relation of obesity with dementia [75, 76]. A higher body mass index (BMI) at middle age was related to an increased risk of dementia in late life [77, 78]. A greater decline in BMI approximately 10 years prior to dementia onset was detected, which is in line with the other studies suggesting an association of accelerated BMI decline with Alzheimer's disease [79, 80]. Low BMI in late life and weight loss may be related to high risk of dementia and Alzheimer's disease [81], but low BMI and weight loss can be interpreted as markers of preclinical Alzheimer's disease, especially when measured less than 10 years prior to clinical diagnosis [25]. In line with these findings, several follow-up studies of older people suggested that accelerated decline in BMI was associated with future development of Alzheimer's disease [79, 82, 83]. Low BMI in late life was related to a higher risk for Alzheimer's disease over a subsequent 5- to 6-year period [81]. Thus, late-life low BMI and weight loss can be interpreted as markers for preclinical Alzheimer's disease, particularly when measured just a few years prior to clinical diagnosis of the disease [17].

4.3.6. Hyperlipidaemia

An association of elevated cholesterol at middle life with increased risk of late-life Alzheimer's disease was reported in some studies [53]. Controversial findings have also been reported on the relation of cholesterol in late life to dementia risk. Some cohort studies found no association or even an inverse association of total cholesterol with dementia risk [84]. A study showed a decline in total cholesterol at least 15 years before dementia onset [85]. Recently, a bidirectional cholesterol-cognition relationship has been reported. High midlife cholesterol was associated with poorer late-life cognition, but decreasing cholesterol after midlife may reflect poorer cognitive status [86].

4.3.7. The metabolic syndrome

Instead of exploring the effect of its subcomponents, several studies have assessed the relationship between metabolic syndrome as a whole and the risk of Alzheimer's disease or cognitive decline. A clustering of interrelated metabolic risk factors such as diabetes, obesity, hypertension and dyslipidaemia has received increasing attention in the past few years. Several components of the metabolic syndrome have been individually related to cognitive outcomes. A prospective study found that the metabolic syndrome contributed to cognitive decline [87]. But this finding was not confirmed in a population of the oldest old. The concept of the metabolic syndrome may be less valid in this age group [88]. Finally, two studies showed that metabolic syndrome was associated with an increased risk of Alzheimer's disease [89, 90].

4.3.8. Alcohol consumption

Excessive alcohol intake can cause alcoholic dementia and may increase the risk of vascular dementia. Heavier alcohol intake at middle age was associated with increased risk of late-life dementia [91]. By contrast, increasing evidence suggests that light to moderate alcohol consumption may be associated with a reduced risk of dementia and cognitive decline [92], a similar effect as observed for cardiovascular disease [25]. In a meta-analysis of 15 prospective studies on the effect of alcohol on dementia risk, light to moderate alcohol consumption was associated with a reduction in the risk of Alzheimer's disease and dementia [93]. However, the role of moderate alcohol consumption in dementia still remains controversial because the inverse association may be due to information bias, the confounding of healthy lifestyles and high socioeconomic status, different approaches in assessments of alcohol consumption, or outcome misclassification.

4.3.9. Cigarette smoking

The relationship between smoking and cognitive decline remains uncertain. Case-control studies have largely suggested that smoking lowers the risk of Alzheimer's disease [13]. Some prospective studies have found an increased risk of Alzheimer's disease associated with smoking [94]. A meta-analysis that examined the association between smoking and Alzheimer's disease while accounting for tobacco-industry affiliation found that the combined results of 18 cross-sectional studies without industry affiliations yielded no association [95]. Analysis of 14 cohort studies without tobacco-industry affiliations yielded a significant increase in the risk of Alzheimer's disease [13]. In the Kungsholmen Project, smoking affected survival in Alzheimer's disease cases more than in non-demented subjects, and the protective effect of smoking on the Alzheimer's disease was no longer present when incident Alzheimer's cases were studied [7] suggesting that previously reported association of cigarette smoking with low prevalence of dementia was probably due to survival bias.

4.3.10. Diet and nutrients

Diets high in fish, fruits and vegetables are high in anti-oxidants and polyunsaturated fatty acids (PUFAs). In some observational studies, high or supplementary intake of vitamins C, E, B6, B12, and folate has been related to a decreased risk of Alzheimer's disease [96, 97]. Indeed, low levels of B12 and folate were found to be related to an increased risk of Alzheimer's disease in a study from the Kungsholmen Project [98]. Investigations on the effect of dietary PUFAs on the risk of cognitive dysfunction proved inconclusive. Several studies showed that the consumption of PUFAs led to reduction in the risk of Alzheimer's disease and dementia, mild cognitive impairment [99]. Population-based studies suggested that moderate to high intake of unsaturated fats at midlife is protective, whereas a moderate intake of saturated fats may increase the risk of dementia and Alzheimer's disease [100, 101], especially among *APOE* ε4 carriers [102, 103]. Fatty acids may affect dementia through various mechanisms such as atherosclerosis and inflammation. Adherence to 'Mediterranean diet' (higher intake of fish, fruits, and vegetables rich in antioxidants) was associated with a reduced risk of Alzheimer's disease independent of vascular pathways [104].

4.4. Psychosocial factors

Psychological factors include social economic status, education attainment in early life, and work complexity in adult-life and leisure activities. Evidence from epidemiological research has been accumulating that some psychosocial factors and healthy lifestyle may postpone the onset of dementia, possibly by enhancing cognitive reserve.

4.4.1. Social economic status

A number of studies have found that higher socioeconomic status (SES) is associated with a reduced risk of developing Alzheimer's disease [105-107]. In most of these studies, SES was assessed based on occupational attainment, current income to reflect socioeconomic level in adulthood, or educational attainment. Findings from a prospective study, however, suggested that early life socioeconomic status assessed at the household or community level was related to level of cognition in late life but not to rate of cognitive decline or risk of Alzheimer's disease [47].

4.4.2. High education

Numerous longitudinal studies have consistently shown that a higher educational achievement in early life is associated with a decreased incidence of dementia, and of Alzheimer's disease in particular. Low dementia prevalence among highly educated persons has been reported by numerous surveys. Educational attainment and lifespan mental activity associated with childhood education may reduce the risk of dementia [25]. The cogntive reserve hypothesis has been proposed to interpret this association such that education could enhance neural and cognitive reserve that may provide compensatory mechanisms to cope with degenerative pathological changes in the brain, and therefore delay onset of the dementia syndrome [17]. Alternatively, educational achievement may be a surrogate or an indicator of intelligent quotient, early life living environments, and occupational toxic exposure experienced over adulthood [108].

4.4.3. Physical activity

Basic science and observational evidence on humans strongly supports the hypothesis that increased physical activity prevents the onset of dementia. Regular exercise, even low-intensity activity such as walking, has been associated with reduced risk of dementia and cognitive decline [109-111]. In the Kungsholmen Project, the component of physical activity presenting in various leisure activities, rather than sports and any specific physical exercise, was related to a decreased dementia risk [110]. A strong protective effect of regular physical activity in middle age against the development of dementia and Alzheimer's disease in late life was reported, especially for persons with the *APOE* ε4 allele [112]. As it may take years to achieve high levels of physical fitness, brief periods of exercise training may not have substantial benefits on cognitive processes, but could still be detectable in the subsets of cognitive domains that are more sensitive to the age related decrements. Physical activity is important not only in promoting general and vascular health, but also in promoting brain plasticity, and it may also affect several gene transcripts and neurotropic factors that are relevant for the maintenance of cognitive functions. There is now increasing amounts of trial evidence to support this hypothesis in terms of cognitive benefits in healthy older adults as well as in people at risk for dementia. However, to date there are no RCTs confirm that increased physical activity prevents dementia.

4.4.4. *Mentally stimulating activity*

Various types of mentally demanding activities have been examined in relation to dementia and AD, including knitting, gardening, dancing, playing board games and musical instruments, reading, social and cultural activities, and watching specific television programs, which often showed a protective effect [113]. Due to the cultural and individual differences in choosing specific activities, some researchers summarize mentally stimulating activities into a composite score, which showed that a cognitive activity score involving participation in seven common activities with information processing as a central component was associated with a reduced risk of AD, even after controlling for APOE ε4 allele, medical conditions, and depressive symptoms [114, 115]. The Swedish Twin Study showed that greater complexity of work, and particularly complex work with people, may reduce the risk of Alzheimer's disease [116]. The Canadian Study of Health and Aging found that high complexity of work appeared to be associated with a reduced risk of dementia, but mostly for vascular dementia [117]. In supporting of these findings, the recent neuroimaging study suggested that a high level of complex mental activity across the lifespan was correlated with a reduced rate of hippocampal atrophy [118].

4.4.5. *Social network and social engagement*

A poor social network or social disengagement in late life was associated with an elevated risk of dementia. Evidence from longitudinal observational studies suggests that a poor social network or social disengagement is associated with cognitive decline and dementia [119, 120]. The risk for dementia and AD was also increased in older people with increasing social isolation and less frequent and unsatisfactory contacts with relatives and friends. Furthermore, low social engagement in late life and a decline in social engagement from middle age to late life were associated with a doubly increased risk of developing dementia and AD in late life. Rich social networks and high social engagement imply better social support, leading to better access to resources and material goods [123]. Rich and large social networks also provide affective and intellectual stimulation that could influence cognitive function and different health outcomes through behavioural, psychological, and physiological pathways [122]. Finally, a recent study suggested that low neuroticism in combination with high extraversion was the personality trait associated with the lowest dementia risk, and among socially isolated individuals even low neuroticism alone seemed to decrease the risk of dementia [121].

4.4.6. *Depression*

Recent evidence suggests a strong relationship between depression and Alzheimer's disease. A lifetime history of major depression has been considered as a risk factor for later development of Alzheimer's disease [124, 125]. The presence of depressive symptoms can affect the conversion of mild cognitive impairment to Alzheimer's disease. Neuronal plaques and neurofibrillary tangles, the two major hallmarks of Alzheimer's disease brain, are more pronounced in the brains of Alzheimer's disease patients with comorbid depression as compared with Alzheimer's disease patients without depression. On the other hand, neurodegenerative phenomena have been observed in different brain regions of patients with a history of depression. Recent evidence suggests that molecular mechanisms and cascades that underlie the pathogenesis of major depression, such as chronic inflammation and hyper-activation of hypothalamic–pituitary–adrenal (HPA) axis, are also involved in the pathogenesis of Alzheimer's disease [125]. A recent study has shown that depression increased the risk of dementia among patients with diabetes [126].

4.5. Other factors

4.5.1. Inflammation

Inflammation is known to be involved in the atherosclerotic process. Thus, serum inflammatory makers may be associated with dementia. Some cohort studies found such an association, and C-reactive protein may be the most promising in predicting dementia risk [127]. In addition, long-term use of non-steroidal anti-inflammatory drugs was suggested to be associated with a lower risk of AD [25].

4.5.2. Hormone replacement therapy

Hormone replacement therapy in postmenopausal women has been frequently reported to be associated with a lower risk of AD. An association between hormone replacement therapy and a reduced risk of dementia and Alzheimer's disease among postmenopausal women had been frequently reported in numerous observational studies until 2004 when, instead of a protective effect, a significantly increased risk of dementia associated with estrogenic therapy was found in the Women's Health Study [128].

4.5.3. Occupational exposures

Manual work involving goods production has been associated with an increased risk of AD and dementia. Occupation and occupational exposures (e.g., electromagnetic fields and heavy metals) may play a role in dementia and Alzheimer's disease [129, 130]. Data from the Kungsholmen Project showed that manual work involving goods production was associated with an increased risk of dementia and Alzheimer's disease [130], and specifically a risk effect was detected with electromagnetic exposure [129]. Occupational exposure to extremely-low-frequency electromagnetic fields (ELF-EMF) has been related to an increased risk of dementia and AD in a number of follow-up studies [129, 131]. The meta-analysis of epidemiological evidence suggests an association between occupational exposure to ELF-EMF and AD [132].

4.5.4. Head trauma and traumatic brain injury

For many years, head trauma has been suggested as a possible risk factor for Alzheimer's disease, and it has been extensively investigated in several studies, but this possible association still remains controversial. Moderate head injuries are associated with twice the risk of developing Alzheimer's compared with no head injuries, and severe head injuries are associated with 4.5 times the risk [133, 134]. Moderate head injury is defined as a head injury resulting in loss of consciousness or post-traumatic amnesia lasting more than 30 minutes; if either of these lasts more than 24 hours, the injury is considered severe. These increased risks have not been shown for individuals experiencing mild head injury or any number of common mishaps, such as bumping one's head while exiting a car. Groups that experienced repeated head injuries, such as boxers, football players and combat veterans, may be at increased risk of dementia, late-life cognitive impairment and evidence of tau tangles (a hallmark of Alzheimer's) at autopsy [135-138]. Additional research is needed to better understand the association between brain injury and increased risk of Alzheimer's disease.

5. Summary of evidence from systematic review

Meta-analyses and systematic reviews have provided robust evidence that cognitive reserve (a concept combining the benefits of education, occupation, and mental activities) [139], physical activity and exercise [140, 141], midlife obesity [142], alcohol intake [93], and smoking [142] are the most important modifiable risk factors for Alzheimer's disease. There is insufficient overall evidence from epidemiological studies to support any association between dietary or supplementary antioxidant or B vitamins and altered risk of incident dementia [143, 144]. Data from several independent time points from a large Swedish epidemiological study suggest that better social networks and social activities might be associated with reduced incidence of Alzheimer's disease [119], but this has not been examined systematically in other large epidemiological cohorts [61].

Many treatable medical conditions have also been associated with an increased risk of Alzheimer's disease, including stroke [145], diabetes [146], midlife hypertension [52], and midlife hypercholesterolemia [147, 148]. Blood pressure and cholesterol both seem to be reduced in late life and in the prodromal to Alzheimer's disease; thus, the difference between midlife and late life is an important distinction. There is probably an important relation between some of these conditions and the lifestyle factors mentioned previously, and interventions to promote healthy living will probably reduce the incidence of diabetes and stroke as well as having other, more direct, effects on dementia. There is limited evidence about the potential effect of management of diabetes or stroke on the risk of subsequent dementia, more intervention trials on this topic are needed (Table 1) [61,149].

Less than two decades have passed since the first incidence data for Alzheimer's disease and other dementias were reported, during which there have been many achievements in the understanding of risk and protective factors of Alzheimer's disease. Accumulated evidence from epidemiological research strongly supports a role for lifestyle and cardiovascular risk factors in the pathogenesis and development of dementia. However, none of these factors has been proven to have a causal relation specifically with Alzheimer's disease. Indeed, this topic is further complicated by the fact that the traditional diagnosis of dementia subtypes has been challenged by population-based neuropathological and neuroimaging studies. Research has shown a range of dementia-associated brain abnormalities from pure vascular lesions at one end to pure Alzheimer's pathologies at the other, with most dementia cases being attributable to both vascular disease and neurodegeneration.

Factors	Systematic review	Results
Overweight and obesity	Meta-analysis of ten studies. Sixteen articles on 15 prospective studies with 3.2-36 years follow-up	Overweight: Dementia RR 1.26 (95% CI 1.10–1.44); Alzheimer's disease 1.35 (95% CI 1·19–1.54) Obesity: Dementia RR 1.64 (95% CI 1.34-2.00); Alzheimer's disease RR 2.04 (95% CI 1.59-2.62)
Smoking	Meta-analysis of four prospective studies with 2–25 years follow-up in over 17 000 people. In the four studies the dementia ORs were 3·17 (95% CI 1.37–7.35), 1.42 (1.07–1.89), 1.60 (1.00–2.57), and 1.63 (1.00–2.67)	Dementia RR 2.2 (95% CI 1.3–3.6)
Physical activity	13 prospective studies focusing on Alzheimer's disease, dementia, or both, with at least 150 000 participants	Dementia RR 0.72 (95% CI 0.60–0.86); Alzheimer's disease 0.55 (95% CI 0.36–0.84)
Cognitive reserve (intelligence, occupation, and education)	22 prospective studies with at least 29 000 participants followed up for a median of 7.1 years	Dementia OR 0.54 (95% CI 0.49–0.59)
Alcohol	15 longitudinal studies with 2–8 years follow-up and at least 14 000 participants	Dementia RR 0.74 (95% CI 0.61–0.91); Alzheimer's disease 0.72 (0.61–0.86)
	Medical conditions	
Midlife hypertension	At least 15 years follow-up in most studies, with at least 16 000 participants	Four of five longitudinal studies focusing on midlife hypertension suggested that it is a significant risk factor for incident dementia (RR 1.24–2.8 in different studies) The biggest differences were reported in studies using 160/95 mm Hg as the threshold for hypertension
Stroke	16 studies with at least 25 000 participants, mainly included patients aged 65 years and over	12 of 16 studies showed significant association between stroke and incident dementia, with overall doubling of incidence
Diabetes	15 prospective cohort studies	Dementia RR 1.47 (95% CI 1.25–1.73); Alzheimer's disease RR 1.39 (95% CI 1.16–1.66)

Factors	Systematic review	Results
Midlife hypercholesterolemia	18 studies, but only five assessed high cholesterol specifically in midlife. All five midlife studies had over 15 years follow-up and a total of over 15 000 participants	Four of five longitudinal studies in midlife suggested a significant positive association between high total cholesterol and incident dementia. For overall difference the RR was 1·4–3·1
	Intervention studies	
Hypertension	12 091 participants between the three trials (SHEP, SYST-EUR, and SCOPE) with mean follow-up of 3·3 years. Only SYST-EUR reported significant benefit	OR 0.89 (95% CI 0.69–1.16) for incident dementia
Statins for prevention of dementia	26 340 participants between the two trials (PROSPER and HPS), with follow-up of 3·2 and 5 years. Cognition was measured with different instruments at different timepoints	Neither of the two trials reported significant benefit of statin therapy
Vitamins B12 or folate	Four trials in older people without existing cognitive impairment	Three trials showed no benefit. One trial (the only that selected participants based on increased homocysteine) reported benefit with respect to global function

RR=relative risk. OR=odds ratio. SHEP=Systolic Hypertension in the Elderly Program. SYST-EUR=Systolic Hypertension in Europe. SCOPE=Study on Cognition and Prognosis in the Elderly. PROSPER=PROspective Study of Pravastatin in the Elderly at Risk. HPS=Heart Protection Study.

Table 1. Meta-analyses or systematic reviews of risk factors for dementia and Alzheimer's disease [61,149]

Population studies have identified many factors that could be important in reducing the risk of dementia, including factors that identify people at risk for dementia (vascular risk factors, depressive symptoms) and factors that may reduce the risk of dementia (cognitive, physical, and social activity, a diet rich in antioxidants and polyunsaturated fatty acids, vascular risk factor control). While early interventional studies have been less conclusive, future trials should continue to examine the effect of risk factor modification on cognitive outcomes. In particular, interventions that combine a number of factors, such as healthy nutrition along with cognitive, social, and physical activity, should be investigated. In the most optimistic view, dementia could be delayed or even prevented by these interventions. At worst, people will improve their overall health, especially their cardiovascular health, and enjoy a more cognitively and socially engaging life.

5.1. Intervention strategies against Alzheimer's disease

Despite the specific challenges posed by neurological disorders, such as Alzheimer's disease and other dementias, interventions need to be implemented to verify findings from the many population-based observational studies, which suggest that preventive and therapeutic interventions have great potential [150].

5.1.1. Vascular factors and related disorders

Most vascular risk factors and related disorders are modifiable or treatable that can serve as targets in the development of primary preventative strategies against dementia. For example, antihypertensive therapy has been shown to reduce the risk of dementia in observational studies, and this finding was partly confirmed by clinical trials. Furthermore, studies have confirmed that obesity and diabetes can be prevented by changing dietary habits and lifestyles, and that health education may help quit smoking. Finally, preventing recurrent cerebrovascular disease and maintaining sufficient cerebral blood perfusion seems to be critical for postponing expression of the dementia syndrome in older people. Thus, controlling high blood pressure and obesity, especially from middle age, and preventing diabetes and recurrent stroke could be the primary preventive measures against late-life dementia.

5.1.2. Intervention towards psychosocial factors and lifestyles

High educational achievements in early life can provide cognitive reserve that benefits the whole life in terms of cognitive health and delaying the onset of late-life dementia. Extensive social networks and active engagements in intellectually stimulating activities such as reading, doing crosswords, and playing board games may significantly lower the risk of dementia by providing cognitive reserve or by reducing psychosocial stress. It is likely that mentally and socially integrated lifestyles could postpone the onset of dementia [119]. Regular physical exercise may reduce the risk of the dementias resulting from cerebral atherosclerosis. Leisure activities with all three components of physical, mental, and social activities may have the most beneficial effect on dementia prevention. Many of the risk factors for dementia, such as hypertension, diabetes, and obesity, may be modified by diet. In addition, a diet high in antioxidants may reduce inflammation, which is associated with the risk of dementia. Thus, it is reasonable to suggest that the risk of dementia itself could be modified by diet. The treatment of depression also seems to improve cognitive function in people who are depressed. Taking together, the most promising strategy for the primary prevention of dementia may be to encourage people implementing multiple preventative measures throughout the life course, including high educational attainment in childhood and early adulthood, an active control of vascular factors (e.g., smoking) and disorders (e.g., hypertension and diabetes) in adulthood, and maintenance of mentally, physically, and socially active lifestyles during middle age and later in life.

6. Conclusions

Alzheimer's disease is a major cause of functional dependence, institutionalisation, and mortality among elderly people. Population-based studies have made a great contribution to our knowledge of Alzheimer's disease. Although many aspects of Alzheimer's disease are

http://dx.doi.org/10.5772/54398

still unclear, we are now able to make more accurate diagnoses than before, and the pattern of dementia distribution has been sufficiently described to guide the planning of medical and social services. Epidemiological studies have shown that vascular risk factors in middle age and later in life significantly contribute to the development and progression of the dementia syndrome, whereas extensive social network and active engagement in social, physical, and mental activities may delay the onset of the dementing disorders. Hence, one of the promising strategies to deal with the tremendous challenge from the epidemic of dementia is to implement appropriate intervention measures from a life-course perspective. Achieving high education in early life and engaging mentally stimulating activity over adulthood to enhance cognitive reserve, and maintaining vascular health by adopting healthy lifestyles and optimally controlling vascular diseases to reduce the burden of vascular lesions in the brain. These preventive measures will enable people to maintain cognitive ability in late life, even though they may have developed a high load of Alzheimer pathologies in their brain.

Acknowledgements

Research grants were received from the Swedish council for working life and social research, the Swedish Research Council in Medicine and the Swedish Brain Power. This study was also supported in part by funds from the Loo and Hans Ostermans Foundation and the Foundation for Geriatric Diseases at Karolinska Institutet, the Gamla Tjänarinnor Foundation, Demensfonden and the Bertil Stohnes Foundation.

Author details

Weili Xu[1,2*], Camilla Ferrari[2,3] and Hui-Xin Wang[2]

*Address all correspondence to: weili.xu@ki.se

1 Department of Epidemiology, Tianjin Medical University, Tianjin, P.R., China

2 Aging Research Center, Karolinska Institutet-Stockholm University, Stockholm, Sweden

3 Department of Neurological and Psychiatric Sciences, University of Florence, Italy

References

[1] From the Centers for Disease Control and Prevention. Public health and aging: trends in aging--United States and worldwide. JAMA 2003;289(11):1371-1373.

[2] Kinsella K, Velkoff VA. The demographics of aging. Aging Clin Exp Res 2002;14(3): 159-169.

[3] Lunenfeld B. An Aging World - demographics and challenges. Gynecol Endocrinol 2008;24(1):1-3.

[4] Bennett DA. Editorial comment on 'Prevalence of dementia in the United States: the aging, demographics, and memory study' by Plassman et al. Neuroepidemiology 2007;29(1-2):133-135.

[5] American Psychiatric Association: Diagnostic and Statistical Manual of Mental Disorders, Third Edition-Revised (DSM-III-R). Washington, DC: American Psychiatric Association; 1987.

[6] American Psychiatric Association: Diagnostic and Statistical Manual of Mental Disorders, Fourth Edition (DSM-IV). Washington, DC: American Psychiatric Association; 1994.

[7] Fratiglioni L, Winblad B, von Strauss E. Prevention of Alzheimer's disease and dementia. Major findings from the Kungsholmen Project. Physiol Behav 2007;92(1-2): 98-104.

[8] Harvey R, Fox N, Rossor M. Dementia Handbook. London: Martin Dunitz; 1999.

[9] Roman GC. Vascular dementia: distinguishing characteristics, treatment, and prevention. J Am Geriatr Soc 2003;51(5 Suppl Dementia):S296-304.

[10] Korczyn AD, Vakhapova V. The prevention of the dementia epidemic. J Neurol Sci 2007;257(1-2):2-4.

[11] Ferri CP, Prince M, Brayne C, Brodaty H, Fratiglioni L, Ganguli M, et al. Global prevalence of dementia: a Delphi consensus study. Lancet 2005;366(9503):2112-2117.

[12] Wimo A, Winblad B, Aguero-Torres H, von Strauss E. The magnitude of dementia occurrence in the world. Alzheimer Dis Assoc Disord 2003;17(2):63-67.

[13] Reitz C, Brayne C, Mayeux R. Epidemiology of Alzheimer disease. Nat Rev Neurol 2011;7(3):137-152.

[14] Lobo A, Launer LJ, Fratiglioni L, Andersen K, Di Carlo A, Breteler MM, et al. Prevalence of dementia and major subtypes in Europe: A collaborative study of population-based cohorts. Neurologic Diseases in the Elderly Research Group. Neurology 2000;54(11 Suppl 5):S4-9.

[15] Plassman BL, Langa KM, Fisher GG, Heeringa SG, Weir DR, Ofstedal MB, et al. Prevalence of dementia in the United States: the aging, demographics, and memory study. Neuroepidemiology 2007;29(1-2):125-132.

[16] Zhang Y, Xu Y, Nie H, Lei T, Wu Y, Zhang L, et al. Prevalence of dementia and major dementia subtypes in the Chinese populations: A meta-analysis of dementia prevalence surveys, 1980-2010. J Clin Neurosci 2012;19(10):1333-1337.

[17] Qiu C, Kivipelto M, von Strauss E. Epidemiology of Alzheimer's disease: occurrence, determinants, and strategies toward intervention. Dialogues Clin Neurosci 2009;11(2):111-128.

[18] Corrada MM, Brookmeyer R, Berlau D, Paganini-Hill A, Kawas CH. Prevalence of dementia after age 90: results from the 90+ study. Neurology 2008;71(5):337-343.

[19] von Strauss E, Viitanen M, De Ronchi D, Winblad B, Fratiglioni L. Aging and the occurrence of dementia: findings from a population-based cohort with a large sample of nonagenarians. Arch Neurology 1999;56(5):587-592.

[20] Kalaria RN, Maestre GE, Arizaga R, Friedland RP, Galasko D, Hall K, et al. Alzheimer's disease and vascular dementia in developing countries: prevalence, management, and risk factors. Lancet Neurol 2008;7(9):812-826.

[21] Llibre Rodriguez JJ, Ferri CP, Acosta D, Guerra M, Huang Y, Jacob KS, et al. Prevalence of dementia in Latin America, India, and China: a population-based cross-sectional survey. Lancet 2008;372(9637):464-474.

[22] Zhang ZX, Zahner GE, Roman GC, Liu J, Hong Z, Qu QM, et al. Dementia subtypes in China: prevalence in Beijing, Xian, Shanghai, and Chengdu. Archives of neurology 2005;62(3):447-453.

[23] Llibre Rodriguez J, Valhuerdi A, Sanchez, II, Reyna C, Guerra MA, Copeland JR, et al. The prevalence, correlates and impact of dementia in Cuba. A 10/66 group population-based survey. Neuroepidemiology 2008;31(4):243-251.

[24] Scazufca M, Menezes PR, Vallada HP, Crepaldi AL, Pastor-Valero M, Coutinho LM, et al. High prevalence of dementia among older adults from poor socioeconomic backgrounds in Sao Paulo, Brazil. Int Psychogeriatr 2008;20(2):394-405.

[25] Qiu C, De Ronchi D, Fratiglioni L. The epidemiology of the dementias: an update. Curr Opin Psychiatry 2007;20(4):380-385.

[26] Fratiglioni L, Launer LJ, Andersen K, Breteler MM, Copeland JR, Dartigues JF, et al. Incidence of dementia and major subtypes in Europe: A collaborative study of population-based cohorts. Neurologic Diseases in the Elderly Research Group. Neurology 2000;54(11 Suppl 5):S10-15.

[27] Kawas C, Gray S, Brookmeyer R, Fozard J, Zonderman A. Age-specific incidence rates of Alzheimer's disease: the Baltimore Longitudinal Study of Aging. Neurology 2000;54(11):2072-2077.

[28] Kukull WA, Higdon R, Bowen JD, McCormick WC, Teri L, Schellenberg GD, et al. Dementia and Alzheimer disease incidence: a prospective cohort study. Arch Neurol 2002;59(11):1737-1746.

[29] Miech RA, Breitner JC, Zandi PP, Khachaturian AS, Anthony JC, Mayer L. Incidence of AD may decline in the early 90s for men, later for women: The Cache County study. Neurology 2002;58(2):209-218.

[30] Matthews F, Brayne C. The incidence of dementia in England and Wales: findings from the five identical sites of the MRC CFA Study. PLoS Med 2005;2(8):e193.

[31] Ravaglia G, Forti P, Maioli F, Martelli M, Servadei L, Brunetti N, et al. Incidence and etiology of dementia in a large elderly Italian population. Neurology 2005;64(9): 1525-1530.

[32] Chandra V, Pandav R, Dodge HH, Johnston JM, Belle SH, DeKosky ST, et al. Incidence of Alzheimer's disease in a rural community in India: the Indo-US study. Neurology 2001;57(6):985-989.

[33] Aguero-Torres H, Qiu C, Winblad B, Fratiglioni L. Dementing disorders in the elderly: evolution of disease severity over 7 years. Alzheimer Dis Assoc Disord 2002;16(4): 221-227.

[34] Aguero-Torres H, Fratiglioni L, Guo Z, Viitanen M, von Strauss E, Winblad B. Dementia is the major cause of functional dependence in the elderly: 3-year follow-up data from a population-based study. Am J Public Health 1998;88(10):1452-1456.

[35] Aguero-Torres H, Fratiglioni L, Guo Z, Viitanen M, Winblad B. Mortality from dementia in advanced age: a 5-year follow-up study of incident dementia cases. J Clin Epidemiol 1999;52(8):737-743.

[36] Cotter VT. The burden of dementia. Am J Manag Care 2007;13 Suppl 8:S193-197.

[37] Wimo A, Jonsson L, Winblad B. An estimate of the worldwide prevalence and direct costs of dementia in 2003. Dement Geriatr Cogn Disord 2006;21(3):175-181.

[38] Qiu C. Epidemiological findings of vascular risk factors in Alzheimer's disease: implications for therapeutic and preventive intervention. Expert Rev Neurother 2011;11(11):1593-1607.

[39] Qiu C, Kivipelto M, Fratiglioni L. Preventing Alzheimer disease and cognitive decline. Ann Inter Med 2011;154(3):211; author reply 212-213.

[40] Ferrari C, Xu WL, Wang HX, Winblad B, Sorbi S, Qiu C, et al. How can elderly apolipoprotein E epsilon4 carriers remain free from dementia? Neurobiol Aging 2012.

[41] Qiu C, Kivipelto M, Aguero-Torres H, Winblad B, Fratiglioni L. Risk and protective effects of the APOE gene towards Alzheimer's disease in the Kungsholmen project: variation by age and sex. J Neurol Neurosurg Psychiatry 2004;75(6):828-833.

[42] D'Introno A, Solfrizzi V, Colacicco AM, Capurso C, Amodio M, Todarello O, et al. Current knowledge of chromosome 12 susceptibility genes for late-onset Alzheimer's disease. Neurobiol Aging 2006;27(11):1537-1553.

[43] Wang HX, Gustafson DR, Kivipelto M, Pedersen NL, Skoog I, Windblad B, et al. Education halves the risk of dementia due to apolipoprotein epsilon4 allele: a collaborative study from the Swedish Brain Power initiative. Neurobiol Aging 2012;33(5):1007 e1001-1007.

[44] Keller L, Xu W, Wang HX, Winblad B, Fratiglioni L, Graff C. The obesity related gene, FTO, interacts with APOE, and is associated with Alzheimer's disease risk: a prospective cohort study. J Alzheimers Dis 2011;23(3):461-469.

[45] Green RC, Cupples LA, Go R, Benke KS, Edeki T, Griffith PA, et al. Risk of dementia among white and African American relatives of patients with Alzheimer disease. JAMA 2002;287(3):329-336.

[46] Fratiglioni L, Ahlbom A, Viitanen M, Winblad B. Risk factors for late-onset Alzheimer's disease: a population-based, case-control study. Ann Neurol 1993;33(3):258-266.

[47] Wilson RS, Scherr PA, Hoganson G, Bienias JL, Evans DA, Bennett DA. Early life socioeconomic status and late life risk of Alzheimer's disease. Neuroepidemiology 2005;25(1):8-14.

[48] Lautenschlager NT, Cupples LA, Rao VS, Auerbach SA, Becker R, Burke J, et al. Risk of dementia among relatives of Alzheimer's disease patients in the MIRAGE study: What is in store for the oldest old? Neurology 1996;46(3):641-650.

[49] Fratiglioni L, Rocca W. Epidemiology of dementia. In: Handbook of Neuropsychology (2nd Edition), Boller F and Cappa SF, eds Elsevier Science B.V.; 2001.

[50] McVeigh C, Passmore P. Vascular dementia: prevention and treatment. Clin Interv Aging 2006;1(3):229-235.

[51] Nelson NW. Differential diagnosis of Alzheimer's dementia and vascular dementia. Dis Mon 2007;53(3):148-151.

[52] Qiu C, Winblad B, Fratiglioni L. The age-dependent relation of blood pressure to cognitive function and dementia. Lancet Neurol 2005;4(8):487-499.

[53] Whitmer RA, Sidney S, Selby J, Johnston SC, Yaffe K. Midlife cardiovascular risk factors and risk of dementia in late life. Neurology 2005;64(2):277-281.

[54] Ruitenberg A, den Heijer T, Bakker SL, van Swieten JC, Koudstaal PJ, Hofman A, et al. Cerebral hypoperfusion and clinical onset of dementia: the Rotterdam Study. Ann Neurol 2005;57(6):789-794.

[55] Qiu C, von Strauss E, Fastbom J, Winblad B, Fratiglioni L. Low blood pressure and risk of dementia in the Kungsholmen project: a 6-year follow-up study. Arch Neurol 2003;60(2):223-228.

[56] Peila R, White LR, Masaki K, Petrovitch H, Launer LJ. Reducing the risk of dementia: efficacy of long-term treatment of hypertension. Stroke 2006;37(5):1165-1170.

[57] Haag MD, Hofman A, Koudstaal PJ, Breteler MM, Stricker BH. Duration of antihypertensive drug use and risk of dementia: A prospective cohort study. Neurology 2009;72(20):1727-1734.

[58] Newman AB, Fitzpatrick AL, Lopez O, Jackson S, Lyketsos C, Jagust W, et al. Dementia and Alzheimer's disease incidence in relationship to cardiovascular disease in the Cardiovascular Health Study cohort. J Am Geriatr Soc 2005;53(7):1101-1107.

[59] Qiu CX, Winblad, B, Marengoni A, Klarin I, Fastbom J, Fratiglioni L. Heart failure and risk of dementia and Alzheimer disease: a population-based cohort study. Arch Intern Med 2006;166:1003-1008.

[60] Purandare N, Burns A, Daly KJ, Hardicre J, Morris J, Macfarlane G, et al. Cerebral emboli as a potential cause of Alzheimer's disease and vascular dementia: case-control study. BMJ 2006;332(7550):1119-1124.

[61] Ballard C, Gauthier S, Corbett A, Brayne C, Aarsland D, Jones E. Alzheimer's disease. Lancet 2011;377(9770):1019-1031.

[62] Arvanitakis Z, Wilson RS, Bennett DA. Diabetes mellitus, dementia, and cognitive function in older persons. J Nutr Health Aging 2006;10(4):287-291.

[63] Cukierman T, Gerstein HC, Williamson JD. Cognitive decline and dementia in diabetes--systematic overview of prospective observational studies. Diabetologia 2005;48(12):2460-2469.

[64] Luchsinger JA, Reitz C, Patel B, Tang MX, Manly JJ, Mayeux R. Relation of diabetes to mild cognitive impairment. Arch Neurol 2007;64(4):570-575.

[65] Arvanitakis Z, Wilson RS, Li Y, Aggarwal NT, Bennett DA. Diabetes and function in different cognitive systems in older individuals without dementia. Diabetes Care 2006;29(3):560-565.

[66] Allen KV, Frier BM, Strachan MW. The relationship between type 2 diabetes and cognitive dysfunction: longitudinal studies and their methodological limitations. Eur J Pharmacol 2004;490(1-3):169-175.

[67] Xu W, Caracciolo B, Wang HX, Winblad B, Backman L, Qiu C, et al. Accelerated Progression from Mild Cognitive Impairment to Dementia in People with Diabetes. Diabetes 2010;59(11):2928-35

[68] Xu W, Qiu C, Gatz M, Pedersen NL, Johansson B, Fratiglioni L. Mid- and late-life diabetes in relation to the risk of dementia: a population-based twin study. Diabetes 2009;58(1):71-77.

[69] Xu WL, Qiu CX, Wahlin A, Winblad B, Fratiglioni L. Diabetes mellitus and risk of dementia in the Kungsholmen project: a 6-year follow-up study. Neurology 2004;63(7):1181-1186.

[70] Xu WL, von Strauss E, Qiu CX, Winblad B, Fratiglioni L. Uncontrolled diabetes increases the risk of Alzheimer's disease: a population-based cohort study. Diabetologia 2009;52(6):1031-1039.

[71] Biessels GJ, Staekenborg S, Brunner E, Brayne C, Scheltens P. Risk of dementia in diabetes mellitus: a systematic review. Lancet Neurol 2006;5(1):64-74.

[72] Roberts RO, Geda YE, Knopman DS, Christianson TJ, Pankratz VS, Boeve BF, et al. Association of duration and severity of diabetes mellitus with mild cognitive impairment. Arch Neurol 2008;65(8):1066-1073.

[73] Strachan MW, Price JF, Frier BM. Diabetes, cognitive impairment, and dementia. Bmj 2008;336(7634):6.

[74] Xu W, Qiu C, Winblad B, Fratiglioni L. The effect of borderline diabetes on the risk of dementia and Alzheimer's disease. Diabetes 2007;56(1):211-216.

[75] Gustafson D. Adiposity indices and dementia. Lancet Neurol 2006;5(8):713-720.

[76] Whitmer RA. The epidemiology of adiposity and dementia. Curr Alzheimer Res 2007;4(2):117-122.

[77] Kivipelto M, Ngandu T, Fratiglioni L, Viitanen M, Kareholt I, Winblad B, et al. Obesity and vascular risk factors at midlife and the risk of dementia and Alzheimer disease. Arch Neurol 2005;62(10):1556-1560.

[78] Xu W, Atti A, Gatz M, Pedersen NL, Johansson B, Fratiglioni L. Midlife overweight and obesity increase dementia risk in old age: a population-based twin study. Neurology 2011;76(18):1568-74.

[79] Buchman AS, Wilson RS, Bienias JL, Shah RC, Evans DA, Bennett DA. Change in body mass index and risk of incident Alzheimer disease. Neurology 2005;65(6): 892-897.

[80] Johnson DK, Wilkins CH, Morris JC. Accelerated weight loss may precede diagnosis in Alzheimer disease. Arch Neurol 2006;63(9):1312-1317.

[81] Atti AR, Palmer K, Volpato S, Winblad B, De Ronchi D, Fratiglioni L. Late-life body mass index and dementia incidence: nine-year follow-up data from the Kungsholmen Project. J Am Geriatr Soc 2008;56(1):111-116.

[82] Johnson DK, Wilkins CH, Morris JC. Accelerated weight loss may precede diagnosis in Alzheimer disease. Arch Neurol 2006;63(9):1312-1317.

[83] Dahl AK, Lopponen M, Isoaho R, Berg S, Kivela SL. Overweight and obesity in old age are not associated with greater dementia risk. J Am Geriatr Soc 2008;56(12): 2261-2266.

[84] Mielke MM, Zandi PP, Sjogren M, Gustafson D, Ostling S, Steen B, et al. High total cholesterol levels in late life associated with a reduced risk of dementia. Neurology 2005;64(10):1689-1695.

[85] Stewart R, White LR, Xue QL, Launer LJ. Twenty-six-year change in total cholesterol levels and incident dementia: the Honolulu-Asia Aging Study. Arch Neurol 2007;64(1):103-107.

[86] Solomon A, Kareholt I, Ngandu T, Wolozin B, Macdonald SW, Winblad B, et al. Serum total cholesterol, statins and cognition in non-demented elderly. Neurobiol Aging 2007.

[87] Yaffe K, Kanaya A, Lindquist K, Simonsick EM, Harris T, Shorr RI, et al. The metabolic syndrome, inflammation, and risk of cognitive decline. JAMA 2004;292(18): 2237-2242.

[88] van den Berg E, Biessels GJ, de Craen AJ, Gussekloo J, Westendorp RG. The metabolic syndrome is associated with decelerated cognitive decline in the oldest old. Neurology 2007;69(10):979-985.

[89] Vanhanen M, Koivisto K, Moilanen L, Helkala EL, Hanninen T, Soininen H, et al. Association of metabolic syndrome with Alzheimer disease: a population-based study. Neurology 2006;67(5):843-847.

[90] Raffaitin C, Gin H, Empana JP, Helmer C, Berr C, Tzourio C, et al. Metabolic syndrome and risk for incident Alzheimer's disease or vascular dementia: the Three-City Study. Diabetes Care 2009;32(1):169-174.

[91] Anttila T, Helkala EL, Viitanen M, Kareholt I, Fratiglioni L, Winblad B, et al. Alcohol drinking in middle age and subsequent risk of mild cognitive impairment and dementia in old age: a prospective population based study. BMJ 2004;329(7465):539.

[92] Stampfer MJ, Kang JH, Chen J, Cherry R, Grodstein F. Effects of moderate alcohol consumption on cognitive function in women. N Engl J Med 2005;352(3):245-253.

[93] Anstey KJ, Mack HA, Cherbuin N. Alcohol consumption as a risk factor for dementia and cognitive decline: meta-analysis of prospective studies. Am J Geriatr Psychiatry 2009;17(7):542-555.

[94] Aggarwal NT, Bienias JL, Bennett DA, Wilson RS, Morris MC, Schneider JA, et al. The relation of cigarette smoking to incident Alzheimer's disease in a biracial urban community population. Neuroepidemiology 2006;26(3):140-146.

[95] Cataldo JK, Prochaska JJ, Glantz SA. Cigarette smoking is a risk factor for Alzheimer's Disease: an analysis controlling for tobacco industry affiliation. J Alzheimers Dis 2010;19(2):465-480.

[96] Luchsinger JA, Mayeux R. Dietary factors and Alzheimer's disease. Lancet Neurol 2004;3(10):579-587.

[97] Morris MC, Evans DA, Bienias JL, Tangney CC, Bennett DA, Aggarwal N, et al. Dietary intake of antioxidant nutrients and the risk of incident Alzheimer disease in a biracial community study. JAMA 2002;287(24):3230-3237.

[98] Wang HX, Wahlin A, Basun H, Fastbom J, Winblad B, Fratiglioni L. Vitamin B(12) and folate in relation to the development of Alzheimer's disease. Neurology 2001;56(9):1188-1194.

[99] Kalmijn S, Launer LJ, Ott A, Witteman JC, Hofman A, Breteler MM. Dietary fat intake and the risk of incident dementia in the Rotterdam Study. Ann Neurol1997;42(5):776-782.

[100] Morris MC, Evans DA, Bienias JL, Tangney CC, Bennett DA, Aggarwal N, et al. Dietary fats and the risk of incident Alzheimer disease. Arch Neurol 2003;60(2):194-200.

[101] Kalmijn S, Launer LJ, Ott A, Witteman JC, Hofman A, Breteler MM. Dietary fat intake and the risk of incident dementia in the Rotterdam Study. Ann Neurol 1997;42(5):776-782.

[102] Laitinen MH, Ngandu T, Rovio S, Helkala EL, Uusitalo U, Viitanen M, et al. Fat intake at midlife and risk of dementia and Alzheimer's disease: a population-based study. Dement Geriatr Cogn Disord 2006;22(1):99-107.

[103] Kivipelto M, Rovio S, Ngandu T, Kareholt I, Eskelinen M, Winblad B, et al. Apolipoprotein E epsilon4 Magnifies Lifestyle Risks for Dementia: A Population Based Study. J Cell Mol Med 2008.

[104] Scarmeas N, Stern Y, Mayeux R, Luchsinger JA. Mediterranean diet, Alzheimer disease, and vascular mediation. Arch Neurol 2006;63(12):1709-1717.

[105] Qiu C, Backman L, Winblad B, Aguero-Torres H, Fratiglioni L. The influence of education on clinically diagnosed dementia incidence and mortality data from the Kungsholmen Project. Arch Neurol 2001;58(12):2034-2039.

[106] Evans DA, Hebert LE, Beckett LA, Scherr PA, Albert MS, Chown MJ, et al. Education and other measures of socioeconomic status and risk of incident Alzheimer disease in a defined population of older persons. Arch Neurol 1997;54(11):1399-1405.

[107] Borenstein AR, Wu Y, Mortimer JA, Schellenberg GD, McCormick WC, Bowen JD, et al. Developmental and vascular risk factors for Alzheimer's disease. Neurobiol Aging 2005;26(3):325-334.

[108] Ngandu T, von Strauss E, Helkala EL, Winblad B, Nissinen A, Tuomilehto J, et al. Education and dementia: what lies behind the association? Neurology 2007;69(14): 1442-1450.

[109] Larson EB, Wang L, Bowen JD, McCormick WC, Teri L, Crane P, et al. Exercise is associated with reduced risk for incident dementia among persons 65 years of age and older. Ann Intern Med 2006;144(2):73-81.

[110] Karp A, Paillard-Borg S, Wang HX, Silverstein M, Winblad B, Fratiglioni L. Mental, physical and social components in leisure activities equally contribute to decrease dementia risk. Dement Geriatr Cogn Disord 2006;21(2):65-73.

[111] Abbott RD, White LR, Ross GW, Masaki KH, Curb JD, Petrovitch H. Walking and dementia in physically capable elderly men. JAMA 2004;292(12):1447-1453.

[112] Rovio S, Kareholt I, Helkala EL, Viitanen M, Winblad B, Tuomilehto J, et al. Leisure-time physical activity at midlife and the risk of dementia and Alzheimer's disease. Lancet Neurol 2005;4(11):705-711.

[113] Crowe M, Andel R, Pedersen NL, Johansson B, Gatz M. Does participation in leisure activities lead to reduced risk of Alzheimer's disease? A prospective study of Swedish twins. J Gerontol B Psychol Sci Soc Sci 2003;58(5):P249-255.

[114] Wilson RS, Bennett DA, Bienias JL, Mendes de Leon CF, Morris MC, Evans DA. Cognitive activity and cognitive decline in a biracial community population. Neurology 2003;61(6):812-816.

[115] Wilson RS, Mendes De Leon CF, Barnes LL, Schneider JA, Bienias JL, Evans DA, et al. Participation in cognitively stimulating activities and risk of incident Alzheimer disease. JAMA 2002;287(6):742-748.

[116] Andel R, Crowe M, Pedersen NL, Mortimer J, Crimmins E, Johansson B, et al. Complexity of work and risk of Alzheimer's disease: a population-based study of Swedish twins. J Gerontol B Psychol Sci Soc Sci 2005;60(5):P251-258.

[117] Kroger E, Andel R, Lindsay J, Benounissa Z, Verreault R, Laurin D. Is complexity of work associated with risk of dementia? The Canadian Study of Health And Aging. American journal of epidemiology 2008;167(7):820-830.

[118] Valenzuela MJ, Sachdev P, Wen W, Chen X, Brodaty H. Lifespan mental activity predicts diminished rate of hippocampal atrophy. PLoS One 2008;3(7):e2598.

[119] Paillard-Borg S, Fratiglioni L, Xu W, Winblad B, Wang HX. An active lifestyle postpones dementia onset by more than one year in very old adults. J Alzheimers Dis Journal 2012;31(4):835-842.

[120] Fratiglioni L, Wang HX, Ericsson K, Maytan M, Winblad B. Influence of social network on occurrence of dementia: a community-based longitudinal study. Lancet 2000;355(9212):1315-1319.

[121] Wang HX, Karp A, Herlitz A, Crowe M, Kareholt I, Winblad B, et al. Personality and lifestyle in relation to dementia incidence. Neurology 2009;72(3):253-259.

[122] Saczynski JS, Pfeifer LA, Masaki K, Korf ES, Laurin D, White L, et al. The effect of social engagement on incident dementia: the Honolulu-Asia Aging Study. Am J Epidemiol 2006;163(5):433-440.

[123] Bennett DA, Schneider JA, Tang Y, Arnold SE, Wilson RS. The effect of social networks on the relation between Alzheimer's disease pathology and level of cognitive function in old people: a longitudinal cohort study. Lancet Neurol 2006;5(5):406-412.

[124] Wilson RS, Schneider JA, Bienias JL, Arnold SE, Evans DA, Bennett DA. Depressive symptoms, clinical AD, and cortical plaques and tangles in older persons. Neurology 2003;61(8):1102-1107.

[125] Caraci F, Copani A, Nicoletti F, Drago F. Depression and Alzheimer's disease: neurobiological links and common pharmacological targets. Eur J Pharmacol 2010;626(1): 64-71.

[126] Katon W, Lyles CR, Parker MM, Karter AJ, Huang ES, Whitmer RA. Association of depression with increased risk of dementia in patients with type 2 diabetes: the Diabetes and Aging Study. Arch Gen Psychiatry 2012;69(4):410-417.

[127] DeLegge MH, Smoke A. Neurodegeneration and inflammation. Nutr Clin Pract 2008;23(1):35-41.

[128] Whitmer RA, Quesenberry CP, Zhou J, Yaffe K. Timing of hormone therapy and dementia: the critical window theory revisited. Annal Neurology 2011;69(1):163-169.

[129] Qiu C, Fratiglioni L, Karp A, Winblad B, Bellander T. Occupational exposure to electromagnetic fields and risk of Alzheimer's disease. Epidemiology 2004;15(6):687-694.

[130] Qiu C, Karp A, von Strauss E, Winblad B, Fratiglioni L, Bellander T. Lifetime principal occupation and risk of Alzheimer's disease in the Kungsholmen project. Am J Ind Med 2003;43(2):204-211.

[131] Feychting M, Jonsson F, Pedersen NL, Ahlbom A. Occupational magnetic field exposure and neurodegenerative disease. Epidemiology 2003;14(4):413-419; discussion 427-418.

[132] Garcia AM, Sisternas A, Hoyos SP. Occupational exposure to extremely low frequency electric and magnetic fields and Alzheimer disease: a meta-analysis. Int J Epidemiol 2008;37(2):329-340.

[133] Plassman BL, Havlik RJ, Steffens DC, Helms MJ, Newman TN, Drosdick D, et al. Documented head injury in early adulthood and risk of Alzheimer's disease and other dementias. Neurology 2000;55(8):1158-1166.

[134] Lye TC, Shores EA. Traumatic brain injury as a risk factor for Alzheimer's disease: a review. Neuropsychol Rev 2000;10(2):115-129.

[135] Roberts GW, Allsop D, Bruton C. The occult aftermath of boxing. J Neurol Neurosurg Psychiatry 1990;53(5):373-378.

[136] Guskiewicz KM, Marshall SW, Bailes J, McCrea M, Cantu RC, Randolph C, et al. Association between recurrent concussion and late-life cognitive impairment in retired professional football players. Neurosurgery 2005;57(4):719-726; discussion 719-726.

[137] Crawford FC, Vanderploeg RD, Freeman MJ, Singh S, Waisman M, Michaels L, et al. APOE genotype influences acquisition and recall following traumatic brain injury. Neurology 2002;58(7):1115-1118.

[138] Groswasser Z, Reider G, II, Schwab K, Ommaya AK, Pridgen A, Brown HR, et al. Quantitative imaging in late TBI. Part II: cognition and work after closed and penetrating head injury: a report of the Vietnam head injury study. Brain Inj 2002;16(8): 681-690.

[139] Valenzuela MJ, Sachdev P. Brain reserve and dementia: a systematic review. Psychol Med 2006;36(4):441-454.

[140] Hamer M, Chida Y. Physical activity and risk of neurodegenerative disease: a systematic review of prospective evidence. Psychol Med 2009;39(1):3-11.

[141] Wang HX, Xu W, Pei JJ. Leisure activities, cognition and dementia. Biochimica et biophysica acta 2012;1822(3):482-491.

[142] Lee Y, Back JH, Kim J, Kim SH, Na DL, Cheong HK, et al. Systematic review of health behavioral risks and cognitive health in older adults. Int Psychogeriatr 2010;22(2):174-187.

[143] Laurin D, Masaki KH, Foley DJ, White LR, Launer LJ. Midlife dietary intake of antioxidants and risk of late-life incident dementia: the Honolulu-Asia Aging Study. Am J Epidemiol 2004;159(10):959-967.

[144] Gray SL, Anderson ML, Crane PK, Breitner JC, McCormick W, Bowen JD, et al. Antioxidant vitamin supplement use and risk of dementia or Alzheimer's disease in older adults. J Am Geriatr Soc 2008;56(2):291-295.

[145] Savva GM, Stephan BC. Epidemiological studies of the effect of stroke on incident dementia: a systematic review. Stroke 2010;41(1):e41-46.

[146] Lu FP, Lin KP, Kuo HK. Diabetes and the risk of multi-system aging phenotypes: a systematic review and meta-analysis. PLoS One 2009;4(1):e4144.

[147] Anstey KJ, Lipnicki DM, Low LF. Cholesterol as a risk factor for dementia and cognitive decline: a systematic review of prospective studies with meta-analysis. Am J Geriatr Psychiatry 2008;16(5):343-354.

[148] Kivipelto M, Solomon A. Cholesterol as a risk factor for Alzheimer's disease - epidemiological evidence. Acta Neurol Scand Suppl 2006;185:50-57.

[149] Anstey KJ, Cherbuin N, Budge M, Young J. Body mass index in midlife and late-life as a risk factor for dementia: a meta-analysis of prospective studies. Obes Rev 2011;12(5):e426-37.

[150] Fratiglionia L, Qiu C. Prevention of cognitive decline in ageing: dementia as the target, delayed onset as the goal. Lancet Neurol 2011;10(9): 819-828.

Chapter 14

Apathy as a Key Symptom in Behavior Disorders: Difference Between Alzheimer's Disease and Subcortical Vascular Dementia

Rita Moretti, Paola Torre, Francesca Esposito,
Enrica Barro, Paola Tomietto and
Rodolfo M. Antonello

Additional information is available at the end of the chapter

http://dx.doi.org/10.5772/54264

1. Introduction

There is currently no consensus on the nosological position of apathy in clinical practice. The clinical significance of negative symptoms such as apathy is increasingly recognized in neurological and psychiatric disorders, particularly those associated with frontal-subcortical dysfunction (Starkstein et al., 2008; Moretti et al., 2012). Apathy is defined as lack of motivation as manifested by diminished goal-directed behavior, reduced goal-directed cognition, and decreased emotional engagement, a reduced interest and participation in normal purposeful behavior, problems in initiation or sustaining an activity, lack of concern or indifference, and a flattening of affect. The prevalence of apathy in neurodegenerative disorders, such as Parkinson's disease vary between 16.5% and 51%, depending upon the instrument for assessment and on the samples examined. Apathy is quite common also in sVAD; different studies try to define its role in AD, but, even the most recent and well-conducted did not distinguish between early and advanced stages of AD, or even between AD and AD with parkinsonism (Starkstein et al., 2008; Stuss et al., 2000; Dujardin et al., 2009). It has been hypothesized that dysfunction of the nigro-striatal pathway may play an important role in the pathophysiology of apathy in neuro-degenerative disorders. In fact, apathy seems to be independent of disease duration, disability and severity of parkinsonism, and levodopa dose in PD, indicating that the brain changes underlying apathy differ from those associated with motor symptoms. Much more interesting is that not all the PD patients become apathetic, indicating that apathy should not entirely be considered a dopamine-dependent syndrome in PD, and is in fact present even in not-purely dopaminergic alterations, such as AD or sVAD (Moretti et al., 2012; Levy et al., 1998; Brown and Pluck, 2000). Existing evidence suggests that apathy can be related to depression, as a key symptom of major depression or side-effect of antidepressant or antipsychotic drugs (Chase et al., 2011). Though, apathy and depression clearly dissociate in specific motor disorders, such as progressive supranuclear palsy, in which there is a high incidence of apathy but a low incidence of depression (Aarsland et al., 2001). Other Authors suggested that apathy might be a consequence of chronic disabling disease and its impact on mobility and opportunity for participation in normal activities. Thus, many Authors used the term "premature social aging" to describe the findings that patients with apathy have little in the way of interests or social activities, spending more time in solitary activities such as watching television or just sitting doing nothing (Starkstein et al., 1992). If apathy is a primary consequence of physical disability or impairment in daily living, then similar changes might be predicted for patients with articular/orthopedic impairment. Surprisingly, the osteoarthritis sample population, despite the motor disability, showed no evidence of apathy. It is thus likely that the physiopathology of apathy is a multifaceted entity. The aim of this preliminary was to assess the behavior spectrum of Alzheimer's Disease (AD) and that of subcortical Vascular Dementia (sVAD), with a particular concern for apathy, and to assess its possible role in the differential clinical diagnosis, as compared to other behavioral changes and different neuropsychological patterns.

We decided to conduct a prospective cohort study, designed to investigate behavioural alterations, and in particular apathy of an AD and of a sVAD population. Therefore, our group recruited 75 men and women aged 65–94 years, entering in Cognitive Disorder Unit Evaluation of the University of Trieste, with Mini-Mental State Examination (MMSE) scores of at least 14 and satisfying DSM-IV for dementia, and suffering from Alzheimer's Disease, according to NINDCS-ADRDA criteria (McKAhn et al., 1984) and 317 patients suffered from from subcortical vascular dementia, in accordance with the NINDS-AIREN criteria (Román et al., 1993); the patients have been selected from June 1st 2008 to June 1st 2011. In order to be enrolled into the study subjects had to show on brain MRI the classical pattern of atrophy of AD (hippocampal atrophy) and display hypoperfusion in temporoparietal and precuneus regions (AD) on HMPAO-SPECT. A patient was diagnosed as having subcortical VaD (sVaD) when the CT/MRI scan showed moderate to severe ischaemic white matter changes (Erkinjuntti et al., 1997) and at least one lacunar infarct. Brain CT-scans or MRI images were randomized and assessed independently, after the radiologist's opinion, by neurologists (RM, PT, RMA). The diagnosis was confirmed after 6 and 12 months of clinical follow-up.

Patients were not included in the study if they showed signs of normal pressure hydrocephalus, previous brain tumours, previous diagnosis of major stroke or brain haemorrhage. We did not include patients with white matter lesions, caused by specific aetiologies, such as multiple sclerosis, brain irradiation, collagen vascular disease, and genetic forms of vascular dementia (such as CADASIL or CARASIL). Patients with previous major psychiatric illness (i.e. schizophrenia, bipolar disorders, psychosis, compulsive-obsessive disorders, etc) or central nervous system disorders and alcoholism were excluded too. Exclusion criteria were, in addition to those provided by the corresponding diagnostic criteria, the absence of an informed caregiver, unavailability of neuroradiological examination, and/or the assumption of psychotropic drugs within two months prior to the clinical assessment. Therefore, five patients were excluded in consequence of lack of a sufficiently informed caregiver and twelve subjects were excluded because they assumed psychotropic drugs during the two months prior to our assessment.

Study subjects underwent a standardized baseline assessment that included a detailed history, a physical examination, laboratory tests and psychiatric evaluations. The physical examination included evaluations of pulse rate and rhythm, blood pressure, heart size and sounds, peripheral pulses, retinal vessel and carotid artery evaluation, electrocardiographic evaluation, and chest X-ray. All patients were followed with periodical neurological and neuropsychological examinations. A complete neuropsychological examination was conducted at baseline, and at 12 months' results were compared.

Main outcomes of the study were: Global performance, which was assessed using the Mini Mental State Examination (Folstein et al., 1975), Frontal Assessment Battery (FAB) (Dubois et al., 2000); Semantic and Phonological Fluency, Digit span subtest (digit span forward and backward) and arithmetic subtest (from Wechsler Adult Intelligent Scale-WAIS; Wechsler, 1981); global behavioral symptoms, assessed by the NeuroPsychiatric Inventory, NPI (Cummings et al., 1994); the caregiver stress, assessed by the Relative Stress Scale, RSS (Green et al., 1992). In addition to these main outcome measures, three further scales were used. The Cornell Scale for Depression in Dementia (Alexopoulos et al., 1988); the Behavioral Pathology in Alzheimer's Disease Rating Scale (BEHAVE-AD) (Greene et al., 1982), and the Clinical Insight Rating Scale (CIR) (Ott et al., 1986) (which provides a measure of its four comprising items – awareness, cognitive deficit, disease progression and functional deficit) were performed. In order to evaluate the apathy, as an independent scale (it is tested as specific item in NPI, and in BEHAVE-AD), we employed the Clinician/Researcher Rated Version of the Apathy Evaluation Scale (AES-C) (Marin et al., 1991). Statistical analyses were performed using the Statistical Package for the Social Sciences (SPSS, version 16.0). Within Groups comparisons were performed by Wilcoxon Signed Rank tests. Between-group comparisons of changes were tested using the marginal homogeneity test, employing the Stewart Maxwell test. This was done for the overall scores for each efficacy variable. In addition, sub-analyses of Spearmann's rho correlation, 2-tailed analyses were performed between behavioral data obtained using the Apathy scores (AES-C), the FAB scores, Cornell's Depression Scores, RSS, CIR, and NPI scores. Results are presented as mean changes from baseline with standard deviations, and P-values are presented where appropriate.

The study subjects were 61 AD patients and 310 sVAD patients. All the patients could be fully studied (mean age 71.1 ± 7.3 years, range= 65-94 years). A synopsis of the cognitive performances obtained by the two groups has been reported in Table 1-2; a synoptic summary of the behavior scores has been reported in Table 3-4; the differential reappraisal of Apathy-scores (AES-C) has been reported in table 5-6. In summary, it can be stated that there are some important cognitive differences in the two groups: AD patients did worse in MMSE; they produced lower in phonological and semantic tasks, in arithmetic calculation and in digit tasks of WAIS; sVAD patients did generally worse in FAB tests. From the behavioral perspective, the following aspects merged from the study: at baseline, the AD group had a worse score of NPI and BEHAVE-AD, and their caregivers did have a heavier stress, as stated by RSS. On the contrary, sVAD patients, at baseline did feel much more depressed (as stated by Cornell'Scale) and did have a better insight in their situation. After 12 months, AD patients showed higher NPI and Behave scores; sVAD patients did show more insight and remained more depressed. Surprisingly, the stress of the caregivers was not significantly different in the two groups. Very interestingly, sVAD patients did manifest more overt apathy, which merged from the AES-C scores, which increase during follow-up and remained a major key point in behavior disturbances of these patients. Spearman's rank correlation analyses indicated that there was a significant correlation between AES-C scores and RSS in sVAD ($r=0.88$, $p<0.01$); a negative correlation with FAB scores ($r=-0.81$, $p<0.01$); analyzing the sub-items, it can be stated a negative relationship between AES-S and C scores and the go/no-go strategies ($r=-0.71$, $p<0.05$); there was no relationship between apathy and depression and insight ratio.

baseline	sVAD	AD	P value (between group)
MMSE	25.8 (2.4)	22.1 (1.9)	<0.05
Word phonological fluency (WAIS)**	34.5 (7.9)	31.2 (3.6)	ns
Semantic category (WAIS)***	37.7 (5.6)	24.5 (3.2)	<0.01
Arithmetic calculations (WAIS) §	6.3 (1.6)	8.6 (1.2)	<0.05
Digit span forward (WAIS)	5.8 (1.5)	5.1 (0.6)	<0.05
Digit span backward (WAIS)	4.4 (2.5)	2.6 (0.8)	<0.05
FAB total score	11.2 (2.1)	10.8 (1.2)	ns
Analogies	2 (0.9)	1.6 (0.2)	ns
Phonemic fluency	1.6 (0.2)	1.8 (0.2)	ns
Motor series	2.2 (0.1)	2.7 (0.4)	ns
Contrast Instructions	2.3 (0.3)	2.2 (0.2)	ns
Go/no-go	0.8 (0.5)	0.9 (0.3)	ns
Comprehension	1.9 (0.1)	0.9 (0.2)	<0.05

Values are mean (SD). NS = not significant.. *Number of items in 45 seconds.; ** Total number of words produced, beginning with T, P, C;

*** Total number of words produced, comprised in the following categories: animal, fruits, professions ; § Number of mistakes

Table 1. Cognitive synoptical results obtained by the two groups studied

12 months follow-up	sVAD within group (12 months vs baseline)	AD within group (12 months vs baseline)	P value (between group)
MMSE	23.8 (2.1) (-2 (.0.3); p<0.05)	17.1 (1.7) (-5 (0.2); p<0.01)	<0.01
Word phonological fluency (WAIS)**	29.5 (2.3) (-5 (5.6); p<0.01)	16.2 (3.1) (-15 (0.5); p<0.01)	<0.01
Semantic category (WAIS)***	27.1 (2.1) (-10.6 (3.5); p<0.01)	12.6 (1.3) (-9.9 (1.9); p<0.01)	<0.01
Arithmetic calculations (WAIS) §	5.4 (1.1) (-0.9 (0.5); ns)	3.4 (1.7) (-5.2 (0.5); p<0.01)	<0.05
Digit span forward (WAIS)	4.1 (1.4) (-1.7 (0.1); p<0.05)	3.2 (0.2) (-1.9 (0.4); p<0.05)	<0.05
Digit span backward (WAIS)	3.6 (0.3) (-0.8 (2.2); ns)	1.9 (0.1) (-0.5 (0.7); p<0.05)	<0.01
FAB total score	5.7 (1.5) (-5.5 (0.6); p<0.01)	7.5 (0.2) (-3.3 (1.0); p<0.05)	<0.01
Analogies	1.2 (0.1) (-0.8 (0.8); p<0.05)	1.4 (0.1) (-0.2 (0.2); ns)	ns
Phonemic fluency	(0.1) (-0.5 (0.1); p<0.05)	1.4 (0.1) (-0.4 (0.1); p<0.05)	ns
Motor series	1.1 (0.3) (-1.1 (0.5); p<0.01)	1.6 (0.2) (-0.9 (0.2); p<0.05)	ns
Contrast Instructions	1.2 (0.5) (-1.1 (0.3); p<0.01)	2.0 (0.1) (-0.2 (0.1); ns)	ns
Go/no-go	0.1 (0.3) (-0.7 (0.2); p<0.05)	0.8 (0.1) (-0.1 (0.2); ns)	ns
Comprehension	1.0 (0.9) (-0.9 (0.8); p<0.05)	0.3 (0.1) (-0.6 (0.1); p<0.05)	<0.05

Values are mean (SD). NS = not significant.. *Number of items in 45 seconds.; ** Total number of words produced, beginning with T, P, C;

*** Total number of words produced, comprised in the following categories: animal, fruits, professions ; § Number of mistakes

In brackets, in each column, comparison within group, 12 months vs baseline, reported as mean, SD, and p

Table 2. Cognitive synoptical results obtained by the two groups studied, at 12 months

baseline	sVAD	AD	P value
RSS	**24.7 (8.7)**	**36.1 (8.5)**	(p<0.01)
NPI	**14.9 (0.3)**	**24.4 (5.2)**	(p<0.01)
CIR	**3 (0.2)**	**2 (0.5)**	(p<0.05)
Cornell	**18.5 (3.5)**	**13.5 (4)**	(p<0.05)
BEHAVE	**9.5 (2.1)**	**12.6 (4.1)**	(p<0.05)

Values are mean (SD). NS = not significant..

Table 3. Behavioral synoptical results

	sVAD	AD	P value
RSS	44.5 (1.6) (+20.2 (5.9), <0.01)	43.9 (2.1) (+7.8 (6.8), <0.05)	ns
NPI	24.1 (0.8) (+10.8 (0.5), <0.01)	56.3 (4.5) (+31.9 (1.1), <0.01)	(p<0.01)
CIR	2.7 (0.3) (+0.3 (0.1), ns)	(0.3) (+1.0 (0.3), <0.05)	(p<0.01)
Cornell	22.1 (1.2) (+4.4 (2.3), <0.05)	12.3 (1.1) (-0.8 (3.1), ns)	(p<0.01)
BEHAVE	22.7 (1.3) (+13.2 (0.8), <0.01)	43.1 (2.3) (+30.5 (0.8), <0.01)	(p<0.01)

Values are mean (SD). NS = not significant.; In brackets, in each column, comparison within group, 12 months vs baseline, reported as mean, SD, and p

Table 4. Behavioral synoptical results

baseline	sVAD	AD	P value
AES-C	48.5 (7.2)	28.0 (4.9)	<0.01

Values are mean (SD). NS = not significant.

Table 5. Apathy scores, by the researcher evaluation (AES-C)

	sVAD	AD	P value
AES-C	67.2 (3.5) (+18.7 (3.7); p<0.01)	33.4 (6.1) (5.4 (1.2); ns)	<0.01

Apathy scores, by the researcher evaluation (AES-C)

Table 6. Values are mean (SD). NS = not significant.. In brackets, in each column, comparison within group, 12 months vs baseline, reported as mean, SD, and p

What merged from this study is a confirmation of the wide known rule, that behavioral disorders are the most problematic in the follow-up of dementia. Among them, apathy is one of the most concerning. Frequency and severity of apathy vary across different dementia subtypes; it is the most common behavioral symptom of behavioral variant of frontotemporal dementia (bvFTD), with reported prevalence ranging from 62 to 89% of patients (Mendez et al., 2008); the prevalence of apathy in AD ranges from 25 to 88% with a trend to increase with disease severity (Starkestein et al., 2006). The prevalence of apathy in other neuro-degenerative disorders, such as Parkinson's disease vary between 16.5% and 51%, depending upon the instrument for assessment and on the samples examined (Moretti et al., 2012). Apathy may be associated with an increased risk of cognitive decline. Symptoms of apathy, but not symptoms of depressive affect, increase the risk of progression from MCI to AD (Richard et al., 2012). Conversely, patients with or without apathy had an increase of similar magnitude in anosognosia scores. In conclusion, anosognosia is a significant predictor of apathy in Alzheimer's disease (Starkstein et al., 2010).

The aim of our study was to assess the behavior spectrum of Alzheimer's Disease (AD) and that of subcortical Vascular Dementia (sVAD), with a particular concern for apathy, and to assess the possible role of apathy in the differential clinical diagnosis, as compared to other behavioral changes and different neuropsychological patterns. Our results showed that there are some important cognitive differences in the two groups. Obviously, the AD patients did worse in MMSE; they produced lower in phonological and semantic tasks, they did many mistakes in arithmetic calculation and their digit span were lower; sVAD patients did generally worse in FAB tests, as a sensitive measure of executive dysfunction. And their behavior problems were different. At baseline, the AD group had a worse score of NPI and BEHAVE-AD, and their caregivers did have a heavier stress, as stated by RSS. On the contrary, sVAD patients, at baseline did feel much more depressed (as stated by Cornell'Scale) and did have a better insight in their situation. After 12 months, AD patients showed higher NPI and Behave scores; sVAD patients did show more insight and remained more depressed. Surprisingly, the stress of the caregivers was not significantly different in the two groups. Very interestingly, sVAD patients did manifest more overt apathy, which merged from the AES-C scores, which increased during follow-up.

So far, it can be argued that sVAD patients have higher insight, more depression and more apathy than AD, and the two last aspects are the major causative factors for an increase of caregiver stress in the one-year follow-up. At that time, the significant difference which was noted at the beginning of the study for the RSS of AD patients, is practically cancelled out, and there is no difference between RSS in AD and sVAD patients. The main reason for what observed is that apathy increases, and caregivers do not know how to manage it. Apathy is one of the greatest stressors for caregivers, and the second most common is disinhibition (Massimo et al., 2009).

As a general observation (Quaranta et al., 2012), the occurrence of apathy is connected to damage of prefrontal cortex (PFC) and basal ganglia (Chase, 2011); "emotional affective" apathy may be related to the orbitomedial PFC and ventral striatum; "cognitive apathy" may be associated with dysfunction of lateral PFC and dorsal caudate nuclei; deficit of "autoactivation" may be due to bilateral lesions of the internal portion of globus pallidus, bilateral paramedian thalamic lesions, or the dorsomedial portion of PFC (Chow et al. 2009). Trying to compare apathy in AD and in the behavior form of Frontal dementia (bvFTD), Quaranta et al (2012) lead to an observation of a different distribution of apathetic symptoms; they stated that subjects affected by bvFTD displayed higher frequency of "affective" symptoms, and a reduction of "auto-activation" (Levy and Dubois, 2006) (or "behavioral apathy," (Marin, 1991)) in comparison with AD sample. The different clinical expression of apathy, among the two groups of patients probably reflects the involvement of different anatomic substrates. Previous studies have reported that in bvFTD apathy is associated with changes in orbitofrontal cortex (Zamboni et al., 2008; Peters et al., 2006), which, in turn, has been postulated to be the anatomical correlate of "affective" apathy (Levy and Dubois, 2006), and with volume loss in the dorsal anterior cingulate and dorsolateral prefrontal cortex (Massimo et al., 2009). Thus, it is possible that the observation by Quaranta et al (2012) may reflect an alteration of orbitofrontal cortex and its connections with subcortical nuclei (ventral striatum), that could be specific of bvFTD. "Affective apathy" may be also regarded as the clinical expression of personality changes in bvFTD; for example, Sollberger et al. (2009) reported that subjects with FTD and semantic dementia displayed a reduction in affiliative behavior (lack of warmth) and showed, in a large sample of subjects aff ected by different neurodegenerative diseases, an association between "warmth" and several cortical and subcortical right hemisphere structures (viz. orbitofrontal cortex, insular cortex, amygdala, and hippocampal and parahippocampal regions). This finding is of particular interest, since the authors reported an association between lack of warmth and cerebral structures related to reward mechanisms, and "affective apathy" has been regarded as consequence of the inability to associate emotions to behaviors (Marin, 1991; 1996). Analogously, affective apathy may be related to an impairment of the so-called prosocial sentiments (such as guilt, pity, and embarrassment), connected to lack of empathy; Moll et al. (2011) reported reduced social sentiments in bvFTD subjects; this deficit was related to hypometabolism in medial frontal polar cortex and septal area.

On the other hand, in AD, apathy severity has been connected to neurofibrillary tangles density in the anterior cingulate gyrus (Marshall et al., 2006) and to grey matter atrophy in the anterior cingulate and in the left medial frontal cortex (Apostolova et al, 2007; Tekin et al., 2001; Marshall et al., 2006). These findings were confirmed by a PET study showing the association of apathy with hypometabolism in the bilateral anterior cingulate gyrus and medial orbitofrontal cortex (Marshall et al., 2007). Many studies tried to identify the neuroanatomical correlates of apathy in AD (Tunnard et al., 2011). Functional imaging studies have tended to find impaired functioning measured by either reduced blood flow or reduced metabolism in the anterior cingulate cortex (ACC) and medial frontal or orbitofrontal cortical (OFC) brain regions (Robert et al., 2006; Lanctot et al., 2007; Marshall et al., 2007). However, it is uncertain whether these regions are unilaterally or bilaterally affected. Others have found reduced function limited to the OFC alone (Holthoff et al., 2005) or the ACC alone (Migneco et al., 2001), suggesting that impaired functioning of both regions is not necessary for apathy to result. MRI studies investigating the structural correlates of apathy in AD patients have, for the most part, replicated findings from functional studies implicating the ACC and OFC most consistently (Apostolova et al., 2007;Laveretsky et al., 2007; Bruen et al., 2008). Additional regions of atrophy in the superior frontal gyrus, specifically BA 9, are also reported (Apostolova et al., 2007; Bruen et al., 2008) as is atrophy of frontopolar (BA 10) and ventrolateral prefrontal regions, including BA 45 (pars triangularis; Bruen et al., 2008).

Also of note, is some evidence that subcortical nuclei which project to prefrontal regions, including the caudate and putamen have shown greater atrophy in apathy in AD (Bruen et al., 2008). Overall then, functional, structural and pathological studies point towards a specific involvement of the ACC and OFC in mediating symptoms of apathy, with a suggestion of wider involvement of frontocortical networks.

One pathophysiological model for apathy in Alzheimer's disease which addresses both structural and biochemical disruption is that of Guimaraes et al. (2008). Their model proposes that the ACC and OFC are part of a broader fronto striatal circuit, which is involved in decision-making. Specifically, these regions are involved in evaluating action and outcomes and, via the basolateral amygdala and nucleus accumbens, feed into an ascending frontostriatal pathway to the dorsolateral prefrontal cortex, which is ultimately responsible for selecting and executing behavioural responses. Damage to the ACC and OFC leads to a disruption of this circuit resulting in impaired decision-making and impaired response initiation, which presents as apathy.

This model resembles quite well our idea of apathy in sVAD. There is good evidence of high levels of apathy subcortical disease, such as Parkinson's Disease, resulting from dysfunction at the striatal level (Pluck and Brown, 2002), and our data suggest than in AD the locus of dysfunction is at the cortical level, namely the ACC and the OFC.

In sVAD, apathy might be the result of a wider prefrontal disease process, or may suggest a putative role for these regions in mediating apathy, namely due to an involvement of the pars triangularis, of the superior frontal gyrus and of the orbital operculum may suggest that degeneration of the OFC is part of. Ventrolateral and superior frontal regions are also involved in the selection and execution of willed action, and so may contribute to the diminished behavioural responses to everyday challenges displayed by apathetic patients. Recently, increased incidence of white matter hyperintensities in the frontal lobe has been associated with apathy (Starkstein et al., 2009); however, some studies have found no evidence of frontal involvement in apathy (Rosen et al., 2005). A recent and well conducted study examined the relationship between behavior alterations and subcortical lesions (white-matter lesions and lacunes) in AD (Palmqvist et al., 2011). Lacunes in the basal ganglia resulted in a 2- to 3-fold increased risk of delusions, hallucinations and depression, when adjusting for cognition and atrophy. This suggests that basal ganglia lesions can contribute to BPSD in patients with AD, independently of the AD process (Palmqvist et al., 2011).

Being that we have chosen sVAD and AD patients, we have tried to avoid the spurious cases of AD/sVAD coexistence. What we have found is a major involvement of subcortical frontal circuits in sVAD, than in AD, and deriving from that, major evidence of apathy in sVAD, than in AD. In normal conditions, one may propose that the prefrontal cortex internalizes the information from the external and internal environments needed to make a decision about possible actions to be elaborated and performed. Neural signals corresponding to the thoughts or actions are then processed by the basal ganglia in order to validate the most relevant signal. Validation processing may be translated into the extraction of the relevant signal from noise to be readdressed to the output target, namely the prefrontal cortex (Levy and Dubois, 2006), where a clear-cut signal can be detected and contributes to disambiguating decision-making and maintaining or modifying the ongoing behaviour. In pathological situations, if there is a focal destruction within the basal ganglia sub-regions, the signal emerging from the basal ganglia is diminished, the ongoing behaviour is not validated (i.e. not amplified) at the level of the cortex and could be difficult to maintain, and the forthcoming one (if it is not reflexive) is not activated (Levy and Dubois, 2006). In sum, an 'auto-activation' deficit results from the inability of voluntary thoughts or actions to reach the activation threshold due to a decreased signal-to-noise ratio at the level of the prefrontal cortex (Levy and Dubois, 2006).

Thus, in that way, we can justify apathy in sVAD due to the major involvement of cortical-subcortical neural pathways. Many studies should be done to differentiate the anatomical, biological, and physiological eventual different substrate in the subcortical vascular forms, and in degenerative disorders, in order to better differentiate them, if necessary, and eventually to treat them.

Acknowledgements

The Authors wish to thank Andrew Wright Smithson, PhD for the careful reading and corrections of the manuscript.

Author details

Rita Moretti[1], Paola Torre[1], Francesca Esposito[1], Enrica Barro[1], Paola Tomietto[2] and Rodolfo M. Antonello[1]

*Address all correspondence to: moretti@univ.trieste.it

1 Medicina Clinica, Ambulatorio Complicanze Internistiche Cerebrali, Dipartimento Universitario Clinico di Scienze Mediche Tecnologiche e Traslazionali, Università degli Studi di Trieste, Italy

2 Reumatologia-Clinica Medica, AOUTS, Ospedale di Cattinara, Italy

References

[1] Aarsland D, Litvan I, Larsen JP. Neuropsychiatric symptoms of patients with progressive supranuclear palsy and Parkinson's disease. J Neuropsychiatry Clin Neurosci 2001;13:42–9.

[2] Alexopoulos GS, Abrams RC, Young RC, Shamoian CA. Cornell Scale for Depression in Dementia. Biol Psychiatry 1988; 23: 271–84.

[3] American Psychiatric Association. DSM-IV (4th ed.) 1994; Washington, DC: American Psychiatric Association.

[4] Brown RG, Pluck G. Negative symptoms: the "pathology" of motivation and goal-directed behaviour. Trends Neurosci 2000;23:412–17.

[5] Cummings JL, Mega M, Gray K, et al. The Neuropsychiatric Inventory: comprehensive assessment of psychopathology in dementia. Neurology 1994; 44: 2308–14.

[6] Dubois B, Slachevsky A, Litvan I, Pillon B. The FAB: a Frontal Assessment Battery at bedside. Neurology. 2000 Dec 12;55(11):1621-6.

[7] Dujardin K, Sockeel P, elliaux M, DESTEE A, Defebvre L. Apathy may herald cognitive decline and dementia in Parkinsons's Disease. Movement Disorders, 2009 (24); 16: 2391-2397.

[8] Erkinjuntti T. Vascular dementia: challenge of clinical diagnosis. Int Psychogeriatr 1997;9: 77–83.

[9] Folstein M, Folstein S, McHugh P. Mini-Mental state. A practical method for grading the cognitive state of patients for the clinician. J Psychiatr Res 1975;12:189–98.

[10] G. McKhann, D. Drachman, M. Folstein, R. Katzman, D. Price, and E. M. Stadlan, "Clinical diagnosis of Alzheimer's disease: Report of the NINCDS-ADRDA Work Group under the auspices of Department of Health and Human Services Task Force on Alzheimer's Disease," Neurology, 1984; 34, 7. 939–944.

[11] Greene JG, Smith R, Gardiner M, Timburg GC. Measuring behavioural disturbance of elderly demented in patients in the community and its effects on relatives: a factor analytic study. Age Ageing 1982; 11: 121–6.

[12] Levy ML, Cummings JL, Fairbanks LA, et al. Apathy is not depression. J Neuropsychiatry Clin Neurosci 1998;10: 314–19.

[13] Marin RS, Biedrzycki RC, Firinciogullari S. Reliability and validity of the apathy evaluation scale. Psychiatr Res 1991; 38:143–62.

[14] Moretti R, Torre P., Antonello RM, Vidus rosin M, Esposito F, Rubelli Furman M, Bellini G. Apathy: a complex symptom, specific to the clinical pattern pf presentation of Parkinson's Disease. Am. J .Alzheimer's Disease and other Dementias, 2012; Volume 27 (3) 2012 pp. 196 - 201.

[15] Ott BR, Lafleche G, Whelihan WM, et al. Impaired awareness of deficits in Alzheimer's Disease. Alzheimer Dis Assoc Disord 1996; 10: 68–76.

[16] Reisberg B, Borenstein J, Salob SP, et al. Behavioral symptoms in Alzheimer's disease: phenomenology and treatment. J Clin Psychiatr 1987; 48(S1): 9–15.

[17] Roman GC, et al. Vascular dementia: Diagnostic criteria for research studies. (Report of the NINDS-AIREN Intemational Workshop) Neurology,1993; 43, 250-260.

[18] Starkstein SE, Leentjens AF. The nosological position of apathy in clinical practice. J Neurol Neurosurg Psychiatr 2008; 10; 202-209.

[19] Starkstein SE, Mayberg SE, Preziosi TJ, et al. Reliability, validity and clinical correlates of apathy in Parkinson's disease. J Neuropsychiatry 1992;4:134–9.

[20] Stuss DT, Van Reekum R, Murphy KJ. Differentiation of states and causes of apathy. In: Borod JC(ed.): The Neuropsychology of emotion. Oxford: Oxford University Press. 2000. Pp. 340--363.

[21] Chase T. N. "Apathy in neuropsychiatric disease: diagnosis, pathophysiology, and treatment," Neurotoxicity Research, 2011; vol. 19, no. 2: pp. 266–278.

[22] Wechsler D. Wechsler adult intelligence scale manual-R. New York: Grune & Stratton. 1981.

[23] Mendez M. F., Lauterbach E. C., Sampson S. M. An evidence-based review of the psychopathology of frontotemporal dementia: a report of the ANPA Committee on Research Journal of Neuropsychiatry and Clinical Neurosciences, 2008; vol. 20, no. 2: 130–149

[24] Starkstein S. E., Jorge R., Mizrahi R., Robinson R. G. A prospective longitudinal study of apathy in Alzheimer's Disease Journal of Neurology, Neurosurgery & Psychiatry, 2006; vol. 77, no. 1: 8–11.

[25] Chow T. W., Binns M. A., Cummings J. L. et al. Apathy symptom profile and behavioral associations in frontotemporal dementia vs dementia of Alzheimer type," Archives of Neurology, 2009; vol. 66, no. 7: 888–893.

[26] Zamboni G., Huey E.D., Krueger F., Nichelli P. F., Grafman J. Apathy and disinhibition in frontotemporal dementia: insights into their neural correlates, Neurology, 2008; vol. 71, no. 10: 736–742.

[27] Peters F., Perani D., Herholz K. et al. Orbitofrontal dysfunction related to both apathy and disinhibition in frontotemporal Dementia. Dementia and Geriatric Cognitive Disorders, 2006; vol. 21, no. 5-6: 373–379.

[28] Massimo L., Powers C., Moore P. et al. Neuroanatomy of apathy and disinhibition in frontotemporal lobar degeneration. Dementia and Geriatric Cognitive Disorders, 2009; vol. 27, no. 1: 96–104.

[29] Marshall G. A., Fairbanks L. A., Tekin S., Vinters H. V., Cummings J. L. Neuropathologic correlates of apathy in Alzheimer's disease. Dementia and Geriatric Cognitive Disorders, 2006; vol. 21, no. 3: 144–147.

[30] Apostolova L.G., Akopyan G. G., Partiali N. et al. Structural correlates of apathy in Alzheimer's disease. Dementia and Geriatric Cognitive Disorders, 2007; vol. 24, no. 2: 91–97.

[31] Marshall G. A., Monserratt L., Harwood D., Mandelkern M., Cummings J. L., Sultzer D. L. Positron emission tomography metabolic correlates of apathy in Alzheimer disease. Archives of Neurology, 2007; vol. 64, no. 7: 1015–1020.

[32] Marin R. S. Apathy: a neuropsychiatric syndrome. Journal of Neuropsychiatry and Clinical Neurosciences, 1991; vol. 3, no. 3: pp. 243–254.

[33] Marin R. S. Apathy: Concept, Syndrome, Neural Mechanisms, and Treatment," Seminars in Clinical Neuropsychiatry, 1996; vol. 1, no. 4: 304–314.

[34] Moll J., Zahn R., de Oliveira-Souza R. et al. Impairment of prosocial sentiments is associated with frontopolar and septal damage in frontotemporal dementia," NeuroImage, 2011; vol. 54, no. 2: 1735–1742.

[35] Quaranta D, Marra C, Rossi C, Gainotti G, Masullo C. Different Apathy Profile in Behavioral Variant of Frontotemporal Dementia and Alzheimer's Disease: A Preliminary Investigation. Current Gerontology and Geriatrics Research, 2012; Article ID 719250, 8 pages; doi:10.1155/2012/719250

[36] Tunnard C., Whitehead D., Hurt C., Wahlund L.O., Mecocci P., Tsolaki M., Vellas B., Spenger C., Kłoszewska I., Soininen H., Lovestone S., Simmons A., on behalf of the AddNeuroMed Consortium. Apathy and cortical atrophy in Alzheimer's disease. Int J Geriatr Psychiatry 2011; 26: 741–748.

[37] Apostolova LG, Akopyan GG, Partiali N, et al. Structural correlates of apathy in Alzheimer's disease. Dement Geriartr Cogn Disord. 2007; 24: 91–97.

[38] Bruen PD, McGeown WJ, Shanks MF, Vennner A. Neuroanatomical correlates of neuropsychiatric sypmptoms in Alzheimer's disease. Brain 2008; 131: 2455–2463.

[39] Guimara˜es HC, Levy R, Teixeira AL, Beato RG, Caramelli P. Neurobiology of apathy in Alzheimer's disease. Arq Neuro-Psiquiatr. 2008; 66: 436–443.

[40] Holthoff VA, Beuthien-Bauman B, Kalbe E, et al. Regional cerebral metabolism in early Alzheimer's disease with clinically significant apathy or depression. Biol. Psychiatry 2005; 57: 412–421.

[41] Lanctot KL, Moosa S, Herrmann N, et al. A SPECT study of apathy in Alzheimer's disease. Dement Geriartr Cogn Disord. 2007; 24: 65–72.

[42] Laveretsky H, Ballmaier M, Pham D, Toga A, Kumar A. Neuroanatomical characteristics of geriatric apathy and depression: a magnetic resonance imaging study. Am J Geriatr Psychiatry 2007; 15: 386–394.

[43] Marshall GA, Fairbanks LA, Tekin S, Vinters HV, Cummings JL. Neuropathologic correlates of apathy in Alzheimer's disease. Dement Geriatr Cogn Disord. 2006; 21: 144–147.

[44] Marshall GA, Monserratt L, Harwood D, et al. Positron emission tomography metabolic correlates of apathy in Alzheimer's disease. Arch Neurol. 2007; 64: 1015–1020.

[45] Migneco O, BenoitM, Koulibaly PM, et al. Perfusion brain SPECT and statistical parametric mapping analysis indicate that apathy is a cingulate syndrome: a study in Alzheimer's disease and nondemented patients. Neuroimage 2001; 13: 896–902.

[46] Pluck GC, Brown RG. Apathy in Parkinson's disease. J Neurol Neurosurg Psychiatr 2002; 73: 636–642.

[47] Robert PH, Darcourt G, Koulibaly MP, et al. Lack of initiative and interest in Alzheimer's disease: a single photon emission computed tomography study. Eur J Neurol 2006; 13: 729–735.

[48] Rosen HJ, Allison SC, Schaeur GF, et al. Neuroanatomical correlates of behavioral disorders in dementia. Brain 2005; 128: 2612–2625.

[49] Starkstein SE, Mizrahi R, Capizzano AA, et al. Neuroimaging correlates of apathy and depression in Alzheimer's Disease. J Neuropsychiatry Clin Neurosci. 2009; 21: 259–265.

[50] Tekin S, Mega MS, Masterman DM, et al. Orbitofrontal and anterior cingulate cortex neurofibrillary tangle burden is associated with agitation in Alzheimer's disease. Ann Neurol 2001; 49: 355–361.

[51] Starkstein SE, Petracca G, Chemerinski E, Kremer J. Syndrome validity of apathy in Alzheimer's disease. Am. J. Psychiatry 2001; 158: 872–577.

[52] Marin RS, Firinciogullari S, Biedrzycki RC. The sources of convergence between measures of apathy and depression. J. Affect. Disord. 1993; 28: 7–14.

[53] Clarke DE, Van Reekum R, Patel J, Simard M, Gomez E, Streiner DL. An appraisal of the psychometric properties of the clinician version of the Apathy Evaluation Scale (AESC)- Int. J. Methods Psychiatr. Res. 2007; 16: 97–110.Resnick B, Zimmerman SI, Magaziner J et al. Use of the Apathy Evaluation Scale as a measure of motivation in elderly people. Rehabil. Nurs. 1998; 23: 141–147.

[54] Tatsch M, Bottino CM, Azevedo D et al. Neuropsychiatric symptoms in Alzheimer disease and cognitively impaired, non-demented elderly from a community-based sample in Brazil: Prevalence and relationship with dementia severity. Am. J. Geriatr. Psychiatry 2006; 14: 438–445.

[55] Jung Hsieh C, Chu H, Jror-Serk Cheng J, Shen WW, Lin CC. Validation of apathy evaluation scale and assessment of severity of apathy in Alzheimer's disease.pcn_Psychiatry and Clinical Neurosciences 2012; 66: 227–234

[56] Starkstein SE, Brockman S, Bruce D, Petracca G. Anosognosia Is a Significant Predictor ofApathy in Alzheimer's Disease. The Journal of Neuropsychiatry and Clinical Neurosciences 2010; 22:378 –383

[57] Richard E, Schmand B, Eikelenboom P, Yang SC, Ligthart SA, Moll van Charante EP, van Gool WA. Symptoms of apathy are associated with progression from mild cogni-

tive impairment to Alzheimer's disease in non-depressed subjects. Dement Geriatr Cogn Disord. 2012;33(2-3):204-9.

[58] Palmqvist S, Sarwari A, Wattmo C, Bronge L, Zhang Y, Wahlund LO, Nägga K. Association between subcortical lesions and behavioral and psychological symptoms in patients with Alzheimer's disease. Dement Geriatr Cogn Disord. 2011;32(6):417-23.

[59] Massimo L, Powers C, Moore P, Vesely L, Avants B, Gee J, Libon DJ, Grossman M. Neuroanatomy of apathy and disinhibition in frontotemporal lobar degeneration. Dement Geriatr Cogn Disord. 2009;27(1):96-104.

[60] Levy R., Dubois B. Apathy and the functional anatomy of the prefrontal cortex-basal ganglia circuits. Cerebral Cortex, 2006; 16, 7: 916–928.

[61] Moretti R, Torre P, Antonello RM (Eds). Basal Ganglia and Thalamus: their role in cognition and behavior. Novascience Editor, NewYork. 2009.

Chapter 15

Predicting Cognitive Decline in Alzheimer's Disease (AD): The Role of Clinical, Cognitive Characteristics and Biomarkers

Mei Sian Chong and Tih-Shih Lee

Additional information is available at the end of the chapter

http://dx.doi.org/10.5772/54289

1. Introduction

Given the rapid ageing of the population worldwide, global estimates of AD - generally considered to be the commonest subtype of dementia - are expected to increase from the current estimated 25 million to 63 million in 2030, and by 2050, a staggering 114 million [1]. Over the last two decades in particular, significant but modest breakthroughs in pharmacological treatment of this devastating condition have occurred. Presently, there is increasing conviction that intervention (especially disease-modifying therapy) will have to be instituted at the earliest possible stage of the illness to confer the greatest benefit.

Prevailing clinical criteria for Mild Cognitive Impairment (MCI) have low to moderate diagnostic accuracy in identifying and predicting progression to dementia. MCI is an unstable clinical construct where some patients convert (MCI-converters) while others remain relatively stable (MCI non-converters). As observed from neuropathological and recent biomarker studies, the accumulation of AD pathology (β-amyloid plaques and neurofibrillary tangles) may precede the onset of clinical disease by as long as 20-30 years [2,3]. This suggests that functional and structural brain changes may occur prior to apparent clinical manifestations of cognitive impairment (Figure 1). However, the current definition of MCI is based primarily on clinical and neuropsychological criteria, and this may have contributed to limited demonstration of efficacy in therapeutic and disease-modifying trials thus far. Supplementing existing criteria with information about biomarkers may enrich the definition of MCI This provided the impetus for the development of reliable biomarkers such as cerebrospinal fluid (CSF), neuroimaging and blood biomarkers to complement clinical approaches in early diagnosis and predicting progression. In support of this, the recent proposed criteria for symptomatic pre-dementia phase of AD (MCI), preclinical AD and presymptomatic AD have included biomarkers reflecting molecular pathology, downstream measures of structural and functional/metabolic changes, and associated biochemical changes in their research diagnostic armamentarium [4].

Longitudinal studies in AD subjects have also noted variability in disease progression. In one study, 11.9% of subjects exhibit rapid cognitive decline while some remained relatively stable [5]. Other studies that utilized parameters such as the decline in Mini Mental State Examination (MMSE) scores [6, 7] (≥3 point decline) also reported a distinctive difference in the clinical course between the fast-progressors and slow-progressors.

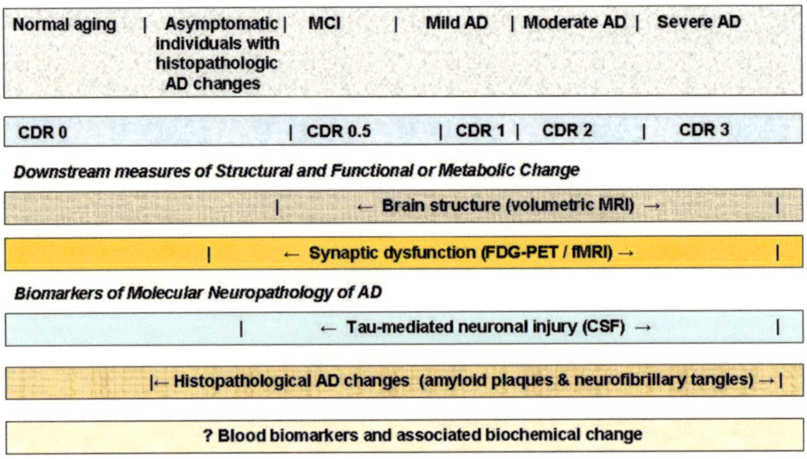

Figure 1. Clinical Continuum of Alzheimer's disease and hypothetical biomarker model

In this chapter, we will review the body of evidence on the use of various clinical and comorbid factors, alone and/or in combination with biomarkers, on predicting rapid cognitive decline across the spectrum of cognitive impairment – defined in terms of AD progression in MCI subjects and rapid cognitive decline in AD subjects. We will also look at longitudinal biomarker measurements as well as their role (alone and/ in combination with clinical and comorbid factors) in predicting cognitive decline and disease trajectories. We will discuss the implications of current research findings to their application in clinical and therapeutic trials. The chapter is not intended to be an exhaustive review of this burgeoning literature, but instead to highlight integrative and potentially novel lines of inquiry.

2. Clinical and cognitive/ behavioural characteristics (table 1)

A number of socio-demographic factors and vascular risk factors have been found to increase risk of development of AD.

Increased risk of cognitive decline in diabetes may reflect a dual pathologic process involving both cerebrovascular damage and neurodegenerative changes. Several possible pathophysiological mechanisms may include hyperglycemia, insulin resistance [8], oxidative stress, advanced glycation end products, and inflammatory cytokines. A shared clinicopathologic study alluded to the potential shared predisposition for developing amyloid in both the pancreas and brain [9]. This is supported by a study of intranasal insulin preventing cognitive decline, cerebral atrophy and white matter changes in mouse models [10]. Diabetes and pre-diabetes have been found to be associated with AD progression in MCI subjects, with progression from MCI to dementia accelerated by 3.18 years[11]. The stronger effect of pre-diabetes on MCI conversion may be caused by high glycemic level in pre-diabetes and increased insulin resistance [12]. Although antihypertensive therapy has been shown to be associated with reduced rate of conversion to AD in midregional proatrial natriuretic peptide-stratified subjects with MCI [13], there has been a paucity of data with regard to the individual effect of hypertension on MCI-converters[14]. A non-significant trend was found for cerebrovascular disease as a risk factor for MCI-converters[15]. Diabetes, hypertension and cerebrovascular disease have been found to be associated with faster progression rate in dementia [16-19]. Although mid-life hypercholesterolemia has been repeatedly shown to increase risk of late-life dementia, there is relatively little evidence of its influence on MCI-converters and the rate of AD decline [20].

Study variable	Population	Results	Key findings
Predicting AD conversion in MCI subjects			
Diabetes and pre-diabetes [11]	302 aMCI and 182 CIND subjects aged ≥ 75 years over 9 years	155 subjects had AD progression	HR 2.87 diabetes (95%CI 1.3-6.34) HR 4.96 pre-diabetes (95% CI 2.27 -10.84) Accelerated progression by 3.18 years
Vascular risk factors [21]	837 MCI subjects followed annually over 5 years	298 converters 352 stable	HR 2.04 (95% CI 1.33-3.11) Hypertension HR 1.84 (95% CI 1.19-2.84) Diabetes HR 1.62 (95% CI 1.00 – 2.62) Hypercholesterolemia HR 1.11 (95% CI 1.04-1.18) Cerebrovascular disease HR 1.60 (95% CI 1,03 – 2.49)
Diabetes, baseline white matter severity, baseline moderate-to-severe carotid stenosis and carotid stenosis change [22]	257 MCI subjects over 3 years	MCI conversion to AD 7.05%/year	Diabetes HR 2.92 (95% CI 1.12-7.6) Baseline WMC severity (mild vs severe) HR 0.04 (95% CI 0.006-0.242) Baseline carotid stenosis (moderate vs mild) HR 8.46 (95% CI 2.1-34.14) Carotid stenosis change HR 124.1 (95% CI 0.95- 16,209.68)
Stroke [15]	121 MCI subjects over 3 years	MCI conversion to AD based on age strata rate (per 100 person-years) Total 2.3 65-69y 0 70-74y 0 75-79 3.1 80-84y 2.0	Stroke RR 4.0 (95% CI 0.92-13.87)
Metabolic syndrome [8]	49 MCI subjects with metabolic syndrome and 72 without metabolic syndrome	Progression to dementia	67.6 (95% CI 35.17 – 129.93) Rate 1000 per person-years
Age [23]	97 amnestic MCI 88 cognitively-unimpaired controls followed up mean 38.8 mths	Annual rate of progression to AD	Odds ratio = 4.5 of AD progression Older age [exp(β)=1.11, SE(β)=0.7, WALD=4.2, p=0.040] predictors of AD conversion
Empirically weighted and Combined neuropsychological battery [42]	43 MCI subjects	14 subsequently converted to AD	Multivariate combinations achieved 84% accuracy, 86% Sn, 83%Sp in predicting AD progression (using episodic memory, speeded executive function, recognition memory (false positives). recognition memory (true positives), speed in visuospatial memory, visuospatial episodic memory
Learning measure and retention measure [43]	607 MCI and HC patients in ADNI cohort divided into 4 groups: (based on learning and retention)	Conversion to AD at 2 years	Low-learning, Low retention OR17.84, 95%CI 7.37-43.10, p<0.001; Low-learning, High retention OR 9.01, 95%CI2.98-27.21,p<0.001; High learning, low retention OR8.48, 95%CI 3.45-20.86, p<0.001 (high learning, high retention as reference group)
MISplus [44]	40MCI subjects	Conversion to to AD at 18 months (n=7)	OR 0.28, 95%CI 0.099-0.79) At cut-off of 2, PPV 71.5%, NPV 91.5%, Accuracy 87%

Hypertension [16]	135 incident AD Patients in Cache Country Dementia Progression Study	Rapid decline on CDR-sum of boxes and MMSE using linear mixed models	Systolic BP ≥160 versus <160mmHg (controlling for other vascular variables) for CDR-SB coeff X time 1.78 (95% CI 1.20-2.36) for MMSE coeff X time -2.38 (-3.23,-1.53)
Hypertension [17]	719 AD patients In multi-center Trial	ADAS-cog increase by ≥1 standard deviation of baseline ADAS-cog score of	OR 6.9 (95% CI 1.5-31.1, p=0.005)
Diabetes [18]	154 AD patients attending Dementia center	Disease progression of decrease of 5 pts or more on MMSE	Crude OR 0.38 (95% CI 0.2-0.9) Multivariate OR 0.36 (95% CI 0.1-0.9)
Cerebrovascular disease[19]	224 AD patients	Decline in MMSE, ADAS-cog and SIB difference	No difference in vascular risk factors except cerebrovascular disease (mean difference in MMSE 13.6 (-14.3—7.6); ADAS-cog 27 (-30.1--13.7); SIB 54.4 (-62.3—29.9)
Vascular risk factors including heart disease, stroke, diabetes, hypertension), smoking, pre-diagnosis blood lipid and LDL-C [20]	156 AD patients living in community mean age 83 y	AD decline using generalized estimating equation models	Only higher LDL-cholesterol was independently associated with faster cognitive decline. Stratified according to APOEε4 showed higher total cholesterol, higher LDL, stroke and heart disease associated with faster decline.
Age [24]	201 Caucasian Probable/Possible AD subjects at ADRC, Pittsburgh	Latent class mixture models of quadratic trajectories includ-Ing random intercept and concomitant variables (MMSE)	Best latent trajectory model: Initial MMSE and age. Parameter estimate 0.85, p<.001 for MMSE, Parameter estimate 0.04,p =0.04 for age.
Education [27]	127 persons in Bronx Aging study developed dementia (out of 488 community dwelling subjects)	Change point models to test predictions of cognitive reserve hypothesis using Buschke Selective Reminding Test (SRT)	Prior to diagnosis, lower levels of formal education associated with poorer performance on memory and verbal fluency. Accelerated decline in SRT shown by estimated annual rates of decline for 16 years, 9.5 years and 4 years of formal education was 3.22, 2.57 and 2.03 points/year respectively.
Neuropsychiatric symptoms [30]	177 memory-clinic AD outpatients	Rapid disease progression defined as loss of ≥1 ability in ADL or drop of ≥ 5 points on MMSE	Affective syndrome increased risk of functional decline (HR2.0, 95%CI 1.1-3.6) AND Manic syndrome (HR 3.2, 95% CI 1.3-7.5)
Pre-progression rate-Clinician estimate of of duration and baseline MMSE [28]	798 probable AD subjects from Alzheimer's Disease and Memory Disorders Centre	Random effects linear regression to calculate pre-progression categories and of change in ADAS-cog, VSAT Time, VSAT Errors, CDR Sum of boxes, PSMS and IADL scores	Slopes of ADAScog and PSMS change for slow pre-progression smaller than fast pre-progression. Rates of change on ADAScog slower for intermediate pre-progression group. Slow progressors survived longer.
Memory and executive Functioning [45]	154 newly diagnosed AD Patients	Rapid progression of ≥ 5MMSE decrease over 2yrs	Memory moderate deficits: HR 1.3 (95%CI: 0.4-4.5); severe deficits: HR 2.3 (95%CI: 0.6-9.0). Executive functions moderate deficits: HR 3.5 (95%CI 0.9-13.7); severe deficits: HR 5.7 (95%CI 1.4-23.2)

HR = Hazards ratio; PPV = Positive predictive value

95% CI= 95% confidence interval; NPV= Negative predictive value

WMC= White matter severity; MMSE =Mini Mental State Examination

RR= Relative risk; SIB = Severe Impairment Battery

OR= Odds ratio

Table 1. Clinical and cognitive/ behavioural characteristics in predicting AD conversion in MCI patients and rapid AD progression/ decline

Vascular risk factors, as a composite entity, have been shown to be associated with MCI conversion [21]. The individual risk factors of hypertension, diabetes, cerebrovascular disease and hypercholesterolemia in the study were associated with high risk of MCI conversion. Treatment of hypertension, diabetes and hypercholesterolemia showed reduced risk of MCI conversion. In the same Chongqing study, the authors showed separately the association of

http://dx.doi.org/10.5772/54289

diabetes, baseline white matter changes (WMC), baseline moderate-to-severe carotid stenosis and carotid stenosis change during follow-up to be predictors of MCI conversion [22]. A separate longitudinal community study (ILSA- Italian Longitudinal Study on Aging) showed MCI progression to AD of 2.3 per 100 person-years with stroke as the only vascular risk factor associated with progression [15].

The heterogeneity of AD syndrome is likely related to, other than amyloid and tau pathology, a number of other factors, such as impaired energy metabolism, oxidative stress, neuro-inflammation, insulin and insulin growth factor (IGF) resistance, and insulin/ IGF-deficiency. These factors are often included as variables of interest in studies attempting to develop diagnostic and therapeutic targets for this disease. Brain insulin resistance promotes oxidative stress, reactive oxygen species (ROS) generation, DA damage and mitochondrial dysfunction, all of which drive pro-apoptosis, pro-inflammatory and pro-AβPP-Aβ cascades. Also, hyperinsulinaemia increases AβPP-Aβ and inflammatory indices in the brain, also promoting formation of advanced glycation end-products which lead to increased generation of ROS. Tau gene expression and phosphorylation are also regulated by insulin and IGF stimulation, where brain insulin and IGF resistance may result in decreased signaling through phosphoinositol-3-kinase (PI3K), Akt and Wnt/β-catenin and increased activation of GSK-3β – which is partly responsible for tau hyperphosphorylation. Hence, the focus on vascular factors in AD is justified based on chronic hyperglycemia, hyperinsulinemia, oxidative stress, advanced glycation end-products and inflammation promoting vascular disease [8].

The metabolic syndrome defined by the Third Adults Treatment Panel of the National Cholesterol Education Program as a combination of three or more of the following components: abdominal obesity (waist circumference >102cm for men and >88 cm for women; elevated plasma triglycerides (≥150mg/dl); low HDL cholesterol (<40mg/dl for men and <50mg/dl for women); high blood pressure (≥130/ ≥85mmHg) or being in hypertensive treatment; and high fasting plasma glucose (≥110mg/dl). This represents a clustering of vascular risk factors for morbidity and mortality. In addition, these factors may interact synergistically to influence cognition in a negative manner. Among MCI patients the presence of metabolic syndrome independently predicted an increased risk of progression to dementia over 3.5 years of follow-up. [23]

Older age has been shown to predict MCI-converters [24]. Latent class modeling methods and disease system analysis approach to characterize trajectories of cognitive decline in AD cohorts have also shown initial MMSE and age to best predict decline [25,26]. However, separate studies using AD clinical trial data with subjects on Donepezil have shown younger age to predict faster decline in placebo-treated patients [27]. Low education is a risk factor for AD. The cognitive reserve hypothesis predicts that persons with higher education delay the onset of accelerated cognitive decline; however, once AD disease process begins, it takes a more rapid course due to increased disease burden [28]. Pre-progression rate (calculated using clinician's standardized assessment of symptom duration in years and baseline MMSE) has also been shown to predict cognitive decline trajectory [29]. Neuropsychiatric symptoms have also been shown to predict faster cognitive and functional decline [25,30,31].

Prospective studies of amnestic MCI (a-MCI) subjects have shown that episodic memory (such as delayed recall of word lists [32-34], spatial short term memory and visual recognition memory [35], and paired-associates learning [36,37]), semantic memory [37,38], attentional processing [39] and mental speed consistently predicted MCI converters. Within a very mild cognitive impairment group, higher CDR-sum of boxes and lower executive function predicted AD conversion [40]. Similarly, in a retrospective study of MCI-converters, verbal and visual memory, associative learning, vocabulary, executive functioning and other verbal tests of general intelligence were impaired at baseline [41]. An empirically weighted and combined set of neuropsychological tests involving domains of episodic memory, speeded executive functioning, recognition memory (false and true positives), visuospatial memory processing speed, and visual episodic memory together were strong predictors of MCI conversion to AD [42]. A recent study demonstrated that MCI individuals with learning deficits on the Rey Auditory Verbal Learning test showed widespread pattern of gray matter loss at baseline, as compared to retention deficits which was associated with more focal gray matter loss. However, impaired learning had modestly better predictive power than impaired retention, highlighting the importance of including learning measures in addition to retention measures when predicting outcomes in MCI subjects [43]. Verbal cued recall measured using the Memory Impairment Screen plus (MISplus) has also been shown to predict MCI conversion [44].

In subjects with AD, rapid disease progression was noted more frequently in subjects with higher education and those with moderate severity of global impairment. More severe memory impairment and executive dysfunctioning were associated with higher probabilities of progression at 2 years [45].

Longitudinally, follow-up of those who developed AD versus those who were non-demented prior to AD diagnosis, showed no evidence for accelerated decline of episodic memory from 6 to 3 years prior to incident dementia diagnosis [46]. Working memory (using digit span backward and forward as well as digit ordering) also did not show temporal change as a potentially useful marker of progression [47].

2.1. Summary

Age, vascular risk factors and metabolic syndrome affect AD conversion in MCI subjects. However, there is currently a lack of data on the effect of intensive vascular risk factor treatment in delaying/ halting the rate of progression in MCI subjects. Educational attainment plays an interesting role in AD. In support of the cognitive reserve hypothesis, higher educational attainment predicts delay of the onset of accelerated cognitive decline; however, once AD disease process begins, it takes a more rapid course due to increased disease burden.

Neuropsychological tests, especially episodic memory and executive functioning tests, seem to predict MCI-converters. When assessing MCI subjects, the inclusion of impaired learning in addition to retention measures may improve predictive power of AD progression from MCI. More severe cognitive impairment is associated with rapid AD progression.

http://dx.doi.org/10.5772/54289

3. Cerebrospinal fluid biomarkers (tables 2)

The most widely studied candidate CSF biomarkers include CSF total tau (t-tau), 42 amino acid form of Aβ ($A\beta_{1\text{-}42}$) and phosphorylated tau protein (p-tau) [48]. They reflect respectively the corresponding central pathogenetic process of neuronal degeneration, amyloid-β peptide deposition in plaques, and hyperphosphorylation of tau with subsequent tangle formation. Fagan et al has also recently demonstrated that CSF Aβ and tau protein measurements, performed using INNOTEST enzyme-linked immunosorbent assay (ELISA) and INNO-BIA AlzBio3, were highly correlated with brain amyloid load, as assessed by PET and Pittsburgh compound B amyloid-imaging (r value from 0.77 to 0.94)[49]. This was further suggested, by a study of antemortem CSF concentrations of $A\beta_{1\text{-}42}$ and t-tau/ $A\beta_{1\text{-}42}$ ratio in an autopsy-confirmed AD cohort, that the standardization of biomarker techniques could potentially replace autopsy-confirmed AD for future diagnosis of definite AD [50].

3.1. Established CSF biomarkers

CSF biomarkers of elevated t-tau [51-56], high p-tau [52,53,57,58], low $A\beta_{1\text{-}42}$ [52,53], and combinations of high t-tau/ p-tau and low $A\beta_{1\text{-}42}$ concentrations [59-64], have been shown to be predictive of MCI-conversion to AD. The consistent feature in all of these studies is that increased CSF t-tau and p-tau concentrations are highly sensitive while low $A\beta_{1\text{-}42}$ concentration is more specific. A recent longitudinal study showed that subjects with the lowest baseline Aβ42, highest tau and and p-tau concentration exhibited the most rapid MMSE decline. In addition, while there was little difference in the levels of these CSF biomarkers between stable MCI and cognitively healthy subjects, MCI-AD converters had the highest total tau concentrations [65].

High CSF t-tau and p-tau concentration (but not Aβ42) was associated with more rapid MMSE decline in a 3-year prospective longitudinal study. This suggests that increased t-tau levels reflect intensity of disease and hence rapidity of AD progression, while Aβ42 is more a diagnostic state marker, not associated with rate or stage of AD [65,66]. Another study showed p-tau to poorly differentiate between AD and vascular dementia, but to correlate with MMSE progression [67]. In contrast, another recent report showed lower Aβ42 levels to be associated with rapid-progressors compared with slow-progressors [68]. Wallin et al showed that AD subjects with a combination of low Aβ42 and very high CSF t-tau and p-tau levels performed worse on baseline cognitive tests, with faster deterioration, poorer outcome to cholinesterase inhibitor treatment and increased mortality [69].

With respect to serial biomarker measurements with disease progression, we found studies showing increasing p-tau 231 levels with disease progression in MCI subjects [70, 71] compared to controls over a period of 12-24 months. No definite trends were observed with Aβ40 and Aβ42 in the same studies [70,71]. A recent longitudinal study showed that nonspecific CSF biomarkers, in particular isoprostane, demonstrated an increase over time, which was correlated with AD conversion in MCI subjects and cognitive decline (as assessed by MMSE) [72].

Study variable	Population	Results	Key findings
Predicting AD conversion in MCI subjects			
Combination CSF biomarkers [64]	137 MCI subjects compared to 39 healthy controls	42% converted to AD	- t-tau >350ng/L & Aβ42 <530 ng/L: Sn: 95%, Sp 83% of AD conversion HR 30, 95% CI 9.32-96.8, p<0.001 - p-tau >60ng/L & Aβ42 <530 ng/L: Sn 95%, Sp 81% of AD conversion HR 26.3, 95% CI 8.16-83.4, p<0.001 - t-tau/ Aβ42 ratio < 6.5 (t-tau>350ng/L) Sn 95%, Sp 87% of AD conversion HR 32.8 (10.2-105.6,p<0.001)
Predicting rapid AD progression/ decline			
CSF biomarker concentration [66]	142 AD subjects followed-up over 5 years	35 subjects had t-tau>800ng/L	- High levels of t-tau correlated with lower baseline MMSE scores. More rapid decline in MMSE score correlated with higher baseline t-tau (r_s=-0.23,p=008). - p-tau>110ng/L showed lower baseline MMSE scores but no difference in progression. - Aβ42 showed no difference in baseline scores or progression.
CSF p-tau concentration [67]	70 AD and VD subjects with 36 age-matched healthy controls	Cognitive decline assessed 12 mth (MMSE ≥ 5 point decline after 1yr)	58% of probable AD patients showed p-tau concentration higher than 36.08ng/L. Cognitive decline correlated with p-tau concentration (x^2 =12.442, p=0.001).
CSF Aβ42 concentration [68]	74 AD subjects	Rapid progressors defined at MMSE decline >4/years	Lower Aβ42 CSF concentration (mean 292 pg/ml) in fast-progressors compared to slow-progressors (mean 453 pg/ml) (p=0.042)
Low CSF Aβ42 and high CSF t-tau and p-tau levels [69]	151 AD subjects	k-means cluster analysis done. Cluster 1 low Aβ42 and low t-tau, p-tau Cluster 2 low Aβ42 and intermediate t-tau, p-tau Cluster 3 low Aβ42 and high t-tau, p-tau	Cluster 3 performed poorer on baseline cognitive tests. They exhibited poorer outcome of cholinesterase inhibitor treatment. Cognition deterioriated faster over time with substantially increased mortality rate.

HR = Hazards ratio

CRP = C-reactive protein

MMSE =Mini Mental State Examination

OR = Odds ratio

Sn = Sensitivity

Sp= Specific

LR+ = positive Likelihood ratio

LR - = negative Likelihood ratio

HR = Hazards ratio

95% CI= 95% confidence interval

Table 2. Cerebrospinal fluid biomarkers in predicting AD conversion in MCI patients and rapid AD progression/ decline

http://dx.doi.org/10.5772/54289

Faster progression of brain atrophy (in terms of regional cortical thinning) has been found in the presence of lower Aβ1-42 levels and higher p-tau in Alzheimer's Disease Neuroimaging Initiative (ADNI) data [73].

3.2. Novel CSF approaches

In a study in which novel CSF biomarkers were identified through mass spectrometry and re-evaluated by ELISA, it was found that NrCAM, YKL-40, chromogranin A and Carnosinase I were potentially able to improve the diagnostic accuracy of existing Aβ42 and tau CSF biomarkers. This could potentially improve characterization of clinic-pathological stages of the cognitive continuum from cognitive normalcy to mild dementia, with the promise of potential utility in clinical trials and monitoring disease progression [74]. Other potential CSF biomarkers include nanoparticle-based amyloid-β-derived diffusible ligands (ADDLs)[75], as well as a multiplexed immunoassay panel of a combination of a subset of markers, in particular, calbindin, which showed significant prognostic potential [76]. Preliminary data have also shown that soluble Aβ oligomers might inhibit long-term potentiation and hence, play an important role in AD pathogenesis. The increasing appreciation of Aβ oligomers (as compared to its native forms) in the pathogenesis of AD may suggest novel pathways to biomarkers, such as anti-oligomer antibodies that are specific for the soluble oligomeric state (as opposed to the fibrillar states). By quantifying Aβ oligomer formation, anti-oligomer antibodies may provide a promising strategy for monitoring disease progression [77,78].

Concerns with CSF biomarkers include measurement variability occurring through lack of standardization of CSF assays [79], high inter-laboratory and between-assay variance, sampling-handling factors, post lumbar-puncture headache, and poor acceptability to patients, especially if repeated measurements are involved. In an attempt to overcome these, the Alzheimer's Association has launched a global quality-control program for AD CSF biomarkers, which will be administrated from the Clinical Neurochemistry Laboratory in Molndal, Sweden. This includes reference samples for use in studies, allowing normalization of biomarker levels and meta-analyses of published papers [80].

3.3. Summary

Elevated CSF total tau, p-tau, low Aβ and high tau: Aβ concentrations have been consistently shown to highly predict MCI-converters and AD progression. CSF Aβ and tau may reach a plateau at a relatively early stage of disease and remain fairly constant thereafter, limiting its utility for longitudinal measurement and in monitoring therapeutic response at the more advanced/ established stage of AD. However, it remains an important biomarker during the preclinical and prodromal stages of AD, reflecting the central pathogenic neurodegenerative process. Novel CSF biomarkers hold promise of circumventing this current limitation, especially Aβ oligomers and their potential use in documenting disease progression as well as being a potential therapeutic target. The invasive nature of lumbar puncture and standardization issues preclude its current routine clinical use.

4. Blood markers (table 3)

Peripheral blood is one of the most convenient sources of biomarkers. While the quest for a marker with high sensitivity and specificity has been ongoing for decades, no single blood-derived biomarker has been particularly outstanding in the diagnosis of AD, in predicting conversion from MCI to AD and in predicting slow and fast progression. The following are some of the most studied biomarkers. One should note that negative studies are usually not published and hence publication bias is possible.

Study variable	Population	Results	Key findings
Predicting AD conversion in MCI subjects			
Abeta Hansson [82]	Cohort 1: 117 MCI subjects followed up for 4 -7 years; Cohort 2: 110 followed up for 2 – 4 years	48 (41%) subjects of cohort 1 developed AD; 15 (14%) subjects of cohort 2 developed AD	No difference in plasma Abeta levels between MCI subjects that subsequently developed AD and HC or stable MCI subjects. HR (per SD decrease adjusted for age, sex): Aβ40 1.08 (0.78-1.51), Aβ42 0.95 (0.71-1.27), Aβ42/42 ratio 0.83 (0.64-1.08)
Koyama [84]	Meta-analysis with 10,303 subjects	Summary risk ratio of 1.60 and 1.67 for AD and dementia respectively	Association of low plasma Abeta42/Abeta40 ratio with AD and dementia.
C Reactive Protein [86]	168 MCI subjects followed up over 2 years	58 subjects developed dementia	Association of high plasma CRP level with accelerated cognitive deterioration and increased risk of AD. MMSE score was significantly lower for patients with high CRP levels than those with low CRP levels (-4.9 ± 5.4 vs -3.2 ±4.2, $p < 0.05$)
APOE [90]	35 prospective cohort studies of MCI subjects, including 6095 subjects over 2.9 years of follow-up	1236 developed AD.	APOE-ε4 allele is associated with a moderately increased risk for progression from MCI to AD-type dementia. OR for MCI subjects with APOE ε4 progression to AD 2.29 (95% CI 1.88 to 2.80).Sn 0.53 (95% CI 0.4 to 0.61), Sp 0.67 (95% CI 0.62 to 0.71), PPV 0.57 (95% CI 0.48 to 0.66), NPV 0.75 (95% CI 0.70 to 0.80). LR+ 1.60 (95% CI 1.48 to 1.72), and LR- 0.75 (95% CI 0.67 t o0.82). Meta-regression showed that Sn,Sp and NPV were dependent on age, APOE-ε4 allele background prevalence or follow-up length
Predicting rapid AD progression/ decline			
APP isoforms in platelets [85]	48 AD subjects followed up over 1 year	Progression of AD	Association of low APPr at baseline in predicting cognitive decline in AD. APPr <0.40, ΔMMSE = -2.8 ± 3.0, $p < 0.05$ APPr ≥0.40, ΔMMSE = -0.9 ±2.3, $p < 0.05$

Combination of Aβ and CRP [87]	122 AD subjects	Followed up 4.2 years	Low plasma levels of Abeta40, Abeta42, and high-sensitivity CRP were associated with a significantly more rapid cognitive decline. Plasma biomarkers contributed to 5-12% variance on Blessed Dementia Scale and Activities of Daily Living.
:eramides [89]	120 probable AD subjects	Follow-up 2.3y	Highest tertiles of DHSM/DHCer and SM/ceramide ratios declined1.35 points (p=0.001) and 1.19 (p=0.004) less per year on the MMSE and increased 3.18 points (p=0.001) and 2.42 (p=0.016) less per year on ADAS-Cog.
APOEε4			
Martins [91]	218 AD subjects	In the non-linear model, possession of an APOEε4 allele was related to earlier and faster cognitive decline. APOEε2 allele related to slower decline.	APOE genotype strongly predicts the rate of cognitive decline in AD. APOEε4 homozygotes showed faster cognitive decline than heterozygotes.
Cosentino [92]	199 population-based incident AD subjects, 215 population-based prevalent AD subjects, 156 clinic-based AD subjects followed up for an average of 4 years	Presence of at least one ε4 allele associated with faster cognitive decline in the population-based incident AD group (p = 0.01). However, this association is absent in prevalent AD subjects in population or clinic based group.	APOEε4 influences cognitive decline most significantly in the earliest stages of AD.

HC = Healthy controls

SD = Standard deviation

OR = Odds ratio

95% CI= 95% confidence interval

Sn = Sensitivity

Sp= Specificity

OR = Odds ratio

PPV = Positive predictive value

NPV= Negative predictive value

LR+ = positive Likelihood Ratio

LR- = negative Likelihood Ratio

Table 3. Blood biomarkers in predicting AD conversion in MCI patients and rapid AD progression/ decline

4.1. Plasma proteins/ peptides

Teleologically the most logical candidate is plasma Amyloid-beta (Aβ) and its derivatives, Aβ40 and Aβ42. They are the most studied of blood markers.

As Aβ accumulation is an early step in AD pathogenesis, such a biomarker would be potentially suitable for identifying patients in the earliest stage of disease process when intervention might be more effective.

Circulating Aβ is composed of Aβ produced by brain and peripheral tissue, and can be transported across the blood-brain barrier. They are derived from the amyloid precursor protein (APP). APP is catabolized via 2 pathways, one of which is amyloidogenic, and involves 3 enzyme systems, alpha, beta and gamma secretases. In the amyloidogenic pathway, APP is first cleaved by beta secretase to generate a secreted form of APP (sAPPbeta) and a C99 fragment. The C99 is then cleaved by gamma secretase to yield Aβ. Different cleavage sites on the C99 fragment produces two forms of Aβ – Aβ40 and Aβ42. While Aβ40 is the more common product, Aβ42 aggregates into amyloid fibrils more rapidly and is contained in both early diffuse plaques and fully formed neuritic plaques. In the non-amyloidogenic pathway, alpha secretase is involved and does not lead to Aβ formation [81].

Since elevation appears to be before or just at the onset of the clinically diagnosed disease, it has been hypothesized that high plasma Aβ42 is an antecedent risk indicator for AD, and its plasma levels declines with onset and progression. There have been many studies involving Aβ40 and Aβ42, though results have been inconclusive and at times contradictory refer to Table 1 [82, 83]. These inconsistent results may reflect variability due to technical reasons, such as timing of sample collection with reference to AD onset, the assay methods, and differential affinities of the antibodies used for different Aβ species. Koyama [84], in a large systematic review, concluded that plasma levels of Aβ40 and Aβ42 individually were not associated with development of AD and dementia. However the *ratio of Aβ42:Aβ40* could predict development of AD and dementia, although the evidence is limited in MCI conversion and AD progression.

APP isoforms in platelets have been suggested to predict cognitive decline. APP metabolism has been found to be altered in the platelets of AD patients, specifically a reduced ratio of the upper (130kDa) to the lower (110-106 kDa) immunoreactivity band (APPr) [85].

The level of plasma C-reactive protein (CRP) rises in response to inflammation. Its role is primarily to activate the complement system. CRP by itself has been reported to be associated with accelerated cognitive deterioration and increased risk of conversion in MCI patients [86]. A combination of raised CRP with low Aβ has been associated with a significantly more rapid cognitive decline [87].

Homocysteine has been reported to be associated with human disease states, notably cardiovascular disease. Deficiencies of the B vitamins – B6(pyridoxine), B9(folic acid) and B12(cobalamin) are associated with high homocysteine levels. However, there is no data on homocysteine with MCI conversion and AD progression.

Clusterin, also called apolipoprotein J and coded by gene CLU, has been reported in genome-wide association studies (GWAS) to be associated with AD [83]. Clusterin is functionally associated with apoptosis and the clearance of cellular debris, including amyloid. Thambiesetty [88] found that higher clusterin levels were associated with slower brain atrophy in normal subjects who developed MCI during a 6-year follow-up. However, there is no current data with MCI conversion and AD progression.

http://dx.doi.org/10.5772/54289

Ceramides are a family of lipid molecules that are made up of sphingosine and a fatty acid. They are also constituent of sphinomyelin (SM). In addition to their structural function, they play a role as signaling molecules in regulating cell differentiation, proliferation, and programmed cell death. Mielke [89] found that high plasma levels of dihydroceramides (DHCer) and ceramide were associated with AD progression, though results did not reach significance. Nevertheless, higher plasma levels of SM, dihydrosphingomyelin (DHSM), SM/ceramide, and DHSM/DHCer ratios were associated with less progression on the MMSE and ADAS-Cog with the ratios being the strongest predictors of clinical progression. There is no current data on MCI progression.

4.2. Genetic and transcriptomic markers

APOEε4 is the best-established genetic risk factor for AD. APOE genotyping is not recommended for the routine diagnosis of AD. However many studies have investigated whether APOEε4 has a predictive value for progression from MCI to AD.

In a large meta-analysis, Elias-Sonnenschein [90] and co-workers found that APOEε4 is associated with a moderately increased risk of progression from MCI to AD.

Martins [91] found that the APOEε4 genotype predicts the age of onset of AD and neuropathic progression in a non-linear fashion. In their non-linear model, possession of an APOEε4 allele was related to earlier and faster cognitive decline, while possession of an APOEε4 was associated with slower decline. Homozygous APOEε4 showed faster cognitive decline than APOEε4 heterozygotes. The linear model was less sensitive and did not detect differences between APOEε4 homo- and heterozygotes.

Cosentino [92] also showed that the presence of at least one allele of APOEε4 was associated with faster decline in the incident population-based AD group. However the findings could not be extrapolated to prevalent AD in population or clinic-based samples. Hence APOEε4 influence may be more stage-dependent, with its effect on cognitive decline most evident in the earliest stages of disease and less so in moderate to severe stages.

Other genetic markers that have been identified in genome-wide association studies (GWAS) have not yet been shown to aid in diagnosis of AD or predict progression of disease in MCI or AD.

Unlike the static genome, the transcriptome comprises the dynamic expression of the genome over the course of the disease. Transcriptomic, or genome-wide gene expression studies, have been used to distinguish AD from healthy controls. One of the genes identified from transcriptomic studies is TOMM40, which has also been identified in GWAS studies [93]. We found that TOMM40 remained significantly downregulated over three time points in a longitudinal study (manuscript submitted for review). Transcriptomic products would ideally be used to track the progression of disease, identify markers that predict conversion of MCI to AD, and distinguish between fast and slow progressors. Hence this is a potential area of biomarker development in predicting MCI conversion and rapid AD progression.

4.3. Multiple marker arrays

Given the disappointing results achieved by single markers despite tremendous efforts, the field has now moved towards multiple markers that are obtained through high throughput technologies, sophisticated statistical analysis and bioinformatics. Ray [94] published a blood plasma-based proteomic screening tool to identify patients with AD and also to identify those likely to progress from MCI to AD. Biological analysis of the 18 proteins points to systemic dysregulation of hematopoiesis, immune responses, apoptosis and neuronal support. However efforts at independent validation of Ray's findings have been discouraging [95].

Based on current literature, no single marker has been found to be significant in all the multiple marker arrays. Moreover one can expect that utilizing high throughput array technology, more multiple marker arrays will appear and dominate the blood biomarker landscape. To sound a note of caution, however, some panels may be derived from 'over-fitting' the dataset and may not survive generalization and independent validation. To date, multiple marker arrays have not been employed to study the conversion of MCI to AD and to differentiate between fast and slow progressors. This would be a logical next step for investigation.

4.4. Summary

Plasma Aβ is an appealing biomarker since many AD interventions under investigation are directed against Aβ. Thus an Aβ-based biomarker is attractive for those who will benefit from such treatments. However, many studies involving various blood biomarkers have conflicting and/or inconclusive results.

APOEε4 influence may be more stage-dependent, with its effect on disease trajectory most evident in the earliest stages of disease and less so in moderate to severe stages. Hence it should be included as a covariate in various clinical progression and therapeutic trials. A major challenge is that the literature thus far has focused on the use of blood biomarkers for diagnosis (requiring the identification of dichotomous - disease versus normal- states), which may not be applicable to the use of such biomarkers for tracking disease progression (for which an effective biomarker must show continuous change rather than merely being present or absent). Nevertheless blood biomarkers should be employed in combination with clinical assessment and neuroimaging to improve diagnostic and prognostic accuracy, especially given the peripheral nature and ease of blood sampling.

5. Neuroimaging (Table 4)

5.1. Structural imaging

Neuroimaging is now one of the most common tools used to aid the diagnosis of AD. It is a huge and burgeoning field and only select modalities and important studies on longitudinal imaging are discussed here.

http://dx.doi.org/10.5772/54289

Study variable	Population	Results	Key findings
Predicting AD conversion in MCI subjects			
<u>Structural Imaging</u>			
Jack et al. [96]	55 NC, 41 MCI, 64 AD subjects; 1-5 years follow-up	Atrophy rates of four structures (hippocampus, entorhinal cortex, whole brain, and ventricle)	Rates of change from serial MRI studies together with standard clinical/psychometric measures can be used as surrogate markers of disease progression in AD. Atrophy rates greater among MCI converters. Atrophy rates greater among AD fast progressors
Jack et al. [97]	133 MCI subjects	52 subjects developed AD (45 were APOEε4 carriers). Mean time to conversion 556 day in APOE carriers.	MRI brain atrophy rate measures can be used as indicators of disease progression in a multi-site therapeutic MCI setting. APC was greater in converters than non-converters. APCs greater in APOE ε4 non-carriers. APCs and changes in cognitive test performance uniformly correlated in expected direction (p<0.000)
Jack et al. [98]	72 aMCI subjects, 91 HC; 1-2 years follow-up.	13 HC developed MCI or AD; 39 MCI subjects developed AD	Larger ventricular APC (HR for a 1-SD increase 1.4, p=0.007) increased risk of AD conversion. Both ventricular APC (HR for a 1-SD increase 1.59, p=0.001) and whole brain APC (HR for 1-SD increase 1.32, p=0.009) provided additional predictive information to covariate-adjusted sectional HC volume at baseline about risk of AD conversion. However, overlap present among those converters and non-converters indicate that these measures are unlikely to provide absolute prognosis for MCI-converters.
Apostolova et al. [99]	20 MCI subjects followed up over 3 years	6 subjects developed AD (MCI-c), 7 remained stable (MCI-nc), and 7 improved (MCI- i).	Smaller hippocampi and specifically CA1 and subicular subfields are associated with increased risk for conversion from MCI to AD. Larger hippocampal volumes and relative preservation of both the subiculum and CA1 are associated with cognitive stability or improvement.
Risascher et al. [101]	339 MCI (277 MCI-stable, 62 MCI-converters) subjects, 206 HC, 148 AD subjects	62 MCI developed AD	Degree of neurodegeneration of MTL structures is the best antecedent MRI marker of imminent conversion, with decreased hippocampal volume (left > right) being the most robust structural MRI feature. Effect sizes of hippocampus (0.6) and MTL structures (0.53) comparing MCI-stable and converters.
Querbes et al. [103]	122 aMCI (50 stable MCI, 72 progressive MCI), 130 HC, 130 AD followed up over 24 months.	72 aMCI developed AD.	Normalised cortical thickness can predict AD conversion with 76% cross-validated accuracy.
<u>Molecular Imaging</u>			
Lo et al. [105]	229 normal ,397 MCI and 193 AD subjects followed up 3 years	Rates of change in CSF Aβ42 , glucose metabolism and hippocampal volume	Amyloid deposition is an early event before hypometabolism or hippocampal atrophy, suggesting that biomarker prediction for cognitive change is stage dependent. Positive APOE4 status accelerated hippocampal atrophy changes in MCI and AD.
Okello et al. [106]	31 aMCI subjects, 26 HC followed up over 3 years	17 out of 31 MCI (55%) had increased [11C]PIB retention at baseline (PIB-positive). 14 of these 17 PIB-positive MCI (82%) developed AD. Half (47%) converted to AD within 1 year.	PIB-positive MCI subjects are more likely to develop AD than PIB-negative subjects. Fast converters have higher PIB retention levels at baseline than slower converters in anterior cingulate, (p=0.027) and frontal cortex (p=0.031). Only 1 out of 14 PIB-negative subjects develop AD. 7 of 17 PIB-positive MCI, APOEε4 carriers associated with faster conversion rates (p=0.035)
Koivunen et al. [107]	29 MCI, 13 HC followed up over 2 years	17 MCI developed AD	Hippocampal atrophy increases and amyloid deposition changes modestly during conversion to AD, suggesting dissociation between the two during evolution of MCI. AD converters had greater [11C]PIB retention at baseline in posterior cingulate (p=0.022), putamen (p=0.041), caudate nucleus (p=0.025). Greater hippocampal atrophy in MCI converters at baseline.

Small et al. [108]	22 HC and 21 MCI followed up over 2 years	Increases in frontal, posterior cingulate, and global binding at follow-up correlated with progression of memory decline (r = -0.32 to -0.37, P = 0.03 to 0.01).	[18F]FDDNP PET scanning may be useful in identifying people at risk for future cognitive decline. Higher [18F]FDDNP binding at baseline is associated with future decline in most cognitive domains (r = -0.31 to -0.56, P = 0.05 to 0.002). Frontal and parietal [18F]FDDNP binding yielded highest diagnostic accuracy. ROC 0.88 (95% CI 0.72-1.00) compared with 0.68 (95% CI 0.45-0.91) for medial temporal binding.
Doraiswamy et al. [109]	51 MCI, 69 HC, and 31 AD followed up over 18 months.	MCI Aβ+ and HC Aβ+ associated with greater clinical worsening on ADAS-Cog and CDR-SB. MCI Aβ+ associated With greater decline in memory, DSS and MMSE (p < 0.05).	Florbetapir PET, which detects Aβ pathology, may be helpful in identifying individuals at increased risk for progression to AD. Higher SUVr in MCI associated with greater decline on ADAS-Cog, CDR-SB, memory measure (DSS) and MMSE (all p<0.05). MCI Aβ+ had higher risk of developing AD.
Ossenkoppele et al. [110]	11 HC, 12 MCI, and 8 AD followed up over 2.5 years.	Global cortical [11C]PIB BPND is significantly increased in MCI subjects, but no changes was observed in AD subjects or HC. Increase most prominent in lateral temporal lobe (p < 0.05). No changes in global [18F] FDDNP.	[11C]PIB and [18F] FDG track molecular changes in different stages of AD. MCI subjects were found to have an increased amyloid load while AD subjects had increased progressive metabolic impairment. [18F]FDDNP is less useful for examining disease progression. Reduction in [18F]FDG uptake at follow-up observed in AD subjects only (esp frontal, parietal, temporal lobes (all p<0.01). Changes in global [11C]PIB binding (p=-0.42, p<0.05) and cingulate [18F]FDG uptake (p=0.43, p<0.01) correlated with changes in MMSE score over time across groups but not for [18F] FDDNP binding (p=-0.18, p=0.35).
Zhang et al. [111]	Meta-analysis of 13 research studies (7 FDG-PET)	FDG-PET pooled estimates: 78.7% Sn (95% CI 68.7-86.6%) 74% Sp (95%CI 67.0-80.3%) PIB-PET pooled estimates: 93.5% Sn (95% CI 71.3-99.9%) 56.2% Sp (95% CI 47.2-64.8%)	Both FDG-PET and PIB-PET are valuable techniques for prediction of AD progression in MCI subjects.
Predicting rapid AD progression/ decline			
Thompson et al. [100]	12 AD subjects, 14 HC	Followed up 3 years	Cortical atrophy occurred in a well defined sequence (temporal- frontal- sensorimotor) as the disease progressed. Mirroring the sequence of neurofibrillary tangle accumulation observed in cross sections at autopsy. Left hemisphere degenerates faster (5.3 ± 2.3% per year in AD v.s. 0.9 ± 0.9% per year in controls; p<0.029) than the right
Kinkingnéhun et al.[103]	23 mild AD subjects and 18 HC followed up	Followed up 3 years	Fast decliners had a more extensive cortical atrophy than slow decliners, especially in the medial occipitoparietal areas (specifically precuneus, Lingual gyrus and cuneus which was not yet detected by clinical and neuropsychological assessment.
<u>Functional Imaging</u>			
Silverman et al. [107]	284 patients presenting symptoms of dementia	Progressive dementia in 59%	In patients presenting symptoms of dementia, regional brain metabolism was a sensitive indicator of AD. A negative PET scan indicated that pathologic progression of cognitive impairment during the mean 3-year follow-up was unlikely to occur. Sn 93%, Sp 76%. –LR 0.1 (95% CI 0.06-0.16) experiencing progressive course after a single negative PET scan.

NC = Normal Controls

MRI = Magnetic Resonance Imaging

APC = Annual percent change

HC = Healthy Controls

SD = Standard deviation

MTL = Medial Temporal Lobe

aMCI = amnestic MCI

PIB = Pittsburgh Compound B

FDDNP = Fluoroethyl)methylamino]-2-napthyl}ethylidene) malononitrile

PET = Positron Emission Tomography

MMSE =Mini Mental State Examination

Sn = Sensitivity

Sp= Specific

-LR = negative Likelihood ratio

Table 4. Neuroimaging methods in predicting AD conversion in MCI patients and rapid AD progression/ decline

With technological advances over the past three decades, MRI is now readily available and relatively economical. Currently it is widely used as a diagnostic tool, to complement clinical assessment and neuropsychological testing. Moreover, MRI has also been considered for longitudinal tracking of the disease progression and to predict whether a MCI patient may go on to develop AD, or whether an AD patient will have an indolent or rapid course. Advances in technology have led to automated data-driven methods, such as automated measurement of whole brain volume over time, voxel-based morphometry (VBM), deformation-based morphometry (DBM) and analysis of cortical thickness. These technologies ameliorate the previous problems associated with manual measurement, inter-rater reliability and difficulties in cross-study comparisons.

In a seminal paper, Jack [96] studied annualized changes in volume of four structures in serial MRI studies: hippocampus, entorhinal cortex, whole brain and ventricles of normal, MCI and AD subjects. All four atrophy rates were greater among MCI-converters compared to non-converters and fast-progressors versus slow progressors. Although the differences in atrophy rates have been replicated consistently in several follow-up studies [97,98], given the overlap among those who did and did not convert, the authors cautioned that these measures were unlikely to provide absolute prognostic information for individual patients.

Using hippocampal volumetry, a prospective longitudinal cohort study found that greater atrophy in the CA1 hippocampal and subicular subfields predicted MCI conversion, whereas larger hippocampal volumes predicted cognitive stability and/or improvement [99].

Employing a 3-dimensional cortical mapping approach, Thompson [100], demonstrated a temporal-frontal-sensorimotor sequence of cortical atrophy with AD progression in a longitudinal series of 12 AD subjects, where left brain was found to degenerate faster than right.

Employing VBM technique, Risacher [101] found that AD and MCI converters demonstrated high atrophy across regions as compared to HC in global and hippocampal grey matter (GM)

density, hippocampal and amygdalar volumes, and cortical thickness values from entorhinal cortex and other temporal and parietal lobe regions. MCI-stable showed intermediate atrophy. Degree of atrophy of medial temporal structures, especially the hippocampi, was found to be the best antecedent MRI marker of imminent conversion.

A separate study also showed that occipitoparietal (specifically precuneus, lingual gyrus and cuneus) atrophy at baseline better anticipated the rate of progression (fast decliners from slow decliners) over 3 years compared to clinical and neuropsychological assessment [102].

Cortical thickness is another measure of interest in structural neuroimaging where a normalized thickness index was computed using a subset of these regions, namely the right medial temporal, left lateral temporal and right posterior cingulate. Normalized thickness index at baseline differed significantly among all the four diagnosis groups (HC, stable MCI, progressive MCI and AD). Furthermore, normalized thickness index also correctly predicted evolution to AD for 76% of aMCI subjects after cross-validation [103].

5.2. Functional and molecular imaging

There are many functional imaging studies for AD though only a few specifically investigate longitudinal progression of MCI and AD using Fluorodeoxyglucose (18F) (FDG)-Positron Emission Tomography (PET) [104].

Lo [105] found that the rate of change of glucose metabolism and hippocampal volume accelerated as cognitive function deteriorated. Moreover, glucose metabolic decline and hippocampal atrophy were significantly slower in subjects with normal cognition compared to those with MCI or AD. Positive APOE4 status was also associated with accelerated hippocampal atrophy.

Molecular imaging utilizes small molecule ligands that bind with nanomolar affinity to amyloid and enters the brain for imaging with PET. It is a measure to detect and quantify cerebral beta-amyloidosis. It should be noted that besides AD, there are other disease conditions that may have cerebral Aβ.The most commonly used ligand is the carbon-11(11C)-based Pittsburgh compound B (PIB), which binds specifically to fibrillar Aβ but exhibits no demonstrable binding to neurofibrillary tangles. However, fluorine-18 (18F)-based tracers, e.g. 2-(1-{6-[(2-fluorine 18-labeled fluoroethyl)methylamino]-2-napthyl}ethylidene) malononitrile ([(18)F]FDDNP) have a considerably longer half-life compared to [11(C)]PIB and some types have been shown to also bind to neurofibrillary tangles.

Okello [106] showed that PIB-positive subjects with MCI are significantly more likely to convert to AD than PIB-negative ones. A separate longitudinal study showed that hippocampal atrophy and amyloid deposition (in posterior cingulate, lateral frontal cortex, temporal cortex, putamen and caudate nucleus) seem to dissociate during the evolution of MCI, the atrophy increasing clearly and [(11)C] PIB retention changing modestly when conversion to AD occurs [107]. Using [(18)F]FDDNP PET, higher baseline binding was associated with future decline in most cognitive domains. Specifically, frontal and parietal [(18)F]FDDNP binding yielded the greatest diagnostic accuracy in identifying MCI-converters versus non-converters [108]. With 18F florbetapir (18F-AV-45) tracer, baseline Aβ + scans were associated with greater

http://dx.doi.org/10.5772/54289

clinical worsening on the AD Assessment Scale-Cognitive subscale (ADAS-Cog) and Clinical Dementia Rating-sum of boxes (CDR-SB). In MCI, Aβ + scans were also associated with greater decline in memory, Digit Symbol Substitution (DSS) and MMSE. Aβ + MCI subjects again tended to convert to AD at a higher rate than Aβ- subjects [109].

In a seminal comparison study of three modalities [110], using [(11)C]PIB, [(18)F]FDDNP and [18F]FDG, there was a significant increase in global cortical [(11)C]PIB binding (most prominent in the lateral temporal lobe) in MCI patients, but no changes in AD patients or controls. Interestingly, [(18)F]FDDNP did not show any changes in global binding potential. Moreover, changes in global [(11)C]PIB binding and posterior cingulate [(18)F]FDG uptake were correlated with changes in MMSE score over time across groups, but not with [(18)F]FDDNP binding. Hence it was postulated that [(11)C]PIB and [(18)F]FDDNP track molecular changes in different stages of AD. There was an increased amyloid load in MCI patients and progressive metabolic impairment in AD patients. The authors opined that [(18)F]FDDNP was less useful for examining disease progression.

To estimate the diagnostic accuracy of FDG-PET and PIB-PET for prediction of short-term conversion to AD in patients with MCI, Zhang [111] and co-workers performed a meta-analysis undertaken with a random-effects model. Overall diagnostic accuracy determined for both FDG-PET and PIB-PET suggests that they are potentially valuable techniques for prediction of progression in patients with MCI. Both have their advantages and their combined use is a promising option.

Villain et al recently published a longitudinal PIB study (testing conducted 18 months apart), showing a significant increase in amyloid-β accumulation in both PIB-positive and negative subjects (significantly higher in PIB-positive individuals) with a bimodal distribution of individual rates of neocortical amyloid- β accumulation [112].

5.3. Summary

MRI volumetry and brain atrophy rates have fairly good diagnostic and predictive value in MCI subjects. Longitudinal data on brain atrophy rates with disease progression are available and hence, can be used for monitoring disease progression in clinical trials. The limitations of structural neuroimaging as a biomarker include problems with the accurate delineation of regions of interest and lack of standardization of imaging and measurement techniques, making it difficult to compare data across the different institutions out of Europe, North America and Australia (all of which have their unified imaging consortiums). The advent of automated data-driven innovations for structural imaging holds promise. FDG-PET appears to be the leading candidate among the functional neuroimaging modalities, with available evidence for MCI diagnosis, prediction of MCI-converters and longitudinal data in monitoring serial progression. To date, [(11]C] PIB is the most extensively studied PET amyloid tracer, although 18F florbetapir proves to be an attractive alternative given the longer half-life. There is emerging evidence for amyloid imaging in the diagnosis of preclinical AD. From the standpoint of clinical trials of anti-amyloid therapy, in-vivo amyloid imaging pre-treatment allows selection of patients with demonstrable cerebral Aβ loads; repeated imaging during ongoing treatment allows detection of decrease in insoluble Aβ load in response to amyloid-clearing drugs such as immunotherapy. Amyloid imaging needs to be more practically accessible and affordable before it can be transferable to the clinical diagnostic routine.

6. Combinational biomarkers

Many of the aforementioned biomarker modalities are not separate discrete entities but have an effect on each other. For example, the association of hypertension with CSF tau and ptau-181, was found to be modified by APOEε4 phenotype, where hypertension is directly related to tau pathology (and not Aβ42) in APOEε4 homozygous carriers [113]. Elevated CSF t-tau and p-tau in presence of APOEε4/ε4 genotype has also been shown to influence faster AD progression in MCI subjects [114].

For the identification of MCI-converters, various literature showing combination biomarkers have been published. They include looking at clinical measures (such as cognitive or neuropsychological tests) in combination with CSF biomarkers [115], neuroimaging measures [116, 117], or in combination with both CSF and neuroimaging measures [118-119].

A combination of CSF and neuroimaging biomarkers [120-4] has found improved predictive accuracy of MCI-converters, supported by slope analyses of annual cognitive decline [120]. Okamura showed that a high ratio between cerebrospinal fluid (CSF) tau and posterior cingulate perfusion on SPECT is useful in identifying MCI converters [125]. Using a machine-learning approach (support vector machines), Furney et al examined the utility of adding cytokine and neuroimaging biomarkers to conventional measures, and found that the combination of cytokine and neuroimaging with clinical and APOEε4 genotype improved accuracy [126]. Recent studies have also looked at multimodal neuroimaging techniques to predict MCI progression [127-129].

Other recent studies have used endophenotype-based approach and found single nucleotide polymorphism (SNP) such as rs1868402 to have strong, replicable association with $CSFptau_{181}$ association with rate of AD progression [130].

7. Conclusion and future directions

Clinical criteria alone, often subjective and dependent on clinical judgment, are insufficient to identify the pre-clinical stages of AD accurately. This has prompted the past decade-long intensive research into the use of more objective neuroimaging and biochemical markers to either replace, or complement, clinical approaches to facilitate an early and accurate diagnosis of the illness [131,132]. The chapter thus far details the rationale (most evident from Table 1) for the combined approach of clinical measures with other biomarkers in predicting AD progression; but in the earlier stages (prodromal and especially preclinical AD stages), biomarkers would play an increasingly important role. Combination biomarker approaches appear to be superior to a single biomarker approach, with the recent focus of researchers being

Subjects	Follow-up (years)	Biomarker	Results
MCI (n=8) NC (n=10) [70]	1	CSF p-tau231	MCI: 5.0; NC: 3.0 *
		CSF Aβ40	MCI: 4.0; NC: 8.0
		CSF Aβ42	MCI: 4.0; NC: 2.0
MCI (n=7) NC (n=9) [71]	2	CSF p-tau231	MCI: 2.0; NC: 20.0 *
		CSF Aβ40	MCI: 0.5; NC: 3.5
		CSFAβ42	MCI: 0.35; NC: 1.5
MCI (n=62) AD (n-68) NC (n=24) [72]	2	CSF isoprostane	NC:-1.9; MCI:-0.4; AD: 5.0 **
		CSF neurofilaments light	NC:-0.18; MCI:-0.79; AD: -0.96
		CSF Aβ40	NC: 0.61; MCI:0.28; AD:0.43
		No change in Aβ42 or p-tau 181.	
MCI (n=57) AD (n=56) [65] NC (n=8)	3	CSF $A\beta_{42}$	MCI(stable): 3.42, MCI (converters):0.78, AD:-11.9**
		CSF tau	MCI(stable):19.7, MCI(converters):17.4, AD: 0.55
		CSFp-tau	MCI(stable):1.24, MCI(converters):-0.21, AD: -2.2
		CSFAβ42/tau	MCI(stable):-0.54.MCI(converters):-0.4,AD: -0.008
		CSFAβ42/ptau	MCI(stable):-0.19, MCI(converters):-0.07,AD:0.18
NC (n=55) MCI (n=41) AD (n=64) [99]	1.2-2.4	Hippocampus*	MCI (stable):-4.4,MCI(converters):-7.8, AD slow -9.4, AD fast -15.4
		Entorhinal cortex	MCI(stable):-15.9, MCI(converters):-16.0, AD slow-20.5, AD fast -22.7
		Whole brain	MCI (stable):-0.8, MCI (converters):-2.5, AD slow -2.4, AD fast -3.6
		Ventricle	MCI (stable):0.8, MCI(converters):1.8, AD slow -6.5, AD fast 1.9
MCI (n=131) [101]	3	Hippocampus *	MCI (converters) -6.78; MCI (non-converters) -3.86
		Entorhinal cortex	MCI (converters) -15.08 ; MCI (non-converters) -8.32
		Whole brain	MCI (converters) -0.88 ; MCI (non-converters) -0.36
		Ventricle	MCI (converters) 5.66 ; MCI (non-converters) 3.33
MCI (n=72) [104]	1-2	Hippocampus *	-3.3 (2.7)
		Entorhinal cortex	-7.0 (4.3)
		Whole brain	-0.7 (1.0)
		Ventricle	3.3 (2.3)
AD (n=32) MCI (n=49) NC (n=103) [116]	1.5	PiB-PET (neocortical PiB rate of change) ($SuVR_{pons}$/year) *	AD: PiB-(acc) +0.06; PiB+(acc) +0.05; PiB (non-acc) -0.01 MCI: PiB-(acc) +0.04; PiB-(non-acc) -0.001; PiB+ (acc) +0.04; PiB (non-acc) -0.01 HC: PiB-(acc)+0.03; PiB- (non-acc) -0.01; PiB+(acc) +0.04; PiB+ (non-acc) -0.004
NC (n=210) MCI (n=357) AD (n=162) [135]	2	CSF $A\beta_{42}$	NC: -0.94; MCI: -1.4; AD; -0.1 *
		CSF tau	NC: 3.45; MCI: 2.34; AD: 1.24
		PIB	NC: 0.098; MCI: -0.008; AD: -0.004
		FDG-PET	NC: -177; MCI: 752; AD: 2993
		Hippocampus	NC: -40; MCI: -80; AD: -116
		Ventricles	NC: 848; MCI: 1551; AD: 2540
		ADAS-Cog total	NC: -0.54; MCI: 1.05; AD: 4.37
		MMSE	NC: 0.0095; MCI:-0.64; AD: -2.4
		CDR-SB	NC: 0.07; MCI 0.63; AD: 1.62
		RAVLT (5 trial total)	NC: 0.29; MCI: -1.37; AD: -3.62

* expressed as % change per year compared to baseline values

** expressed as annual change β

MCI = Mild Cognitive Impairment

NC = Normal Controls

AD = Alzheimer's Disease

CSF = Cerebrospinal fluid

PIB = Pittsburgh Compound B

FDG-PET = Fluorodeoxyglucose (18F)-Positron Emission Tomography

MMSE = Mini Mental State Examination

CDR-SB = Clinical Dementia Rating – Sum of Boxes

RAVLT = Rey Auditory Verbal Learning Tes

Table 5. Longitudinal biomarker studies

on multimodal approach using various systems biology and multivariate modeling methods. Additionally, multi-site prospective studies, such as the Alzheimer's Disease Neuroimaging Initiative (ADNI), allow for global summary of results and patterns of change observed in clinical measures and candidate biomarkers [133] (Table 5). It must also be highlighted that some of the heterogeneity of biomarker findings thus far is related to the different periods of follow-up and hence AD conversion rates in MCI subjects.

The dynamic biomarker model, in the AD pathological cascade first proposed by Jack in 2010 [134], has been an area of intense interest. However, this inverse relationship between fibrillar amyloid plaque burden (on PIB imaging) and corresponding decrease in CSF Aβ42 and elevated tau, has led to the simplistic interpretation that the AD pathological cascade is purely driven by the amyloid cascade (Figure 1). This is partly due to extrapolation from cross-sectional studies, where in fact, longitudinal studies are required to determine the temporal order of the appearance of various pathogenic processes involved in this complex disease. Storandt et al [135] has recently demonstrated in a community cohort that CSF Aβ42 and tau were minimally correlated, suggesting that they represent independent processes. Additionally, they accounted for only 60% of variance on PIB imaging, suggesting that a third process may be related to brain atrophy or plaque formation [136].

In addition, understanding longitudinal biomarker change allows its potential inclusion in clinical trials, with recent studies advocating the use of neuroimaging biomarkers [137,138], CSF biomarkers [139] and/or combination biomarkers [137,140] to boost the power of clinical trials and decrease sample size in MCI trials. An integrated analyses approach using patient (age) severity- and disease-related (severe baseline cognitive, global or behavioural status) factors in established AD has been shown, with the potential of symptomatic AD therapy, to decrease likelihood of faster decline [141].

Further work on biomarkers is important because of their multiple potential roles. Biomarkers have the potential to be used as a prognostic tool for the prediction of AD conversion in MCI subjects and rapid AD progression, with translation into clinical practice by using a most practical algorithm, and as a diagnostic tool in prodromal/ preclinical stages of AD. Biomarkers may also lead to a deeper understanding of the complex pathogenesis of AD disease – including stage-specific and stage-independent processes. There is also currently an unfulfilled potential in biomarker-enriched clinical trials and the use of biomarkers in preclinical AD, especially in the advent of newer therapeutic targets. Finally there is also potential to extrapolate biomarker findings 'backwards' into the earliest stages of disease so that we may be able to identify those at risk and consider instituting interventions. This would enable earliest therapeutic intervention for at-risk subjects most amenable to disease-modifying treatments, and exclude those for whom the possible risks from investigational treatment would be more difficult to justify. At the very least, it would identify those who might benefit most from intensive monitoring and management of clinical factors, e.g. blood pressure, diabetes and lipids, and also non-invasive interventions, e.g. cognitive training. This vital work can only been done through multi-center studies and standardized evaluation techniques using various systems biology and statistical modeling approaches.

http://dx.doi.org/10.5772/54289

Author details

Mei Sian Chong[1] and Tih-Shih Lee[2]

1 Department of Geriatric Medicine, Tan Tock Seng Hospital, Singapore

2 Duke University Medical School, USA

References

[1] Wimo A, Winbald B, Aguero Torres H, von Strauss E. The magnitude of dementia occurrence in the world. Alz Dis Assoc Disord 2003; 17: 63-67.

[2] Price JL, Morris JC. Tangles and plaques in nondemented aging and preclinical Alzheimer disease. Ann Neurol 1999; 45:358-68.

[3] Bateman RJ, Xiong C, Benzinger TL, Fagan AM, Goate A, Fox NC, Marcus DS, Cairns NJ, Xie X, Blazey TM, Holtzman DM, Santacruz A, Buckles V, Oliver A, Moulder K, Aisen PS, Ghetti B, Klunk WE, McDade E, Martins RN, Masters CL, Mayeux R, Ringman JM, Rossor MN, Schofield PR, Sperling RA, Salloway S, Morris JC; the Dominantly Inherited Alzheimer Network. Clinical and Biomarker Changes in Dominantly Inherited Alzheimer's Disease. N Engl J Med. 2012 Jul 11.

[4] Jack CR Jr, Albert MS, Knopman DS, McKhann GM, Sperling RA, Carrillo MC, Thies B, Phelps CH. Introduction to the recommendations from the National Institute on Aging-Alzheimer's Association workgroups on diagnostic guidelines for Alzheimer's disease. Alzheimers Dement. 2011 May;7(3):257-62. Epub 2011 Apr 21.

[5] Cores F, Nourhashemi F, Guerin O et al. Prognosis of Alzheimer's disease today : a two-year prospective study in 686 patients from the REAL-FR Study. Alzheimers Dement 2008; 4(1): 22-29.

[6] Roselli F, Tartaglione B, Federico F, Lepore V, Defazio G, Livrea P. Rate of MMSE score change in Alzheimer's disease: Influence of education and vascular risk factors. Clin Neurol Neurosurg 2009; 111(4):327-30.

[7] Soto ME, Anrieu S, Cantet C, Reynish E et al. Predictive value of rapid decline in Mini Mental State Examination in clinical practice for prognosis in Alzheimer's disease. Dement Geriatr Cogn Disord 2008; 26(2): 109-16.

[8] de la Monte SM. Contributions of Brain Insulin Resistance and Deficiency in Amyloid-Related Neurodegeneration in Alzheimer's disease. Drugs 2012; 73(1):49-66.

[9] Janson J, Laedtke T, Parisi JE, O/Brien P et al. Increased risk of type 2 diabetes in Alzheimer disease. Diabetes 2004; 53:474-481.

[10] Francis GJ, Martinez JA, Liu WQ, Xu K, Ayer A, Fine J, Tuor UI, Glazner G, Hanson, LR, Frey WH 2nd, Toth C. Intranasal insulin prevents cognitive decline, cerebral

atrophy and white matter changes in murine type I diabetic encephalopathy. Brain 2008;131(Pt 12):3311-34.

[11] Xu E, Caracciolo B, Wang H, Winblad B et a. Accelerated progression from Mild Cognitive Impairment to Dementia in People with Diabetes. Diabetes 2010; 59:2928-2935.

[12] Cole AR, Astell A, Green C, Sutherland C. Molecular connexions between dementia and diabetes. Neurosci Biobehav Rev 2007; 31:1046-63.

[13] Schenider P, Buerger K, Teipel S, Uspenskaya O, Harmann O et al. Antihypertension Therapy is associated with reduced rate of conversion to Alzheimer's disease in midregional proatrial natriuretic peptide strateified subjects with mild cognitive impairment. Biol Psy 2011; 70:145-51.

[14] Siuda J, Gorzkowska A, Patalong-Ogiewa M, Krzystanek E, Czech E et al. From mild cognitive impairment to Alzheimer's disease - influence of homocysteine, vitamin B12 and folate on cognition over time: results from one-year follow-up. Neurol Neurochir Pol. 2009 Jul-Aug;43(4):321-9.

[15] Solfrizzi V, Panza F, Colacicco Am, D'Introno A et al. Vascular risk factors, incidence of MCI, and rates of progression to dementia. Neurology 2004; 63(10): 1882-91.

[16] Mielke MM, Rosenberg PB, Tschanz J et al. Vascular factors predict rate of progression in Alzheimer disease. Neurology 2007; 69:1850-58.

[17] Musicco M, Palmer K, Salamone G, Lupo F, Perri R et al. Predictors of progression of cognitive decline in Alzheimer's disease: the role of vascular and sociodemographic factors." J Neurol. 2009 Aug;256(8):1288-95.

[18] Bellew KM, Pigeon JG, Fleischman W, Gardner RM, Baker WW. Hypertension and the Rate of Cognitive Decline in Patients with Dementia of the Alzheimer Type. Alzheimer Dis Assoc Disord 2004; 18(4): 208-213.

[19] Regan C, Katona C, Walker Z, Hooper J, Donovan J et al. Relationship of vascular risk to the progression of Alzheimer disease. Neurology 2006; 67:1357-62.

[20] Helzner EP, Luchsinger JA, Scarmeas N et al. Contribution of vascular risk factors to disease progressionn in Alzheimer's Disease. Arch Neurol 2009; 66(3):343-48.

[21] Li J, Wang YJ, Zhang M, Xu ZQ et al. Vascular risk factors promote conversion from mild cognitive impairment to Alzheimer disease. Neurology 2011; 76:1485-91.

[22] Li L, Wang Y, Yan J, Chen Y, Zhou R et al. Clinical predictors of cognitive decline in patients with mild cognitive impairment: the Chongqing aging study. J Neurol 2012; 259:1303-1311.

[23] Solfrizzi V, Scafato E, Capurso C, D'Introno A, Colacicco AM, Frisardi V,Vendemiale G, Baldereschi M, Crepaldi G, Di Carlo A, Galluzzo L, Gandin C,Inzitari D, Maggi S, Capurso A, Panza F; Italian Longitudinal Study on Aging Working Group.Metabolic

http://dx.doi.org/10.5772/54289

syndrome, mild cognitive impairment, and progression to dementia. The Italian Longitudinal Study on Aging. Neurobiol Aging 2011;32(11):1932-41.

[24] Forlenza OV, Diniz BS, Talib LL, Radanovic M et al. Clinical and biologic predictors of Alzheimer's disease in patients with amnestic mild cognitive impairment. Revista Brasilerira de Psiquiatria 2010; 32(3):216-22.

[25] Wilkosz PA, Seltman HJ, Devlin B, Weamer EA, Lopez OL et al. Trajectories of Cognitive Decline in Alzheimer's disease. Int Psychogeriatr 2010; 22(2):281-90.

[26] Gomeni R, Simeoni M, Zvartau-Hind M, Irizarry MC, Austin D, Gold M. Modeling Alzheimer's disease progression using the disease system analysis approach. Alz Dement 2012; 8:39-50.

[27] Lopez OL, Schwam E, Cummings J, Gauthier S, Jones R, Wilkinson D et al. Predicting cognitive decline in Alzheimer's disease: An integrated analysis. Alz Dement 2010; 6:431-39.

[28] Hall CB, Derby C, LeValley A, Katz MH, Verghese J, Lipton RB. Education delays accelerated decline on a memory test in persons who develop dementia. Neurology 2007; 69:1657-64.

[29] Doody RS, Pavlik V, Massman P, Rountree S et al. Predicting progression of Alzheimer's disease. Alzheimer's Res Therapy 2010;2:2.

[30] Buccione I, Perri R, Carlesimo GA, Fadda L et al. Cognitive and behavioural predictors of progression rates in Alzheimer's disease. Eur J Neurology 2007; 14:440-6.

[31] Palmer K, Lupo F, Perri R, Salamone G et al. Predicting Disease progression in Alzheimer's disease: The role of Neuropsychiatric syndromes on functional and cognitive decline. J Alz Dis 2011; 24:35-45.

[32] De Jaeger CA, Hoegevorst E, Combrinck M, Budge MM. Sensitivity and specificity of neuropsychological tests for mild cognitive impairment, vascular cognitive impairment and Alzheimer's disease. Psychological Medicine 2003; 33:1039–50.

[33] Albert M, Blacker D, Moss MB, Tanzi R, McArdle JJ. Longitudinal change in cognitive performance among individuals with mild cognitive impairment. Neuropsychology 2007; 21(2):158-69.

[34] Pozueta A, Rodriguez-Rodriguez E, Vazquez-Higuera J, Mateo I et al. Detection of early Alzheimer's disease in MCI patients by combination of MMSE and an episodic memory test. BMC Neurology 2011; 11:78.

[35] Gavett BE, Ozonoff A, Doktor V, Palmisano J et al. Predicting cognitive decine and conversion to Alzheimer's disease in older adults using the NAB List Learning test. J Int Neuropsychol Soc 2010; 16(4): 651-60.

[36] PJ Nestor, P Scheltens, JR Hodges. Advances in the early detection of Alzheimer's disease. Nat Med. 2004 Jul;10 Suppl:S34–41. Review.

[37] Fowler KS, Salling MM, Conway El, Semple JM, Louis WJ. Paired associate performance in the early detection of DAT. J Int Neuropsychol Soc 2002; 8(1):58-71.

[38] DeCarli C, Mungas D, Harvey D, Reed B, Weiner M, Chui H, Jagust WC. Memory impairment, but not cerebrovascular disease, predicts progression of MCI to dementia. Neurology 2004; 63:220–7.

[39] Amieva H, Letenneur L, Dartigues JF, Rouch-Leroyer I, Sourgen C, D Alchee-Biree F, Dib M, Barbeger-Gateau P, Orgogozo JM, Fabrigoule C. Annual Rate and Predictors of Conversion to Dementia in Subjects Presenting Mild Cognitive Impairment Criteria Defined according to a Population-Based Study. Dement Geriatr Cogn Disord 2004; 18:87–93.

[40] Dickerson BC, Sperling RA, Hyman BT, Albert MS, Blacker D. Clinical Prediction of Alzheimer Disease Dementia across the spectrum of mild cognitive impairment. Arch Gen Psychiatry 2007; 64(12):1443-50.

[41] Guarch J, Marcos T, Salamero M, Blesa R. Neuropsychological markers of dementia in patients with memory complaints. Int J Geriatr Psychiatry 2004; 19:352–58.

[42] Chapman RM, Mapstone M, McCrary JW, Gardner MN, Porsteinnson AP et al. Predicting conversion from Mild Cognitive Impairment to Alzheimer's disease using neuropsychological tests and multivariate methods. J Clin Exp Neuropsychol 2011; 33(2): 187-99.

[43] Chan Y, Bondi MW, Fennema-Notestine C, McEvoy LK et al. Brain substrates of learning and retention in mild cognitive impairment diagnosis and progression to Alzheimer's disease. Neuropsychologia 2010; 48(5):1237-47.

[44] Dierckx E, Engelborghs S, De Raedt R, Van Buggenhout M, De Deyn PP et al. Verba; cued recall as a predictor of conversion to Alzheimer's disease in Mild Cognitive Impairment. Int J Geriatr Psy 2009;24:1094-1100.

[45] Musicco M, Salamone G, Caltagirone C, Cravello L et al. Neuropsychological Predictors of Rapidly Progressing Patients with Alzheimer's disease. Dement Geriatr Cogn Disord 2010; 30:219-28.

[46] Backman L, Small BJ, Fratiglioni L. Stability of the preclinical memory deficit in Alzheimer's disease. Brain 2001; 124:96-102.

[47] Bennett DA, Wilson RS, Schneider JA, Evans DA et al. Natural history of mild cognitive impairment in older persons. Neurology 2002; 59:198-205.

[48] Blennow K, Hampal H. CSF markers for incipient Alzheimer's disease. Lancet Neurol 2003; 2:605-13.

[49] Fagan AM, Shaw LM, Xiong C, Vanderstichele H et al. Comparison of Analytical Platforms for cerebrospinal fluid measures of β-amyloid 1-42, total tau, and P-tau_{181} for identifying Alzheimer Disease Amyloid Plaque Pathology. Arch neurol doi:10.1001/archneurol.2011.105

[50] Shaw LM, Vanderstichele H, Knapik-Czajka M et al. Qualification of the analytical and clinical performance of CSF biomarker analyses in ADNI. Acta Neuropathol 2011; 121:597-609.

[51] Arai H, Nakagawa T, Kosaka Y et al. Elevated cerebrospinal fluid tau protein as a predictor of dementia in memory-impaired patients. Alzheimer's Res 1997; 3:211-3.

[52] Andreasen N, Vanmechelen E, Vanderstichele H, Davidsson P, Blennow K. Cerebrospinal fluid levels of total-tau, phosphor-tau and Aβ42 predicts development of Alzheimer's disease in patients with mild cognitive impairment. Acta Neurol Scand 2003; 107(suppl 179):47-51.

[53] Hampel H, Teipel SJ, Fuchsberger T, Andreasen N, Wiltfang J, Otto M, Shen Y, Dodel R, u Y, Farlow M, Moller HJ et al. Value of CSF beta-amyloid1-42 and tau as predictors of Alzheimer's disease in patients with mild cognitive impairment. Mol Psychiatry 2004; 9:705-10.

[54] Maruyama M, Arai H, Sugita M, Tanji H, Higuchi M, Okamura N, Matsui T, Higuchi S, Matsushita S, Yoshida H, Sasaki H. Cerebrospinal fluid amyloid $\beta_{1\text{-}42}$ in the mild cognitive impairment stage of Alzheimer's disease. Exp Neurol 2001; 172:433-6.

[55] Mattson N et al. CSF biomarkers and incipient Alzheimer disease in patients with mild cognitive impairment. JAMA 2009; 302:485-93.

[56] Visser PJ et al. Prevalence and prognostic value of CSF markers of Alzheimer's disease pathology in patients with subjective cognitive impairment or mild cognitive impairment in the DESCRIPA study: a prospective cohort study. Lancet Neurol 2009; 8:619-27.

[57] Arai H, Idhiguro K, Ohno H, Moriyama M, Itoh N, Okamura N, Matsui T, Morikawa Y, Horikawa E, Kohno H, Sasaki H et al. CSF phosphorylated tau protein and mild cognitive impairment: a prospective study. Exp Neurol 2000; 1666:201-3.

[58] Buerger K, Teipel SJ, Zinkoiwski R, Blennow K, Arai H, Engel R, Hofmann-Keiffer K, McCulloch C, Ptok U, Heun R, Andreasen N et al. CST tau protein phosphorylated at threonine 231 correlates with cognitive decline in MCI subjects. Neurology 2002; 59:627-9.

[59] Riemenscheneider M, Lautenschlager N, Wagenpfeil S, Diehl J, Drzezga A, Kurz A. Cerebrospinal fluid tau and beta-amyloid 42 proteins identify Alzheimer disease in subjects with mild cognitive impairment. Arch Neurol 2002; 59:1729-34.

[60] Andreasen N, Minthon L, Vanmechelen E, Vanderstichele H, Davidsson P, Winblad B, Blennow K. Cerebrospinal fluid tau and Aβ42 as predictors of development of Alzheimer's disease in patients with mild cognitive impairment. Neurosci Letters 1999; 273:5-8.

[61] Herruka S, Hallikainen M, Soininen H, Pirttila T. CSF Aβ42 and tau or phosphorylated tau and prediction of progressive mild cognitive impairment. Neurology 2005; 64:1294-7.

[62] Zetterberg H, Wahlund LO, Blennow K. Cerebrospinal fluid markers for prediction of Alzheimer's disease. Neurosci Letters 2003; 352: 67-9.

[63] Parnetti L, Lanari A, Silvestrelli G, Saggese E, Reboldi P. Diagnosing prodromal Alzheimer's disease: Role of CSF biochemical markers. Mechan Ageing Dev 2005 [EPub]

[64] Hansson O, Zetterberg H, Buchhave P, Londos E, Blennow K, Minthon L. Association between CSF biomarkers and incipient Alzheimer's disease in patients with mild cognitive impairment: a follow-up study. Lancet Neurol 2006:5:228-34.

[65] Seppala TT, Koivisto AM, Hartikainen P et al. Longitudinal changes of CSF Biomarkers in Alzheimer's disease. J Alz Iis 2011; 24:583-94.

[66] Samgard K, Zetterberg H, Blennow K, Hansson O et al. Cerebrospinal fluid total tau as a marker of Alzheimer's disease intensity. Int J Geriatr Psy 2010: 25:403-10.

[67] Ravaglia S, Bini P, Sinforiani E, Franciotta D et al. Cerebrospinal fluid levels of tau phosphrylated at threonine 181 in patients with Alzheimer's disease and vascular dementia. Neurol Sci 2008; 29:417-23.

[68] Vlachos GSm Oarasjevas GP, Naoumis D, Kapaki E. Cerebrospinal fluid β-amyloid$_{1-42}$ correlates with rate of progression in Alzheimer's disease. J Neural Transm 2012; 119:799-804.

[69] Wallin AK, Blennow K, Zetterberg J, Londos E et al. CSF biomarkers predict a more malignant course in Alzheimer disease. Neurology 2010; 74(19): 1531-7.

[70] deLeon MJ, Segal S, Tarshish CY, DeSanti S, Zinkowski R, Mehta PD, Convit A, Caraos C, Rusinek H, Tsui W, Saint Louis LA et al. Longitudinal cerebrospinal fluid tau load increases in mild cognitive impairment. Neurosci Letters 2002; 333:183-6.

[71] Leon MJ, Desanti S, Zinkowski R, Mehta PD, Pratico D, Segal S, Rusinek H, Li J, Tsui W, Saint Louis LA, Clark CM et al. Longitudinal CSF and MRI biomarkers improve the diagnosis of mild cognitive impairment. Neurobiol Aging. 2005 Aug 25.

[72] Kester ML, Scheffer PG, Koel-Simmelink MJ, Twaalfhoven H et al. Serial CSF sampling in Alzheimer's disease: specific versus non-specific markers. Neurobiol Aging 2012; 33:1591-98.

[73] Rosun D, Schuff N, Shaw LM, Trojanowski JQ, Weiner MW et al. Relationship between CSF biomarkers of Alzheimer's disease and Rates of Regional Cortical Thinning in ADNI data. J Alzheimer's Dis 2011; 26:77-90.

[74] Perrin RJ, Craig-Schapiro R, Malone JP, Shah AR, Gilmore P et al. Identification and Validation of Novel Cerebrospinal fluid biomarkers for staging early Alzheimer's Disease. PLOS One 2011; 6(1):e16032.

[75] Georganopoulou DG, Chang L, Nam J, Thaxton CS et al. Nanoparticle-based detection in cerebral spinal fluid of a soluble pathogenic biomarker for Alzheimer's disease. PNAS 2005; 102(7):2273-6.

[76] Craig-Scharpiro R, Kuhn M, Xiong C, Pickering Eh et al. Multiplexed Immunoassay Panel identified Novel CSF Biomarkers for Alzheimer's Disease Diagnosis and Prognosis. PLOS One 2011; 6(4):e18850.

[77] Glabe CG, Kayed R. Common structure and toxic function of amyloid oligomers implies a common mechanism of pathogenesis. Neurology 2006; 66(Suppl 1): S74-78.

[78] Lemere CA, Maier M, Jiang L, Peng Y, Seabrook TJ. Amyloid-Beta Immunotherapy for the Prevention and Treatment of Alzheimer Disease: Lessons from mice, monkeys and humans. Rejuvenation Res 2006; 9(1): 77-84.

[79] Olsson A et al. Simultaneous measurement of β-amyloid$_{(1\text{-}42)}$, total tau, and phosphorylated tau (Thr^{181}) in cerebrospinal fluid by xMAP technology. Lin Chem 2005; 51:336-345.

[80] Mattsson N, Zetterberg H, Blennow K. Lessons from multicenter studies on CSF biomarkers for Alzheimer's disease. Int J Alz Dis 2010. doi:10.4061/2010/610613.

[81] Lee TS, Chua SM, Ly P, Song W. Genomic and molecular characterization of Alzheimer Disease. Current Psych Reviews, 2010, 6, 104-113.

[82] Hansson O, Zetterberg H, Vanmechelen E, Vanderstichele H, Andreasson U, Londos E, Wallin A, Minthon L, Blennow K. Evaluation of plasma Abeta(40) and Abeta(42) as predictors of conversion to Alzheimer's disease in patients with mild cognitive impairment. Neurobiol Aging. 2010 Mar;31(3):357-67. Epub 2008 May 19.

[83] Mayeux R, Schupf N.Mayeux Blood-based biomarkers for Alzheimer's disease: plasma Aβ40 and Aβ42, and genetic variants. Neurobiol Aging. 2011 Dec;32 Suppl 1:S10-9. Review.

[84] Koyama A, Okereke OI, Yang T, Blacker D, Selkoe DJ, Grodstein F. Plasma Amyloid-β as a Predictor of Dementia and Cognitive Decline: A Systematic Review and Meta-analysis.Arch Neurol. 2012 Mar 26.

[85] Borroni B, Colciaghi F, Archetti S, Marcello E, Caimi L, Di Luca M, Padovani A. Predicting cognitive decline in Alzheimer disease. Role of platelet amyloid precursor protein. Alzheimer Dis Assoc Disord. 2004 Jan-Mar;18(1):32-4.

[86] Xu G, Zhou Z, Zhu W, Fan X, Liu X. Plasma C-reactive protein (CRP) is related to cognitive deterioration and dementia in patients with mild cognitive impairment (Xu 2009) Neurol Sci. 2009 Sep 15;284(1-2):77-80. Epub 2009

[87] Locascio JJ, Fukumoto H, Yap L, Bottiglieri T, Growdon JH, Hyman BT, Irizarry MC. Plasma amyloid beta-protein and C-reactive protein in relation to the rate of progression of Alzheimer disease. Arch Neurol. 2008 Jun;65(6):776-85

[88] Thambisetty M, An Y, Kinsey A, Koka D, Saleem M, Güntert A, Kraut M, Ferrucci L, Davatzikos C, Lovestone S, Resnick SM. Plasma clusterin concentration is associated with longitudinal brain atrophy in mild cognitive impairment. Neuroimage. 2012 Jan 2;59(1):212-7. Epub 2011 Jul 28.

[89] Mielke MM, Haughey NJ, Bandaru VV, Weinberg DD, Darby E, Zaidi N, Pavlik V, Doody RS, Lyketsos CG. Plasma sphingomyelins are associated with cognitive progression in Alzheimer's disease. J Alzheimers Dis. 2011;27(2):259-69.

[90] Elias-Sonnenschein LS, Viechtbauer W, Ramakers IH, Verhey FR, Visser PJ. Predictive value of APOE-ε4 allele for progression from MCI to AD-type dementia: a meta-analysis. J Neurol Neurosurg Psychiatry. 2011 Oct;82(10):1149-56. Epub 2011 Apr 14.

[91] Martins CA, Oulhaj A, de Jager CA, Williams JH. APOE alleles predict the rate of cognitive decline in Alzheimer disease: a nonlinear model. Neurology. 2005 Dec 27;65(12):1888-93.

[92] Cosentino S, Scarmeas N, Helzner E, Glymour MM, Brandt J, Albert M, Blacker D, Stern Y.APOE epsilon 4 allele predicts faster cognitive decline in mild Alzheimer disease. Neurology. 2008 May 6;70(19 Pt 2):1842-9. Epub 2008 Apr 9

[93] Lee TS, Goh L, Chong MS, Chua SM, Chen GB, Feng L, Lim WS, Chan M, Ng TP, Krishnan KR. Downregulation of TOMM40 expression in the blood of Alzheimer disease subjects compared with matched controls. J Psychiatr Res. 2012 Jun;46(6): 828-30. Epub 2012 Apr 1.

[94] Ray S, Britschgi M, Herbert C, Takeda-Uchimura Y, Boxer A, Blennow K, Friedman LF, Galasko DR, Jutel M, Karydas A, Kaye JA, Leszek J, Miller BL, Minthon L, Quinn JF, Rabinovici GD, Robinson WH, Sabbagh MN, So YT, Sparks DL, Tabaton M, Tinklenberg J, Yesavage JA, Tibshirani R, Wyss-Coray T. Nat Med. Classification and prediction of clinical Alzheimer's diagnosis based on plasma signaling proteins. 2007 Nov; 13(11):1359-62. Epub 2007 Oct 14.

[95] Soares HD, Chen Y, Sabbagh M, Roher A, Schrijvers E, Breteler M. Identifying early markers of Alzheimer's disease using quantitative multiplex proteomic immunoassay panels. Ann N Y Acad Sci. 2009 Oct;1180:56-67.

[96] Jack CR Jr, Shiung MM, Gunter JL, O'Brien PC, Weigand SD, Knopman DS, Boeve BF, Ivnik RJ, Smith GE, Cha RH, Tangalos EG, Petersen RC. Comparison of different MRI brain atrophy rate measures with clinical disease progression in AD. Neurology. 2004 Feb 24;62(4):591-600.

[97] Jack CR Jr, Petersen RC, Grundman M, Jin S, Gamst A, Ward CP, Sencakova D, Doody RS, Thal LJ; Members of the Alzheimer's Disease Cooperative Study (ADCS). Longitudinal MRI findings from the vitamin E and donepezil treatment study for MCI. Neurobiol Aging. 2008 Sep;29(9):1285-95. Epub 2007 Apr 23.

[98] Jack CR Jr, Shiung MM, Weigand SD, O'Brien PC, Gunter JL, Boeve BF, Knopman DS, Smith GE, Ivnik RJ, Tangalos EG, Petersen RC. Brain atrophy rates predict subsequent clinical conversion in normal elderly and amnestic MCI. Neurology. 2005 Oct 25;65(8): 1227-31.

[99] Apostolova LG, Dutton RA, Dinov ID, Hayashi KM, Toga AW, Cummings JL, Thompson PM Conversion of mild cognitive impairment to Alzheimer disease predicted by hippocampal atrophy maps. Arch Neurol. 2006 May;63(5):693-9.

[100] Thompson PM, Hayashi KM, de Zubicaray G, Janke AL, Rose SE, Semple J, Herman D, Hong MS, Dittmer SS, Doddrell DM, Toga AW. Dynamics of gray matter loss in Alzheimer's disease. J Neurosci. 2003 Feb 1;23(3):994-1005.

[101] Risacher SL, Saykin AJ, West JD, Shen L, Firpi HA, McDonald BC; Alzheimer's Disease Neuroimaging Initiative (ADNI). Baseline MRI predictors of conversion from MCI to probable AD in the ADNI cohort. Curr Alzheimer Res. 2009 Aug;6(4):347-61.

[102] Kinkingnéhun S, Sarazin M, Lehéricy S, Guichart-Gomez E, Hergueta T, Dubois B.VBM anticipates the rate of progression of Alzheimer disease: a 3-year longitudinal study. Neurology. 2008 Jun 3;70(23):2201-11. Epub 2008 Apr 30.

[103] Querbes O, Aubry F, Pariente J, Lotterie JA, Démonet JF, Duret V, Puel M, Berry I, Fort JC, Celsis P; Alzheimer's Disease Neuroimaging Initiative. Early diagnosis of Alzheimer's disease using cortical thickness: impact of cognitive reserve. Brain. 2009 Aug;132(Pt 8):2036-47. Epub 2009 May 12.

[104] Silverman DH, Small GW, Chang CY, Lu CS, Kung De Aburto MA, Chen W, Czernin J, Rapoport SI, Pietrini P, Alexander GE, Schapiro MB, Jagust WJ, Hoffman JM, Welsh-Bohmer KA, Alavi A, Clark CM, Salmon E, de Leon MJ, Mielke R, Cummings JL, Kowell AP, Gambhir SS, Hoh CK, Phelps ME. Positron emission tomography in evaluation of dementia: Regional brain metabolism and long-term outcome. JAMA. 2001 Nov 7;286(17):2120-7.

[105] Lo RY, Hubbard AE, Shaw LM, Trojanowski JQ, Petersen RC, Aisen PS, Weiner MW, Jagust WJ; Alzheimer's Disease Neuroimaging Initiative. Longitudinal change of biomarkers in cognitive decline. Arch Neurol. 2011 Oct;68(10):1257-66. Epub 2011 Jun 13.

[106] Okello A, Koivunen J, Edison P, Archer HA, Turkheimer FE, Någren K, Bullock R, Walker Z, Kennedy A, Fox NC, Rossor MN, Rinne JO, Brooks DJ. Conversion of amyloid positive and negative MCI to AD over 3 years: an 11C-PIB PET study. Neurology. 2009 Sep 8;73(10):754-60. Epub 2009 Jul 8.

[107] Koivunen J, Scheinin N, Virta JR, Aalto S, Vahlberg T, Någren K, Helin S, Parkkola R, Viitanen M, Rinne JO. Amyloid PET imaging in patients with mild cognitive impairment: a 2-year follow-up study. Neurology. 2011 Mar 22;76(12):1085-90. Epub 2011 Feb 16.

[108] Small GW, Siddarth P, Kepe V, Ercoli LM, Burggren AC, Bookheimer SY, Miller KJ, Kim J, Lavretsky H, Huang SC, Barrio JR.Prediction of cognitive decline by positron emission tomography of brain amyloid and tau. Arch Neurol. 2012 Feb;69(2):215-22.

[109] Doraiswamy PM, Sperling RA, Coleman RE, Johnson KA, Reiman EM, Davis MD, Grundman M, Sabbagh MN, Sadowsky CH, Fleisher AS, Carpenter A, Clark CM, Joshi

AD, Mintun MA, Skovronsky DM, Pontecorvo MJ; For the AV45-A11 Study Group. Amyloid-β assessed by florbetapir F 18 PET and 18-month cognitive decline: A multicenter study. Neurology. 2012 Aug 1.

[110] Ossenkoppele R, Tolboom N, Foster-Dingley JC, Adriaanse SF, Boellaard R, Yaqub M, Windhorst AD, Barkhof F, Lammertsma AA, Scheltens P, van der Flier WM, van Berckel BN. Longitudinal imaging of Alzheimer pathology using [11C]PIB, [18F]FDDNP and [18F]FDG PET. Eur J Nucl Med Mol Imaging. 2012 Jun;39(6):990-1000. Epub 2012 Mar 23.

[111] Zhang S, Han D, Tan X, Feng J, Guo Y, Ding Y. Diagnostic accuracy of 18 F-FDG and 11 C-PIB-PET for prediction of short-term conversion to Alzheimer's disease in subjects with mild cognitive impairment. Int J Clin Pract. 2012 Feb;66(2):185-98. doi: 10.1111/j. 1742-1241.2011.02845.x.

[112] Villain N, Chetelat G, Grassiot B, Bourgeat P et al. Regional dynamics of amyloid- β deposition in healthy elderly, mild cognitive impairment and Alzheimer's disease: a voxelwise PiB-PET longitudinal study. Brain 2012; doi:10.1093/brain/aws125.

[113] Kester MI, van der Lier WM, Mandic G, Blankenstein MA et al. Joint effect of hypertension and APOE genotype on CSF biomarkers for Alzheimer's disease. J Alz IDis 2010;20:1083-90.

[114] Blom ES, Gledraitis V, Zetterberg H, Fukumoto H et al. Rapid progression from mild cognitive impairment to Alzheimer's Disease in subjects with elevated levels of tau in cerebrospinal fluid and the APOE e4/e4 genotype. Dement Geriatr Cogn Disord 2009; 27:458-464.

[115] Palmqvist S, Hertze J, Minthon L, Wattmo C et al. Comparison of Brief Cognitive Tests and CSF biomarkers in prediciting Alzheimer's disease in mild cognitive impairment: Six-year follow-up study. PLOS one 2012; 7(6):e38639

[116] Ewers M, Walsh C, Trojanowski JQ, Shaw LM et al. Prediction of conversion from mild cognitive impairment to Alzheimer's disease dementia based upon biomarkers and neuropsychological test performance. Neurobiol Aging 2012; 33(7):1203-14.

[117] Cui Y, Liu B, Luo S, Zhen X et al. Identification of Conversion from mild cognitive impairment to Alzheimer's disease using multivariate predictors. PLOS One 2011; 6(7):e21896.

[118] El Fakhri G, Kijewski MF, Johnson KA, Syrkin G, Killany RJ, Becker JA, Zimmerman RE, Albert MS. MRI-guided SPECT perfusion measures and volumetric MRI in Prodromal Alzheimer Disease. Arch Neurol 2003; 60:1066-72.

[119] Huang C, Wahlund LO, Almkvist O, Elehu D, Svensson L, Jonsson T, Winblad B, Julin P. Voxel- and VOI-based analysis of SPECT CBF in relation to clinical and psychological heterogeneity of mild cognitive impairment. Neuroimage. 2003 Jul;19(3):1137-44.

[120] Stephanie V, van Rossum I, Burns L, KNol D et al. Test sequence of CSF and MRI biomarkers for prediction of AD in subjects with MCI. Neurobiol Aging 2012; 33:2272-81.

[121] Vemuri P, Wiste HJ, Weigand SD, Shaw LM et al. MRI and CSF biomarkers in normal, MCI and AD subjects. Neurology 2009;73:294-301.

[122] Eckerstrom C, Andreasson U, Olsson E, Rolstad S, Blennow K et al. Combination of hippocampal volume and cerebrospinal fluid biomarkers improves predictive value in mild cognitive impairment. Dement Geriatr Cogn Disord 2010; 29:294-300.

[123] Davatzikos C, Bhatt P, Shaw LM, Batmanghelich KN, Trojanowski JQ. Prediction of MCI to AD conversion, via MRI, CSF biomarkers and pattern classification. Neurobiol Aging 2011; 2322.e19-2322.e27

[124] Hansson O, Buchhave P, Zetterberg H, Blennow K et al. Combined rCBF and CSF biomarkers predict preogression from mild cognitive impairment to Alzheimer's disease. Neurobiol Aging 2009;30:165-173.

[125] Okamura N, Arai H, Maruyama M et al. Combined analysis of CSF tau levels and [(123)I]Iodoamphetamine SPECT in mild cognitive impairment: implications for a novel predictor of Alzheimer's disease. Am J Psychiatry 2002; 159:474-76.

[126] Furney SJ, Kronenberg D, Simmons A, Guntert A, Dobson RJ et al. Combinatorial markers of mild cognitive impairment conversion to Alzheimer's disease – cytokines and MRI measures together predict disease progression. J Alz Dis 2011; 26:395-405.

[127] Zhang D, Shen D, Alzheimer's Disease Neuroimaging Initiative. Predicting future clinical changes of MCI patients using Longitudinal and Multimodal Biomarkers. PLOS One 2012; 7(3):e33182.

[128] Zhang D, Wang Y, Zhou L, Yuan H et al. Multimodal classification of Alzheimer's disease and mild cognitive impairment. Neuroimage 2011; 55:856-67.

[129] Hinrichs C, Singh V, Xu G, Johnson SC et al. Predictive markers for AD in a multi-modality Framework: An Analysis of MCI progression in the ADNI population. Neuroimage 2011; 55(2): 574-89.

[130] Cruchaga C, Kauwe JSK, Mayo K, Spiegel N et al. SNPs associated with cerebrospinal fluid phosphor-tau levels influence rate of decline in Alzheimer Disease. PLOS Genetics 2010; 6(9):e1001101.

[131] Chong MS, Sahadevan S. Preclinical Alzheimer's disease: diagnosis and prediction of progression. Lancet Neurol 2005; 4: 576-79.

[132] Chong MS, Lim WS, Sahadevan S. Biomarkers in prediction of progression of preclinical Alzheimer's disease. Current Opinion in Investigational Drugs 2006: 7(7): 600-607.

[133] Beckett LA, Harvey DJ, Gamst A, Donohue M et al. The Alzheimer's Disease Neuroimaging Initiative: Annual Change in Biomarkers and Clinical Outcomes. Alz Dement 2010; 6(3): 257-64.

[134] Jack CR, Knopman DS, Jagust WJ, et al. Hypothetical model of dynamic biomarkers of the Alzheimer's pathological cascade. Lancet Neurol 2010; 9:119-28

[135] Storandt M, Head D, Fagan AM, Holtzman DM, Morris JC. Toward a multifactorial model of Alzheimer disease. Neurobiol Aging 2012; 33:2262-71.

[136] Rowe CC, Ellisa KA, Rimajova M, Bourgeat P et al. Amyloid imaging results from the Australian Imaging, Biomarkers and Lifestyle (AIBL) study of aging. Neurobiol Aging 2010; 31:1275-83.

[137] Kohannim O, HUa X, Hibar DP, Lee S, Chou U, Toga AW et al. Boosting power for clinical trials using classifiers based on multiple biomarkers. Neurobiol Aging 2010; 31:1429-42.

[138] Lorenzi M, Donohue M, Paternico D, Scarpazza C et al. Enrichment through biomarkers in clinical trials of Alzheimer's drugs in patients with mild cognitive impairment. Neurobiol Aging 2010; 31:1443-51.

[139] van Rossum IA, Vos S, Handels R, Visser PJ. Biomarkers as Predictors for Conversion from Mild Cognitive Impairment to Alzheimer-Type Dementia: Implications for Trial Design. J Alz Dis 2010; 20:881-91.

[140] Yu P, Dean RA, Hall SD, Qi Y et al. Enriching Amnestic Mild Cognitive Impairment Populations for Clinical Trials: Optimal Combination of Biomarkers to Predict Conversion to Dementia. J Alz Dis; doi 10.3233/JAD-2012-120832.

[141] Lopez OL, Schqam E, Cummings J, Gautheir S, Jones R et al. Predicting cognitive decline in Alzheimer's diseae: An integrated analysis. Alz Dement 2010; 6:431-9.

Chapter 16

Alzheimer's Disease and Diabetes

Brent D. Aulston, Gary L. Odero, Zaid Aboud and
Gordon W. Glazner

Additional information is available at the end of the chapter

http://dx.doi.org/10.5772/54913

1. Introduction

"I have lost myself"

- *Auguste Deter, the first patient diagnosed with Alzheimer's Disease, 1906*

Identification of Alzheimer's Disease Alois Alzheimer was a German neuropathologist and among the first to identify and describe the hallmarks of what is known today as Alzheimer's disease (AD). In November of 1901, Dr. Alzheimer was presented with 51 year-old Auguste Deter who was suffering from mental incompetence, aphasia, disorientation, paranoia, and unprovoked bursts of anger. Deter's emotional and mental devastation became evident when she confided to Dr. Alzheimer "I have lost myself."

Symptoms similar to Deter's had been observed in patients for years and were considered a natural part of aging. However, it was unusual for such a pointed disease state to occur in someone so young. Over the next four and half years, Deter became increasingly demented, until her death at the age of 55. Upon examination of Deter's brain, Dr. Alzheimer found microscopic strands of protein which he described as "tangled bundles of fibrils" (neurofibrillary tangles) in addition to "miliary foci" (amyloid plaques). In 1906, at the 37th Conference of South-West German Psychiatrists in Tübingen, Alois Alzheimer presented Deter's case as, "a peculiar disease of the cerebral cortex."

To this day both the cause of and treatment for AD remain a mystery. AD is a multifaceted disease of great complexity, however, over 100 years of research has provided clues to its mechanisms. Of particular recent interest is the emerging realization that another rapidly growing disease, type 2 diabetes mellitus (T2DM), is linked to development of AD [1].

This chapter examines the current state of knowledge regarding the association of T2DM to vascular changes in the brain and the implications these changes have in AD development.

Other factors that contribute to AD such as insulin resistance and accumulation of the neurotoxic peptide amyloid beta (Aβ) are also examined. It's likely that no central cause of AD exists but rather, the disease represents a breakdown of several critical components involved in the general health and function of the brain.

Epidemiology of AD and T2DM AD is the most common form of dementia [2] and remains incurable. While the cause of AD remains unknown, several risk factors have been identified that may provide insight into the fundamentals of AD pathogenesis.

T2DM is a known risk factor for AD [1] suggesting that insulin signaling abnormalities play a central role in AD pathology. Moreover, AD brains show decreased insulin levels, decreased activity of insulin receptors and signs of compensatory mechanisms such as increased insulin receptor density [3] indicating AD as "type 3 diabetes" [4, 5].

Loss of insulin signaling in diabetes can occur by either type 1 or type 2 processes. Type 1 diabetes mellitus (T1DM) is characterized as an autoimmune disease that results in the destruction of insulin producing β cells found in the pancreas. In contrast, T2DM is a state of insulin resistance in which insulin levels are normal or elevated but tissues are unresponsive to its effects. While both T1DM and T2DM can lead to cognitive deficits, T2DM poses a greater risk for AD development [6, 7] and as a result the parallels between T2DM and AD are studied more vigorously than T1DM associations. Therefore, the majority of information presented here pertains to type 2 diabetic pathologies.

In addition to insulin resistance, T2DM is associated with the development of vascular dysfunction in the brain [8, 9]. T2DM is a risk factor for microvascular complications as well as macrovascular defects [10] such as stroke [11]. Vascular abnormalities are strongly associated with AD [12-16] implying further involvement of T2DM in disease onset.

2. Type 2 diabetes, vascular changes and Alzheimer's disease

Insulin signaling in the vasculature Activation of the insulin receptor (IR) leads to phosphorylation of insulin receptor substrate (IRS) which serve as docking proteins for phosphatidylinositol 3-kinase (PI3K). PI3K generates phosphatidyl-3,4,5-triphosphate (PIP_3) which then phosphorylates 3-phosphoinositide-dependent protein kinase-1 (PDK-1). Finally, PDK-1 phosphorylates Akt and stimulates endothelial nitric oxide synthase (eNOS) resulting in the production of nitric oxide (NO) and vascular relaxation [17, 18]. Interestingly, insulin receptor activation can also mediate vasoconstriction. Activation of IR can also lead to phosphorylation of Shc which then binds Grb-2 resulting in activation of Sos. This complex then activates Ras leading to phosphorylation Raf which results in activation of MAPK. Activation of MAPK stimulates release of endothelin-1 (ET-1), a vasoconstrictor [19-21]. By mediating vascular properties, insulin signaling plays a significant role in glucose and oxygen availability to the brain. Conversely, dysfunction in insulin signaling, as observed in T2DM, has profound detrimental effects on hemodynamics and, thus, maintenance of normative brain function.

http://dx.doi.org/10.5772/54913

Vascular complications associated with type 2 diabetes It is estimated that approximately 200 million people worldwide have diabetes and by 2025 the number is expected to increase to 333 million [22]. Epidemiological studies have indicated that patients with T2DM have a greater incidence of cardiovascular disease, cerebrovascular disease (CVD), hypertension and renal disease relative to the general population [8, 9]. In addition, a large number of population-based studies have identified diabetes as a risk factor for dementia [23-25], primarily as a result of CVD [26, 27]. At only 3% of body weight, the brain uses ~20% of the body's oxygen and ~25% of the body's blood glucose [28, 29], demonstrating that it is by far the most metabolically active organ. This oxygen and glucose consumption is constantly required, since brain neurons are obligate aerobic cells and have no other source of energy. The majority of this energy is used to maintain cellular ionic homeostasis, and thus when cerebral blood flow (CBF) ceases, brain function ends within seconds and damage to neurons occurs within minutes [30].

The vascular complications associated with diabetes can be divided into two classes based on the vascular etiology of their pathology: macrovascular (hypertension, coronary artery disease, atherosclerosis, stroke) and microvascular (neuropathy, retinopathy, nephropathy). Macrovascular complications are those that affect the larger (non-capillary) blood vessels. Statistics show that diabetes increases the risk of stroke and atherosclerosis [31]. Atherosclerosis accounts for 70% of morbidity associated with T2DM [32], while other studies have shown an association between the degree of hyperglycemia and increased risk of myocardial infarction and stroke [33-36]. While macrovascular complications themselves represent important pathological consequences of T2DM, they have also been shown to provide the etiological link between T2DM and the development of Alzheimer's disease.

Link between type 2 diabetes and Alzheimer's disease AD is an age-related disorder characterized by progressive cognitive decline and dementia. An estimated 5.3 million people in the United States are currently affected and represents the sixth-leading cause of death. Significant evidence has been provided that links T2DM to AD. For example, a comprehensive meta-analysis showed that the aggregate relative risk of AD for people with diabetes was 1.5 (95%-CI 1.2 to 1.8) [37]. Studies have shown that T2DM, impaired fasting glucose and increased islet amyloid deposition are more common in patients with Alzheimer's disease than in control subjects [38, 39]. Unsurprisingly, insulin signaling provides an important mechanistic link between T2DM and AD.

Ischemic CVD caused by T2DM is positively associated with AD through shared pathological mechanisms such as hyperinsulinemia, impaired insulin signaling, oxidative stress, inflammatory mechanisms and advanced glycation end-products (AGEs) [40]. Defective insulin signaling is associated with decreased cognitive ability and development of dementa, including AD [41], rendering signaling neurons more vulnerable to metabolic stress and accelerating neuronal dysfunction [42]. In vitro insulin-stimulated Akt phosphorylation is decreased in hyperinsulinemic conditions in cortical neurons [43]. Finally, all forms of amyloid beta (Aβ) (monomers, oligomers and Aβ-derived diffusible ligands (ADDLs)) can inhibit insulin signaling by directly binding to the insulin receptor and inhibit insulin signaling [44].

Mechanisms of macrovascular complications of diabetes A central pathological mechanism in diabetic-related macrovascular disease is atherosclerosis, which leads to the hardening of arterial walls throughout the body resulting in impaired blood flow. Although the mechanism for the susceptibility of diabetic patients to ischemic heart disease remains unclear, accumulating lines of evidence implicate hyperglycemia, hyperlipidemia and inflammation as playing key roles in the development of this disorder [45]. This link between obesity and both T2DM and atherosclerosis implicates elevated amounts of glucose oxidized LDL and free fatty acids (FFAs) in disease pathogenesis, potentially as triggers for the production of pro-inflammatory cytokines by macrophages [32].

In the insulin resistant state, there is a specific impairment in the vasodilatory PI3K pathway, whereas the Ras/MAPK-dependent pathway is unaffected [46, 47]. This results in decreased production of NO and an increased secretion of ET-1 in humans [48] leading to increased vasoconstriction. The decrease in NO production is significant in that NO protects blood vessels from endogenous injury by mediating molecular signals that prevent platelet and leukocyte interaction with the vascular wall and inhibit vascular smooth muscle cell proliferation and migration [49, 50]. Decreased production of NO allows for increased expression of proinflammatory transcription factor NF-κB, and subsequent expression of leukocyte adhesion molecules and production of chemokines and cytokines [51]. Activation of these proteins promote monocyte and vascular smooth muscle cell migration into the intima and formation of macrophage foam cells, initiating the morphological changes associated with the onset of atherosclerosis [52, 53].

High levels of FFAs are found in insulin-resistant individuals. FFAs generated by increased activity of hormone-sensitive lipase that contribute to and result in insulin resistance [54-56]. In vitro vascular endothelial cell culture treated with FFA resulted in decreased insulin-stimulated eNOS activity and NO production [57]. It is believed that FFA increases cellular levels of diacylglycerols, ceramide, and long-chain fatty acyl coenzyme A (CoA), all of which have been shown to activate protein kinase C (PKCβ1). Activation of PKCβ1 results in increased phosphorylation of IRS-1 that leads to reduced Akt and eNOS resulting in decreased vasodilatory capacity [58, 59]. Increase in FFAs result in an increase in reactive oxygen species (ROS) from NADPH and the mitochondrial electron transport chain [60]. The increase in ROS results in increased PKC which activates the hexosamine biosynthetic pathway leading to increased AGEs and subsequent decrease in endothelial-derived NO [60]. Hyperglycemia has been found to decrease activation of Akt and eNOS via O-GlcNAC of eNOS at the Akt phosphorylation sites [61, 62]. Hyperglycemia increases activation of PKCα, PKCβ, PKCδ resulting in decreased eNOS and concomitant increase in endothelial ET-1 [60]. T2DM is associated with vascular dysfunction as a result of increased atherosclerosis and decreased cerebral blood flow. The combination of both processes is decreased glucose and oxygen supply to vital organs such as the brain. The biochemical events leading to the macrovascular impairment has particular significance to brain health as the risk of stroke is a major complication of T2DM.

Type 2 diabetes and cardiovascular disease T2DM has been shown to be associated with an increased risk of coronary heart disease and stroke [63-66]. Insulin resistance, the mechanism underlying T2DM, has also been linked to a higher incidence and recurrence of stroke [67]. Two key pathological mediators of stroke observed in T2DM are intracranial stenosis [68] and

http://dx.doi.org/10.5772/54913

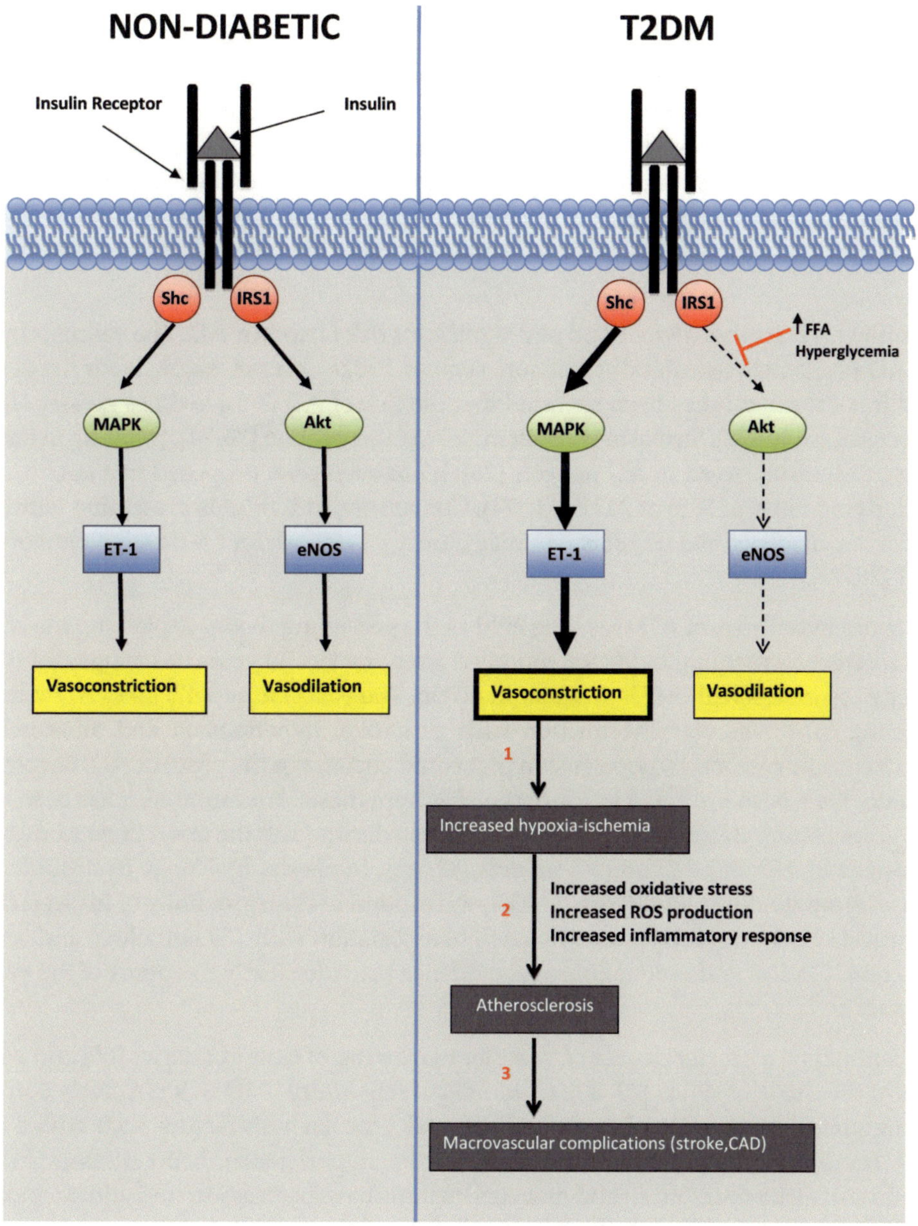

Figure 1. Pathways leading to macrovascular complications of type 2 diabetes mellitus (T2DM). In non-diabetic individuals (*left*), activation of the insulin receptor can result in activation of both vasodilatation and vasoconstriction. Under normative conditions, there is a balance of both processes to regulate the immediate metabolic requirements of various tissues. In type 2 diabetic patients (*right*), factors such as an increase in free fatty acids and hyperglycemia have been shown to specifically inhibit the Akt pathway while the MAPK pathway remains unaffected. This leads to an imbalance in homeostatic regulation of vascular function and hemodynamics (*1*). The resultant decrease in nutrient availability to affected tissues results in an increase in oxidative stress and ROS production and an increased inflammatory response (*2*). Released pro-inflammatory cytokines and macrophage recruitment instigates the onset of atherosclerosis, ultimately leading to macrovascular complications (*3*).

carotid atherosclerosis [69]. Insulin resistance has been associated with elevated expression of the fibrinolytic inhibitor plasminogen activator inhibitor 1 [70] resulting in decreased fibrinoyltic capacity and concurrent increased thrombosis due, in part, to an increase in platelet activation [71]. Insulin resistance has also been shown to induce endothelial dysfunction and inflammation [71], adversely affecting vascular function and initiating atherosclerosis, respectively. Collectively, these data implicate insulin resistance to the impairment of normative cerebrovascular function resulting in the activation of pathways that encourage the onset of stroke. Stroke could, in turn, exacerbate and/or initiate the onset of another disorder such as AD.

Pre-existing CVD has been identified as a significant risk factor for AD. The vascular hypothesis of AD posits that vascular dysfunction, such as stroke, is a pre-requisite for the development of this disorder. It has been reported that the risk of AD is three times greater after the occurrence of stroke [72]. Stroke may result in neurodegeneration [73, 74], resulting in the rapid cognitive decline observed in AD patients [75]. It has even been proposed that stroke may be the underlying cause of 50% of AD cases [74]. Conversely, individuals presenting with severe cognitive impairments, and possibly AD, may be at a greater risk for the development of stroke or CVD [76, 77].

The amyloid hypothesis of AD was long held as the prevailing theory explaining the etiology of AD. However, emerging evidence compiled from the last 20 years has suggested that the pathology associated with AD is vascular in origin. The vascular hypothesis of AD states that pre-existing cardiovascular dysfunction such as stroke, hypertension and atherosclerosis results in chronic cerebral hypoperfusion that could encourage the onset of AD. Several lines of evidence have been provided in support of this hypothesis. For example, it has been shown that cerebrovascular dysfunction precedes cognitive decline and the onset of neurodegenerative changes in AD and AD animal models [12, 13]. In rhesus monkeys, dystrophic axons labeled with amyloidogenic enzyme, BACE1, were found in close proximity or in direct contact with cortical blood vessels [78], asserting a tight association with AD pathology and vascular dysfunction. Clinical and epidemiological evidence provides further support of the vascular hypothesis.

AD patients show a greater degree of vascular narrowing of carotid arteries [65] and cerebral arteries of the Circle of Willis [79, 80]. In addition, large artery CVD was positively correlated to the frequency of neuritic plaques [81]. Several vascular risk factors such stroke (silent infarcts, transient ischemic attacks), atherosclerosis, hypertension, heart disease (coronary artery disease, atrial fibrillation) and diabetes mellitus have been associated with an increased risk AD-type dementia [82]. Between 60 to 90% of AD patients exhibit various cerebrovascular pathologies including White matter lesions, cerebral amyloid angiopathy (CAA), microinfarcts, small infarcts, hemorrhages and microvascular degeneration [12-16]. It believed that cardiovascular dysfunctions act as a nidus for accelerated Aβ deposition resulting in the onset of AD [83].

Aberrant blood brain barrier (BBB) function exposes neurons to neurotoxic substances. Chronic cerebral hypoperfusion is believed to render the brain more vulnerable to various insults, resulting in AD and associated cognitive loss [84]. Clinical observations in AD patients have revealed extensive degeneration of endothelium [85] and features indicative of BBB breakdown [86]. At the cellular level, AD is known to cause abnormal structural changes to arterioles and capillaries, swelling and increased number of pinocytotic vesciles in endothelial cells, decreased mitochondrial content, increased deposition of proteins of the basement membrane, reduced microvascular density and occasional swelling of astrocyte endfeet [87-92]. Aβ trafficking across the BBB deposition is also dependent on mechanisms of influx and efflux. Increased expression of receptor for advanced glycation endproducts (RAGE) may be responsible for Aβ influx from the blood to the brain has been reported in addition to a decrease in LRP1 receptors that are responsible for clearing Aβ from the brain to the blood [12, 93].

A functional consequence associated with BBB dysfunction is the resultant impairment in cerebral hemodynamics. AD impairs autoregulation, the mechanism that is responsible for the stabilization of blood flow to the brain in response to changes in cerebral perfusion pressure [94]. In an APP x PS1 mouse model neurovascular coupling, the process in which activation of a brain region evokes a local increase in blood flow, was impaired [95]. Finally, AD has shown to adversely affect vasomotor/vascular reactivity, the process that mediates vasodilatory or vasoconstrictor responses of cerebral blood vessels to hypercapnic or hypocapnic stimuli (ie. global or regional brain blood flow response to systemic changes in arterial CO_2) [96-98]. Cumulatively, the impairment of these processes adversely affects cerebral blood regulation that, in turn, would negatively affect nutrient availability to neurons. This would result in cerebral hypoperfusion, a process that is widely believed to initiate the onset of AD pathology.

There are a number of known direct links between biochemical pathways central to AD and hypoxia/ischemia. A rat model for vascular cognitive impairment has been developed referred to as the two-vessel occlusion model of cerebral ischemia. Studies found decreased cerebral blood flow up to 4 weeks, cognitive deficits, APP proteolysis to form Aβ-sized fragments [99-101]. Other studies have observed an overexpression of Aβ persisting for up to 3 months after surgery [102] and cognitive impairment [103], strongly suggesting that decreased CBF is a key mediator in the pathophysiology of AD. Several studies have been able to identify some of the molecular mechanisms as to how hypoxia/ischemia exerts its effects on AD-related genes.

APP expression increases following chronic cerebral hypoperfusion and ischemia [104, 105], and a greater proportion of APP is proteolytically cleaved by increased activity of amyloidogenic enzyme, BACE1, which is concurrently increased in AD following ischemic events [106]. Hypoxia inducible factor-1α (HIF-1α) plays an essential role in cellular and systemic responses to low oxygen and has been found to increase BACE1 mRNA expression [107]. Furthermore, BACE1 stabilization is enhanced in AD in addition to a decrease in its trafficking [108, 109]. Increased BACE results in greater γ-secretase-mediated production of Aβ [110]. In an APP overexpressing mouse model, chronic cerebral hypoperfusion as the result of cerebral amyloid angiopathy (pathological deposition of $A\beta_{1-40}$ in brain blood vessels) was followed by an increased rate of leptomeningeal Aβ precipitating the risk of microinfarcts [111]. Hypoxia/

ischemia not only causes increased amyloidogenic cleavage of APP and greater Aβ production, but also impairs Aβ degradation and trafficking [12, 112].

Decreased Aβ-degrading enzymes in response to hypoxic conditions increase the likelihood of developing pathological levels of Aβ in the brain [113-115]. Aβ serves not only as the end result of a pathological cascade, but Aβ itself has been found to contribute to dysfunction in components of the neurovascular unit. In endothelial cells Aβ was observed to decrease endothelial cell proliferation and accelerate senescence of endothelial cells in vivo and in vitro, inhibit VEGF-induced activation of Akt and eNOS in endothelial cells [116, 117]. Aβ has been found to decrease eNOS (via PKC-dependent pathway) resulting in decreased vascular tonus and decreased substance P-induced vasodilation of the basilar artery[118, 119]. In vascular smooth muscle cells (VSMCs), Aβ affects cellular morphological changes [120] and increases expression of transcription factors, serum response factor and myocardin, resulting in decreased Aβ clearance by downregulating LRP expression [12]. Finally, Aβ has been shown to cause retraction and swelling of astrocyte endfeet in an AD mouse model with CAA [121] as well as increase cholinergic denervation of cortical microvessels which, taken together, results in impaired functional hyperemia [122].

Type 2 diabetes and vascular dementia A significant number of population-based studies have indicated an increased risk for the development of dementia attributed to T2DM [23-25]. Due to the importance of insulin in the regulation of several cardiovascular functions, it is unsurprising that insulin resistance plays a role in the cerebrovascular mechanisms of T2DM-induced dementia. The presence of brain infarcts in demented diabetics who did not have AD has been reported 123. Interestingly, the association between T2DM and the development of AD and VaD has been found to be independent of hypertension and hypercholesterolemia [23] indicating that is CVD alone is not sufficient to initiate dementia. Non-cerebrovascular mechanisms such as peripheral hyperinsulinemia and generation of advanced glycation end-products also play in the etiology of T2DM-related dementia [124]. Studies have shown that the increased risk of developing vascular dementia was greater than developing AD in type 2 diabetics [7, 125, 126], indicating that although symptomatically similar and frequently confused [127], their etiologies are distinct.

Vascular dementia versus Alzheimer's dementia The leading cause of dementia is Alzheimer's disease accounting for 70-90% of all cases [127], while vascular dementia (VaD) accounts for the majority of the remaining incidents of dementia [128]. They share common risk factors including hypertension, diabetes mellitus, and hyperlipidemia. [129], highlighting the tight association between these two forms of dementia. In fact, it is now widely believed that AD and VaD are frequently present in the same brain. So-called "mixed dementia" has been observed in elderly people with cardiovascular risk factors in addition to slow progressive cognitive decline [130].

Differing clinical manifestations separate VaD from AD dementia. For example, VaD progression appears more varied than AD in relation to symptoms, its rate of progression and the disease outcome [131]. Increased damage to the ganglia-thalamo-cortical circuits specific to VaD results in problems with attention and the planning and speed of mental processing whereas the primary impairments characteristic of AD are memory and language-related

[132]. It has been suggested that differences in the clinical observations in AD and VaD patients may be due to the type, severity and location of vascular damage [133-135]. Furthermore, perturbations in vascular hemodynamics have been observed in VaD and AD [136, 137], however, AD patients had comparatively less impairment in cerebral perfusion than those with VaD [138] suggesting that hemodynamic disturbances may underlie different types of dementia [138]. While the precise mechanism that vascular risk factors initiate cognitive decline remains elusive [139], T2DM have been identified as an important contributing factor to the development of VaD.

Associations between vascular dementia and Alzheimer's dementia While regarded as two separate conditions, AD and VaD share common cerebrovascular pathologies such as CAA, endothelial cell and vascular smooth muscle cell degeneration, macro- and microinfarcts, hemorrhage and white matter changes [140-142]. These shared pathologies have been shown epidemiologically with almost 35% of AD patients showing evidence of cerebral infarction at autopsy [143, 144], and, conversely, VaD patients display AD-like pathology in the absence of pre-existing AD [145]. It has been postulated that CVD, thought to be the etiology of both disorders, not only result in dementia but also increase the likelihood of individuals with AD-related lesions for developing dementia [146, 147].

3. Insulin signaling in the brain

Insulin/IGF-1 pathway activation. The brain is a major metabolic organ that accounts for ~25% of the body's total glucose use [28, 29]. While glucose uptake in peripheral tissues requires insulin, in the brain this is considered to be an insulin-independent process. Insulin, however, along with Insulin-like Growth Factor-1 (IGF-1), are required for proper brain function as they provide critical neurotrophic support for neurons. IGF-1 and insulin share similar amino acid sequences/ tertiary structures [148] and are known to bind to and activate one anothers' receptors [149]. Both insulin and IGF-1 receptors are tyrosine kinases [150-152] that, when activated, phosphorylate substrate proteins such as IRS. IRS phosphorylation leads to down-stream activation of PI3K and Akt, a serine/threonine kinase and key mediator of insulin/ IFG-1's neurotrophic effects. Neuronal processes known to be, at least in part, under the control of insulin/IGF-1 include regulation of apoptotic proteins, transcription of both survival and pro-death genes, neurite outgrowth, and activity of metabolic proteins.

The source of brain insulin remains controversial. While preproinsulin mRNA has been reported in the neurons [153-155], very little insulin is synthesized in the brain [156]. Additionally, glial cells have been found not to be involved in insulin production [157], therefore, it is recognized that the majority of insulin in the brain is produced by pancreatic β cells [158-161]. In contrast, IGF-1 is produced locally in the brain and does not depend on growth hormone influence as is the case of liver and other tissues [148].

Neuronal insulin receptors are different than those found in the periphery [162]. Insulin receptors are present in one of two isoforms; the IR-A isoform that lacks exon 11 that the other isoform, IR-B, expresses [163, 164]. A major functional difference between the two isoforms is that IR-A has a higher affinity for the neurotrophic factor Insulin-like Growth Factor – 2 (IGF-II) [165] and a slightly higher affinity for insulin [166] and has also been shown to associate/dissociate with insulin quicker than IR-B [149]. Brain specific insulin receptors are mainly the IR-A isoform and as result of differential glycosylation have a lower molecular weight than their peripheral counterparts [162].

Structurally, the insulin receptor is a homodimer composed 2α chains and 2β chains held together with disulphide bonds [167-169]. Insulin receptor binding of insulin/IGF-1 results in a conformational change that activates the catalytic tyrosine kinase activity of the β subunits [170]. This activation of the insulin receptor results in autophosphorylation at multiple tyrosine residues [171, 172] including tyrosine 960 in the juxtamembrane region of the β subunit [173, 174]. Phosphorylation at this site is a vital component of the insulin signaling cascade because it provides a binding motif for the phospho-tyrosine binding (PTB) domain of IRS [173, 174]. Once docked to the insulin receptor, IRS is phosphorylated on tyrosine residues [170].

Tyrosine phosphorylation of IRS proteins creates binding sites for Src homology 2 (SH2) domain containing proteins such as PI3K [175]. PI3K catalyzes the production of 3′phosphoinositide secondary messengers which are critical to the insulin signaling cascade. PI3K is composed of a catalytic p110 subunit and a regulatory p85 subunit that contains SH2 domains that interact with activated IRS [176]. Formation of the IRS/PI3K complex increases the catalytic activity of the p110 subunit [177].

3′phosphoinositides produced by PI3K are important signal conductors that bind to PH (pleckstrin homology) domains on proteins such as IRS [177] and Akt [178]. This interaction is needed to bring IRS and AKT proteins towards the inner layer of the plasma membrane near the juxtamembrane region of the insulin receptor [179] and in close proximity to activating kinases, respectively [180-185]. Furthermore, binding of 3′phosphoinositides is required for Akt to be competent for phosphorylation [184, 186-188].

Akt has two phosphorylation sites, Thr 308 and Ser 473, capable of inducing catalytic activity [189]. PDK1, which also depends on 3′phosphoinosites for its function, phosphorylates Akt at Thr 308 [189, 190].While overexpression of PDK1 has been shown to activate Akt [186], optimal activation of Akt requires additional phosphorylation at Ser 473 by mTORC2 [191] which stabilizes the conformation state of Akt [192].

Akt mediates the neurotrophic effects of insulin/IGF-1, in part, by inhibiting pro-apoptotic machinery [193] and concomitantly activating anti-apoptotic proteins [194-198]. Akt's role in neurotrophic support also involves the regulation of survival transcription factors such as NF-κB [199] and CREB [198] as well as those involved in pro-death gene expression such as the FoxO family [200-202]. Moreover, Akt is involved in production of the neurotrophin BDNF [198], activation of proteins involved in neurite outgrowth (for review see: [203]) and regulation of the metabolic protein GSK-3β [204].

Akt and Bcl-2 family members The Bcl-2 family is a structurally related group of proteins that regulate cell death through effects on the mitochondria [205] (for review see [206, 207]). Bcl-2 members include the pro-apoptotic proteins BID, BIM, PUMA, BAD, NOXA, BAX, and BAK [205] along with anti-apoptotic mediators such as Bcl-2 and Bcl-xL [205]. Because Bcl-2 proteins

http://dx.doi.org/10.5772/54913

possess the ability to form heterodimers with one another [208-210], their regulation of apoptosis can be described as a balancing act in which an increase of anti-apoptotic members leads to survival while increased pro-death proteins result in apoptosis.

Mitochondrial stress incurred by ROS can lead to elevated Ca^{2+} levels in the mitochondrial matrix [211, 212] resulting in increased mitochondrial membrane permeability and release of pro-apoptotic factors such as Cytochrome c, and AIF (apoptosis inducing factor) [213]. Bcl-xL is an anti-apoptotic Bcl-2 family member that prevents Ca^{2+} induced mitochondrial permeability [214]. In the absence of insulin/IGF-1 stimulation, the survival effects of Bcl-xL are blocked as Bcl-xL is complexed with the pro-death Bcl-2 family member Bad [215-217]. Akt liberates Bcl-xL by phosphorylating Bad [195-197, 218] allowing for mitochondrial stabilization.

Mitochondrial permeability marks a critical event in the cell death cascade. Akt promotes cell survival prior to Cytochrome c release through Bcl-xL activity but has also been found to act post apoptotic factor release. When Cytochrome c is released from the mitochondria, it will associate with Apaf-1, dATP and Caspase-9 forming a structure known as the apoptosome (For review see [219]). Formation of the apoptosome activates the proteolytic activity of caspase-9 which cleaves and activates other caspases critical to the apoptotic process [220, 221]. Akt blocks apoptosome formation by phosphorylating Caspase 9 [193].

Bcl-2 is another anti-apoptotic protein under the control of Akt [222]. Bcl-2's role in cell survival is similar to that of Bcl-xL in that in maintains mitochondrial membrane integrity [223]. Mitochondrial permeability has been linked to an oxidized shift in the mitochondria [224] while Bcl-2 has been shown to promote a more reduced state [225]. Up-regulation of Bcl-2 may lead to higher cell reductive capacity [224] which is supported by the observation that Bcl-2 overexpressing cells show increased amounts of NADPH and are resistant to ROS generation [226].

The Bcl-2 promoter contains a cAMP response element site (CRE) that can enhance Bcl-2 expression by binding the transcription factor CREB. Akt is known to phosphorylate CREB which results in increased CREB binding to CBP and increased transcriptional activity [198]. Therefore, the ability of Akt to promote cell survival is mediated, in part, by influence over gene expression such as the up-regulation of Bcl-2 [227-230] and through direct protein interactions such as Bad phosphorylation resulting in Bcl-xL liberation [194-197].

Akt and transcription factor regulation Also under CREB transcriptional control is the neurotrophic factor BDNF [231, 232] which is essential for neuronal development, differentiation, synaptic plasticity, neuroprotection and restoration against a broad range of cellular insults [233]. BDNF has been a focus of AD research for its ability to stimulate non-amyloidogenic APP processing pathways [234, 235] in addition to protecting neuronal cultures against the cytotoxic effects of Aβ [236]. This indicates that decreased insulin signaling resulting in reduced BDNF production may be a contributing factor in AD development. In accordance, AD patients have decreased serum BDNF concentrations compared to healthy, elderly subjects [237-241] while reduced BDNF levels were associated with decreased cognitive performance in healthy individuals [242].

The transcription factor NF-κB is also under Akt control [199]. Like CREB, NF-κB plays critical roles in neuron survival [201, 243, 244] and is also involved in neurite outgrowth, myelin formation and axonal regeneration [245]. Genes for antioxidant proteins such as MnSOD [246] and Cu/ZnSOD [247] and anti-apoptotic proteins Bcl-2 and Bcl-xL are targets of NF-κB [248].

In its inactive form, NF-κB is bound to IκB proteins that sequester it to the cytosol (for review see [249, 250]). NF-κB is activated when IκB proteins are phosphorylated by IκB Kinase (IKK) complexes and targeted for degradation which allows NF-κB to translocate to the nucleus where it binds to regulatory DNA sequences [251]. The IKK complex consists of catalytic IKKα and IKKβ subunits and a regulatory IKKγ subunit [251]. Akt facilitates NF-κB activation by phosphorylating IKKα at a critical regulatory site that promotes IKK activation [252] and subsequent IκB degradation.

Akt influence is not limited to only survival transcription factors but extends to pro-death modulators as well [253, 254].The forkhead box class O (FoxO) family of transcription factors contribute to apoptosis through the induction of pro-death genes such as Fas L [201, 255, 256] and the Bcl-2 member BIM-1 [257]. Fas L facilitates apoptosis by activation of caspases [258] while BIM-1 activates the pro-apoptotic Bcl-2 family memeber BAX [259]. In the absence of Akt, FoxO transcription factors are transcriptionally active in the nucleus [200-202]. Akt phosphorylates FoxO family members at a conserved c-terminal sequence [253] which leads to nuclear exclusion and inhibition of transcriptional activity.

p53,another pro-death transcription factor known to be inactivated by Akt, [260] induces the expression of the pro-apoptotic Bcl-2 family member BAX. BAX proteins form oligomers that insert into the outer mitochondrial membrane which provide a passageway for Cytochrome c and other pro-apoptotic proteins to escape through [261]. Increased p53 activity leading to BAX expression has been linked to neuronal deprivation of neurotrophic factors [262].

Akt and neurite outgrowth Akt effects extend beyond apoptosis regulation as Akt also contributes to neurite outgrowth (for review see [203]). In hippocampal neurons Akt enhances characteristics such as dendritic length/complexity, caliber, and branching [263-267] with similar effects, excluding dendritic length, observed in dorsal root ganglia neurons [268-271]. Akt substrates implicated in neurite outgrowth include GSK-3β [272, 273], CREB [198], mTOR [274], peripherin [275], and β-catenin [276]. Akt may also work in conjunction with other pathways involved in neurite outgrowth. For example, Akt has been found to be complexed with Hsp-27 (heat shock protein) in spinal motor neurons following nerve injury [277] as well as in areas of regeneration following sciatic nerve axotomy [278].

Akt and GSK-3β Activity of the metabolic protein GSK-3β is also influenced by Akt. GSK-3β was originally identified for decreasing glycogen production through inhibition of glycogen synthase [272, 279-281]. However, GSK-3β is also involved in protein synthesis, cell proliferation/differentiation, microtubule dynamics, cell motility and apoptosis. Of particular interest, GSK-3β has also been shown to phosphorylate cytoskeletal associated tau proteins [282] which, in a diseased state, result in protein aggregates known as neurofibrillary tangles [283]. Neurofibrillary tangles have been linked to increased oxidative stress, mitochondrial dysfunction and apoptosis [284, 285] and are the most significant structural correlates of

http://dx.doi.org/10.5772/54913

dementia in AD [286, 287]. IGF-1 protects neurons from ischemic damage by reducing GSK-3β activity [288] which implies a critical role of Akt in GSK- 3β regulation. Indeed, Akt has been shown to inhibit GSK-3β [204] thus demonstrating a direct role of insulin/IGF-1 signaling in the prevention of AD pathology.

Loss of insulin signaling While not a cause of death on its own, loss of insulin signaling in the brain leaves neurons vulnerable to a myriad of insults. Insulin signaling is known to protect against oxidative stress, mitochondrial collapse, over-activity of GSK-3β leading to hyperphosphorylation of tau, activation of death promoting transcription factors and formation of apoptotic structures. Insulin also results in increased BDNF neurotrophic support as well as increased neurite outgrowth.

The mitochondrial permeability transition mediates apoptosis through the release of pro apoptotic factors. Insulin signaling maintains mitochondrial membrane integrity by increasing levels and activity of anti-apoptotic Bcl-2 family members [194-197, 227-230]. In the absence of insulin signaling, the balance of Bcl-2 proteins tips in favor of pro-apoptotic members resulting in cell death. Post mitochondrial collapse, normal insulin signaling can still prevent apoptosis by blocking formation of apoptotic complexes [193, 229] while a state of insulin resistance allows this process to continue unimpeded.

Even under normal circumstances, ROS are produced in respiratory chain reactions in the mitochondria [289]. However, if not properly managed, ROS can cause oxidative damage to proteins, lipids, and nucleic acids. Insulin supplies cells with antioxidant proteins capable of diffusing the oxidative effects of ROS by activating protective transcription factors such as NF-κB [246, 247, 263]. Insulin resistance not only results in reduced antioxidants but also leaves cells susceptible to ROS mediated mitochondrial collapse because of the before mentioned lack of anti-apoptotic Bcl-2 members.

The FoxO family of transcription factors is known to play a role in the cell's response to oxidative stress, however, their prolonged activation results in apoptosis [290]. Insulin signaling inactivates FoxO transcription factors through phosphorylation by Akt. Absence of insulin signaling allows FoxO members to remain in the nucleus and sustain transcription of pro-death genes [201, 255-257].

Insulin resistance is linked to structural changes in AD by overactive GSK-3β. Neurofibrillary tangles are a pathological hallmark of AD [283] and produced by hyperphosphorylation of tau by GSK-3β. Under normal insulin signaling, GSK-3β is inactivated by Akt. Neurofibrillary tangles are one of two significant pathological characteristics of AD the other being accumulation of Aβ [291]. Aβ toxicity and aggregation into plaques has devastating consequences in the brain such as synaptic disruption [292] and inhibition of LTP [293], interference of detoxifying enzymes [294], increased ROS and oxidative stress [295], increased vulnerability to calcium overload [296] and the before mentioned effects on brain vasculature. Aβ also depresses insulin signaling [297] which results in further loss of neurotrophic support. Insulin signaling, on the other, hand is involved in Aβ clearance [298] introducing a convoluted relationship between insulin and Aβ.

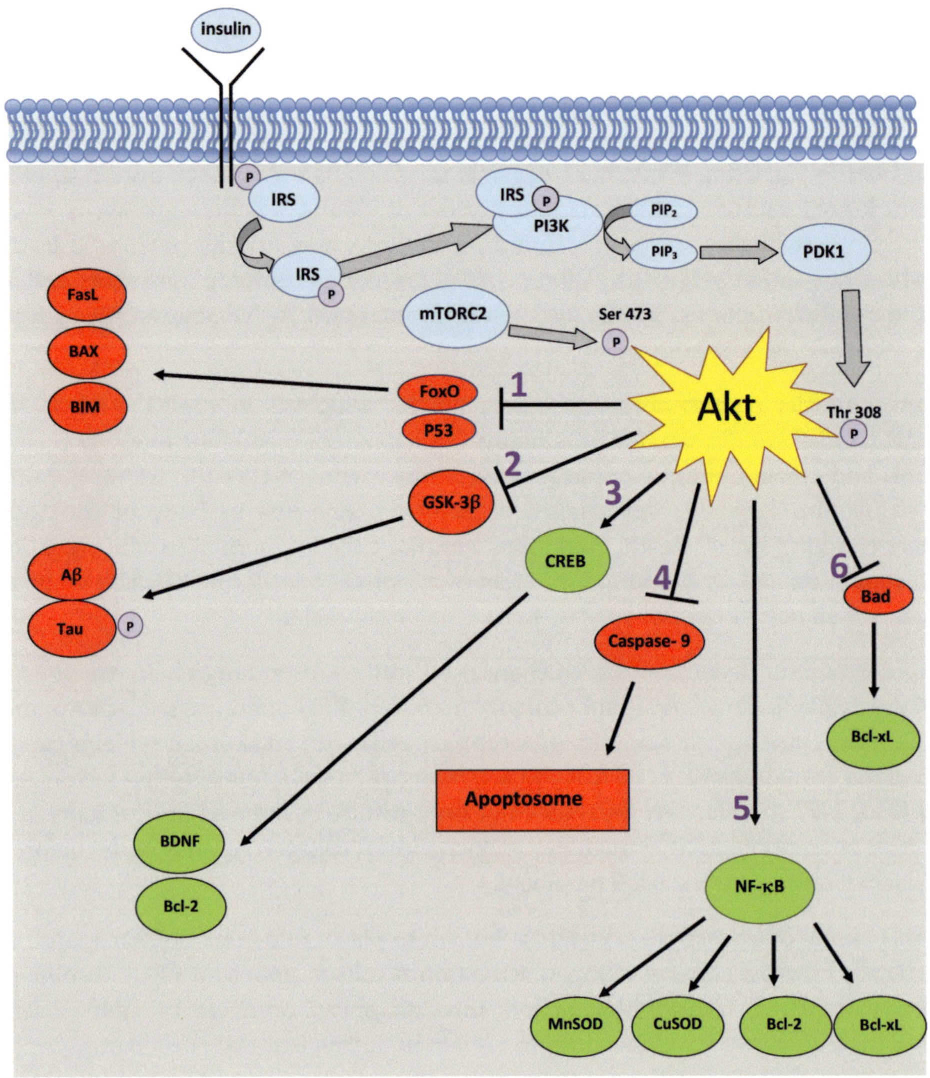

Figure 2. Insulin receptor binding of insulin triggers a complex signaling cascade (in blue) leading to activation of the serine/threonine kinase Akt. Upon binding of insulin, insulin receptors are autophophorylated and subsequently bind IRS proteins. IRS proteins are then phsophorylated by activated insulin receptors and complex with PI3K resulting in PI3K activation. Activated PI3K produces phospholipid secondary messengers by catalyzing the conversion of phosphatidylinositol 4,5-bisphosphate (PIP_2) to phosphatidylinositol 3,4,5-trisphosphate (PIP_3). PIP_3 messengers activate PDK1 which phosphorylates Akt at Threonine 308. Akt is further activated by phosphorylation at Ser 473 by mammalian target of rapamyicin 2 (mTORC2). Targets of activated Akt include pro-apoptotic mediators (in red) as well as pro-survival machinery (in green). Loss of insulin signaling (at sites labeled with numbers 1-6 in purple) allows FoxO and p53 transcription factors to remain active and (1) transcribe genes for pro-apoptotic proteins such as BIM, BAX and FasL. Akt inhibits the activity of GSK-3β that, when active, (2) causes increased amyloidogenic processing and hyperphosphorylation of tau. Other pro-apoptotic proteins inhibited by Akt include (3) caspase-9, which forms an apoptotic structure known as the apoptosome, and (6) Bad, which blocks activity of the ant-apoptotic protein Bcl-xL. Pro-survival modulators regulated by Akt include CREB and NF-κB. Reduction of CREB transcriptional activity as a result of a loss of insulin signaling leads to (4) decreased BDNF and Bcl-2 expression while inhibition of NF-κB leads to (5) reduced expression of anti-oxidants such as MnSOD and CuSOD as well as anti-apoptotic Bcl-2 family members.

4. Generation of Aβ

Background Aβ is a small peptide 38-43 amino acids in size long believed to have a major role in neurodegeneration and pathology of AD (for review see [299]). In sporadic AD (sAD), which accounts for over 90% of AD cases, Aβ's role in pathogensis is still under heavy investigation. The cause of familial AD (fAD), however, has been linked to 3 mutations involved in Aβ processing; presinilins 1 and 2 (PS1/PS2), which are part of Aβ producing complexes, and amyloid precursor protein (APP) from which Aβ is derived [300]. Successive cleavages of APP by β- and γ-secretases produce toxic Aβ peptides (for review see [301]) while cleavage by α-secretase produces the neuroprotective product Secreted APP alpha (sAPPα) [302].

While the physiological role of APP remains unknown, it has been suggested that APP plays a part in neurite outgrowth, synaptogenesis, neuronal trafficking along the axon, transmembrane signal transduction, cell adhesion and calcium metabolism, all of which still require in vivo evidence (for review see [303]). APP concentrations are elevated in the brain during the prenatal period in mice which implies a role of APP in brain development [304]. In the adult brain, APP is expressed in regions of synaptic modification [304] and has been shown to increase hippocampal neuronal response to glutamate [305].

APP belongs to a family of transmembrane proteins that includes APP-like protein 1 and 2 (APPLP1/APPLP2). All APP family members are processed in a similar fashion by α, β, and γ secretases [306-308], however the Aβ domain is unique to APP. Three isoforms of APP have been identified consisting of 695, 751, or 770 amino acids which arise from alternative splicing of the same gene located on chromosome 21 [309]. APP 751 and APP 770 are expressed in most tissues and contain a 56 amino acid Kunitz Protease inhibitor (KPI) domain not found in the neuron specific 695 isoform [310, 311]. mRNA levels of the 2 KPI containing isoforms are elevated in AD brains and are associated with Aβ deposition [312].

Synthesis of APP occurs in the endoplasmic reticulum where it is then transported through the golgi apparatus to the trans golgi network where the highest concentrations of APP are found in neurons [313-315]. From there, APP can be transported in secretory vesicles to the cell surface where α-secretases are located, however, Aβ production occurs within the trans golgi network where γ-secretase complexes are thought to reside [315-318].

APP cleavage Aβ generation requires cleavage of APP by β-secretase which has been indentified to be BACE1 [319-322]. Several studies have found that regions of the brain affected by AD have elevated BACE1 activity and levels [319, 320]. Once identified, BACE1 became a popular therapeutic target for AD treatment. However, BACE1 knockout mice have shown reduced survivability after birth and were smaller than wild-type littermates [323]. BACE1 knockouts also present with hyperactive behavior [323] and other abnormalities such as hypomyelination of peripheral nerves, reduced grip strength and elevated pain sensitivity [324].

APP cleavage by BACE1 results in two fragments: sAPPβ and Beta Carboxyl Terminal Fragment (βCTF) [301, 325]. sAPPβ has been identified as a ligand for Death Receptor 6 which mediates axonal pruning and neuronal death [326]. The remaining βCTF can be cleaved by

γ secretase to produce Aβ [301]. γ-secretase is a complex composed of at least 4 components: PS1 or PS2, nicastrin, anterior pharynx defective-1 (APH-1) and presenilin enhancer-2 (PEN-2) [327, 328]. βCTF cleavage by γ secretase produces either $A\beta_{40}$ or $A\beta_{42}$ peptides [301]. $A\beta_{42}$ is the more hydrophic and amyloidogenic of the 2 species and makes up about 10% of Aβ produced [329]. An increased $A\beta_{42}/A\beta_{40}$ ratio has consistently been shown in fAD patients suggesting that $A\beta_{42}$ is critical to AD pathogensis [330, 331].

5. Aβ and insulin resistance

Aβ depresses insulin signaling Insulin resistance is recognized as a contributing factor in development of AD to the point that AD has been referred to as "type 3 diabetes" [4, 5]. This coincides with Aβ being a pathological hallmark of AD as Aβ contributes to insulin resistance [297]. Aβ oligomers are known impair insulin signaling in neurons [332] by competing with insulin for receptor binding sites [297] and studies have linked Aβ oligomers to decreased insulin receptor numbers [332].

Development of insulin resistance provides neurons with a dangerous dilemma as neurons rely on insulin signaling for Aβ clearance and inhibition of amyloidogenic processing. Insulin increases Aβ trafficking from the trans golgi-network leading to secretion [333]. Secretion of Aβ may be important in preventing neurodegeneration as intraneural Aβ accumulations have been found in brain regions prone to early AD in patients with mild cognitive impairment [334] and studies done with transgenic mice indicate that intracellular Aβ accumulation is an early event of the neuropathological phenotype [335-337]. Insulin signalling protects against Aβ toxicity [298] and inhibits GSK-3β activity [204] which, in addition to hyperphosphorylating tau, promotes amyloidogenic APP cleavage [160, 338].

Insulin signaling pathways in the brain are complex and depend on a delicate balance of cell activity to function properly. Accumulation of Aβ perturbs this balance resulting in insulin resistance and formation of a vicious cycle as insulin signaling is no longer able to clear and regulate Aβ. As Aβ oligomers increase, insulin resistance worsens. This cycle is perpetuated by competition between insulin and Aβ as substrates for IDE.

Insulin, Aβ and insulin degrading enzyme IDE is responsible for insulin degradation but has also been shown to degrade Aβ peptides [339-341], a process known to be decreased in AD brains [318]. Studies have shown that increased insulin signaling can increase levels of IDE [44] which can be abolished by pharmacological inhibition of PI3K. Aβ can decrease PI3K activity, [342] and thus is able to prevent its own degradation. In cases of hyperinsulinemia, excess insulin blocks IDE binding sites which further diminishes Aβ degradation [115].

In summary, Aβ contributes to insulin resistance [297, 332] by occupying binding sites on insulin receptors [297] and is associated with decreased insulin receptor numbers in neurons [332]. Decreases in insulin signaling result in increased Aβ processing as well as activation of GSK-3β which promotes Aβ processing [160, 338]. Insulin signaling impairment also leads to decreased IDE, which is needed to degrade Aβ [339-341, 343]. IDE deficiencies are exacerbated in hyperinsulinemic conditions as IDE binding sites are overloaded with excess insulin and made unavailable for Aβ [115]. Lack of insulin signaling and IDE availability allows for continued accumulation of Aβ, further depression of insulin signaling systems, increased neuronal vulnerability and further neurodegeneration.

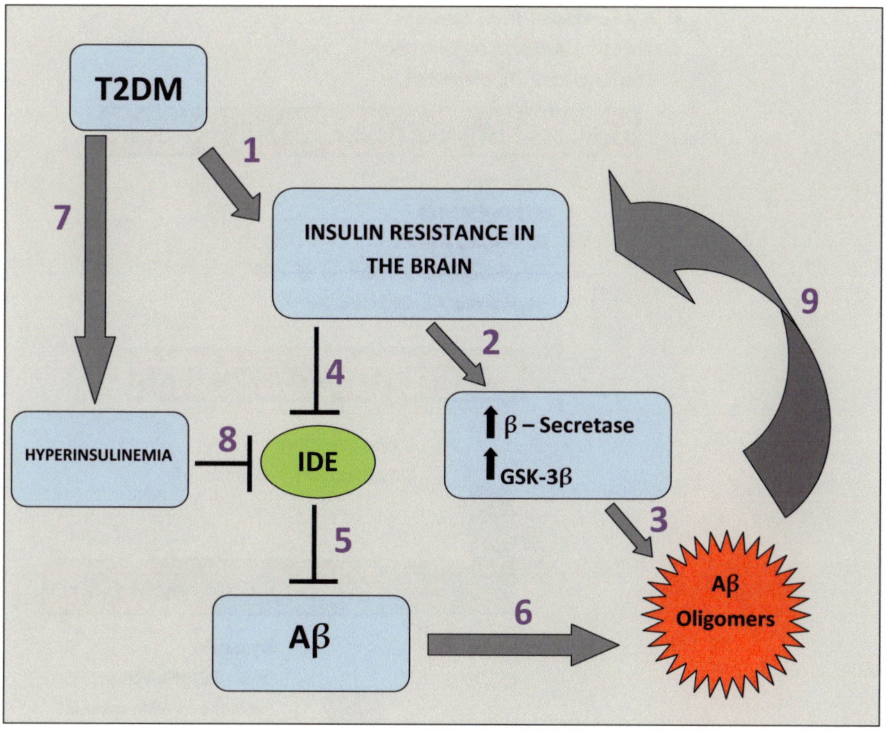

Figure 3. T2DM can lead to the induction of insulin resistance in the brain. (2) Reduction of insulin signaling in the brain increases the activities of GSK-3β and β secretases which (3) increase levels of toxic Aβ oligomers. Furthermore, (4) insulin resistance lowers the expression of Aβ-degrading IDE. (5) Reduced IDE then leads to increased Aβ and (6) accumulation of Aβ oligomers. T2DM also causes (7) hyperinsulinemia which exacerbates IDE deficiencies because (8) excess insulin occupies IDE binding sites rendering them unavailable for Aβ. The increased amyloidogenic processing that occurs in insulin resistance combined with decreased Aβ clearance by IDE results in a deleterious positive-feedback cycle as (9) Aβ oligomers contribute to insulin resistance in the brain. As Aβ levels continue to rise, insulin resistance worsens leading to further production of the toxic peptide.

6. Conclusion

By 2050 it's estimated that over 100 million people worldwide will have AD [344] causing a substantial financial burden for health care systems. In that same time span, the annual cost of treating AD is predicated to exceed $1 trillion in the United States alone [345]. These crippling social and economical effects place increased priority for advancement of AD research.

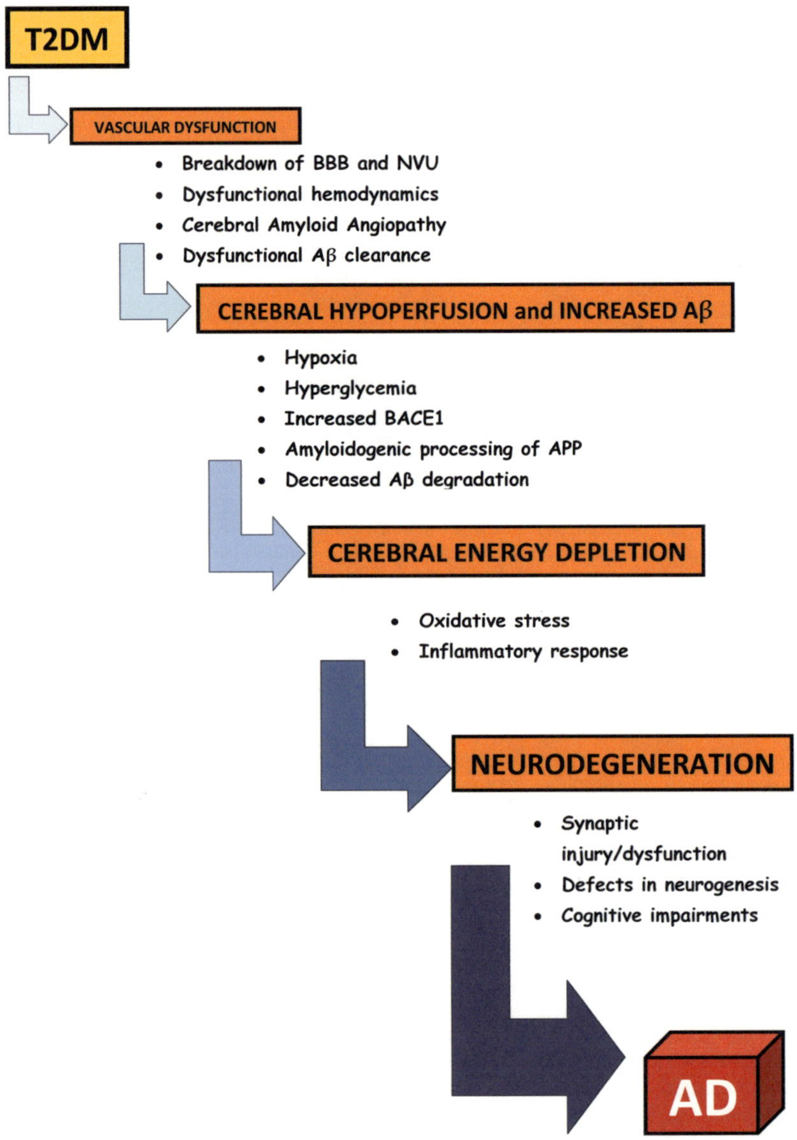

Figure 4. Vascular hypothesis of AD. The vascular complications have been casually linked to the progression of AD. Vascular dysfunction resulting from type 2 diabetes results in a state of cerebral hypoperfusion, leading to significant energy depletion in the brain. Neurodegeneration results in cognitive impairments and ultimately AD.

While AD remains a disease of more questions than answers, a wide array of evidence suggests a close relationship between AD and T2DM. T2DM has been characterized as having both macrovascular and microvascular complications that result in CVD. It is the vasculature that provides the tangible pathological link between T2DM and AD. Significant data has been collected in favor of the vascular hypothesis of AD, which is founded on the idea that pre-existing CVD sets into motion pathological cascades that ultimately result in AD.

AD and T2DM also share commonality in the form of insulin resistance. Lack of insulin neurotrophic support in the brain leaves neurons defenseless against oxidative stress, Aβ toxicity and apoptosis. Aβ is especially dangerous to neurons because it further depresses insulin signaling and can alter levels of protective enzymes involved in its degradation such as IDE. AD is a disease that not only causes death in weakened cells but also further depresses protective mechanisms making recovery unattainable.

Because AD affects multiple structures and pathways, it is likely that successful treatment will involve a comprehensive battery of therapeutics rather than a single therapy. T2DM plays a major role in vascular abnormalities and insulin resistance which parallel AD pathologies. As a result, further exploration of the relationship between T2DM and AD may be a promising direction of future research. Moreover, preventative measures against T2DM such as proper diet and dedication to an active lifestyle may take center stage as a means of curbing the AD epidemic.

Author details

Brent D. Aulston[1,2], Gary L. Odero[1], Zaid Aboud[1,2] and Gordon W. Glazner[1,2]

1 St. Boniface Hospital Research Centre, Winnipeg, MB, Canada

2 Department of Pharmacology and Therapeutics, University of Manitoba, Winnipeg, MB, Canada

References

[1] Ott, A, et al. Diabetes mellitus and the risk of dementia: The Rotterdam Study. Neurology, (1999)., 1937-1942.

[2] Ritchie, K, & Lovestone, S. The dementias. Lancet, (2002)., 1759-1766.

[3] Frolich, L, et al. A disturbance in the neuronal insulin receptor signal transduction in sporadic Alzheimer's disease. Ann N Y Acad Sci, (1999)., 290-293.

[4] Rivera, E. J, et al. Insulin and insulin-like growth factor expression and function deteriorate with progression of Alzheimer's disease: link to brain reductions in acetylcholine. J Alzheimers Dis, (2005)., 247-268.

[5] Steen, E, et al. Impaired insulin and insulin-like growth factor expression and signaling mechanisms in Alzheimer's disease--is this type 3 diabetes? J Alzheimers Dis, (2005)., 63-80.

[6] Sinclair, A. J, Girling, A. J, & Bayer, A. J. Cognitive dysfunction in older subjects with diabetes mellitus: impact on diabetes self-management and use of care services. All Wales Research into Elderly (AWARE) Study. Diabetes Res Clin Pract, (2000). , 203-212.

[7] Peila, R, Rodriguez, B. L, & Launer, L. J. Type 2 diabetes, APOE gene, and the risk for dementia and related pathologies: The Honolulu-Asia Aging Study. Diabetes, (2002). , 1256-1262.

[8] Kannel, W. B, & Mcgee, D. L. Diabetes and cardiovascular disease. The Framingham study. JAMA, (1979). , 2035-2038.

[9] Stratton, I. M, et al. Association of glycaemia with macrovascular and microvascular complications of type 2 diabetes (UKPDS 35): prospective observational study. BMJ, (2000). , 405-412.

[10] Defronzo, R. A. Pharmacologic therapy for type 2 diabetes mellitus. Ann Intern Med, (2000). , 73-74.

[11] Buse, J. B, et al. Primary prevention of cardiovascular diseases in people with diabetes mellitus: a scientific statement from the American Heart Association and the American Diabetes Association. Diabetes Care, (2007). , 162-172.

[12] Bell, R. D, et al. SRF and myocardin regulate LRP-mediated amyloid-beta clearance in brain vascular cells. Nat Cell Biol, (2009). , 143-153.

[13] De La Torre, J. C. Is Alzheimer's disease a neurodegenerative or a vascular disorder? Data, dogma, and dialectics. Lancet Neurol, (2004). , 184-190.

[14] Formichi, P, et al. CSF Biomarkers Profile in CADASIL-A Model of Pure Vascular Dementia: Usefulness in Differential Diagnosis in the Dementia Disorder. Int J Alzheimers Dis, 2010. (2010).

[15] Jagust, W. J, et al. The Alzheimer's Disease Neuroimaging Initiative positron emission tomography core. Alzheimers Dement, (2010). , 221-229.

[16] Pakrasi, S, & Brien, J. T. O. Emission tomography in dementia. Nucl Med Commun, (2005). , 189-196.

[17] Kahn, A. M, et al. Insulin acutely inhibits cultured vascular smooth muscle cell contraction by a nitric oxide synthase-dependent pathway. Hypertension, (1997). , 928-933.

[18] Bolotina, V. M, et al. Nitric oxide directly activates calcium-dependent potassium channels in vascular smooth muscle. Nature, (1994). , 850-853.

[19] Potenza, M. A, et al. Insulin resistance in spontaneously hypertensive rats is associated with endothelial dysfunction characterized by imbalance between NO and ET-1 production. Am J Physiol Heart Circ Physiol, (2005). , H813-H822.

[20] Potenza, M. A, et al. Treatment of spontaneously hypertensive rats with rosiglitazone and/or enalapril restores balance between vasodilator and vasoconstrictor actions of

insulin with simultaneous improvement in hypertension and insulin resistance. Diabetes, (2006)., 3594-3603.

[21] Formoso, G, et al. Dehydroepiandrosterone mimics acute actions of insulin to stimulate production of both nitric oxide and endothelin 1 via distinct phosphatidylinositol 3-kinase- and mitogen-activated protein kinase-dependent pathways in vascular endothelium. Mol Endocrinol, (2006)., 1153-1163.

[22] Wild, S, et al. Global prevalence of diabetes: estimates for the year 2000 and projections for 2030. Diabetes Care, (2004)., 1047-1053.

[23] Biessels, G. J, et al. Risk of dementia in diabetes mellitus: a systematic review. Lancet Neurol, (2006)., 64-74.

[24] Lu, F. P, Lin, K. P, & Kuo, H. K. Diabetes and the risk of multi-system aging phenotypes: a systematic review and meta-analysis. PLoS One, (2009)., e4144.

[25] Profenno, L. A, Porsteinsson, A. P, & Faraone, S. V. Meta-analysis of Alzheimer's disease risk with obesity, diabetes, and related disorders. Biol Psychiatry, (2012). , 505-512.

[26] Ahtiluoto, S, et al. Diabetes, Alzheimer disease, and vascular dementia: a population-based neuropathologic study. Neurology, (2010)., 1195-1202.

[27] Kalaria, R. N. Neurodegenerative disease: Diabetes, microvascular pathology and Alzheimer disease. Nat Rev Neurol, (2009)., 305-306.

[28] Zlokovic, B. V. The blood-brain barrier in health and chronic neurodegenerative disorders. Neuron, (2008)., 178-201.

[29] Zlokovic, B. V. Neurovascular pathways to neurodegeneration in Alzheimer's disease and other disorders. Nat Rev Neurosci, (2011)., 723-738.

[30] Moskowitz, M. A, Lo, E. H, & Iadecola, C. The science of stroke: mechanisms in search of treatments. Neuron, (2010)., 181-198.

[31] Beckman, J. A, Creager, M. A, & Libby, P. Diabetes and atherosclerosis: epidemiology, pathophysiology, and management. JAMA, (2002)., 2570-2581.

[32] Masters, S. L, Latz, E, & Neill, L. A. O. The inflammasome in atherosclerosis and type 2 diabetes. Sci Transl Med, (2011)., 81ps17.

[33] Klein, R. Hyperglycemia and microvascular and macrovascular disease in diabetes. Diabetes Care, (1995)., 258-268.

[34] Turner, R. C, et al. Risk factors for coronary artery disease in non-insulin dependent diabetes mellitus: United Kingdom Prospective Diabetes Study (UKPDS: 23). BMJ, (1998)., 823-828.

[35] Kuusisto, J, et al. NIDDM and its metabolic control predict coronary heart disease in elderly subjects. Diabetes, (1994)., 960-967.

[36] Lehto, S, et al. Predictors of stroke in middle-aged patients with non-insulin-dependent diabetes. Stroke, (1996). , 63-68.

[37] Cheng, G, et al. Diabetes as a risk factor for dementia and mild cognitive impairment: a meta-analysis of longitudinal studies. Intern Med J, (2012). , 484-491.

[38] Janson, J, et al. Increased risk of type 2 diabetes in Alzheimer disease. Diabetes, (2004). , 474-481.

[39] Leibson, C. L, et al. Risk of dementia among persons with diabetes mellitus: a population-based cohort study. Am J Epidemiol, (1997). , 301-308.

[40] Pansari, K, Gupta, A, & Thomas, P. Alzheimer's disease and vascular factors: facts and theories. Int J Clin Pract, (2002). , 197-203.

[41] De La Monte, S. M. Insulin resistance and Alzheimer's disease. BMB Rep, (2009). , 475-481.

[42] Kim, B, & Feldman, E. L. Insulin resistance in the nervous system. Trends Endocrinol Metab, (2012). , 133-141.

[43] Kim, B, et al. Cortical neurons develop insulin resistance and blunted Akt signaling: a potential mechanism contributing to enhanced ischemic injury in diabetes. Antioxid Redox Signal, (2011). , 1829-1839.

[44] Zhao, Z, et al. Insulin degrading enzyme activity selectively decreases in the hippocampal formation of cases at high risk to develop Alzheimer's disease. Neurobiol Aging, (2007). , 824-830.

[45] Stocker, R, & Keaney, J. F. Jr., Role of oxidative modifications in atherosclerosis. Physiol Rev, (2004). , 1381-1478.

[46] Jiang, Z. Y, et al. Characterization of selective resistance to insulin signaling in the vasculature of obese Zucker (fa/fa) rats. J Clin Invest, (1999). , 447-457.

[47] Cusi, K, et al. Insulin resistance differentially affects the PI 3-kinase- and MAP kinase-mediated signaling in human muscle. J Clin Invest, (2000). , 311-320.

[48] Piatti, P. M, et al. Hypertriglyceridemia and hyperinsulinemia are potent inducers of endothelin-1 release in humans. Diabetes, (1996). , 316-321.

[49] Sarkar, R, et al. Nitric oxide reversibly inhibits the migration of cultured vascular smooth muscle cells. Circ Res, (1996). , 225-230.

[50] Kubes, P, Suzuki, M, & Granger, D. N. Nitric oxide: an endogenous modulator of leukocyte adhesion. Proc Natl Acad Sci U S A, (1991). , 4651-4655.

[51] Zeiher, A. M, et al. Nitric oxide modulates the expression of monocyte chemoattractant protein 1 in cultured human endothelial cells. Circ Res, (1995). , 980-986.

[52] Nomura, S, et al. Significance of chemokines and activated platelets in patients with diabetes. Clin Exp Immunol, (2000). , 437-443.

[53] Collins, T, & Cybulsky, M. I. NF-kappaB: pivotal mediator or innocent bystander in atherogenesis? J Clin Invest, (2001). , 255-264.

[54] Petersen, K. F, & Shulman, G. I. Etiology of insulin resistance. Am J Med, (2006). Suppl 1): , S10-S16.

[55] Roden, M, et al. Mechanism of free fatty acid-induced insulin resistance in humans. J Clin Invest, (1996). , 2859-2865.

[56] Steinberg, H. O, & Baron, A. D. Vascular function, insulin resistance and fatty acids. Diabetologia, (2002). , 623-634.

[57] Wang, X. L, et al. Free fatty acids inhibit insulin signaling-stimulated endothelial nitric oxide synthase activation through upregulating PTEN or inhibiting Akt kinase. Diabetes, (2006). , 2301-2310.

[58] Naruse, K, et al. Activation of vascular protein kinase C-beta inhibits Akt-dependent endothelial nitric oxide synthase function in obesity-associated insulin resistance. Diabetes, (2006). , 691-698.

[59] Kim, F, et al. Free fatty acid impairment of nitric oxide production in endothelial cells is mediated by IKKbeta. Arterioscler Thromb Vasc Biol, (2005). , 989-994.

[60] Muniyappa, R, et al. Cardiovascular actions of insulin. Endocr Rev, (2007). , 463-491.

[61] Du, X. L, et al. Hyperglycemia inhibits endothelial nitric oxide synthase activity by posttranslational modification at the Akt site. J Clin Invest, (2001). , 1341-1348.

[62] Schnyder, B, et al. Rapid effects of glucose on the insulin signaling of endothelial NO generation and epithelial Na transport. Am J Physiol Endocrinol Metab, (2002). , E87-E94.

[63] Barba, R, et al. Poststroke dementia : clinical features and risk factors. Stroke, (2000). , 1494-1501.

[64] Breteler, M. M. Vascular risk factors for Alzheimer's disease: an epidemiologic perspective. Neurobiol Aging, (2000). , 153-160.

[65] Hofman, A, et al. Atherosclerosis, apolipoprotein E, and prevalence of dementia and Alzheimer's disease in the Rotterdam Study. Lancet, (1997). , 151-154.

[66] Barnes, D. E, & Yaffe, K. The projected effect of risk factor reduction on Alzheimer's disease prevalence. Lancet Neurol, (2011). , 819-828.

[67] Arenillas, J. F, et al. Metabolic syndrome and resistance to IV thrombolysis in middle cerebral artery ischemic stroke. Neurology, (2008). , 190-195.

[68] De Angelis, M, et al. Prevalence of carotid stenosis in type 2 diabetic patients asymptomatic for cerebrovascular disease. Diabetes Nutr Metab, (2003). , 48-55.

[69] Letonja, M. S, et al. Association of the C242T polymorphism in the NADPH oxidase phox gene with carotid atherosclerosis in Slovenian patients with type 2 diabetes. Mol Biol Rep, (2012). , 22.

[70] Palomo, I, et al. Hemostasis alterations in metabolic syndrome (review). Int J Mol Med, (2006). , 969-974.

[71] Alessi, M. C, & Juhan-vague, I. Metabolic syndrome, haemostasis and thrombosis. Thromb Haemost, (2008). , 995-1000.

[72] Kalaria, R. N, & Ballard, C. Overlap between pathology of Alzheimer disease and vascular dementia. Alzheimer Dis Assoc Disord, (1999). Suppl 3: , S115-S123.

[73] Henon, H, et al. Preexisting dementia in stroke patients. Baseline frequency, associated factors, and outcome. Stroke, (1997). , 2429-2436.

[74] Kokmen, E, et al. Dementia after ischemic stroke: a population-based study in Rochester, Minnesota (1960-1984). Neurology, (1996). , 154-159.

[75] Pasquier, F, Leys, D, & Scheltens, P. The influence of coincidental vascular pathology on symptomatology and course of Alzheimer's disease. J Neural Transm Suppl, (1998). , 117-127.

[76] Ferrucci, L, et al. Cognitive impairment and risk of stroke in the older population. J Am Geriatr Soc, (1996). , 237-241.

[77] Gale, C. R, Martyn, C. N, & Cooper, C. Cognitive impairment and mortality in a cohort of elderly people. BMJ, (1996). , 608-611.

[78] Cai, Y, et al. beta-Secretase-1 elevation in aged monkey and Alzheimer's disease human cerebral cortex occurs around the vasculature in partnership with multisystem axon terminal pathogenesis and beta-amyloid accumulation. Eur J Neurosci, (2010). , 1223-1238.

[79] Beach, T. G, et al. Circle of Willis atherosclerosis: association with Alzheimer's disease, neuritic plaques and neurofibrillary tangles. Acta Neuropathol, (2007). , 13-21.

[80] Roher, A. E, et al. Circle of willis atherosclerosis is a risk factor for sporadic Alzheimer's disease. Arterioscler Thromb Vasc Biol, (2003). , 2055-2062.

[81] Honig, L. S, Kukull, W, & Mayeux, R. Atherosclerosis and AD: analysis of data from the US National Alzheimer's Coordinating Center. Neurology, (2005). , 494-500.

[82] Grammas, P. Neurovascular dysfunction, inflammation and endothelial activation: implications for the pathogenesis of Alzheimer's disease. J Neuroinflammation, (2011). , 26.

[83] Kawai, M, et al. The relationship of amyloid plaques to cerebral capillaries in Alzheimer's disease. Am J Pathol, (1990). , 1435-1446.

[84] Kalaria, R. N. The role of cerebral ischemia in Alzheimer's disease. Neurobiol Aging, (2000). , 321-330.

[85] Kalaria, R. N, & Hedera, P. Differential degeneration of the cerebral microvasculature in Alzheimer's disease. Neuroreport, (1995). , 477-480.

[86] De La Torre, J. C. Cerebromicrovascular pathology in Alzheimer's disease compared to normal aging. Gerontology, (1997). , 26-43.

[87] Buee, L, et al. Pathological alterations of the cerebral microvasculature in Alzheimer's disease and related dementing disorders. Acta Neuropathol, (1994). , 469-480.

[88] Christov, A, et al. Structural changes in Alzheimer's disease brain microvessels. Curr Alzheimer Res, (2008). , 392-395.

[89] Davies, D. C, & Hardy, J. A. Blood brain barrier in ageing and Alzheimer's disease. Neurobiol Aging, (1988). , 46-48.

[90] Kalaria, R. N, & Pax, A. B. Increased collagen content of cerebral microvessels in Alzheimer's disease. Brain Res, (1995). , 349-352.

[91] Masters, C. L, & Beyreuther, K. The blood-brain barrier in Alzheimer's disease and normal aging. Neurobiol Aging, (1988). , 43-44.

[92] Claudio, L. Ultrastructural features of the blood-brain barrier in biopsy tissue from Alzheimer's disease patients. Acta Neuropathol, (1996). , 6-14.

[93] Yan, S. D, et al. RAGE and amyloid-beta peptide neurotoxicity in Alzheimer's disease. Nature, (1996). , 685-691.

[94] Van Beek, A. H, et al. Cerebral autoregulation: an overview of current concepts and methodology with special focus on the elderly. J Cereb Blood Flow Metab, (2008). , 1071-1085.

[95] Rancillac, A, Geoffroy, H, & Rossier, J. Impaired neurovascular coupling in the APPxPS1 mouse model of Alzheimer's disease. Curr Alzheimer Res, (2012).

[96] Claassen, J. A, et al. Transcranial Doppler estimation of cerebral blood flow and cerebrovascular conductance during modified rebreathing. J Appl Physiol, (2007). , 870-877.

[97] Lee, S. T, Jung, K. H, & Lee, Y. S. Decreased vasomotor reactivity in Alzheimer's disease. J Clin Neurol, (2007). , 18-23.

[98] Menendez-gonzalez, M, et al. Vasomotor reactivity is similarly impaired in patients with Alzheimer's disease and patients with amyloid hemorrhage. J Neuroimaging, (2011). , e83-e85.

[99] Barone, F. C, et al. Vascular cognitive impairment: dementia biology and translational animal models. Curr Opin Investig Drugs, (2009). , 624-637.

[100] Farkas, E, Luiten, P. G, & Bari, F. Permanent, bilateral common carotid artery occlusion in the rat: a model for chronic cerebral hypoperfusion-related neurodegenerative diseases. Brain Res Rev, (2007). , 162-180.

[101] Vicente, E, et al. Astroglial and cognitive effects of chronic cerebral hypoperfusion in the rat. Brain Res, (2009). , 204-212.

[102] Liu, H, et al. Regulation of beta-amyloid level in the brain of rats with cerebrovascular hypoperfusion. Neurobiol Aging, (2011). e31-42., 826.

[103] Zhiyou, C, et al. Upregulation of BACE1 and beta-amyloid protein mediated by chronic cerebral hypoperfusion contributes to cognitive impairment and pathogenesis of Alzheimer's disease. Neurochem Res, (2009). , 1226-1235.

[104] Kalaria, R. N, et al. The amyloid precursor protein in ischemic brain injury and chronic hypoperfusion. Ann N Y Acad Sci, (1993). , 190-193.

[105] Stephenson, D. T, Rash, K, & Clemens, J. A. Amyloid precursor protein accumulates in regions of neurodegeneration following focal cerebral ischemia in the rat. Brain Res, (1992). , 128-135.

[106] Wen, Y, et al. Increased beta-secretase activity and expression in rats following transient cerebral ischemia. Brain Res, (2004). , 1-8.

[107] Zhang, X, et al. Hypoxia-inducible factor 1alpha (HIF-1alpha)-mediated hypoxia increases BACE1 expression and beta-amyloid generation. J Biol Chem, (2007). , 10873-10880.

[108] Tesco, G, et al. Depletion of GGA3 stabilizes BACE and enhances beta-secretase activity. Neuron, (2007). , 721-737.

[109] Zhang, Y, et al. Mutant ubiquitin-mediated beta-secretase stability via activation of caspase-3 is related to beta-amyloid accumulation in ischemic striatum in rats. J Cereb Blood Flow Metab, (2010). , 566-575.

[110] Li, L, et al. Hypoxia increases Abeta generation by altering beta- and gamma-cleavage of APP. Neurobiol Aging, (2009). , 1091-1098.

[111] Okamoto, Y, et al. Cerebral hypoperfusion accelerates cerebral amyloid angiopathy and promotes cortical microinfarcts. Acta Neuropathol, (2012). , 381-394.

[112] Deane, R, et al. RAGE mediates amyloid-beta peptide transport across the blood-brain barrier and accumulation in brain. Nat Med, (2003). , 907-913.

[113] Miners, J. S, et al. Decreased expression and activity of neprilysin in Alzheimer disease are associated with cerebral amyloid angiopathy. J Neuropathol Exp Neurol, (2006). , 1012-1021.

[114] Weeraratna, A. T, et al. Alterations in immunological and neurological gene expression patterns in Alzheimer's disease tissues. Exp Cell Res, (2007). , 450-461.

[115] Qiu, W. Q, & Folstein, M. F. Insulin, insulin-degrading enzyme and amyloid-beta peptide in Alzheimer's disease: review and hypothesis. Neurobiol Aging, (2006). , 190-198.

[116] Hayashi, S, et al. Alzheimer disease-associated peptide, amyloid beta40, inhibits vascular regeneration with induction of endothelial autophagy. Arterioscler Thromb Vasc Biol, (2009). , 1909-1915.

[117] Donnini, S, et al. Abeta peptides accelerate the senescence of endothelial cells in vitro and in vivo, impairing angiogenesis. FASEB J, (2010). , 2385-2395.

[118] Gentile, M. T, et al. Mechanisms of soluble beta-amyloid impairment of endothelial function. J Biol Chem, (2004). , 48135-48142.

[119] Huang, Z, et al. Enlarged infarcts in endothelial nitric oxide synthase knockout mice are attenuated by nitro-L-arginine. J Cereb Blood Flow Metab, (1996). , 981-987.

[120] Christie, R, et al. Structural and functional disruption of vascular smooth muscle cells in a transgenic mouse model of amyloid angiopathy. Am J Pathol, (2001). , 1065-1071.

[121] Merlini, M, et al. Vascular beta-amyloid and early astrocyte alterations impair cerebrovascular function and cerebral metabolism in transgenic arcAbeta mice. Acta Neuropathol, (2008). , 293-311.

[122] Tong, P, et al. Insulin-induced cortical actin remodeling promotes GLUT4 insertion at muscle cell membrane ruffles. J Clin Invest, (2001). , 371-381.

[123] Arvanitakis, Z, et al. Diabetes is related to cerebral infarction but not to AD pathology in older persons. Neurology, (2006). , 1960-1965.

[124] Luchsinger, J. A. Type 2 diabetes, related conditions, in relation and dementia: an opportunity for prevention? J Alzheimers Dis, (2010). , 723-736.

[125] Curb, J. D, et al. Longitudinal association of vascular and Alzheimer's dementias, diabetes, and glucose tolerance. Neurology, (1999). , 971-975.

[126] Xu, W. L, et al. Diabetes mellitus and risk of dementia in the Kungsholmen project: a 6-year follow-up study. Neurology, (2004). , 1181-1186.

[127] Brookmeyer, R, Gray, S, & Kawas, C. Projections of Alzheimer's disease in the United States and the public health impact of delaying disease onset. Am J Public Health, (1998). , 1337-1342.

[128] Clark, C. M, et al. Earlier onset of Alzheimer disease symptoms in latino individuals compared with anglo individuals. Arch Neurol, (2005). , 774-778.

[129] Korczyn, A. D. Mixed dementia--the most common cause of dementia. Ann N Y Acad Sci, (2002). , 129-134.

[130] Goldberg, I, et al. Microembolism, silent brain infarcts and dementia. J Neurol Sci, (2012).

[131] Erkinjuntti, T. Clinical deficits of Alzheimer's disease with cerebrovascular disease and probable VaD. Int J Clin Pract Suppl, (2001). , 14-23.

[132] Roman, G. C, & Royall, D. R. Executive control function: a rational basis for the diagnosis of vascular dementia. Alzheimer Dis Assoc Disord, (1999). Suppl 3: , S69-S80.

[133] Barber, R, et al. White matter lesions on magnetic resonance imaging in dementia with Lewy bodies, Alzheimer's disease, vascular dementia, and normal aging. J Neurol Neurosurg Psychiatry, (1999). , 66-72.

[134] Cordonnier, C, et al. Prevalence and severity of microbleeds in a memory clinic setting. Neurology, (2006). , 1356-1360.

[135] Zarei, M, et al. Regional white matter integrity differentiates between vascular dementia and Alzheimer disease. Stroke, (2009). , 773-779.

[136] Cacabelos, R, et al. Cerebrovascular risk factors in Alzheimer's disease: brain hemodynamics and pharmacogenomic implications. Neurol Res, (2003). , 567-580.

[137] Gorelick, P. B. Risk factors for vascular dementia and Alzheimer disease. Stroke, (2004). Suppl 1): , 2620-2622.

[138] Sabayan, B, et al. Cerebrovascular hemodynamics in Alzheimer's disease and vascular dementia: a meta-analysis of transcranial Doppler studies. Ageing Res Rev, (2012). , 271-277.

[139] Altman, R, & Rutledge, J. C. The vascular contribution to Alzheimer's disease. Clin Sci (Lond), (2010). , 407-421.

[140] Vinters, H. V. Cerebral amyloid angiopathy. A critical review. Stroke, (1987). , 311-324.

[141] Kalaria, R. N, et al. Production and increased detection of amyloid beta protein and amyloidogenic fragments in brain microvessels, meningeal vessels and choroid plexus in Alzheimer's disease. Brain Res Mol Brain Res, (1996). , 58-68.

[142] Kosunen, O, et al. Diagnostic accuracy of Alzheimer's disease: a neuropathological study. Acta Neuropathol, (1996). , 185-193.

[143] Olichney, J. M, et al. Cerebral infarction in Alzheimer's disease is associated with severe amyloid angiopathy and hypertension. Arch Neurol, (1995). , 702-708.

[144] Premkumar, D. R, et al. Apolipoprotein E-epsilon4 alleles in cerebral amyloid angiopathy and cerebrovascular pathology associated with Alzheimer's disease. Am J Pathol, (1996). , 2083-2095.

[145] Kalaria, R. Similarities between Alzheimer's disease and vascular dementia. J Neurol Sci, (2002). , 29-34.

[146] Frisoni, G. B, et al. Apolipoprotein E epsilon 4 allele in Alzheimer's disease and vascular dementia. Dementia, (1994). , 240-242.

[147] Snowdon, D. A, et al. Brain infarction and the clinical expression of Alzheimer disease. The Nun Study. JAMA, (1997). , 813-817.

[148] Bondy, C. A, & Cheng, C. M. Signaling by insulin-like growth factor 1 in brain. Eur J Pharmacol, (2004). , 25-31.

[149] Yamaguchi, Y, et al. Ligand-binding properties of the two isoforms of the human insulin receptor. Endocrinology, (1993). , 1132-1138.

[150] Kasuga, M, Karlsson, F. A, & Kahn, C. R. Insulin stimulates the phosphorylation of the 95,000-dalton subunit of its own receptor. Science, (1982). , 185-187.

[151] Jacobs, S, et al. Somatomedin-C stimulates the phosphorylation of the beta-subunit of its own receptor. J Biol Chem, (1983). , 9581-9584.

[152] Rubin, J. B, Shia, M. A, & Pilch, P. F. Stimulation of tyrosine-specific phosphorylation in vitro by insulin-like growth factor I. Nature, (1983). , 438-440.

[153] Schechter, R, et al. Developmental regulation of insulin in the mammalian central nervous system. Brain Res, (1992). , 27-37.

[154] Schechter, R, et al. Preproinsulin I and II mRNAs and insulin electron microscopic immunoreaction are present within the rat fetal nervous system. Brain Res, (1996). , 16-27.

[155] Schechter, R, & Abboud, M. Neuronal synthesized insulin roles on neural differentiation within fetal rat neuron cell cultures. Brain Res Dev Brain Res, (2001). , 41-49.

[156] Coker, G. T, et al. Analysis of tyrosine hydroxylase and insulin transcripts in human neuroendocrine tissues. Brain Res Mol Brain Res, (1990). , 93-98.

[157] Devaskar, S. U, et al. Insulin gene expression and insulin synthesis in mammalian neuronal cells. J Biol Chem, (1994). , 8445-8454.

[158] Banks, W. A. The source of cerebral insulin. Eur J Pharmacol, (2004). , 5-12.

[159] Burns, J. M, et al. Peripheral insulin and brain structure in early Alzheimer disease. Neurology, (2007). , 1094-1104.

[160] Salkovic-petrisic, M, & Hoyer, S. Central insulin resistance as a trigger for sporadic Alzheimer-like pathology: an experimental approach. J Neural Transm Suppl, (2007). , 217-233.

[161] Erol, A. An integrated and unifying hypothesis for the metabolic basis of sporadic Alzheimer's disease. J Alzheimers Dis, (2008). , 241-253.

[162] Park, C. R. Cognitive effects of insulin in the central nervous system. Neurosci Biobehav Rev, (2001). , 311-323.

[163] Ebina, Y, et al. The human insulin receptor cDNA: the structural basis for hormone-activated transmembrane signalling. Cell, (1985). , 747-758.

[164] Ullrich, A, et al. Human insulin receptor and its relationship to the tyrosine kinase family of oncogenes. Nature, (1985). , 756-761.

[165] Frasca, F, et al. Insulin receptor isoform A, a newly recognized, high-affinity insulin-like growth factor II receptor in fetal and cancer cells. Mol Cell Biol, (1999). , 3278-3288.

[166] Mosthaf, L, et al. Functionally distinct insulin receptors generated by tissue-specific alternative splicing. Embo J, (1990). , 2409-2413.

[167] Hedo, J. A, et al. Direct demonstration of glycosylation of insulin receptor subunits by biosynthetic and external labeling: evidence for heterogeneity. Proc Natl Acad Sci U S A, (1981). , 4791-4795.

[168] Massague, J, Pilch, P. F, & Czech, M. P. A unique proteolytic cleavage site on the beta subunit of the insulin receptor. J Biol Chem, (1981). , 3182-3190.

[169] Siegel, T. W, et al. Purification and properties of the human placental insulin receptor. J Biol Chem, (1981). , 9266-9273.

[170] Kanzaki, M. Insulin receptor signals regulating GLUT4 translocation and actin dynamics. Endocr J, (2006). , 267-293.

[171] Frattali, A. L, & Pessin, J. E. Relationship between alpha subunit ligand occupancy and beta subunit autophosphorylation in insulin/insulin-like growth factor-1 hybrid receptors. J Biol Chem, (1993). , 7393-7400.

[172] Lee, J, et al. Insulin receptor autophosphorylation occurs asymmetrically. J Biol Chem, (1993). , 4092-4098.

[173] Lee, J, & Pilch, P. F. The insulin receptor: structure, function, and signaling. Am J Physiol, (1994). Pt 1):, C319-C334.

[174] White, M. F, et al. Mutation of the insulin receptor at tyrosine 960 inhibits signal transmission but does not affect its tyrosine kinase activity. Cell, (1988). , 641-649.

[175] White, M. F. The IRS-signalling system: a network of docking proteins that mediate insulin action. Mol Cell Biochem, (1998). , 3-11.

[176] Myers, M. G, et al. IRS-1 activates phosphatidylinositol 3′-kinase by associating with src homology 2 domains of Proc Natl Acad Sci U S A, (1992). p. 10350-4., 85.

[177] Virkamaki, A, Ueki, K, & Kahn, C. R. Protein-protein interaction in insulin signaling and the molecular mechanisms of insulin resistance. J Clin Invest, (1999). , 931-943.

[178] Mayer, B. J, et al. A putative modular domain present in diverse signaling proteins. Cell, (1993). , 629-630.

[179] Yenush, L, et al. The pleckstrin homology domain is the principal link between the insulin receptor and IRS-1. J Biol Chem, (1996)., 24300-24306.

[180] Coffer, P. J, & Woodgett, J. R. Molecular cloning and characterisation of a novel putative protein-serine kinase related to the cAMP-dependent and protein kinase C families. Eur J Biochem, (1991)., 475-481.

[181] Burgering, B. M, & Coffer, P. J. Protein kinase B (c-Akt) in phosphatidylinositol-3-OH kinase signal transduction. Nature, (1995)., 599-602.

[182] Andjelkovic, M, et al. Activation and phosphorylation of a pleckstrin homology domain containing protein kinase (RAC-PK/PKB) promoted by serum and protein phosphatase inhibitors. Proc Natl Acad Sci U S A, (1996)., 5699-5704.

[183] Kohn, A. D, Takeuchi, F, & Roth, R. A. Akt, a pleckstrin homology domain containing kinase, is activated primarily by phosphorylation. J Biol Chem, (1996)., 21920-21926.

[184] Bellacosa, A, et al. Akt activation by growth factors is a multiple-step process: the role of the PH domain. Oncogene, (1998)., 313-325.

[185] Soskic, V, et al. Functional proteomics analysis of signal transduction pathways of the platelet-derived growth factor beta receptor. Biochemistry, (1999)., 1757-1764.

[186] Alessi, D. R, et al. Phosphoinositide-dependent protein kinase-1 (PDK1): structural and functional homology with the Drosophila DSTPK61 kinase. Curr Biol, (1997)., 776-789.

[187] Stokoe, D, et al. Dual role of phosphatidylinositol-3,4,5-trisphosphate in the activation of protein kinase B. Science, (1997)., 567-570.

[188] Currie, R. A, et al. Role of phosphatidylinositol 3,4,5-trisphosphate in regulating the activity and localization of 3-phosphoinositide-dependent protein kinase-1. Biochem J, (1999). Pt 3):, 575-583.

[189] Alessi, D. R, et al. Mechanism of activation of protein kinase B by insulin and IGF-1. EMBO J, (1996)., 6541-6551.

[190] Alessi, D. R, et al. Characterization of a 3-phosphoinositide-dependent protein kinase which phosphorylates and activates protein kinase Balpha. Curr Biol, (1997)., 261-269.

[191] Sarbassov, D. D, et al. Phosphorylation and regulation of Akt/PKB by the rictor-mTOR complex. Science, (2005)., 1098-1101.

[192] Yang, J, et al. Crystal structure of an activated Akt/protein kinase B ternary complex with GSK3-peptide and AMP-PNP. Nat Struct Biol, (2002)., 940-944.

[193] Cardone, M. H, et al. Regulation of cell death protease caspase-9 by phosphorylation. Science, (1998)., 1318-1321.

[194] Datta, S. R, et al. Akt phosphorylation of BAD couples survival signals to the cell-intrinsic death machinery. Cell, (1997)., 231-241.

[195] del PesoL., et al., Interleukin-3-induced phosphorylation of BAD through the protein kinase Akt. Science, (1997). , 687-689.

[196] Blume-jensen, P, Janknecht, R, & Hunter, T. The kit receptor promotes cell survival via activation of PI 3-kinase and subsequent Akt-mediated phosphorylation of Bad on Ser136. Curr Biol, (1998). , 779-782.

[197] Wang, H. G, et al. Ca2+-induced apoptosis through calcineurin dephosphorylation of BAD. Science, (1999). , 339-343.

[198] Du, K, & Montminy, M. CREB is a regulatory target for the protein kinase Akt/PKB. J Biol Chem, (1998). , 32377-32379.

[199] Kane, L. P, et al. Induction of NF-kappaB by the Akt/PKB kinase. Curr Biol, (1999). , 601-604.

[200] Biggs, W. H, et al. Protein kinase B/Akt-mediated phosphorylation promotes nuclear exclusion of the winged helix transcription factor FKHR1. Proc Natl Acad Sci U S A, (1999). , 7421-7426.

[201] Brunet, A, et al. Akt promotes cell survival by phosphorylating and inhibiting a Forkhead transcription factor. Cell, (1999). , 857-868.

[202] Kops, G. J, et al. Direct control of the Forkhead transcription factor AFX by protein kinase B. Nature, (1999). , 630-634.

[203] Read, D. E, & Gorman, A. M. Involvement of Akt in neurite outgrowth. Cell Mol Life Sci, (2009). , 2975-2984.

[204] Bhat, R. V, et al. Regulation and localization of tyrosine216 phosphorylation of glycogen synthase kinase-3beta in cellular and animal models of neuronal degeneration. Proc Natl Acad Sci U S A, (2000). , 11074-11079.

[205] Llambi, F, et al. A unified model of mammalian BCL-2 protein family interactions at the mitochondria. Mol Cell, (2011). , 517-531.

[206] Green, D. R, & Reed, J. C. Mitochondria and apoptosis. Science, (1998). , 1309-1312.

[207] Reed, J. C. Bcl-2 family proteins. Oncogene, (1998). , 3225-3236.

[208] Pastorino, J. G, et al. Functional consequences of the sustained or transient activation by Bax of the mitochondrial permeability transition pore. J Biol Chem, (1999). , 31734-31739.

[209] Antonsson, B, et al. Bax oligomerization is required for channel-forming activity in liposomes and to trigger cytochrome c release from mitochondria. Biochem J, (2000). Pt 2: , 271-278.

[210] Rong, Y, & Distelhorst, C. W. Bcl-2 protein family members: versatile regulators of calcium signaling in cell survival and apoptosis. Annu Rev Physiol, (2008). , 73-91.

[211] Lemasters, J. J, et al. Mitochondrial calcium and the permeability transition in cell death. Biochim Biophys Acta, (2009). , 1395-1401.

[212] Paradies, G, et al. Role of cardiolipin peroxidation and Ca2+ in mitochondrial dysfunction and disease. Cell Calcium, (2009). , 643-650.

[213] Bossy-wetzel, E, & Green, D. R. Apoptosis: checkpoint at the mitochondrial frontier. Mutat Res, (1999). , 243-251.

[214] Tornero, D, Posadas, I, & Cena, V. Bcl-x(L) blocks a mitochondrial inner membrane channel and prevents Ca2+ overload-mediated cell death. PLoS One, (2011). , e20423.

[215] Yang, E, et al. Bad, a heterodimeric partner for Bcl-XL and Bcl-2, displaces Bax and promotes cell death. Cell, (1995). , 285-291.

[216] Ottilie, S, et al. Dimerization properties of human BAD. Identification of a BH-3 domain and analysis of its binding to mutant BCL-2 and BCL-XL proteins. J Biol Chem, (1997). , 30866-30872.

[217] Zha, J, et al. BH3 domain of BAD is required for heterodimerization with BCL-XL and pro-apoptotic activity. J Biol Chem, (1997). , 24101-24104.

[218] Datta, S. R, Brunet, A, & Greenberg, M. E. Cellular survival: a play in three Akts. Genes Dev, (1999). , 2905-2927.

[219] Tsujimoto, Y. Role of Bcl-2 family proteins in apoptosis: apoptosomes or mitochondria? Genes Cells, (1998). , 697-707.

[220] Cryns, V, & Yuan, J. Proteases to die for. Genes Dev, (1998). , 1551-1570.

[221] Pettmann, B, & Henderson, C. E. Neuronal cell death. Neuron, (1998). , 633-647.

[222] Merry, D. E, & Korsmeyer, S. J. Bcl-2 gene family in the nervous system. Annu Rev Neurosci, (1997). , 245-267.

[223] Murphy, A. N, et al. Bcl-2 potentiates the maximal calcium uptake capacity of neural cell mitochondria. Proc Natl Acad Sci U S A, (1996). , 9893-9898.

[224] Vercesi, A. E, et al. The role of reactive oxygen species in mitochondrial permeability transition. Biosci Rep, (1997). , 43-52.

[225] Ellerby, L. M, et al. Shift of the cellular oxidation-reduction potential in neural cells expressing Bcl-2. J Neurochem, (1996). , 1259-1267.

[226] Esposti, M. D, et al. Bcl-2 and mitochondrial oxygen radicals. New approaches with reactive oxygen species-sensitive probes. J Biol Chem, (1999). , 29831-29837.

[227] Singleton, J. R, Dixit, V. M, & Feldman, E. L. Type I insulin-like growth factor receptor activation regulates apoptotic proteins. J Biol Chem, (1996). , 31791-31794.

[228] Minshall, C, et al. IL-4 and insulin-like growth factor-I inhibit the decline in Bcl-2 and promote the survival of IL-3-deprived myeloid progenitors. J Immunol, (1997). , 1225-1232.

[229] Tamatani, M, Ogawa, S, & Tohyama, M. Roles of Bcl-2 and caspases in hypoxia-induced neuronal cell death: a possible neuroprotective mechanism of peptide growth factors. Brain Res Mol Brain Res, (1998). , 27-39.

[230] Pugazhenthi, S, et al. Insulin-like growth factor-I induces bcl-2 promoter through the transcription factor cAMP-response element-binding protein. J Biol Chem, (1999). , 27529-27535.

[231] Shieh, P. B, et al. Identification of a signaling pathway involved in calcium regulation of BDNF expression. Neuron, (1998). , 727-740.

[232] Tao, X, et al. Ca2+ influx regulates BDNF transcription by a CREB family transcription factor-dependent mechanism. Neuron, (1998). , 709-726.

[233] Hu, Y, & Russek, S. J. BDNF and the diseased nervous system: a delicate balance between adaptive and pathological processes of gene regulation. J Neurochem, (2008). , 1-17.

[234] Fu, W, Lu, C, & Mattson, M. P. Telomerase mediates the cell survival-promoting actions of brain-derived neurotrophic factor and secreted amyloid precursor protein in developing hippocampal neurons. J Neurosci, (2002). , 10710-10719.

[235] Rohe, M, et al. Brain-derived neurotrophic factor reduces amyloidogenic processing through control of SORLA gene expression. J Neurosci, (2009). , 15472-15478.

[236] Arancibia, S, et al. Protective effect of BDNF against beta-amyloid induced neurotoxicity in vitro and in vivo in rats. Neurobiol Dis, (2008). , 316-326.

[237] Laske, C, et al. BDNF serum and CSF concentrations in Alzheimer's disease, normal pressure hydrocephalus and healthy controls. J Psychiatr Res, (2007). , 387-394.

[238] Lee, J. G, et al. Decreased serum brain-derived neurotrophic factor levels in elderly korean with dementia. Psychiatry Investig, (2009). , 299-305.

[239] Forlenza, O. V, Diniz, B. S, & Gattaz, W. F. Diagnosis and biomarkers of predementia in Alzheimer's disease. BMC Med, 20108: , 89.

[240] Forlenza, O. V, et al. Clinical and biological predictors of Alzheimer's disease in patients with amnestic mild cognitive impairment. Rev Bras Psiquiatr, (2010). , 216-222.

[241] Forlenza, O. V, et al. Effect of brain-derived neurotrophic factor Val66Met polymorphism and serum levels on the progression of mild cognitive impairment. World J Biol Psychiatry, (2010). , 774-780.

[242] Gunstad, J, et al. Serum brain-derived neurotrophic factor is associated with cognitive function in healthy older adults. J Geriatr Psychiatry Neurol, (2008). , 166-170.

[243] Maggirwar, S. B, et al. Nerve growth factor-dependent activation of NF-kappaB contributes to survival of sympathetic neurons. J Neurosci, (1998). , 10356-10365.

[244] Riccio, A, et al. Mediation by a CREB family transcription factor of NGF-dependent survival of sympathetic neurons. Science, (1999). , 2358-2361.

[245] Mincheva, S, et al. The canonical nuclear factor-kappaB pathway regulates cell survival in a developmental model of spinal cord motoneurons. J Neurosci, (2011). , 6493-6503.

[246] Maehara, K, Hasegawa, T, & Isobe, K. I. A NF-kappaB subunit is indispensable for activating manganese superoxide: dismutase gene transcription mediated by tumor necrosis factor-alpha. J Cell Biochem, (2000). p. 474-86., 65.

[247] Rojo, A. I, et al. Regulation of Cu/Zn-superoxide dismutase expression via the phosphatidylinositol 3 kinase/Akt pathway and nuclear factor-kappaB. J Neurosci, (2004). , 7324-7334.

[248] Tamatani, M, et al. Tumor necrosis factor induces Bcl-2 and Bcl-x expression through NFkappaB activation in primary hippocampal neurons. J Biol Chem, (1999). , 8531-8538.

[249] May, M. J, Ghosh, S, Rel, N. F-k. a. p. p. a B, Kappa, I, & Proteins, B. an overview. Semin Cancer Biol, (1997). , 63-73.

[250] Mercurio, F, & Manning, A. M. Multiple signals converging on NF-kappaB. Curr Opin Cell Biol, (1999). , 226-232.

[251] Perkins, N. D. Integrating cell-signalling pathways with NF-kappaB and IKK function. Nat Rev Mol Cell Biol, (2007). , 49-62.

[252] Ozes, O. N, et al. NF-kappaB activation by tumour necrosis factor requires the Akt serine-threonine kinase. Nature, (1999). , 82-85.

[253] Van Der Heide, L. P, Hoekman, M. F, & Smidt, M. P. The ins and outs of FoxO shuttling: mechanisms of FoxO translocation and transcriptional regulation. Biochem J, (2004). Pt 2): , 297-309.

[254] Miyashita, T, & Reed, J. C. Tumor suppressor is a direct transcriptional activator of the human bax gene. Cell, (1995). p. 293-9., 53.

[255] Reif, K, Burgering, B. M, & Cantrell, D. A. Phosphatidylinositol 3-kinase links the interleukin-2 receptor to protein kinase B and S6 kinase. J Biol Chem, (1997). p. 14426-33., 70.

[256] Stahl, M, et al. The forkhead transcription factor FoxO regulates transcription of and Bim in response to IL-2. J Immunol, (2002). p. 5024-31., 27Kip1.

[257] Dijkers, P. F, et al. Expression of the pro-apoptotic Bcl-2 family member Bim is regulated by the forkhead transcription factor FKHR-L1. Curr Biol, (2000). , 1201-1204.

[258] Graham, S. H, & Chen, J. Programmed cell death in cerebral ischemia. J Cereb Blood Flow Metab, (2001). , 99-109.

[259] Yamaguchi, H, & Wang, H. G. Bcl-XL protects BimEL-induced Bax conformational change and cytochrome C release independent of interacting with Bax or BimEL. J Biol Chem, (2002). , 41604-41612.

[260] Yamaguchi, A, et al. Akt activation protects hippocampal neurons from apoptosis by inhibiting transcriptional activity of J Biol Chem, (2001). p. 5256-64., 53.

[261] Kowaltowski, A. J, Vercesi, A. E, & Fiskum, G. Bcl-2 prevents mitochondrial permeability transition and cytochrome c release via maintenance of reduced pyridine nucleotides. Cell Death Differ, (2000). , 903-910.

[262] Aloyz, R. S, et al. is essential for developmental neuron death as regulated by the TrkA and p75 neurotrophin receptors. J Cell Biol, (1998). p. 1691-703., 53.

[263] Jaworski, J, et al. Control of dendritic arborization by the phosphoinositide-3′-kinase-Akt-mammalian target of rapamycin pathway. J Neurosci, (2005). , 11300-11312.

[264] Kumar, V, et al. Regulation of dendritic morphogenesis by Ras-PI3K-Akt-mTOR and Ras-MAPK signaling pathways. J Neurosci, (2005). , 11288-11299.

[265] Yoshimura, T, et al. Ras regulates neuronal polarity via the PI3-kinase/Akt/GSK-3beta/CRMP-2 pathway. Biochem Biophys Res Commun, (2006). , 62-68.

[266] Lim, C. S, & Walikonis, R. S. Hepatocyte growth factor and c-Met promote dendritic maturation during hippocampal neuron differentiation via the Akt pathway. Cell Signal, (2008). , 825-835.

[267] Zheng, J, et al. Clathrin-dependent endocytosis is required for TrkB-dependent Akt-mediated neuronal protection and dendritic growth. J Biol Chem, (2008). , 13280-13288.

[268] Markus, A, Zhong, J, & Snider, W. D. Raf and akt mediate distinct aspects of sensory axon growth. Neuron, (2002). , 65-76.

[269] Mills, J, et al. Role of integrin-linked kinase in nerve growth factor-stimulated neurite outgrowth. J Neurosci, (2003). , 1638-1648.

[270] Tucker, B. A, Rahimtula, M, & Mearow, K. M. Laminin and growth factor receptor activation stimulates differential growth responses in subpopulations of adult DRG neurons. Eur J Neurosci, (2006). , 676-690.

[271] Tucker, B. A, Rahimtula, M, & Mearow, K. M. Src and FAK are key early signalling intermediates required for neurite growth in NGF-responsive adult DRG neurons. Cell Signal, (2008). , 241-257.

[272] Cross, D. A, et al. Inhibition of glycogen synthase kinase-3 by insulin mediated by protein kinase B. Nature, (1995). , 785-789.

[273] Salas, T. R, et al. Alleviating the suppression of glycogen synthase kinase-3beta by Akt leads to the phosphorylation of cAMP-response element-binding protein and its transactivation in intact cell nuclei. J Biol Chem, (2003). , 41338-41346.

[274] Asnaghi, L, et al. Bcl-2 phosphorylation and apoptosis activated by damaged microtubules require mTOR and are regulated by Akt. Oncogene, (2004). , 5781-5791.

[275] Konishi, H, et al. Identification of peripherin as a Akt substrate in neurons. J Biol Chem, (2007). , 23491-23499.

[276] Kim, H, et al. Delta-catenin-induced dendritic morphogenesis. An essential role of interaction through Akt1-mediated phosphorylation. J Biol Chem, (2008). p. 977-87., 190RhoGEF.

[277] Konishi, H, et al. Activation of protein kinase B (Akt/RAC-protein kinase) by cellular stress and its association with heat shock protein Hsp27. FEBS Lett, (1997). , 493-498.

[278] Murashov, A. K, et al. Crosstalk between Hsp25 and Akt in spinal motor neurons after sciatic nerve injury. Brain Res Mol Brain Res, (2001). p. 199-208., 38.

[279] Frame, S, & Cohen, P. GSK3 takes centre stage more than 20 years after its discovery. Biochem J, (2001). Pt 1): , 1-16.

[280] Grimes, C. A, & Jope, R. S. The multifaceted roles of glycogen synthase kinase 3beta in cellular signaling. Prog Neurobiol, (2001). , 391-426.

[281] Doble, B. W, & Woodgett, J. R. GSK-3: tricks of the trade for a multi-tasking kinase. J Cell Sci, (2003). Pt 7): , 1175-1186.

[282] Hooper, C, Killick, R, & Lovestone, S. The GSK3 hypothesis of Alzheimer's disease. J Neurochem, (2008). , 1433-1439.

[283] Iqbal, K, et al. Mechanisms of tau-induced neurodegeneration. Acta Neuropathol, (2009). , 53-69.

[284] Mandelkow, E. M, et al. Clogging of axons by tau, inhibition of axonal traffic and starvation of synapses. Neurobiol Aging, (2003). , 1079-1085.

[285] Brewster, J. L, et al. Endoplasmic reticulum stress and trophic factor withdrawal activate distinct signaling cascades that induce glycogen synthase kinase-3 beta and a caspase-9-dependent apoptosis in cerebellar granule neurons. Mol Cell Neurosci, (2006). , 242-253.

[286] Duyckaerts, C, Delatour, B, & Potier, M. C. Classification and basic pathology of Alzheimer disease. Acta Neuropathol, (2009). , 5-36.

[287] Takashima, A. Amyloid-beta, tau, and dementia. J Alzheimers Dis, (2009). , 729-736.

[288] Wang, J. M, et al. Reduction of ischemic brain injury by topical application of insulin-like growth factor-I after transient middle cerebral artery occlusion in rats. Brain Res, (2000). , 381-385.

[289] St-pierre, J, et al. Topology of superoxide production from different sites in the mitochondrial electron transport chain. J Biol Chem, (2002). , 44784-44790.

[290] Barthel, A, Schmoll, D, & Unterman, T. G. FoxO proteins in insulin action and metabolism. Trends Endocrinol Metab, (2005). , 183-189.

[291] Zetterberg, H, Wahlund, L. O, & Blennow, K. Cerebrospinal fluid markers for prediction of Alzheimer's disease. Neurosci Lett, (2003). , 67-69.

[292] Lacor, P. N, et al. Synaptic targeting by Alzheimer's-related amyloid beta oligomers. J Neurosci, (2004). , 10191-10200.

[293] Walsh, D. M, et al. Naturally secreted oligomers of amyloid beta protein potently inhibit hippocampal long-term potentiation in vivo. Nature, (2002). , 535-539.

[294] Tillement, L, Lecanu, L, & Papadopoulos, V. Alzheimer's disease: effects of beta-amyloid on mitochondria. Mitochondrion. 11(1): , 13-21.

[295] Abramov, A. Y, Canevari, L, & Duchen, M. R. Calcium signals induced by amyloid beta peptide and their consequences in neurons and astrocytes in culture. Biochim Biophys Acta, (2004). , 81-87.

[296] Mattson, M. P, et al. beta-Amyloid peptides destabilize calcium homeostasis and render human cortical neurons vulnerable to excitotoxicity. J Neurosci, (1992). , 376-389.

[297] Xie, L, et al. Alzheimer's beta-amyloid peptides compete for insulin binding to the insulin receptor. J Neurosci, (2002). , RC221.

[298] Messier, C, & Teutenberg, K. The role of insulin, insulin growth factor, and insulin-degrading enzyme in brain aging and Alzheimer's disease. Neural Plast, (2005). , 311-328.

[299] Thinakaran, G, & Koo, E. H. Amyloid precursor protein trafficking, processing, and function. J Biol Chem, (2008). , 29615-29619.

[300] Rocchi, A, et al. Causative and susceptibility genes for Alzheimer's disease: a review. Brain Res Bull, (2003). , 1-24.

[301] Zhang, Y. W, et al. APP processing in Alzheimer's disease. Mol Brain. 4: , 3.

[302] De Strooper, B, & Annaert, W. Proteolytic processing and cell biological functions of the amyloid precursor protein. J Cell Sci, (2000). Pt 11): , 1857-1870.

[303] Zheng, H, & Koo, E. H. The amyloid precursor protein: beyond amyloid. Mol Neurodegener, (2006). , 5.

[304] Loffler, J, & Huber, G. Beta-amyloid precursor protein isoforms in various rat brain regions and during brain development. J Neurochem, (1992). , 1316-1324.

[305] Tominaga-yoshino, K, et al. Neurotoxic and neuroprotective effects of glutamate are enhanced by introduction of amyloid precursor protein cDNA. Brain Res, (2001). , 121-130.

[306] Wasco, W, et al. Isolation and characterization of APLP2 encoding a homologue of the Alzheimer's associated amyloid beta protein precursor. Nat Genet, (1993)., 95-100.

[307] Wasco, W, et al. Identification of a mouse brain cDNA that encodes a protein related to the Alzheimer disease-associated amyloid beta protein precursor. Proc Natl Acad Sci U S A, (1992)., 10758-10762.

[308] Coulson, E. J, et al. What the evolution of the amyloid protein precursor supergene family tells us about its function. Neurochem Int, (2000)., 175-184.

[309] Goate, A, et al. Segregation of a missense mutation in the amyloid precursor protein gene with familial Alzheimer's disease. Nature, (1991)., 704-706.

[310] Rohan de SilvaH.A., et al., Cell-specific expression of beta-amyloid precursor protein isoform mRNAs and proteins in neurons and astrocytes. Brain Res Mol Brain Res, (1997)., 147-156.

[311] Kang, J, & Muller-hill, B. Differential splicing of Alzheimer's disease amyloid A4 precursor RNA in rat tissues: PreA4(695) mRNA is predominantly produced in rat and human brain. Biochem Biophys Res Commun, (1990)., 1192-1200.

[312] Menendez-gonzalez, M, et al. APP processing and the APP-KPI domain involvement in the amyloid cascade. Neurodegener Dis, (2005)., 277-283.

[313] Xu, H, et al. Generation of Alzheimer beta-amyloid protein in the trans-Golgi network in the apparent absence of vesicle formation. Proc Natl Acad Sci U S A, (1997)., 3748-3752.

[314] Hartmann, T, et al. Distinct sites of intracellular production for Alzheimer's disease A beta40/42 amyloid peptides. Nat Med, (1997)., 1016-1020.

[315] Greenfield, J. P, et al. Endoplasmic reticulum and trans-Golgi network generate distinct populations of Alzheimer beta-amyloid peptides. Proc Natl Acad Sci U S A, (1999)., 742-747.

[316] Cupers, P, et al. The discrepancy between presenilin subcellular localization and gamma-secretase processing of amyloid precursor protein. J Cell Biol, (2001)., 731-740.

[317] Kovacs, D. M, et al. Alzheimer-associated presenilins 1 and 2: neuronal expression in brain and localization to intracellular membranes in mammalian cells. Nat Med, (1996)., 224-229.

[318] Perez, A, et al. Degradation of soluble amyloid beta-peptides 1-40, 1-42, and the Dutch variant 1-40Q by insulin degrading enzyme from Alzheimer disease and control brains. Neurochem Res, (2000)., 247-255.

[319] Sinha, S, et al. Purification and cloning of amyloid precursor protein beta-secretase from human brain. Nature, (1999)., 537-540.

[320] Vassar, R, et al. Beta-secretase cleavage of Alzheimer's amyloid precursor protein by the transmembrane aspartic protease BACE. Science, (1999). , 735-741.

[321] Yan, R, et al. Membrane-anchored aspartyl protease with Alzheimer's disease beta-secretase activity. Nature, (1999). , 533-537.

[322] Lau, K. F, et al. X11 alpha and x11 beta interact with presenilin-1 via their PDZ domains. Mol Cell Neurosci, (2000). , 557-565.

[323] Dominguez, D, et al. Phenotypic and biochemical analyses of BACE1- and BACE2-deficient mice. J Biol Chem, (2005). , 30797-30806.

[324] Hu, X, et al. Bace1 modulates myelination in the central and peripheral nervous system. Nat Neurosci, (2006). , 1520-1525.

[325] Chow, V. W, et al. An overview of APP processing enzymes and products. Neuromolecular Med. 12(1):, 1-12.

[326] Nikolaev, A, et al. APP binds DR6 to trigger axon pruning and neuron death via distinct caspases. Nature, (2009). , 981-989.

[327] Kimberly, W. T, et al. Gamma-secretase is a membrane protein complex comprised of presenilin, nicastrin, Aph-1, and Pen-2. Proc Natl Acad Sci U S A, (2003). , 6382-6387.

[328] Takasugi, N, et al. The role of presenilin cofactors in the gamma-secretase complex. Nature, (2003). , 438-441.

[329] Burdick, D, et al. Assembly and aggregation properties of synthetic Alzheimer's A4/ beta amyloid peptide analogs. J Biol Chem, (1992). , 546-554.

[330] Scheuner, D, et al. Secreted amyloid beta-protein similar to that in the senile plaques of Alzheimer's disease is increased in vivo by the presenilin 1 and 2 and APP mutations linked to familial Alzheimer's disease. Nat Med, (1996). , 864-870.

[331] Borchelt, D. R, et al. Familial Alzheimer's disease-linked presenilin 1 variants elevate Abeta1-42/1-40 ratio in vitro and in vivo. Neuron, (1996). , 1005-1013.

[332] Zhao, W. Q, et al. Amyloid beta oligomers induce impairment of neuronal insulin receptors. FASEB J, (2008). , 246-260.

[333] Gasparini, L, et al. Stimulation of beta-amyloid precursor protein trafficking by insulin reduces intraneuronal beta-amyloid and requires mitogen-activated protein kinase signaling. J Neurosci, (2001). , 2561-2570.

[334] Gouras, G. K, et al. Intraneuronal Abeta42 accumulation in human brain. Am J Pathol, (2000). , 15-20.

[335] Oddo, S, et al. Triple-transgenic model of Alzheimer's disease with plaques and tangles: intracellular Abeta and synaptic dysfunction. Neuron, (2003). , 409-421.

[336] Oddo, S, et al. A dynamic relationship between intracellular and extracellular pools of Abeta. Am J Pathol, (2006). , 184-194.

[337] Oakley, H, et al. Intraneuronal beta-amyloid aggregates, neurodegeneration, and neuron loss in transgenic mice with five familial Alzheimer's disease mutations: potential factors in amyloid plaque formation. J Neurosci, (2006). , 10129-10140.

[338] Phiel, C. J, et al. GSK-3alpha regulates production of Alzheimer's disease amyloid-beta peptides. Nature, (2003). , 435-439.

[339] Farris, W, et al. Partial loss-of-function mutations in insulin-degrading enzyme that induce diabetes also impair degradation of amyloid beta-protein. Am J Pathol, (2004). , 1425-1434.

[340] Vekrellis, K, et al. Neurons regulate extracellular levels of amyloid beta-protein via proteolysis by insulin-degrading enzyme. J Neurosci, (2000). , 1657-1665.

[341] Farris, W, et al. Insulin-degrading enzyme regulates the levels of insulin, amyloid beta-protein, and the beta-amyloid precursor protein intracellular domain in vivo. Proc Natl Acad Sci U S A, (2003). , 4162-4167.

[342] Takashima, A, et al. Exposure of rat hippocampal neurons to amyloid beta peptide (25-35) induces the inactivation of phosphatidyl inositol-3 kinase and the activation of tau protein kinase I/glycogen synthase kinase-3 beta. Neurosci Lett, (1996). , 33-36.

[343] Zhao, L, et al. Insulin-degrading enzyme as a downstream target of insulin receptor signaling cascade: implications for Alzheimer's disease intervention. J Neurosci, (2004). , 11120-11126.

[344] Brookmeyer, R, et al. Forecasting the global burden of Alzheimer's disease. Alzheimers Dement, (2007). , 186-191.

[345] Vellas, B, et al. Disease-modifying trials in Alzheimer's disease: a European task force consensus. Lancet Neurol, (2007). , 56-62.

Chapter 17

Prevention of Alzheimer's Disease: Intervention Studies

Francesca Mangialasche, Weili Xu and
Miia Kivipelto

Additional information is available at the end of the chapter

http://dx.doi.org/10.5772/55034

1. Introduction

The aging of the population is a worldwide phenomenon, and studying age-related diseases has become a relevant issue from both a scientific and a public health perspective. Dementia is a syndrome characterised by loss of cognitive abilities in multiple domains that results in impairment in normal activities of daily living and loss of independence [1]. Both prevalence and incidence of dementia rise exponentially with advancing age, and 70% of all dementia cases occur in people aged 75+ years [2]. The worldwide increase in the number of older adults, more pronounced in the 80+ age group, explains the epidemic proportions assumed by dementia. According to the World Alzheimer Report, there were 35.6 million people living with dementia worldwide in 2010, a number that will increase to 65.7 million by 2030 and 115.4 million by 2050 unless effective means reducing the disease incidence are introduced [3]. Dementia is a major cause of disability and institutionalization of elderly people and because of its increased prevalence this disorder is becoming an emerging public health issue not only in developed countries but also in less developed regions of the world. The total estimated worldwide costs of dementia were US$604 billion in 2010, including the costs of informal care (unpaid care provided by family and others), direct costs of social care (provided by community care professionals, and in residential home settings) and the direct costs of medical care (the costs of treating dementia and other conditions in primary and secondary care) [3].

Alzheimer's disease (AD) is considered the most common cause of dementia, accounting for 60–70% of all dementia cases. The hallmarks of AD neuropathology in the brain are the presence of extracellular plaques composed of amyloid-β (Aβ) and intracellular neurofibrillary tangles (NFTs) composed of hyperphosphorylated aggregates of the microtubule-associated tau protein [4].

Vascular dementia (VaD), mainly due to cerebrovascular diseases (CVD), is the second most frequent type of dementia [5, 6]. This current classification of dementia types is being reconsidered in light of recent neuropathological and neuroimaging studies, which have shown a range of dementia-associated brain abnormalities from pure vascular lesions at one end to pure AD pathologies at the other, with most dementia cases being attributable to both CVD and AD. In fact, AD and CVD-related changes often coexist in the brain of older adults with dementia and mild cognitive impairment (MCI) [7, 8]. Also, both types of lesions are detected in the brain of cognitively normal elderly people, highlighting the importance of mixed pathologies in increasing the risk of late-life dementia [9]. The co-occurrence of AD and CVD is consistent with the evidence that AD and VaD share several risk and protective factors, including cardiovascular and lifestyle related factors. Overall, this implies that dementia syndrome is a valid target for prevention, especially from the public health perspective.

Prevention is traditionally divided into three levels: primary, secondary, and tertiary prevention. Primary prevention aims to reduce the incidence of the disease by eliminating or treating specific risk factors, which may decrease or delay the development of dementia. Secondary prevention aims to early detection of the disease, before any symptom has emerged, when treatment could stop its progression. Tertiary prevention aims to reduce the impact of complications and disability of long-term diseases.

Regarding primary prevention, both observational and interventional epidemiological studies have been conducted for dementia and AD. On the other hand, in the field of AD the development of pharmacological interventions has been mainly limited to a tertiary prevention level, since the diagnostic criteria currently in use for AD (National Institute of Neurological and Communicative Disorders and Stroke-Alzheimer's Disease and Related Disorders Association, NINCDS-ADRDA - criteria) identify the presence of the disease only when AD is severe enough to cause a dementia syndrome [10]. Thus, the majority of anti-AD drugs have been tested in subjects already in the symptomatic stage of the disease, and so far no drug has shown the ability to stop the disease progression (i.e. disease-modifying effect) [11]. However, several studies have shown that the pathophysiological process of AD begins years, if not decades, before the diagnosis of Alzheimer's dementia and individuals generally experience a gradual impairment of cognitive functions, which can progress to a dementia syndrome [12-14].

Recent advances in neuroimaging, cerebrospinal fluid (CSF) assays, and other techniques now provide the ability to detect evidence of the AD pathophysiological process in vivo, but the diagnostic criteria currently in use do not take into account these biomarkers. Three international workgroups promoted by the American National Institute of Aging (NIA) and the American Alzheimer's Association recently proposed new diagnostic guidelines to identify dementia due to AD, MCI due to AD, and preclinical AD [15-17]. These new criteria formalize the different clinical stages of AD and incorporate biomarkers (genetic, biochemical, neuroimaging) that can be detected in vivo and are believed to reflect AD pathology. These diagnostic criteria are now being validated and can be revised as long as new findings from research on biomarkers in AD will clarify the link between AD pathophysiology and the AD clinical syndrome. These criteria offer the opportunity to identify subjects who can be target of secondary prevention in order to halt the progression of the brain damage and prevent or delay the onset of cognitive symptoms. A step in this direction has been done by planning randomized controlled trials (RCTs) testing anti-amyloid drugs in older adults with evidence of brain amyloid accumulation. The same type of intervention will also be tested in subjects at risk of early onset AD due to genetic mutations associated with familial AD.

This chapter summarizes the major findings concerning primary prevention of late onset dementia and AD, based on current epidemiological evidence from observational and interventional studies. Preventive strategies for early onset AD are also mentioned. Although many aspects of the dementias are still unclear, some risk and protective factors have been identified. It is also possible to delineate some preventative strategies. Ongoing interventional studies testing the effect of preventive measures for dementia and AD are discussed, and methodological challenges in designing dementia prevention trials are summarized.

2. Observational studies

Several community-based prospective studies of aging and health have been carried out in different countries since the 80s'. These studies have provided relevant information on the aetiology of dementia and AD, and have led to the identification of possible preventive strategies. Evidence from these observational studies has shown that dementia is a multifactorial disorder caused by several interrelated mechanisms in which the interaction of genetic and environmental factors plays the major role (Table 1). The pathways that lead from different risk factors to dementia are not fully understood, but several etiological hypotheses have been proposed: the vascular hypothesis, inflammatory hypothesis, oxidative-stress hypothesis, toxic hypothesis and psychosocial hypothesis [18, 19]. These theories highlight potential links of various risk factors to both the vascular and the neurodegenerative brain pathologies that can cause dementia, supporting the validity of dementia syndrome as target for prevention [6, 20].

2.1. Non-modifiable risk factors for Alzheimer's disease

Both modifiable and non-modifiable risk factors have been identified for dementia and AD, and while for some factors the scientific evidence is quite robust, for others the results are still inconclusive.

2.1.1. Age

Increasing age is a well-established risk factor for dementia, which is a common disorders after 75 years of age, but rare before age 60. The incidence rates of dementia increase exponentially with advancing age. In Europe, approximately two per 1,000 person-years become demented among people aged 65-69 years, and the incidence increases to 70 to 80 per 1,000 person-years for people 90 years or over [21, 22]. It is still unclear if the incidence of dementia continues to increase even in the oldest old or reaches a plateau at a certain age. The Cache County Study found that the incidence of dementia increased with age, peaked, and then started to decline at extreme old ages for both men and women. However, some meta-analyses and large-scale studies in Europe provided no evidence for the potential decline in the incidence of dementia among the oldest old [21, 22].

Risk factors	Protective factors	Combined effects
Age **Genetic** Familial aggregation *APOE* ε4 *APP* *GSK3β* *DYRK1A* *Tau* *CLU* *TOMM40* *PICALM* *CR1* **Vascular** Cerebrovascular lesions Cardiovascular diseases Diabetes mellitus and pre-diabetes *Midlife positive association but late-life negative association* Hypertension High BMI (overweight and obesity) High serum cholesterol **Lifestyle** Smoking High alcohol intake **Diet** Saturated fats Homocysteine **Others** Depression Occupational exposure Traumatic brain injury Infective agents (Herpes Simplex Virus Type I, Clamydophila pneumoniae, Spirochetes)	**Genetic** *APP* **Psychosocial factors** High education and SES High work complexity Rich social network and social engagement Mentally stimulating activity **Lifestyle** Physical activity **Diet** Mediterranean diet Polyunsaturated (PUFA) and fish-related fats Vitamin B_6, B_{12}, folate Antioxidant vitamins (A, C, E) Vitamin D **Drugs** Statins Antihypertensive drugs HRT NSAIDs	**Increased risk** *Genetic and environmental factors in midlife* *APOE*ε4 magnifies the effect of high alcohol intake, smoking, physical inactivity and high intake of saturate fat *Vascular factors in midlife* Hypertension, obesity, hypercholesterolemia and physical inactivity have an additive effect when they co-occur *Vascular factors/diseases in late-life* Higher risk in individuals with brain hypoperfusion profile: chronic heart failure, low pulse pressure, low diastolic pressure Higher risk in individuals with atherosclerosis profile: high systolic pressure, diabetes mellitus or prediabetes, stroke **Decreased risk** *Genetic and environmental factors in midlife* High education reduces the negative effect of *APOE*ε4 Physical activity counteracts the risk due to *APOE*ε4 *Environmental factors in midlife* High work complexity modulates the increased dementia risk due to low education *Genetic and environmental factors in late-life* Active leisure activities or absence of vascular risk factors reduces the risk due to *APOE*ε4

APOE: apolipoprotein E. BMI: body mass index. *CLU*: clusterin. *CR1*: complement component receptor 1. *DYRK1A*: dual-specificity tyrosine-(Y)-phosphorylation regulated kinase 1A. *GSK3β*: glycogen synthase kinase-3beta. HRT: hormone replacement therapy. NSAIDs: nonsteroidal anti-inflammatory drugs. *PICALM*: phosphatidylinositol binding clathrin assembly protein. PUFA: polyunsaturated fatty acid. SES: socioeconomic status. *TOMM40*: translocase of outer mitochondrial membrane 40 homolog.

Table 1. Proposed risk and protective factors for dementia and Alzheimer's disease

2.1.2. *Familial aggregation*

Familial aggregation is another important risk factor for late life dementia and AD. First-degree relatives of AD patients have a higher lifetime risk for developing AD than relatives of non-demented people or the general population (Table 1) [21, 22]. It is likely that shared genetic and environmental factors contribute to the familial aggregation. The amount of risk of AD that is attributable to genetics is estimated to be around 70% [25].

2.1.3. *Genes*

The Apolipoprotein E *(APOE)* ε4 allele is the only established genetic risk factor for both early- and late-onset AD; it is a susceptibility gene, being neither necessary nor sufficient for the development of AD. The risk of AD increases with increasing number of the ε4 alleles in a dose-dependent manner, but the risk effect decreases with increasing age. Individuals with two *APOE* ε4 alleles have a more than seven times increased risk of developing AD compared with those with *APOE* ε3 alleles and approximately 15 to 20 percent of AD cases are attributable to the *APOE* ε4 allele [25-28].

Other genes have been related to increased risk of late life AD, but the association is less consistent. These are mainly genes involved in the metabolism and processing of the amyloid precursor protein (APP) and Aβ, as well as tau protein, including the *GSK3β*, *DYRK1A*, *Tau*, and *CLU* genes [25]. Until now, mutations in APP have not been implicated in the late-onset form of AD, with the exception of the rare variant, N660Y, which was recently identified in one case from a late-onset AD family [29]. A recent study identified a mutation in the *APP* gene that can be protective against AD and age-related cognitive decline. This mutation is associated with a reduced production of amyloidogenic peptides [30]. Other genes that have been associated with increased risk of AD are *TOMM40*, *CR1* and *PICALM*. The *TOMM40* gene is located in a region of chromosome 19, which is in linkage disequilibrium with *APOE*, and its polymorphism affects the age on onset of AD in subjects with an *APOE* genotype [31]. *CR1* is involved in the complement cascade, while *PICALM* encodes a protein that is involved in clathrin-mediated endocytosis, an essential step in the intracellular trafficking of proteins and lipids such as nutrients, growth factors and neurotransmitters [32].

Several aspects challenge the identification of genetic risk factors for late life AD, including the fact that risk conferred by a single gene is generally small, and for some genes is the combination of risk alleles that is relevant for a significant change of the overall risk. Also, the heterogeneous and mixed nature of brain pathology causing dementia, particularly coexisting CVD, makes it more difficult to identify genetic risk factors for AD. Nevertheless, the identification of genetic risk factors for late onset AD can have implication for preventive and therapeutic strategies. In fact, it has been shown that the *APOE ε4* allele can modulate the effect of lifestyle related risk factors [33] and influence the effect of pharmacological treatment for AD [34]. It is thus possible that future preventive and therapeutic measures will be tailored according to specific genetic risk profiles.

2.2. Modifiable risk and protective factors for Alzheimer's disease

Different modifiable factors have been proposed to play a role in late life dementia and AD, including nutritional factors (i.e., diet and nutritional supplements), social or economic factors, medical conditions and lifestyle related factors (e.g., smoking habit, physical activity, etc.) (Table 1). A report commissioned by the National institute of Health (NIH) to the Agency for Healthcare Research and Quality (AHRQ) was published in 2010, and concluded that current research evidence on many risk and protective factors for cognitive decline and AD is not of sufficient strength, thus recommendations for preventing these conditions cannot be made [35, 36]. Another previous review yielded similar conclusions [37]. These negative perspectives have been criticized, since there is consistent and robust epidemiological evidence that use of antihypertensive medications, cessation of smoking and increasing physical activity produces cognitive benefits in older adults [38]. Furthermore, the analytical strategy used in the Evidence Based Review carried out by the AHRQ did not take into account the life-course perspective [39]. Observational longitudinal studies have shown that the risk of late-life dementia and AD is determined by exposures to multiple factors experienced over the life-span and that the effect of specific risk/protective factors largely depends on age [39]. Thus, a life-course perspective is relevant for chronic disorders with a long latent period (such as dementia). It allows the identification of time windows when exposures have their greatest effect on outcome and assessment of whether cumulative exposures could have multiplicative or additive effects over the life course [40]. Age-dependent associations with AD have been suggested for several aging-related medical conditions. For example, elevated blood pressure, body mass index (BMI) and total cholesterol levels at a young age and in middle age (<65 years) have been associated with an increased risk of dementia and AD, whereas having lower values in late life (age >75 years) has been also associated with subsequent development of dementia/ AD [41-46].

2.2.1. Risk factors

1. **Vascular risk factors and disorders**: An association of elevated blood pressure in midlife with an increased risk of dementia and AD later in life has been reported in several population-based studies [41, 47], while follow-up studies of late-life blood pressure and risk of dementia yield mixed results, largely depending on the length of follow-up. The short-term follow-up studies (e.g., less than 3 years) often found no association or even an inverse association between blood pressure and risk of dementia and AD [41]. However, studies of very old people (i.e., 75 + years) with a longer follow-up period (i.e., more than 6 years) also revealed an increased risk of dementia associated with low blood pressure [48], suggesting that among very old people low blood pressure may also contribute to the development of dementia, possibly by influencing cerebral blood perfusion.

   For BMI, the bidirectional association with dementia and AD has been shown in several studies, and longitudinal studies of elderly people have associated accelerated decline in BMI with subsequent development of dementia. This implies that low BMI and weight loss in advanced age can be interpreted as markers for preclinical dementia [45, 46, 49-55].

http://dx.doi.org/10.5772/55034

Regarding serum total cholesterol, the importance of the pattern of change in cholesterol levels after midlife has been shown by two studies with a long follow-up, reporting that a decline in plasma total cholesterol after midlife may be associated with the risk of cognitive decline, dementia and AD in late life [56, 57]. These findings suggest that high total serum cholesterol in midlife seems to be a risk factor for dementia and AD in advanced age, while decreasing serum cholesterol after midlife may reflect ongoing disease processes and represent a marker of early stages in the development of dementia and AD. The use of statins (cholesterol-lowering drugs) in relation to dementia has been investigated in several community studies, with mixed findings. Some observational studies suggest a protective effect, while others did not, and clinical trials using statins for prevention of cognitive decline or dementia mainly reported no effects [6, 58]. Diabetes mellitus has been associated with increased risk of dementia and AD over adult life, but the risk is stronger when diabetes occurs in mid-life than in late-life [59]. Also pre-diabetes, impaired glucose regulation, and impaired insulin secretion have been associated with and increased risk of dementia and AD [60].

Cerebrovascular lesions and cardiovascular diseases have been shown to be risk factors for dementia and AD. Several population-based studies reveal an approximately two- to four-fold increased risk of incident dementia associated with clinical stroke (post-stroke dementia) [61, 62]. It is probable that an association of clinical stroke with AD is rarely reported due to the fact that a history of stroke is part of the current criteria for excluding the diagnosis of AD. However, asymptomatic cerebrovascular lesions such as silent brain infarcts and white matter lesions have been associated with an increased risk of dementia and AD [63, 64], although the association with AD is likely to be due to the inclusion of mixed dementia cases. The Cardiovascular Health Study found that cardiovascular disease was associated with an increased incidence of dementia, with the highest risk seen among people with peripheral arterial disease, suggesting that extensive peripheral atherosclerosis is a risk factor for dementia [65]. Atrial fibrillation, heart failure, and severe atherosclerosis measured with ankle-to-brachial index are also associated with the increased risk of dementia and AD [66-69].

2. **Environmental and other factors**: Current smoking is another major risk factor for dementia and AD, and based on the worldwide prevalence of smoking, about 14% of all AD cases are potentially attributable to this risk factor [70]. Although it is not entirely clear whether depression is a risk factor for or a preclinical symptom of dementia, studies with long-term follow-up support the risk-factor hypothesis [71]. Other conditions have been proposed as risk factors for dementia and AD, but the evidence is still sparse. These include occupational exposure, traumatic brain injury and infections. Occupational exposure to heavy metals such as aluminum and mercury has been suggested to be a risk factor for AD; even high consumption of aluminum from drinking water has been associated with an elevated risk of AD and dementia [6, 72]. In addition, occupational exposure to extremely-low-frequency electromagnetic fields (ELF-EMFs) has been related to an increased risk of dementia and AD [73, 74].

Traumatic brain injury has been extensively investigated as a possible risk factor for AD. The meta-analysis of case-control studies supported an association between a history of head injury and the increased risk of AD [75]. In contrast, some longitudinal studies found that AD was not associated with head trauma or only associated with severe traumatic head injury [76]. The role of viral and bacterial organisms in the development of chronic neurodegeneration is long established. Thus, Treponema pallidum and HIV, in particular, have been associated with the development of dementia. Other infections in the central nervous system (CNS), particularly Herpes Simplex Virus Type 1, Chlamydophila pneumoniae and several types of Spirochetes, have been suggested as possible aetiological agents in the development of sporadic AD, but with little consistent evidence. It has also been suggested that peripheral infections may have a role in accelerating neurodegeneration in AD by activating already primed microglial cells within the CNS [77].

2.2.2. Protective factors

1. **Psychosocial factors**: Protective factors for dementia and AD have also been identified, including high education and socioeconomic status (SES) in early life as well as a number of factors in adult life: high work complexity, rich social network, social engagement, mentally-stimulating activity, non-smoking and regular physical exercise [6, 78, 79]. Living with a partner during mid-life has been associated with reduced risk of cognitive impairment and dementia later in life, suggesting that being in a relationship entails cognitive and social challenges that can increase the cognitive reserve [80]. Even at old ages the active engagement in mental, physical and social activities may postpone the onset of dementia, possibly by increasing the cognitive reserve [81].

2. **Lifestyle and diet**: In addition, several follow-up studies reported a decreased risk of dementia and AD associated with healthy dietary patterns and nutritional factors, such as high adherence to a Mediterranean diet or dietary intake of antioxidants (e.g., vitamins E and C) and ω-3 polyunsaturated fatty acid (PUFA, often measured as fish consumption) [82-86], although some negative results have been also reported [87-90]. Light-to-moderate alcohol intake (e.g., 1-3 drinks per day) has been associated to a reduced incidence of dementia and AD [6, 91, 92], while heavy alcohol consumption at midlife has been associated to an increased risk of dementia/AD, especially among *APOE* ε4 carriers [93]. Alcohol may have beneficial influences on several cardiovascular factors, including lipid and lipoprotein levels, inflammatory and hemostatic factors. Indeed, moderate alcohol drinking has been related to a reduced risk of cardiovascular diseases, and may be associated with fewer brain infarcts [6]. However, it has been also suggested that the apparent cognitive benefits of light-to-moderate alcohol intake could be due to potential biases that result from methodological limitations of the observational studies such as information bias, confounding of socioeconomic status and healthy lifestyles, and inconsistent approaches of alcohol assessments [6].

3. **Vitamins**: The micronutrient vitamin E is the main lipid-soluble, chain-breaking, non-enzymatic antioxidant in the human body [94], and is essential for normal neurological functions [95]. Vitamin E includes eight natural congeners: four tocopherols and four

tocotrienols, named as α, β, γ, and δ [96]. Each congener shows different biological properties potentially relevant for neuroprotection. These include antioxidant and anti-inflammatory activity and modulation of signaling pathways involved in neurodegeneration [96, 97]. Most investigation of vitamin E in relation to dementia and AD has focused primarily only on α-tocopherol, with conflicting findings. Overall, studies investigating vitamin E intake only from supplements found no association with dementia/AD risk [89, 98-101], or a reduced incidence was found only for the combined use of vitamin E and C supplements [102, 103]. On the other hand, studies examining vitamin E dietary intake consistently report a reduced risk of dementia/AD in individuals with high vitamin E intake [84, 85, 104-106]. This might be explained by the fact that while vitamin E supplements contain only α-tocopherol, dietary intake can provide a balanced combination of different forms of vitamin E, which can be more relevant for neuroprotection. Recent studies seem to support this hypothesis: a multicenter European study found that both AD and MCI were associated with low plasma tocopherols and tocotrienols levels [107]. Further, in the Swedish Kungsholmen Project a decreased AD risk was found in subjects with high plasma levels of total tocopherols and total tocotrienols [108].

Vitamin B12 and folate are essential micronutrients that are part of the homocysteine metabolic cycle, and both vitamin B12 and folate deficiencies can result in increased total homocysteine levels, which may lead to a variety of disorders including cardiovascular and cerebrovascular conditions. Several studies reported and increased risk of dementia/AD, worse cognitive functioning and structural brain changes in individuals with low levels of vitamin B12, holotranscobalamin (the biologically active fraction of vitamin B12) or folate, or high levels of total homocysteine [109-115]. Other studies did not confirm these findings, but methodological differences (e.g., different follow-up duration, implementing the study after mandatory folic acid fortification, etc.) could account for the discrepancy [116-119]. Reviews of RCTs concluded that supplementations of folic acid and vitamin B12 had no benefits on cognition in healthy or cognitively impaired older people, although they were effective in reducing serum homocysteine levels [120, 121]. A more recent RCT testing the efficacy of B vitamins (B6, B12, folate) in subjects with MCI reported beneficial effects of the supplementation, in terms of reduced rate of brain atrophy and cognitive decline, which were more evident in subjects with elevated homocysteine levels [122, 123].

Vitamin D is a secosteroid hormone that is suggested to have neuroprotective effects that include regulation of neuronal calcium homeostasis, as well as antioxidant, neurotrophic and anti-inflammatory properties. Few recent longitudinal studies found a reduced risk of cognitive decline or AD in subjects with higher blood levels or higher dietary intake of vitamin D [124-126]. Despite the epidemiological evidence is still weak vitamin D is already being tested as a therapeutic agent in AD [127].

2.2.3. Combined effect

Cumulative and combined exposure to different risk factors can lead to modified effects on dementia/AD risk (Table 1). In the Finnish Cardiovascular Risk Factors, Aging, and Dementia study (CAIDE), the risk of dementia has been evaluated in relation to a score (CAIDE Dementia Risk Score) combining mid-life risk factors, including low education and cardiovascular factors (i.e., hypertension, obesity, hypercholesterolemia, physical inactivity). The risk of dementia increased as the score increased in a dose-response trend, making it possible to identify individuals who can greatly benefit from preventive intervention that targets vascular risk factors [128]. Similar findings have been reported for late-life exposures: in the Swedish Kungsholmen Project, the cumulative effect of vascular risk factors and vascular diseases on dementia/AD risk has been investigated in people aged 75+ years. These factors were aggregated according to two pathophysiological hypotheses: the brain hypoperfusion profile, defined by chronic heart failure, low pulse pressure, and low diastolic pressure, and the atherosclerosis profile, which included high systolic pressure, diabetes mellitus or prediabetes, and stroke. In both profiles, dementia/AD risk increased with increasing scores in a dose-response manner, suggesting a synergy of vascular risk factors in promoting dementia/AD also in advanced age [129]. The American Cardiovascular Health Cognition Study developed a Late-life Dementia Risk Index, and also its brief version, which groups older adults in the three categories of low, moderate, and high risk of developing dementia. Both versions of the index support the cumulative effect of different factors in determining the risk of dementia after the age of 65 years. These indices include information from different domains, including demographic factors (age), genetic (presence of the *APOE* ε4 allele), lifestyle (BMI<18.5, lack of alcohol consumption), comorbid vascular conditions (internal carotid artery thickening, angina, coronary artery by-pass surgery, stroke, peripheral artery disease), evidence of brain abnormalities showed by magnetic resonance imaging (MRI) (white matter diseases or enlarged ventricles), cognitive test scores and physical performances [130, 131].

The combined effect of genetic-environmental or environmental-environmental joint exposures may also lead to the attenuation of the dementia risk. Population-based studies suggest an effect modification for the *APOE* ε4 allele, the most important genetic risk factor for sporadic AD. *APOE* ε4 carriers seem more vulnerable to risk factors like alcohol drinking, smoking, physical inactivity and high intake of saturate fat, indicating that people with genetic susceptibility may reduce their initial AD risk by lifestyle interventions (i.e., physical activity, sufficient intake of PUFA, and avoiding excess alcohol drinking and smoking) [33]. The protective effect of lifestyle in *APOE* ε4 carriers seem to be present also in advanced age: in the Swedish Kungsholmen Project, subjects aged 75+ years who were *APOE* ε4 carriers, but with high education, active leisure activities, or good vascular health (i.e., absence of vascular risk factors), had a reduced risk of dementia and AD, as well as a delayed time of onset of the disease [132]. Further, it has been shown that high education may reduce dementia risk among *APOE* ε4 allele carriers [133].

Regarding the interactions among modifiable risk factors, results from the Kungsholmen Project suggested that complexity of work with data and people was related to a decreased dementia risk and that the highest level of work complexity may modulate the increased dementia risk due to low education [78].

In conclusion, even though the evidence for some risk and protective factors in dementia and AD is still scarce, and their role needs to be further clarified, findings from observational studies points at different modifiable factors that can be managed in order to prevent or delay dementia onset. Moreover, epidemiological findings strongly suggest that the life-course approach model and the multifactorial nature of dementia and AD should be considered when planning any preventive strategy.

3. Interventional studies

3.1. Current evidence

Different medications, including statins, antihypertensive drugs, estrogens alone or in combination with progestin (hormone replacement therapy, HRT), nonsteroidal anti-inflammatory drugs (NSAIDs), and nutraceuticals (vitamin B12, C, E, folate, Ginkgo biloba) have been tested as primary or secondary prevention measures for dementia and AD in subjects with normal cognition or MCI. In general, for all these compounds the protective effects suggested by observational studies have not been confirmed in RCTs, the results of which are inconsistent or even suggest a detrimental effect on cognition (e.g., NSAIDs, HRT) [120, 134-136]. Few interventional studies implementing non-pharmacological approaches have been carried out. Among them some RCTs on cognitive training and physical activity provided encouraging results, which need further confirmation [134, 137]. It is possible that the negative results from the RCTs done so far reflect the real inefficacy of the tested strategies in preventing dementia and AD. However, the apparent contradiction of results from observational and interventional studies could be explained by several factors:

1. The intervention was done outside the time-window when management of a risk factor would reduce dementia risk: several risk factors exert their effect mainly during mid-life, whereas RCTs have been done in older adults. This is the case for vascular risk factors, which seem to be more relevant when the exposure occurs during mid-life. Moreover, the HRT research suggests that estrogens may have beneficial, neutral, or detrimental effects on the brain depending on age at treatment, type of menopause (natural versus medically or surgically induced) or stage of menopause [138]. This concept, called the "window of opportunity hypothesis" is in agreement with the life-course approach model. There is evidence of neuroprotective effects of estrogens in women before the age of natural menopause and in the early postmenopausal stage (50-60 years), while estrogens initiated in late postmenopause (65-79 years) increase the risk of cognitive impairment and dementia [138-142]. The large-scale RCT of the Women's Health Initiative Memory Study (WHI-MS) showed that estrogens therapy alone or in combination with progestin was associated with a two-fold increased risk for dementia and MCI [139, 140]. The WHI-MS study enrolled women aged 65-79 years, who were given the HRT many years after the onset of natural or surgical menopause. In contrast, the Kronos Early Estrogen Prevention Study (KEEPS) tested the HRT in recently menopausal women (mean age 53 years; enrolment within three years after menopause), reporting beneficial effects [141]. In fact, the use of the HRT in the KEEPS participants has been associated with the improvement of markers of cardiovascular risk, anxiety and depression, without adverse effects on

cognition [141]. Overall these results suggest that the role of the HRT in age-related cognition and dementia needs to be further investigated, taking into account the time-window when the treatment is administered.

2. Short treatment and follow-up: many studies were of relatively short length. Thus, interventions have been implemented for a period that is not long enough to determine a neuroprotective effect, and the limited follow-up duration of many RCTs would not allow detection of differences in dementia incidence.

3. The statistical power was inadequate, since some RCTs had small samples and dementia has been considered a secondary endpoint in most clinical trials (e.g., antihypertensive therapy), in which clear benefits for primary endpoints (e.g., coronary heart disease and stroke) are shown usually in a short period of observation.

4. The choice of compounds tested in RCTs using nutraceuticals was not optimal: although several products have been tested, supplements composition is still a debated issue. For instance, whereas observational studies suggested that a balanced intake of different forms of vitamin E can be important for reducing dementia/AD risk, only one form (α-tocopherol) has been tested in RCTs, with conflicting findings [84, 85, 107, 108, 143]. Moreover, intake of high doses of α-tocopherol supplements has been associated with increased hemorrhagic stroke and mortality risk [144]. Regarding the studies on vitamins B, while the majority of RCTs done so far did not find evidence of benefit [120, 121], a recent RCT reported favourable effects in subjects with MCI, especially individuals with elevated homocysteine levels. In this latter RCT supplementation was done using a combination of vitamins B (B6, B12, folate) at high doses, suggesting that refining the type of supplements (i.e. composition, concentration) might increases the possibility to achieve beneficial effects in selected populations [122, 123].

5. Despite the multifactorial nature of dementia and the importance of combined risk exposures, most studies were based on a mono-intervention approach, almost always testing single agents or lifestyle interventions. In multifactorial conditions, a small reduction in multiple risk factors can substantially decrease overall risk.

In conclusion, despite the discrepancies between findings of observational and interventional studies and the disappointing results of intervention studies on dementia and AD, methodological issues of the RCTs carried out thus far suggest that a valid evaluation of the efficacy of preventive measures has yet to be undertaken.

3.2. Ongoing multidomain intervention studies

The disappointing results of previous trials, testing the effects of mono-intervention strategies in cognitively normal elderly or already cognitively impaired persons, have pointed out some key issues: i) timing – starting earlier may lead to better effects; ii) target group – a healthy, young population would require long follow-up times, large sample sizes and considerable financial resources; iii) lack of consistent and uniformly applied definitions of MCI has lead to enrolment of heterogeneous groups underpowering the studies; iv) outcome measures – cognitive impairment may be a better endpoint than conversion to dementia; v) ethical issues are also important, as placebo-controlled trials for high blood pressure and cholesterol are not possible due to their known protective effects regarding cardio- and cerebrovascular disease. Furthermore, a critical aspect that needs to be taken into account when planning preventive measures for dementia and AD, is the multifactorial nature of these disorders, which require multiple prevention approaches. Intervention studies combining several different approaches have not been conducted for AD so far, and the knowledge derived from the previously described observational and interventional studies has paved the way for some ongoing RCTs on prevention of cognitive decline and dementia. In Europe there are three large ongoing RCTs: FINGER, MAPT and PreDIVA [145, 146] (Table 2). The common denominator of these studies is the multidomain approach, which aims to target simultaneously several risk factors for dementia and AD in older adults, mainly by promoting lifestyle changes and adherence to medical treatments for vascular risk factors and vascular diseases. All RCTs exclude individuals with dementia or substantial cognitive decline, and use clinical evaluation and neuropsychological tests to detect cognitive changes and dementia incidence as main outcomes. Further, secondary outcomes include functional status, mood disorders, quality of life, adherence to the intervention programs and health resources utilization. These two latter aspects are essential from a public health perspective, since they provide information on feasibility and cost effectiveness of prevention strategies. Additionally, both FINGER and MAPT include ancillary studies on neuroimaging (morphological and functional), CSF and blood markers related to AD pathophysiology in order to investigate the effect of the interventions on brain morphology and metabolism, clarify mechanisms underlying preventive measures and identify biomarkers that can be used to monitor effects of interventions.

The Finnish Geriatric Intervention Study to Prevent Cognitive Impairment and Disability (FINGER, NCT01041989) is a multicenter RCT aiming to prevent cognitive impairment, dementia and disability in 60-77 year-old people. The study population is represented by 1282 individuals at increased risk of dementia, selected according to the CAIDE Dementia Risk Score and the CERAD neuropsychological test battery [128, 145]. The 2-year multidomain intervention includes nutritional guidance, physical activity, cognitive training, increased social activity and intensive monitoring and management of metabolic and vascular risk factors (hypertension, dyslipidemia, obesity, impaired glucose tolerance). Individuals in the reference group are given general public health advice on lifestyle and vascular risk factors. FINGER participants are recruited from previous population-based observational surveys (i.e., FINRISK, FIN-D2D) with detailed retrospective information on lifestyle and vascular factors [145]. Thus, differences in these variables can be taken into account, which is normally not possible in RCTs. The primary outcome is cognitive decline measured by a sensitive Neuropsychological Test Battery (NTB) and the Stroop and Trail Making tests, which can depict early cognitive impairment typical for AD and VaD. The planned 7-year extended follow-up will allow detection of differences in dementia/AD incidence. Two earlier intervention trials in Finland were important sources of inspiration for the FINGER study. The Diabetes Prevention Study (now completed) is a landmark RCT showing the effectiveness and feasibility of physical exercise and dietary interventions as preventive measures in people with impaired glucose tolerance. In this RCT lifestyle intervention in people at high risk for type 2 diabetes resulted in sustained lifestyle changes and a reduction in diabetes incidence, which remained after the individual lifestyle counselling was stopped [147, 148]. The four-year exercise and dietary intervention study Dose-Responses to Exercise Training (DRs EXTRA) had a drop-out rate of only 8% after two years, and preliminary results suggested a potential benefit of higher physical fitness on cognition [149].

RCT **Country**	**FINGER** **Finland**	**MAPT** **France**	**Pre-DIVA** **Netherlands**
Sample size	1282	1680	3534
Main inclusion criteria	Dementia Risk Score >6 and mild degree of cognitive impairment	Frail elderly people (subjective memory complaint, slow walking speed, limitation in IADL)	All elderly within GP practices, non demented (MMSE >23)
Age at enrolment, yrs	60 -77	≥ 70	70-78
Study design	Multi-center, randomized, single-blind, parallel-group	Multi-center, randomized, controlled trial	Multi-site, open, cluster-randomized parallel group
Multi-domain intervention	Nutritional guidance, physical activity, cognitive training, increased social activity and intensive monitoring and management of metabolic and vascular risk factors	Vascular care, nutritional advice, exercise advice, cognitive training, and/or DHA 800 mg/day	Nurse-led vascular care including medical treatment of risk factors, diet advice, exercise advice
Intervention period	2 yrs	3 yrs	6 yrs
Follow-up period	7 yrs	5 ysr	6 yrs
Primary outcome	Neuropsychological test battery, Trail Making test, Stroop test, Dementia	Change in cognitive function (Grober and Buschke memory test)	Dementia, Disability
Study Completion	2013	2013	2016

DHA: docosahexaenoic acid acid. IADL: Instrumental Activities of Daily Living. MMSE: Mini Mental State Examination

Table 2. Ongoing multi-domain prevention RCTs on dementia

The Multidomain Alzheimer Preventive Trial (MAPT, NCT00672685) is a French multicenter RCT evaluating the efficacy of isolated supplementation with ω-3 fatty acid, isolated multidomain intervention, or their combination in the prevention of cognitive decline in frail individuals aged ≥70 years. 1680 community-dwelling participants have been enrolled, using a definition of frailty that includes three components: presence of memory complaints, limitation in one instrumental activity of daily living (IADL) and slow walking speed. The 3-year multidomain intervention consists of group training sessions (physical exercise, cognitive training and nutritional advice) and yearly personalized preventive consultations that aim to identify dementia and frailty risk factors (vascular risk factors, nutritional problems, sensory deficits, mood disorders, walking difficulties) and promote their management in collaboration with the general practitioner. Follow-up is 5 years, and the main outcome measure is the 3-year change in cognitive function assessed with a neuropsychological test (Grober and Buschke) [145, 150].

The Prevention of Dementia by Intensive Vascular Care (PreDIVA) study is a Dutch multi-center, open, cluster-RCT comparing standard and intensive care of cardiovascular risk factors in preventing dementia and disability in elderly people. The study includes 3534 community-dwellers aged 70-78 years, recruited from primary care practices. The standard care is based on guidelines for Dutch general practice, while the multi-component intensive vascular care addresses hypertension, hypercholesterolemia, smoking habits, overweight, physical inactivity and diabetes mellitus, which are strictly controlled with medication and lifestyle interventions. Study duration is 6 years, and primary outcomes are incident dementia assessed according to standard criteria and disability as measured with the AMC Linear Disability Scale (ALDS) [146].

Researchers involved in these large European trials (FINGER, MAPT and PreDIVA) recently started the European Dementia Prevention Initiative (EDPI), an international collaboration to improve preventive strategies against dementia [151]. Collaboration and data sharing within the EDPI will allow refining methodological aspects of prevention trials, including identification of target populations; improvement of intervention methods (i.e., type, intensity, duration); and development and standardization of relevant outcome measures and prognostic and monitoring tools that can be easily implemented in large populations. This will help planning larger and international prevention trials able to provide robust evidence on dementia/AD prevention.

3.3. Presymptomatic Alzheimer's disease treatment: Anti-amyloid drugs

Presymptomatic (or preclinical) AD treatments have been defined as "those interventions that are initiated before apparent cognitive decline and are intended to reduce the chance of developing AD-related symptoms" [152]. The proposed term refers to an intervention whether it is started before or after biological evidence of the underlying disease, and whether it postpones the onset, partially reduces the risk of, or completely prevents symptomatic AD [153]. The progress on the knowledge about the AD phenotype, particularly on the biomarkers which have been incorporated in the new diagnostic criteria for dementia and MCI due AD, as well preclinical AD, has provided the basis for intervention studies evaluating pharmacological interventions in asymptomatic subjects who are at risk of AD, because of an established biomarker burden or a specific genetic profile. Three RCTs are planned to start in 2013 to verify safety and efficacy of anti-amyloid drugs as preventive measure in AD (Table 3). The Alzheimer's Prevention Initiative (API) and the Dominantly Inherited Alzheimer's Network (DIAN) studies will enrol subjects who carry genetic mutations for dominantly inherited AD: mutations in the *APP*, presenilin-1 (*PSEN1*), and presenilin-2 (*PSEN2*) genes can cause early-onset familial AD that accounts for no more than 5 percent of all cases [154].

Data from the DIAN study have shown that different phenotypic changes can be detected several years before the onset of cognitive symptoms in individual with autosomal dominant AD: it has been shown that CSF levels of Aβ42 decline 25 years before expected symptom onset, and brain deposition of Aβ can be detected 15 years before. Further, increased concentrations of tau protein in the CSF and brain atrophy are visible 15 years before expected symptom onset, while cerebral hypometabolism can be observed 10 years before [155]. The API RCT will focus on the world largest early-onset AD kindred in Antioquia, Columbia. Of about 5000 individuals in this kindred, approximately 1500 carry a mutation in the *PSEN1* gene (E280A) causing early onset AD (mean age of onset: 45 years) [156, 157]. The trial will also include a small number of individuals in the United States, recruited in collaboration with researchers from the DIAN study [158]. The drug used in the API study is the anti-amyloid antibody crenezumab, which has been chosen based on the evidence of its ability to remove from the brain different forms of Aβ and its safety profile (low risk of cerebral vasogenic oedema and microhaemorrhages) [157]. The trial within the DIAN cohort will include people with mutations in any of the three genes linked to early-onset AD: *PSEN1*, *PSEN2*, and *APP*. Three different anti-amyloid compounds will be evaluated in the first phase of the study (2 years): the beta-secretase inhibitor LY2886721, which limits the production of Aβ; and two anti-amyloid antibodies (Gantenerumab, Solanezumab) which promote Aβ removal from the brain. The more effective drug(s) will be further tested in a 3 years extension phase of the study. A third trial, the Anti-Amyloid Treatment of Asymptomatic Alzheimer's (A4) RTC, aims to prevent sporadic AD and will evaluate the effect of an anti-amyloid compound in older adults with evidence of brain amyloid accumulation at neuroimaging evaluation. The study is sponsored by the Alzheimer's Disease Cooperative Study, and also in this case the drug candidate still needs to be identified among anti-amyloid compounds. The study is expected to detect differences in the rate of cogntive decline, while it has not enough statistical power to detect a difference in dementia incidence. The A4 study will also include an ethics arm examining the psychological impact of disclosing information to individuals about their risk of developing AD [157].

Overall, these studies provide the opportunity to test the efficacy of AD-modifying treatments in an earlier stage of AD compared to the pharmacological RCTs done so far. While testing these compounds in young, healthy individuals would require enormous financial resources and too long follow up, the recruitment strategies implemented in these studies allow testing the benefit of anti-amyloid drugs earlier than otherwise possible. This approach provides also the opportunity to further verify the amyloid hypothesis, which has been reconsidered many times over the past decades and criticized in light of the recent failures of RCTs testing anti-amyloid drugs in subjects with mild-to-moderate AD. A possible interpretation of these failures is that the anti-amyloid therapies have missed their "window of opportunity", since

http://dx.doi.org/10.5772/55034

they have been provided too late. The preventive RCTs on anti-amyloid drugs are based on the assumption that an earlier interference on amyloid accumulation, before irreversible brain damage occurs, would exert a significant disease-modifying effect. These prevention studies will also allow determining the ability of different biomarkers to predict a clinical benefit, information needed to help qualify biomarker endpoints for use in prevention trials. These studies offer great hope, but also safety concerns, since anti-amyloid compounds will be tested in subjects with no cognitive problems and the long-term risk associated with the use of anti-amyloid drugs is yet unknown.

RCT	**API** **Alzheimer's Prevention Initiative**	**DIAN** **Dominantly Inherited Alzheimer Network**	**A4** **Anti-Amyloid Treatment of Asymptomatic AD**
Sample size	300 members of Colombian families. A small number of individuals from USA (collaboration with the DIAN network) will also be included	240 members of families with early-onset AD	1500 older adults with no cognitive impairment
Main inclusion criteria	Carriers of a mutated *PSEN1* gene. Non-carriers will also be included, to ensure double-blinding about the genetic status	Carriers of mutation in *PSEN1,* or *PSEN2,* or *APP*. Non-carriers will also be included, to ensure double-blinding about the genetic status	Evidence of brain amyloid accumulation. Subject with no evidence of amyloid burden will also be included
Age at enrolment, yrs	≥ 30	NA	≥ 70
Study design	Randomized, double blind, placebo controlled trial	Randomized, double blind, placebo controlled trial	Randomized, double blind, placebo controlled trial
Intervention	Anti-amyloid antibody Crenezumab (Genentech)	Three anti-amyloid therapies: the beta-secretase inhibitor LY2886721 (Lilly), and the anti-amyloid antibodies Gantenerumab (Roche) and Solanezumab (Lilly)	One anti-amyloid therapy (to be determined)
Duration	5 yrs, (interim analysis at 2 yrs)	2 yrs + 3 yrs extension	3 yrs + 2 yrs extension
Outcomes	Primary: cognitive function Secondary: biomarkers, including brain amyloid load and brain atrophy	Initial phase (2 yrs): biomarkers analysis, to identify the most promising drug candidate Follow-up phase (3 yrs): cognitive function	Primary: cognitive function Secondary: biomarkers

APP: amyloid precursor protein. *PSEN1*: presenilin 1. *PSEN2*: presenilin 1

Table 3. Alzheimer's prevention trials based on anti-amyloid treatments

4. Conclusion

Prevention is a newer area in dementia/AD research, and the shift from observation to action has occurred only in the last decade, with several intervention studies now ongoing, and other RCTs starting soon. Although the pathogenesis of dementia is not fully elucidated, primary prevention seems possible, as most factors involved in dementia onset and progression are modifiable or amenable to management. The recent AHRQ/NIH report shows that development of successful preventive strategies requires a more refined knowledge on risk and protective factors for dementia and AD, as well as a validation of the observational studies with large intervention studies [19]. AD and VaD share several risk factors, and most dementia cases are attributable to both vascular and neurodegenerative brain damage. Furthermore, population-based neuropathological studies have shown that both subclinical neurodegenerative (amyloid plaques, neurofibrillary tangles, Lewy bodies) and vascular lesions are common in the brains of cognitively normal elderly individuals, as is their co-occurrence [9]. In light of this, preventive strategies aiming to postpone the onset of dementia syndrome have great potential.

Epidemiological research suggests that the most effective strategy may be to encourage the implementation of multiple preventive measures throughout the life course, including high educational attainment in childhood and early adulthood; active control of vascular factors and disorders over adulthood; and maintenance of mentally, physically, and socially active lifestyles during middle age and later in life. It has been estimated that half of AD cases worldwide are potentially attributable to modifiable risk factors, and a 10-25% reduction in these factors could potentially prevent 3 million AD cases worldwide, with a reduction in all risk factors having the greatest impact on dementia prevalence [70]. However, RCTs are indispensable to confirm the effect of risk reduction strategies targeting multiple risk factors. Multidomain interventional RCTs are now ongoing and will provide new insights into prevention of cognitive impairment and dementia. Full implementation of the life-course approach is more challenging, due to the difficulties of carrying out RCTs over many decades. Such long-term studies would require very large sample sizes and huge financial resources, and a pragmatic way to assess the effect of long-term interventions within a RCT has not yet been established. Furthermore, several risk and protective factors are not appropriate for intervention trials, due to unethical reasons, thus evidence about these factors rely on conducting rigorous observational studies (e.g., placebo-controlled trials for high blood pressure or cholesterol are not possible because such treatments are known to protect against cardio/cerebrovascular diseases) [35]. Methodological alternatives to RCTs have been proposed to obtain robust evidence on AD and dementia prevention [37, 159].

Platforms for early intervention could be established by incorporating the classical clinical trial approach to disease into a public health model, with long-term longitudinal databases including large populations. Establishing comprehensive databases for studies on aging can create the opportunity to formulate and validate tools for early detection of people who are at increased risk of late-life cognitive impairment, to identify important targets (risk factors) for preventive interventions, and to test such interventions in RCTs.

The first initiatives with an international perspective have already been established, for example the Leon Thal Symposia [160], Prevent Alzheimer's Disease by 2020 (PAD2020, http://www.pad2020.org), and the European Dementia Prevention Initiative (EDPI, http://www.edpi.org). It has been suggested that a worldwide database could be built by integrating and expanding already existing cohorts and registries [160].

The ongoing RTCs on dementia prevention will have to take into account the "window of opportunity hypothesis" when evaluating the results of interventions. In fact, efficacy of preventive actions may vary by age. Thus, implementation of interventions at the appropriate time in the life course is crucial for successful prevention. Refining of prognostic tools, which can be used for early detection of subjects at risk of dementia in the general population, will also help to better plan intervention studies. Also, when targeting elderly individuals, the frequent coexistence of chronic diseases needs to be considered, since it can negatively impact cognitive performance and limit adherence to preventive interventions. On the other hand, appropriate management of morbidity can help improve cognitive performance and delay dementia onset. For instance, although stroke is a known risk factor for dementia, it has been recently reported that about 25% of stroke patients discontinued one or more of their prescribed secondary prevention medications within 3 months of hospitalization for acute stroke [161-163]. Improving long-term adherence to post-stroke treatment can prevent recurrent cerebrovascular diseases and contribute to preventing or delaying clinical expression of dementia syndrome. Additionally, there is evidence of inadequate management of hypertension and hypercholesterolemia in the older adults [146]. Similar situations exist for heart failure, which increases the risk of dementia among older adults [68], and diabetes mellitus, which accelerates the progression from mild cognitive impairment to dementia by more than 3 years [164]. Preliminary results from the PreDIVA study showed that 87% of the study participants have at least one modifiable risk factor amenable to intervention, proving the presence of a window of opportunity for improved risk management [146].

In conclusion, prevention of dementia is now moving from observational to interventional studies to verify hypotheses and define tools that can be applied in the general population. Epidemiological and preclinical studies will continue to provide new information on risk/protective factors and pathological mechanisms. The international collaboration among research teams involved in ongoing multidomain RCTs will allow the sharing of experiences and discussions on methodological aspects of these studies. This can help in interpretation of results, identification and solution of problems related to intervention strategies, and refinement of preventative approaches. The multidomain intervention RCTs are at one end of the current spectrum of intervention trials in AD/cognitive impairment. At the other end are RCTs testing disease-modifying drugs (i.e. anti-amyloid therapy) in genetically at-risk groups or those with established biomarker burden. The shift towards pre-symptomatic and pre-dementia stages of AD has brought prevention and treatment RCTs much closer to each other than before. Since a cure for dementia is not yet available, finding effective preventive strategies is essential for a sustainable society in an aging world. As dementia, cardiovascular diseases, stroke and diabetes mellitus – all major public health problems – share several risk factors, public health efforts promoting healthier lifestyle have the potential to enhance health status in advanced age.

Acknowledgements

This work has been supported by: the Swedish Research Council for Medical Research; Academy of Finland; La Carita Foundation, Finland; Alzheimer's Association (USA); the Swedish Foundations Ragnhild och Einar Lundströms-Minne-Lindhés, Stohnes-Stiftelse and Gamla-Tjänarinnor.

Author details

Francesca Mangialasche[1,2*], Weili Xu[1,3] and Miia Kivipelto[1,4]

*Address all correspondence to: francesca.mangialasche@ki.se

1 Aging Research Center, Karolinska Institutet-Stockholm University, Stockholm, Sweden

2 Institute of Gerontology and Geriatrics, Department of Clinical and Experimental Medicine, University of Perugia, Perugia, Italy

3 Department of Epidemiology, Tianjin Medical University, Tianjin, P.R., China

4 Department of Neurology, University of Eastern Finland, Kuopio, Finland

References

[1] American Psychiatric AssociationDiagnostic and statistic manual of mental disorders 3rd ed., revised (DSM-III-R). Association AP, editor. Washington D.C.(1987).

[2] Fratiglioni, L, Launer, L. J, Andersen, K, Breteler, M. M, Copeland, J. R, Dartigues, J. F, et al. Incidence of dementia and major subtypes in Europe: A collaborative study of population-based cohorts. Neurologic Diseases in the Elderly Research Group. Neurology. (2000). Suppl 5):S, 10-5.

[3] Alzheimer's Disease International, World Alzheimer Report. The Global Economic Impact of Dementia. 2010; Available from: http://www.alz.co.uk/research/files/WorldAlzheimerReport2010ExecutiveSummary.pdf.

[4] Jack, C. R. Jr., Albert MS, Knopman DS, McKhann GM, Sperling RA, Carrillo MC, et al. Introduction to the recommendations from the National Institute on Aging-Alz-

heimer's Association workgroups on diagnostic guidelines for Alzheimer's disease. Alzheimers Dement. (2011). May;, 7(3), 257-62.

[5] Fratiglioni, L, & Qiu, C. Prevention of common neurodegenerative disorders in the elderly. Experimental gerontology. (2009). Jan-Feb;44(1-2):46-50.

[6] Qiu, C, Kivipelto, M, & Von Strauss, E. Epidemiology of Alzheimer's disease: occurrence, determinants, and strategies toward intervention. Dialogues in clinical neuroscience. (2009). , 11(2), 111-28.

[7] Stephan, B. C, Matthews, F. E, Ma, B, Muniz, G, Hunter, S, Davis, D, et al. Alzheimer and vascular neuropathological changes associated with different cognitive States in a non-demented sample. J Alzheimers Dis. (2012). , 29(2), 309-18.

[8] Schneider, J. A, Arvanitakis, Z, Bang, W, & Bennett, D. A. Mixed brain pathologies account for most dementia cases in community-dwelling older persons. Neurology. (2007). Dec 11;, 69(24), 2197-204.

[9] Sonnen, J. A. Santa Cruz K, Hemmy LS, Woltjer R, Leverenz JB, Montine KS, et al. Ecology of the aging human brain. Archives of neurology. (2011). Aug;, 68(8), 1049-56.

[10] Mckhann, G, Drachman, D, Folstein, M, Katzman, R, Price, D, & Stadlan, E. M. Clinical diagnosis of Alzheimer's disease: report of the NINCDS-ADRDA Work Group under the auspices of Department of Health and Human Services Task Force on Alzheimer's Disease. Neurology. (1984). Jul;, 34(7), 939-44.

[11] Mangialasche, F, Solomon, A, Winblad, B, Mecocci, P, & Kivipelto, M. Alzheimer's disease: clinical trials and drug development. Lancet neurology. (2010). Jul;, 9(7), 702-16.

[12] Morris, J. C. Early-stage and preclinical Alzheimer disease. Alzheimer disease and associated disorders. (2005). Jul-Sep;, 19(3), 163-5.

[13] Petersen, R. C, Doody, R, Kurz, A, Mohs, R. C, Morris, J. C, Rabins, P. V, et al. Current concepts in mild cognitive impairment. Arch Neurol. (2001). Dec;, 58(12), 1985-92.

[14] Harvey, R, Fox, N, & Rossor, M. Dementia Handbook. London: Martin Dunitz; (1999).

[15] Albert, M. S, Dekosky, S. T, Dickson, D, Dubois, B, Feldman, H. H, Fox, N. C, et al. The diagnosis of mild cognitive impairment due to Alzheimer's disease: recommendations from the National Institute on Aging-Alzheimer's Association workgroups on diagnostic guidelines for Alzheimer's disease. Alzheimers Dement. (2011). May;, 7(3), 270-9.

[16] Mckhann, G. M, Knopman, D. S, Chertkow, H, Hyman, B. T, & Jack, C. R. Jr., Kawas CH, et al. The diagnosis of dementia due to Alzheimer's disease: recommendations from the National Institute on Aging-Alzheimer's Association workgroups on diag-

nostic guidelines for Alzheimer's disease. Alzheimers Dement. (2011). May;, 7(3), 263-9.

[17] Sperling, R. A, Aisen, P. S, Beckett, L. A, Bennett, D. A, Craft, S, Fagan, A. M, et al. Toward defining the preclinical stages of Alzheimer's disease: recommendations from the National Institute on Aging-Alzheimer's Association workgroups on diagnostic guidelines for Alzheimer's disease. Alzheimers Dement. (2011). May;, 7(3), 280-92.

[18] Qiu, C, & Fratiglioni, L. Epidemiology of the dementias. In: McNamara P, editor. Dementia History and Incidence. Santa Barbara, CA: ABC-CLIO PRESS, INC; (2011).

[19] Fratiglioni, L, & Qiu, C. Prevention of cognitive decline in ageing: dementia as the target, delayed onset as the goal. Lancet neurology. (2011). Sep;, 10(9), 778-9.

[20] Kivipelto, M, & Solomon, A. Preventive neurology: on the way from knowledge to action. Neurology. (2009). Jul 21;, 73(3), 168-9.

[21] Fratiglioni, L, Von Strauss, E, & Qiu, C. Epidemiology of the dementias of old age. In: Dening T, R. Jacoby, C. Oppenheimer, and A. Thomas., editor. The Oxford Textbook of Old Age Psychiatry. London: Oxford University Press; (2008). , 391-406.

[22] Matthews, F, & Brayne, C. The incidence of dementia in England and Wales: findings from the five identical sites of the MRC CFA Study. PLoS medicine. (2005). Aug; 2(8):e193.

[23] Green, R. C, Cupples, L. A, Go, R, Benke, K. S, Edeki, T, Griffith, P. A, et al. Risk of dementia among white and African American relatives of patients with Alzheimer disease. Jama. (2002). Jan 16;, 287(3), 329-36.

[24] Seshadri, S, & Wolf, P. A. Lifetime risk of stroke and dementia: current concepts, and estimates from the Framingham Study. Lancet neurology. (2007). Dec;, 6(12), 1106-14.

[25] Ballard, C, Gauthier, S, Corbett, A, Brayne, C, Aarsland, D, & Jones, E. Alzheimer's disease. Lancet. [Research Support, Non-U.S. Gov't Review]. (2011). Mar 19;, 377(9770), 1019-31.

[26] Qiu, C, Kivipelto, M, Aguero-torres, H, Winblad, B, & Fratiglioni, L. Risk and protective effects of the APOE gene towards Alzheimer's disease in the Kungsholmen project: variation by age and sex. J Neurol Neurosurg Psychiatry. (2004). Jun;, 75(6), 828-33.

[27] Slooter, A. J, Cruts, M, Kalmijn, S, Hofman, A, Breteler, M. M, Van Broeckhoven, C, et al. Risk estimates of dementia by apolipoprotein E genotypes from a population-based incidence study: the Rotterdam Study. Archives of neurology. (1998). Jul;, 55(7), 964-8.

[28] Corder, E. H, Saunders, A. M, Strittmatter, W. J, Schmechel, D. E, Gaskell, P. C, Small, G. W, et al. Gene dose of apolipoprotein E type 4 allele and the risk of Alz-

heimer's disease in late onset families. Science (New York, NY. (1993). Aug 13;, 261(5123), 921-3.

[29] Cruchaga, C, Haller, G, Chakraverty, S, Mayo, K, Vallania, F. L, Mitra, R. D, et al. Rare variants in APP, PSEN1 and PSEN2 increase risk for AD in late-onset Alzheimer's disease families. PloS one. (2012). e31039.

[30] Jonsson, T, Atwal, J. K, Steinberg, S, Snaedal, J, Jonsson, P. V, Bjornsson, S, et al. A mutation in APP protects against Alzheimer's disease and age-related cognitive decline. Nature. (2012). Aug 2;, 488(7409), 96-9.

[31] Roses, A. D, Lutz, M. W, Amrine-madsen, H, Saunders, A. M, Crenshaw, D. G, Sundseth, S. S, et al. A TOMM40 variable-length polymorphism predicts the age of late-onset Alzheimer's disease. The pharmacogenomics journal. Oct;, 10(5), 375-84.

[32] Harold, D, Abraham, R, Hollingworth, P, Sims, R, Gerrish, A, Hamshere, M. L, et al. Genome-wide association study identifies variants at CLU and PICALM associated with Alzheimer's disease. Nature genetics. (2009). Oct;, 41(10), 1088-93.

[33] Kivipelto, M, Rovio, S, Ngandu, T, Kareholt, I, Eskelinen, M, Winblad, B, et al. Apolipoprotein E epsilon4 magnifies lifestyle risks for dementia: a population-based study. Journal of cellular and molecular medicine. (2008). Dec;12(6B):, 2762-71.

[34] Salloway, S, Sperling, R, Gilman, S, Fox, N. C, Blennow, K, Raskind, M, et al. A phase 2 multiple ascending dose trial of bapineuzumab in mild to moderate Alzheimer disease. Neurology. (2009). Dec 15;, 73(24), 2061-70.

[35] Williams, J. W, Plassman, B. L, Burke, J, Holsinger, T, & Benjamin, S. Preventing Alzheimer's Disease and Cognitive Decline. Evidence Report/Technology Assessment Prepared by the Duke Evidence-based Practice Center under Contract No. HHSA 290-(2007). I.). Rockville, MD: Agency for Healthcare Research and Quality.: AHRQ Publication No. E0052010.(193), 10.

[36] NIHConsensus Development Conference Statement on Preventing Alzheimer's Disease and Cognitive Decline. Bethesda, MD (2010).

[37] Hughes, T. F, & Ganguli, M. Modifiable Midlife Risk Factors for Late-Life Cognitive Impairment and Dementia. Current psychiatry reviews. (2009). May 1;, 5(2), 73-92.

[38] Flicker, L, Liu-ambrose, T, & Kramer, A. F. Why so negative about preventing cognitive decline and dementia? The jury has already come to the verdict for physical activity and smoking cessation. British journal of sports medicine. (2010). May;, 45(6), 465-7.

[39] Qiu, C, Kivipelto, M, & Fratiglioni, L. Preventing Alzheimer disease and cognitive decline. Annals of internal medicine. (2011). Feb 1;154(3):211; author reply , 2-3.

[40] Whalley, L. J, Dick, F. D, & Mcneill, G. A life-course approach to the aetiology of late-onset dementias. Lancet Neurol. (2006). Jan;, 5(1), 87-96.

[41] Qiu, C, Winblad, B, & Fratiglioni, L. The age-dependent relation of blood pressure to cognitive function and dementia. Lancet Neurol. (2005). Aug;, 4(8), 487-99.

[42] Qiu, C, Xu, W, & Fratiglioni, L. Vascular and psychosocial factors in Alzheimer's disease: epidemiological evidence toward intervention. J Alzheimers Dis. (2010). , 20(3), 689-97.

[43] Kivipelto, M, Helkala, E. L, Laakso, M. P, Hanninen, T, Hallikainen, M, Alhainen, K, et al. Apolipoprotein E epsilon4 allele, elevated midlife total cholesterol level, and high midlife systolic blood pressure are independent risk factors for late-life Alzheimer disease. Annals of internal medicine. (2002). Aug 6;, 137(3), 149-55.

[44] Mielke, M. M, Zandi, P. P, Sjogren, M, Gustafson, D, Ostling, S, Steen, B, et al. High total cholesterol levels in late life associated with a reduced risk of dementia. Neurology. (2005). May 24;, 64(10), 1689-95.

[45] Atti, A. R, Palmer, K, Volpato, S, Winblad, B, De Ronchi, D, & Fratiglioni, L. Late-life body mass index and dementia incidence: nine-year follow-up data from the Kungsholmen Project. J Am Geriatr Soc. (2008). Jan;, 56(1), 111-6.

[46] Kivipelto, M, Ngandu, T, Fratiglioni, L, Viitanen, M, Kareholt, I, Winblad, B, et al. Obesity and vascular risk factors at midlife and the risk of dementia and Alzheimer disease. Arch Neurol. (2005). Oct;, 62(10), 1556-60.

[47] Alonso, A, & Mosley, T. H. Jr., Gottesman RF, Catellier D, Sharrett AR, Coresh J. Risk of dementia hospitalisation associated with cardiovascular risk factors in midlife and older age: the Atherosclerosis Risk in Communities (ARIC) study. Journal of neurology, neurosurgery, and psychiatry. (2009). Nov;, 80(11), 1194-201.

[48] Qiu, C, Winblad, B, & Fratiglioni, L. Low diastolic pressure and risk of dementia in very old people: a longitudinal study. Dementia and geriatric cognitive disorders. (2009). , 28(3), 213-9.

[49] Dahl, A. K, Lopponen, M, Isoaho, R, Berg, S, & Kivela, S. L. Overweight and obesity in old age are not associated with greater dementia risk. Journal of the American Geriatrics Society. (2008). Dec;, 56(12), 2261-6.

[50] West, N. A, & Haan, M. N. Body adiposity in late life and risk of dementia or cognitive impairment in a longitudinal community-based study. The journals of gerontology. (2009). Jan;, 64(1), 103-9.

[51] Hughes, T. F, Borenstein, A. R, Schofield, E, Wu, Y, & Larson, E. B. Association between late-life body mass index and dementia: The Kame Project. Neurology. (2009). May 19;, 72(20), 1741-6.

[52] Fitzpatrick, A. L, Kuller, L. H, Lopez, O. L, Diehr, P, Meara, O, Longstreth, E. S, Jr, W. T, et al. Midlife and late-life obesity and the risk of dementia: cardiovascular health study. Archives of neurology. (2009). Mar;, 66(3), 336-42.

[53] Rosengren, A, Skoog, I, Gustafson, D, & Wilhelmsen, L. Body mass index, other cardiovascular risk factors, and hospitalization for dementia. Archives of internal medicine. (2005). Feb 14;, 165(3), 321-6.

[54] Whitmer, R. A, Gunderson, E. P, Barrett-connor, E, & Quesenberry, C. P. Jr., Yaffe K. Obesity in middle age and future risk of dementia: a 27 year longitudinal population based study. BMJ (Clinical research ed. (2005). Jun 11;330(7504):1360.

[55] Hassing, L. B, Dahl, A. K, Thorvaldsson, V, Berg, S, Gatz, M, Pedersen, N. L, et al. Overweight in midlife and risk of dementia: a 40-year follow-up study. International journal of obesity ((2005). Aug;, 33(8), 893-8.

[56] Solomon, A, Kareholt, I, Ngandu, T, Winblad, B, Nissinen, A, Tuomilehto, J, et al. Serum cholesterol changes after midlife and late-life cognition: twenty-one-year follow-up study. Neurology. (2007). Mar 6;, 68(10), 751-6.

[57] Stewart, R, White, L. R, Xue, Q. L, & Launer, L. J. Twenty-six-year change in total cholesterol levels and incident dementia: the Honolulu-Asia Aging Study. Arch Neurol. (2007). Jan;, 64(1), 103-7.

[58] Cramer, C, Haan, M. N, Galea, S, Langa, K. M, & Kalbfleisch, J. D. Use of statins and incidence of dementia and cognitive impairment without dementia in a cohort study. Neurology. (2008). Jul 29;, 71(5), 344-50.

[59] Xu, W, Qiu, C, Gatz, M, Pedersen, N. L, Johansson, B, & Fratiglioni, L. Mid- and late-life diabetes in relation to the risk of dementia: a population-based twin study. Diabetes. (2009). Jan;, 58(1), 71-7.

[60] Xu, W, Qiu, C, Winblad, B, & Fratiglioni, L. The effect of borderline diabetes on the risk of dementia and Alzheimer's disease. Diabetes. (2007). Jan;, 56(1), 211-6.

[61] Pendlebury, S. T, & Rothwell, P. M. Prevalence, incidence, and factors associated with pre-stroke and post-stroke dementia: a systematic review and meta-analysis. Lancet neurology. (2009). Nov;, 8(11), 1006-18.

[62] Savva, G. M, & Stephan, B. C. Epidemiological studies of the effect of stroke on incident dementia: a systematic review. Stroke; a journal of cerebral circulation. (2010). Jan;41(1):e, 41-6.

[63] Troncoso, J. C, Zonderman, A. B, Resnick, S. M, Crain, B, Pletnikova, O, & Brien, O. RJ. Effect of infarcts on dementia in the Baltimore longitudinal study of aging. Annals of neurology. (2008). Aug;, 64(2), 168-76.

[64] Vermeer, S. E, & Prins, N. D. den Heijer T, Hofman A, Koudstaal PJ, Breteler MM. Silent brain infarcts and the risk of dementia and cognitive decline. N Engl J Med. (2003). Mar 27;, 348(13), 1215-22.

[65] Newman, A. B, Fitzpatrick, A. L, Lopez, O, Jackson, S, Lyketsos, C, Jagust, W, et al. Dementia and Alzheimer's disease incidence in relationship to cardiovascular dis-

ease in the Cardiovascular Health Study cohort. J Am Geriatr Soc. (2005). Jul;, 53(7), 1101-7.

[66] Laurin, D, Masaki, K. H, White, L. R, & Launer, L. J. Ankle-to-brachial index and dementia: the Honolulu-Asia Aging Study. Circulation. (2007). Nov 13;, 116(20), 2269-74.

[67] Ott, A, Breteler, M. M, De Bruyne, M. C, Van Harskamp, F, Grobbee, D. E, & Hofman, A. Atrial fibrillation and dementia in a population-based study. The Rotterdam Study. Stroke; a journal of cerebral circulation. (1997). Feb;, 28(2), 316-21.

[68] Qiu, C, Winblad, B, Marengoni, A, Klarin, I, Fastbom, J, & Fratiglioni, L. Heart failure and risk of dementia and Alzheimer disease: a population-based cohort study. Arch Intern Med. (2006). May 8;, 166(9), 1003-8.

[69] Van Oijen, M, De Jong, F. J, Witteman, J. C, Hofman, A, Koudstaal, P. J, & Breteler, M. M. Atherosclerosis and risk for dementia. Annals of neurology. (2007). May;, 61(5), 403-10.

[70] Barnes, D. E, & Yaffe, K. The projected effect of risk factor reduction on Alzheimer's disease prevalence. Lancet neurology. (2011). Sep;, 10(9), 819-28.

[71] Ownby, R. L, Crocco, E, Acevedo, A, John, V, & Loewenstein, D. Depression and risk for Alzheimer disease: systematic review, meta-analysis, and metaregression analysis. Archives of general psychiatry. (2006). May;, 63(5), 530-8.

[72] Rondeau, V, Jacqmin-gadda, H, Commenges, D, Helmer, C, & Dartigues, J. F. Aluminum and silica in drinking water and the risk of Alzheimer's disease or cognitive decline: findings from 15-year follow-up of the PAQUID cohort. American journal of epidemiology. (2009). Feb 15;, 169(4), 489-96.

[73] Feychting, M, Jonsson, F, Pedersen, N. L, & Ahlbom, A. Occupational magnetic field exposure and neurodegenerative disease. Epidemiology. [Research Support, Non-U.S. Gov't]. (2003). Jul;discussion 27-8., 14(4), 413-9.

[74] Garcia, A. M, Sisternas, A, & Hoyos, S. P. Occupational exposure to extremely low frequency electric and magnetic fields and Alzheimer disease: a meta-analysis. International journal of epidemiology. (2008). Apr;, 37(2), 329-40.

[75] Fleminger, S, Oliver, D. L, Lovestone, S, Rabe-hesketh, S, & Giora, A. Head injury as a risk factor for Alzheimer's disease: the evidence 10 years on; a partial replication. Journal of neurology, neurosurgery, and psychiatry. (2003). Jul;, 74(7), 857-62.

[76] Himanen, L, Portin, R, Isoniemi, H, Helenius, H, Kurki, T, & Tenovuo, O. Longitudinal cognitive changes in traumatic brain injury: a 30-year follow-up study. Neurology. (2006). Jan 24;, 66(2), 187-92.

[77] Holmes, C, & Cotterell, D. Role of infection in the pathogenesis of Alzheimer's disease: implications for treatment. CNS drugs. (2009). Dec;, 23(12), 993-1002.

[78] Karp, A, Andel, R, Parker, M. G, Wang, H. X, Winblad, B, & Fratiglioni, L. Mentally stimulating activities at work during midlife and dementia risk after age 75: follow-up study from the Kungsholmen Project. Am J Geriatr Psychiatry. (2009). Mar;, 17(3), 227-36.

[79] Rovio, S, Kareholt, I, Helkala, E. L, Viitanen, M, Winblad, B, Tuomilehto, J, et al. Leisure-time physical activity at midlife and the risk of dementia and Alzheimer's disease. Lancet neurology. (2005). Nov;, 4(11), 705-11.

[80] Hakansson, K, Rovio, S, Helkala, E. L, Vilska, A. R, Winblad, B, Soininen, H, et al. Association between mid-life marital status and cognitive function in later life: population based cohort study. BMJ (Clinical research ed. (2009). b2462.

[81] Paillard-borg, S, Fratiglioni, L, Winblad, B, & Wang, H. X. Leisure activities in late life in relation to dementia risk: principal component analysis. Dementia and geriatric cognitive disorders. (2009). , 28(2), 136-44.

[82] Barberger-gateau, P, Raffaitin, C, Letenneur, L, Berr, C, Tzourio, C, Dartigues, J. F, et al. Dietary patterns and risk of dementia: the Three-City cohort study. Neurology. (2007). Nov 13;, 69(20), 1921-30.

[83] Morris, M. C, Evans, D. A, Bienias, J. L, Tangney, C. C, Bennett, D. A, Aggarwal, N, et al. Dietary fats and the risk of incident Alzheimer disease. Arch Neurol. (2003). Feb;, 60(2), 194-200.

[84] Devore, E. E, Grodstein, F, Van Rooij, F. J, Hofman, A, Stampfer, M. J, Witteman, J. C, et al. Dietary antioxidants and long-term risk of dementia. Archives of neurology. (2010). Jul;, 67(7), 819-25.

[85] Morris, M. C, Evans, D. A, Tangney, C. C, Bienias, J. L, Wilson, R. S, Aggarwal, N. T, et al. Relation of the tocopherol forms to incident Alzheimer disease and to cognitive change. The American journal of clinical nutrition. (2005). Feb;, 81(2), 508-14.

[86] Scarmeas, N, Stern, Y, Tang, M. X, Mayeux, R, & Luchsinger, J. A. Mediterranean diet and risk for Alzheimer's disease. Annals of neurology. (2006). Jun;, 59(6), 912-21.

[87] Devore, E. E, Grodstein, F, Van Rooij, F. J, Hofman, A, Rosner, B, Stampfer, M. J, et al. Dietary intake of fish and omega-3 fatty acids in relation to long-term dementia risk. The American journal of clinical nutrition. (2009). Jul;, 90(1), 170-6.

[88] Kroger, E, Verreault, R, Carmichael, P. H, Lindsay, J, Julien, P, Dewailly, E, et al. Omega-3 fatty acids and risk of dementia: the Canadian Study of Health and Aging. The American journal of clinical nutrition. (2009). Jul;, 90(1), 184-92.

[89] Gray, S. L, Anderson, M. L, Crane, P. K, Breitner, J. C, Mccormick, W, Bowen, J. D, et al. Antioxidant vitamin supplement use and risk of dementia or Alzheimer's disease in older adults. Journal of the American Geriatrics Society. (2008). Feb;, 56(2), 291-5.

[90] Feart, C, Samieri, C, Rondeau, V, Amieva, H, Portet, F, Dartigues, J. F, et al. Adherence to a Mediterranean diet, cognitive decline, and risk of dementia. Jama. (2009). Aug 12;, 302(6), 638-48.

[91] Anstey, K. J, Mack, H. A, & Cherbuin, N. Alcohol consumption as a risk factor for dementia and cognitive decline: meta-analysis of prospective studies. Am J Geriatr Psychiatry. (2009). Jul;, 17(7), 542-55.

[92] Peters, R, Peters, J, Warner, J, Beckett, N, & Bulpitt, C. Alcohol, dementia and cognitive decline in the elderly: a systematic review. Age and ageing. (2008). Sep;, 37(5), 505-12.

[93] Anttila, T, Helkala, E. L, Viitanen, M, Kareholt, I, Fratiglioni, L, Winblad, B, et al. Alcohol drinking in middle age and subsequent risk of mild cognitive impairment and dementia in old age: a prospective population based study. Bmj. (2004). Sep 4;329(7465):539.

[94] Parks, E, & Traber, M. G. Mechanisms of vitamin E regulation: research over the past decade and focus on the future. Antioxidants & redox signaling. (2000). Fall;, 2(3), 405-12.

[95] Muller, D. P, & Goss-sampson, M. A. Neurochemical, neurophysiological, and neuropathological studies in vitamin E deficiency. Critical reviews in neurobiology. (1990). , 5(3), 239-63.

[96] Reiter, E, Jiang, Q, & Christen, S. Anti-inflammatory properties of alpha- and gamma-tocopherol. Molecular aspects of medicine. (2007). Oct-Dec;28(5-6):668-91.

[97] Sen, C. K, Khanna, S, Rink, C, & Roy, S. Tocotrienols: the emerging face of natural vitamin E. Vitamins and hormones. (2007). , 76, 203-61.

[98] Luchsinger, J. A, Tang, M. X, Shea, S, & Mayeux, R. Antioxidant vitamin intake and risk of Alzheimer disease. Archives of neurology. (2003). Feb;, 60(2), 203-8.

[99] Laurin, D, Foley, D. J, Masaki, K. H, White, L. R, Launer, L. J, Vitamin, E, & Supplements, C. and risk of dementia. Jama. (2002). Nov 13;, 288(18), 2266-8.

[100] Fillenbaum, G. G, Kuchibhatla, M. N, Hanlon, J. T, Artz, M. B, Pieper, C. F, Schmader, K. E, et al. Dementia and Alzheimer's disease in community-dwelling elders taking vitamin C and/or vitamin E. The Annals of pharmacotherapy. (2005). Dec;, 39(12), 2009-14.

[101] Maxwell, C. J, Hicks, M. S, Hogan, D. B, Basran, J, & Ebly, E. M. Supplemental use of antioxidant vitamins and subsequent risk of cognitive decline and dementia. Dement Geriatr Cogn Disord. (2005). , 20(1), 45-51.

[102] Zandi, P. P, Anthony, J. C, Khachaturian, A. S, Stone, S. V, Gustafson, D, Tschanz, J. T, et al. Reduced risk of Alzheimer disease in users of antioxidant vitamin supplements: the Cache County Study. Archives of neurology. (2004). Jan;, 61(1), 82-8.

[103] Masaki, K. H, Losonczy, K. G, Izmirlian, G, Foley, D. J, Ross, G. W, Petrovitch, H, et al. Association of vitamin E and C supplement use with cognitive function and dementia in elderly men. Neurology. (2000). Mar 28;, 54(6), 1265-72.

[104] Engelhart, M. J, Geerlings, M. I, Ruitenberg, A, Van Swieten, J. C, Hofman, A, Witteman, J. C, et al. Dietary intake of antioxidants and risk of Alzheimer disease. Jama. (2002). Jun 26;, 287(24), 3223-9.

[105] Corrada, M. M, Kawas, C. H, Hallfrisch, J, Muller, D, & Brookmeyer, R. Reduced risk of Alzheimer's disease with high folate intake: the Baltimore Longitudinal Study of Aging. Alzheimers Dement. (2005). Jul;, 1(1), 11-8.

[106] Li, F. J, Shen, L, & Ji, H. F. Dietary Intakes of Vitamin E, Vitamin C, and beta-Carotene and Risk of Alzheimer's Disease: A Meta-Analysis. J Alzheimers Dis. (2012). Apr 27.

[107] Mangialasche, F, Xu, W, Kivipelto, M, Costanzi, E, Ercolani, S, Pigliautile, M, et al. Tocopherols and tocotrienols plasma levels are associated with cognitive impairment. Neurobiology of aging. (2012). Oct;, 33(10), 2282-90.

[108] Mangialasche, F, Kivipelto, M, Mecocci, P, Rizzuto, D, Palmer, K, Winblad, B, et al. High plasma levels of vitamin E forms and reduced Alzheimer's disease risk in advanced age. J Alzheimers Dis. (2010). , 20(4), 1029-37.

[109] Hooshmand, B, Solomon, A, Kareholt, I, Leiviska, J, Rusanen, M, Ahtiluoto, S, et al. Homocysteine and holotranscobalamin and the risk of Alzheimer disease: a longitudinal study. Neurology. (2011). Oct 19;, 75(16), 1408-14.

[110] Hooshmand, B, Solomon, A, Kareholt, I, Rusanen, M, Hanninen, T, Leiviska, J, et al. Associations between serum homocysteine, holotranscobalamin, folate and cognition in the elderly: a longitudinal study. Journal of internal medicine. (2010). Feb;, 271(2), 204-12.

[111] Dufouil, C, Alperovitch, A, Ducros, V, & Tzourio, C. Homocysteine, white matter hyperintensities, and cognition in healthy elderly people. Annals of neurology. (2003). Feb;, 53(2), 214-21.

[112] Garcia, A, Haron, Y, Pulman, K, Hua, L, & Freedman, M. Increases in homocysteine are related to worsening of stroop scores in healthy elderly persons: a prospective follow-up study. The journals of gerontology. (2004). Dec;, 59(12), 1323-7.

[113] Nurk, E, Refsum, H, Tell, G. S, Engedal, K, Vollset, S. E, Ueland, P. M, et al. Plasma total homocysteine and memory in the elderly: the Hordaland Homocysteine Study. Annals of neurology. (2005). Dec;, 58(6), 847-57.

[114] Seshadri, S, Beiser, A, Selhub, J, Jacques, P. F, Rosenberg, I. H, & Agostino, D. RB, et al. Plasma homocysteine as a risk factor for dementia and Alzheimer's disease. The New England journal of medicine. (2002). Feb 14;, 346(7), 476-83.

[115] Wang, H. X, Wahlin, A, Basun, H, Fastbom, J, Winblad, B, Fratiglioni, L, & Vitamin, B. and folate in relation to the development of Alzheimer's disease. Neurology. (2001). May 8;, 56(9), 1188-94.

[116] Kado, D. M, Karlamangla, A. S, Huang, M. H, Troen, A, Rowe, J. W, Selhub, J, et al. Homocysteine versus the vitamins folate, B6, and B12 as predictors of cognitive function and decline in older high-functioning adults: MacArthur Studies of Successful Aging. The American journal of medicine. (2005). Feb;, 118(2), 161-7.

[117] Kang, J. H, Irizarry, M. C, & Grodstein, F. Prospective study of plasma folate, vitamin B12, and cognitive function and decline. Epidemiology (Cambridge, Mass. (2006). Nov;, 17(6), 650-7.

[118] Mooijaart, S. P, Gussekloo, J, Frolich, M, Jolles, J, Stott, D. J, Westendorp, R. G, et al. Homocysteine, vitamin B-12, and folic acid and the risk of cognitive decline in old age: the Leiden 85-Plus study. The American journal of clinical nutrition. (2005). Oct;, 82(4), 866-71.

[119] Tangney, C. C, Tang, Y, Evans, D. A, & Morris, M. C. Biochemical indicators of vitamin B12 and folate insufficiency and cognitive decline. Neurology. (2009). Jan 27;, 72(4), 361-7.

[120] Malouf, R. Grimley Evans J. Folic acid with or without vitamin B12 for the prevention and treatment of healthy elderly and demented people. Cochrane database of systematic reviews (Online). (2008). CD004514.

[121] Dangour, A. D, Whitehouse, P. J, Rafferty, K, Mitchell, S. A, Smith, L, Hawkesworth, S, et al. B-vitamins and fatty acids in the prevention and treatment of Alzheimer's disease and dementia: a systematic review. J Alzheimers Dis. (2010). , 22(1), 205-24.

[122] De Jager, C. A, Oulhaj, A, Jacoby, R, Refsum, H, & Smith, A. D. Cognitive and clinical outcomes of homocysteine-lowering B-vitamin treatment in mild cognitive impairment: a randomized controlled trial. International journal of geriatric psychiatry. (2011). Jun;, 27(6), 592-600.

[123] Smith, A. D, Smith, S. M, De Jager, C. A, Whitbread, P, Johnston, C, Agacinski, G, et al. Homocysteine-lowering by B vitamins slows the rate of accelerated brain atrophy in mild cognitive impairment: a randomized controlled trial. PloS one. (2010). e12244.

[124] Slinin, Y, Paudel, M. L, Taylor, B. C, Fink, H. A, Ishani, A, Canales, M. T, et al. Hydroxyvitamin D levels and cognitive performance and decline in elderly men. Neurology. (2010). Jan 5;, 74(1), 33-41.

[125] Annweiler, C, Rolland, Y, Schott, A. M, Blain, H, Vellas, B, Herrmann, F. R, et al. Higher Vitamin D Dietary Intake Is Associated With Lower Risk of Alzheimer's Disease: A Year Follow-up. The journals of gerontology. (2012). Apr 13., 7.

[126] Llewellyn, D. J, Lang, I. A, Langa, K. M, Muniz-terrera, G, Phillips, C. L, Cherubini, A, et al. Vitamin D and risk of cognitive decline in elderly persons. Archives of internal medicine. (2010). Jul 12;, 170(13), 1135-41.

[127] Annweiler, C, & Beauchet, O. Possibility of a new anti-alzheimer's disease pharmaceutical composition combining memantine and vitamin D. Drugs & aging. (2012). Feb 1;, 29(2), 81-91.

[128] Kivipelto, M, Ngandu, T, Laatikainen, T, Winblad, B, Soininen, H, & Tuomilehto, J. Risk score for the prediction of dementia risk in 20 years among middle aged people: a longitudinal, population-based study. Lancet neurology. (2006). Sep;, 5(9), 735-41.

[129] Qiu, C, Xu, W, Winblad, B, & Fratiglioni, L. Vascular risk profiles for dementia and Alzheimer's disease in very old people: a population-based longitudinal study. J Alzheimers Dis. (2010)., 20(1), 293-300.

[130] Barnes, D. E, Covinsky, K. E, Whitmer, R. A, Kuller, L. H, Lopez, O. L, & Yaffe, K. Predicting risk of dementia in older adults: The late-life dementia risk index. Neurology. (2009). Jul 21;, 73(3), 173-9.

[131] Barnes, D. E, Covinsky, K. E, Whitmer, R. A, Kuller, L. H, Lopez, O. L, & Yaffe, K. Commentary on "Developing a national strategy to prevent dementia: Leon Thal Symposium 2009." Dementia risk indices: A framework for identifying individuals with a high dementia risk. Alzheimers Dement. (2010). Mar;, 6(2), 138-41.

[132] Ferrari, C, Xu, W. L, Wang, H. X, Winblad, B, Sorbi, S, Qiu, C, et al. How can elderly apolipoprotein E epsilon4 carriers remain free from dementia? Neurobiol Aging. (2012). Apr 11.

[133] Wang, H. X, Gustafson, D, Kivipelto, M, Pedersen, N. L, Skoog, I, Winblad, B, et al. Education halves the risk of dementia due to apolipoprotein ε4 allele: a collaborative study from the Swedish Brain Power initiative. Neurobiol Aging. (2012). May; 33(5): 1007.e1-7.

[134] Daviglus, M. L, Bell, C. C, Berrettini, W, Bowen, P. E, & Connolly, E. S. Jr., Cox NJ, et al. National Institutes of Health State-of-the-Science Conference statement: preventing alzheimer disease and cognitive decline. Annals of internal medicine. (2011). Aug 3;, 153(3), 176-81.

[135] Solomon, A, & Kivipelto, M. Cholesterol-modifying strategies for Alzheimer's disease. Expert review of neurotherapeutics. (2009). May;, 9(5), 695-709.

[136] Wald, D. S, Kasturiratne, A, & Simmonds, M. Effect of folic acid, with or without other B vitamins, on cognitive decline: meta-analysis of randomized trials. The American journal of medicine. (2010). Jun;e2., 123(6), 522-7.

[137] Komulainen, P, Kivipelto, M, Lakka, T. A, Savonen, K, Hassinen, M, Kiviniemi, V, et al. Exercise, fitness and cognition- A randomised controlled trial in older individuals: The DR's EXTRA study. European Geriatric Medicine. (2010)., 1(5), 266-72.

[138] Rocca, W. A, Grossardt, B. R, & Shuster, L. T. Oophorectomy, menopause, estrogen treatment, and cognitive aging: clinical evidence for a window of opportunity. Brain research. (2011). Mar 16;, 1379, 188-98.

[139] Shumaker, S. A, Legault, C, Kuller, L, Rapp, S. R, Thal, L, Lane, D. S, et al. Conjugated equine estrogens and incidence of probable dementia and mild cognitive impairment in postmenopausal women: Women's Health Initiative Memory Study. Jama. (2004). Jun 23;, 291(24), 2947-58.

[140] Shumaker, S. A, Legault, C, Rapp, S. R, Thal, L, Wallace, R. B, Ockene, J. K, et al. Estrogen plus progestin and the incidence of dementia and mild cognitive impairment in postmenopausal women: the Women's Health Initiative Memory Study: a randomized controlled trial. Jama. (2003). May 28;, 289(20), 2651-62.

[141] Kronos Longevity Research Institute. Hormone Therapy Has Many Favorable Effects in Newly Menopausal Women: Initial Findings of the Kronos Early Estrogen Prevention Study (KEEPS). (2012). October 3, 2012]; Available from: http://www.menopause.org/docs/agm/general-release.pdf?sfvrsn=0.

[142] Whitmer, R. A, Quesenberry, C. P, Zhou, J, & Yaffe, K. Timing of hormone therapy and dementia: the critical window theory revisited. Annals of neurology. (2011). Jan;, 69(1), 163-9.

[143] Isaac, M. G, Quinn, R, & Tabet, N. Vitamin E for Alzheimer's disease and mild cognitive impairment. Cochrane database of systematic reviews (Online). (2008). CD002854.

[144] Schurks, M, Glynn, R. J, Rist, P. M, Tzourio, C, & Kurth, T. Effects of vitamin E on stroke subtypes: meta-analysis of randomised controlled trials. BMJ (Clinical research ed. (2010). c5702.

[145] Andrieu, S, Aboderin, I, Baeyens, J. P, Beard, J, Benetos, A, Berrut, G, et al. IAGG Workshop: Health Promotion Program on Prevention of Late Onset Dementia. The journal of nutrition, health & aging. (2011). , 15(7), 562-75.

[146] Richard, E. Van den Heuvel E, Moll van Charante EP, Achthoven L, Vermeulen M, Bindels PJ, et al. Prevention of dementia by intensive vascular care (PreDIVA): a cluster-randomized trial in progress. Alzheimer disease and associated disorders. (2009). Jul-Sep;, 23(3), 198-204.

[147] Lindstrom, J, Ilanne-parikka, P, Peltonen, M, Aunola, S, Eriksson, J. G, Hemio, K, et al. Sustained reduction in the incidence of type 2 diabetes by lifestyle intervention: follow-up of the Finnish Diabetes Prevention Study. Lancet. (2006). Nov 11;, 368(9548), 1673-9.

[148] Tuomilehto, J, Lindstrom, J, Eriksson, J. G, Valle, T. T, Hamalainen, H, Ilanne-parikka, P, et al. Prevention of type 2 diabetes mellitus by changes in lifestyle among subjects with impaired glucose tolerance. N Engl J Med. (2001). May 3;, 344(18), 1343-50.

[149] Komulainen, P, Kivipelto, M, Lakka, T. A, Savonen, K, Hassinen, M, Kiviniemi, V, et al. Exercise, fitness and cognition- A randomised controlled trial in older individuals: The DR's EXTRA study. European Geriatric Medicine (2012). , 1(2), 266-72.

[150] Gillette-guyonnet, S, Andrieu, S, Dantoine, T, Dartigues, J. F, Touchon, J, & Vellas, B. Commentary on "A roadmap for the prevention of dementia II. Leon Thal Symposium 2008." The Multidomain Alzheimer Preventive Trial (MAPT): a new approach to the prevention of Alzheimer's disease. Alzheimers Dement. (2009). Mar;, 5(2), 114-21.

[151] Richard, E, Andrieu, S, Solomon, A, Mangialasche, F, Ahtiluoto, S, Moll van Charante, et al. Methodological challenges in designing dementia prevention trials - the European Dementia Prevention Initiative (EDPI). J Neurol Sci. (2012). Nov 15;322(1-2):64-70.

[152] Reiman, E. M, Langbaum, J. B, & Tariot, P. N. Alzheimer's prevention initiative: a proposal to evaluate presymptomatic treatments as quickly as possible. Biomarkers in medicine. (2010). Feb;, 4(1), 3-14.

[153] Reiman, E. M, Langbaum, J. B, Fleisher, A. S, Caselli, R. J, Chen, K, Ayutyanont, N, et al. Alzheimer's Prevention Initiative: a plan to accelerate the evaluation of presymptomatic treatments. J Alzheimers Dis. (2011). Suppl , 3, 321-9.

[154] Blennow, K, De Leon, M. J, & Zetterberg, H. Alzheimer's disease. Lancet. (2006). Jul 29;, 368(9533), 387-403.

[155] Bateman, R. J, Xiong, C, Benzinger, T. L, Fagan, A. M, Goate, A, Fox, N. C, et al. Clinical and biomarker changes in dominantly inherited Alzheimer's disease. The New England journal of medicine. (2012). Aug 30;, 367(9), 795-804.

[156] Lopera, F, Ardilla, A, Martinez, A, Madrigal, L, Arango-viana, J. C, Lemere, C. A, et al. Clinical features of early-onset Alzheimer disease in a large kindred with an E280A presenilin-1 mutation. Jama. (1997). Mar 12;, 277(10), 793-9.

[157] Miller, G. Alzheimer's research. Stopping Alzheimer's before it starts. Science (New York, NY. (2012). Aug 17;, 337(6096), 790-2.

[158] Alzheimer's Prevention Initiative, Treatment Trials. (2012). October 2012; Available from: http://endalznow.org/about-api/treatment-trials.aspx.

[159] West, S. G, Duan, N, Pequegnat, W, & Gaist, P. Des Jarlais DC, Holtgrave D, et al. Alternatives to the randomized controlled trial. American journal of public health. (2008). Aug;, 98(8), 1359-66.

[160] Khachaturian, Z. S, Petersen, R. C, Snyder, P. J, Khachaturian, A. S, Aisen, P, De Leon, M, et al. Developing a global strategy to prevent Alzheimer's disease: Leon Thal Symposium 2010. Alzheimers Dement. (2011). Mar;, 7(2), 127-32.

[161] Zhu, L, Fratiglioni, L, Guo, Z, Basun, H, Corder, E. H, Winblad, B, et al. Incidence of dementia in relation to stroke and the apolipoprotein E epsilon4 allele in the very

old. Findings from a population-based longitudinal study. Stroke; a journal of cerebral circulation. (2000). Jan;, 31(1), 53-60.

[162] Honig, L. S, Tang, M. X, Albert, S, Costa, R, Luchsinger, J, Manly, J, et al. Stroke and the risk of Alzheimer disease. Archives of neurology. (2003). Dec;, 60(12), 1707-12.

[163] Bushnell, C. D, Zimmer, L. O, Pan, W, Olson, D. M, Zhao, X, Meteleva, T, et al. Persistence with stroke prevention medications 3 months after hospitalization. Archives of neurology. (2010). Dec;, 67(12), 1456-63.

[164] Xu, W, Caracciolo, B, Wang, HX, Winblad, B, Bäckman, L, Qiu, C, et al. Accelerated progression from mild cognitive impairment to dementia in people with diabetes. Diabetes. 2010 Nov;59(11):2928-35